Evidence-based Rheumatology

Evidence-based Rheumatology

Edited by

Peter Tugwell

Professor of Medicine, and Epidemiology and Community Medicine, Institute of Population Health, University of Ottawa, Ottawa, Canada

Beverley Shea

Director of Research Operations, Institute of Population Health, University of Ottawa, Ottawa, Canada

Maarten Boers

Professor of Clinical Epidemiology, Department of Clinical Epidemiology and Biostatistics, VU University Medical Centre, Amsterdam, the Netherlands

Peter Brooks

Professor and Executive Dean, Department of Health Sciences, University of Queensland, St Lucia, Australia

Lee S Simon

Associate Professor of Medicine, Beth Israel Deaconess Medical Centre, Harvard Medical School, Boston, USA

Vibeke Strand

Clinical Professor, Division of Immunology, Stanford University, Portola Valley, USA

George Wells

Professor and Chair, Department of Epidemiology and Community Medicine, and Institute of Population Health, University of Ottawa, Ottawa, Canada

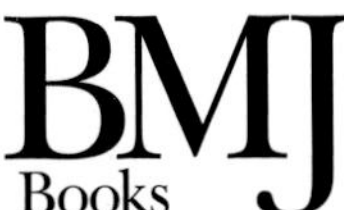

First published in 2004
by BMJ Books, BMA House, Tavistock Square,
London WC1H 9JR

www.bmjbooks.com
www.evidbasedrheum.com

British Library Cataloguing in Publication Data

A catalogue record for this book is available from the British Library

ISBN 0 7279 1446 4

Typeset by SIVA Math Setters, Chennai, India
Printed and bound in Malaysia by Times Offset

Contents

Contributors

Authors and Editors

Rick Adachi
Department of Medicine,
St Joseph's Hospital, McMaster University,
Hamilton, Canada

Maarten Boers
Department of Clinical Epidemiology and Biostatistics,
VU University Medical Center,
Amsterdam, the Netherlands

Annelies Boonen
Department of Medicine, Division of Rheumatology,
University Hospital Maastricht,
Maastricht, the Netherlands

Peter Brooks
Department of Health Sciences,
University of Queensland,
St Lucia, Australia

Rachelle Buchbinder
Department of Clinical Epidemiology,
Monash University, *and*
Department of Epidemiology and Preventive Medicine,
Cabrini Hospital,
Malvern, Australia

Eliza Chakravarty
Division of Immunology and Rheumatology,
Stanford University School of Medicine,
Palo Alto, USA

Phil Clements
Department of Medicine, Division of Rheumatology,
University of California, Los Angeles (UCLA),
Los Angeles, USA

Ann Cranney
Division of Rheumatology,
Queen's University,
Kingston, Canada

Maxime Dougados
Cochin Hospital,
René Descartes University,
Paris, France

Paul Emery
Department of Rheumatology,
University of Leeds,
Leeds, UK

Marlene Fransen
Institute for International Health,
Newtown, Australia

Daniel E Furst
Department of Medicine, Division of Rheumatology,
University of California, Los Angeles (UCLA),
Los Angeles, USA

Sherine E Gabriel
Department of Health Sciences Research, Division of Epidemiology,
Mayo Clinic,
Rochester, USA

Sally Green
Monash Institute of Health Services,
Monash University,
Clayton, Australia

Gordon Guyatt
Department of Clinical Epidemiology and Biostatistics,
McMaster University,
Hamilton, Canada

Hilal Maradit Kremers
Department of Health Sciences Research, Division of Epidemiology,
Mayo Clinic,
Rochester, USA

Suzanne E Lane
Department of Rheumatology,
Addenbrooke's Hospital,
Cambridge, UK

France Légaré
Department of Family Medicine,
Laval University,
Québec, Canada

Jessie McGowan
Institute of Population Health,
University of Ottawa,
Ottawa, Canada

Carina Mihai
Department of Internal Medicine and Rheumatology,
Cantacuzino Hospital, Carol Davila University of Medicine and Pharmacy,
Bucharest, Romania

Annette M O'Connor
Faculty of Health Sciences,
University of Ottawa,
Clinical Epidemiology Program,
Ottawa Health Research Institute,
Ottawa, Canada

Manathip Osiri
Department of Medicine, Division of Rheumatology,
Chulalongkorn University,
Bangkok, Thailand

Thao Pham
Service de Rhumatologie Sud,
Hôpital la Conception,
Marseille, France

Janet Pope
Rheumatology Centre,
St Joseph's Health Care London,
London, Canada

Philippe Ravaud
Department of Epidemiology, Biostatistic and Clinical Research,
Bichat Hospital,
Paris, France

Nancy Santesso
Institute of Population Health,
University of Ottawa,
Ottawa, Canada

Joel Schiffenbauer
Centre for Drug Evaluation and Research (CDER),
Food and Drug Administration (FDA),
Rockville, USA

Naomi Schlesinger
Department of Medicine, Rheumatology Section,
UMDNJ/NJ Medical School,
Newark, USA

Ralph Schumacher
Arthritis Research,
Philadelphia VA Medical Center,
Philadelphia, USA

David GI Scott
Norfolk and Norwich University Hospital,
Norwich, UK

Beverley Shea
Institute of Population Health,
University of Ottawa,
Ottawa, Canada

Lee S Simon
Beth Israel Deaconess Medical Center,
Harvard Medical School,
Boston, USA

Dawn Stacey
Population Health PhD Program,
University of Ottawa and Ottawa Health Research Institute,
Ottawa, Canada

Vibeke Strand
Division of Immunology,
Stanford University,
Portola Valley, USA

Maria E Suarez-Almazor
Baylor College of Medicine and Houston Center for Quality and Utilization Studies,
Department of Medicine,
Veteran Affairs Medical Center,
Houston, USA

Peter Tugwell
Faculty of Medicine, Department of Epidemiology and Community Medicine and Institute of Population Health, University of Ottawa,
Ottawa, Canada

Richard A Watts
Ipswich Hospital NHS Trust,
Ipswich, UK

George Wells
Department of Epidemiology and Community Medicine,
and Institute of Population Health, University of Ottawa,
Ottawa, Canada

Sjef van der Linden
Department of Medicine, Division of Rheumatology,
University Hospital Maastricht,
Maastricht, the Netherlands

Astrid van Tubergen
Department of Medicine, Division of Rheumatology,
University Hospital Maastricht,
Maastricht, the Netherlands

Other Contributors

Consumers
Cheryln Kohen
Ann Qualman
Fergus J Rogers
Joyce Gordon

Ottawa Methods Group
Daniel Francis
Maria Judd
Jessie McGowan
Annette O'Connor
Joan Peterson
Vivian Robinson
Nancy Santesso
Beverley Shea
Dawn Stacey
Peter Tugwell
George Wells

Acknowledgements
Ashley Porter
Candyce Hamel
Chris Cates
Peter Cates
Adam Shea
Elizabeth Lacasse
Mary Banks
Christina Karaviotis
Elaine Leek
Thelma Hasson
Ninke Smidt
Willem Assendelft
Petrus Struijs

We would like to thank the Institute of Population Health (IPH) and the University of Ottawa for their in-kind contribution, without which the publication of this book would not have been possible.

Introduction

Peter Tugwell, Beverley Shea, Maarten Boers, Peter Brooks, Lee S Simon, Vibeke Strand, George Wells

This is one of a series of evidence-based books from BMJ Books – others have included texts on cardiology, gastroenterology and hepatology, dermatology, ophthalmology, oncology, and pediatrics and child health.

Over the past three decades, the emergence of evidence-based health care (EBHC) has had a substantial impact on clinical practice. In the first half of the twentieth century, treatments, usually based on a strong scientific rationale and experimental work in animals, were routinely introduced into clinical care without adequate and appropriate scientific proof of efficacy in people. Fortunately, the need for a more critical approach to medical practice was recognized. In 1948 the first randomised controlled trial (RCT) in humans was performed under the direction of the British Medical Research Council.[1] Epidemiologists and statisticians, notably Sir Richard Doll and Sir Bradford Hill, provided scientific leadership to the medical community, which responded with improvements in the quality of clinical research. The use of randomised allocation to control confounding variables, and to minimise bias, was recognised as invaluable for the performance of valid studies of treatments. The initiation of these landmark experiments defined a new era in clinical research; the RCT soon became the benchmark for the evaluation of medical and surgical interventions.

Rheumatologists played an important part in these early days. In 1955, the Empire Rheumatism Council reported on perhaps the first randomised trial in the discipline of rheumatology.[2] They showed that cortisone was more effective than salicylates in the treatment of rheumatoid arthritis. As noted in Chapter 9 on rheumatoid arthritis, this treatment has stood the test of time.

Researchers currently understand the need for rigorous approaches to minimising the potential biases that may lead to erroneous conclusions. In addition, they are becoming increasingly aware that the "users" of research must share this understanding if they are to make evidence-based decisions on health and health care. The original "critical appraisal" movement was oriented to the clinician user.[3] This evolved into the evidence-based medicine movement that has been increasingly adopted by clinicians and incorporated into medical curricula. The "user" also includes others such as policymakers,[4] consumers,[5,6] and journalists.[7] We hope that evidence-based texts such as this BMJ series will speed up such change in practice.

What is evidence-based rheumatology?

The term "evidence-based medicine" was coined at McMaster Medical School in the 1980s;[8] it refers to the process of systematically finding, appraising, and using contemporaneous research findings as the basis for clinical decisions. There are typically five steps: formulation of a clear clinical question from a patients' problem; searching the literature for relevant clinical articles; evaluating using critical appraisal criteria, the evidence for its validity and usefulness; implementing these findings in clinical practice; and continuous evaluation of the previous steps. Thus, evidence-based rheumatology is the application of the most valid scientific information to the care of patients with rheumatic diseases. Physicians who treat patients with musculoskeletal diseases must provide their patients with the most effective and safest therapy. To meet this high standard, individual clinicians must have access to, and be able to evaluate, scientific evidence. Although many practitioners argue that this has always been the standard of care in clinical medicine, a great deal of evidence exists to the contrary.

In rheumatology, the appreciation and application of the advances in psychometrics and clinimetrics has not been adopted quickly. In the 1970s, only "objective" outcomes, that is laboratory tests (such as the erythrocyte sedimentation rate (ESR)) or clinician findings (such as joint counts performed by physicians) were judged sufficiently credible for regulatory approval. Patient reported outcomes (PROs) have always had face validity but had to await the demonstration of adequate psychometric and clinimetric performances. This was a major stimulus for the involvement of the six OMERACT (Outcome Measures in Rheumatology) meetings to date.

OMERACT brings the key constituencies together to achieve consensus on establishing "core sets" of outcomes in the main rheumatologic conditions (ankylosing spondylitis, lupus, osteoarthritis, osteoporosis, rheumatoid arthritis, systemic sclerosis) that meet the methodological requirements of validity, responsiveness, and feasibility.[9] Patient reported outcomes, such as pain and disability, are now accepted as major endpoints in these conditions by clinicians and regulatory agencies.

Relevant outcomes are necessary but not sufficient. The choice of outcomes is but one of the elements of study design that is needed to arrive at the best estimates of benefits and harms for therapeutic interventions. There is now a general acceptance that randomised trials, when feasible, will provide the most rigorous estimates (and where these are available this text will restrict itself to them). Although randomized controlled trials (RCT) are the most valuable source of data for evaluating healthcare interventions, other kinds of evidence must sometimes be used. In some instances, most obviously in studies of toxicity when looking for rare or delayed effects, it is neither possible nor ethical to perform RCTs. Here, data from methodologically rigorous observational studies are extremely valuable. Examples include the increased risk of vertebral fractures with corticosteroids. Finally, case series can provide compelling evidence for the adoption of a new therapy in the absence of data from RCTs, if the natural history of disease is both well characterised and severe. An example is the use of hip replacement as a dramatically effective intervention for patients with disabling osteoarthritis of the joint.[10]

The Cochrane Collaboration

The number of trials of therapy has grown too large for any individual to keep abreast of them. In response to this, the Cochrane Library was established to provide systematic, up-to-date reviews of all relevant RCTs of health care. This was named in honour of Archie Cochrane. In an influential book published in 1972,[11] Archie Cochrane, a British epidemiologist, drew attention to our great collective ignorance about the effects of health care. He recognised that people who want to make more informed decisions about health care do not have ready access to reliable reviews of the available evidence. In 1979, he wrote: "*It is surely a great criticism of our profession that we have not organised a critical summary, by specialty or subspecialty, adapted periodically, of all relevant randomised controlled trials.*"[12]

This suggestion inspired Iain Chalmers and others to establish the Cochrane Collaboration, an international initiative to facilitate the availability on a website (and CDs) of systematic reviews of trials of interventions across all areas of health care.[11,13]

The Cochrane Musculoskeletal Group (CMSG), established in 1993, consists of over 200 individuals representing healthcare professionals, researchers, and consumers. The coverage of musculoskeletal conditions includes: gout, lupus erythematosus, osteoarthritis, osteoporosis, pediatric rheumatology, rheumatoid arthritis, soft tissue conditions, spondylo-arthropathy, systemic sclerosis, and vasculitis. This forms the scope of *Evidence-based Rheumatology*.

Good decisions about health care rely on more than good reviews of the results of research. The Cochrane Collaboration will make the results of research assessing the effects of health care more easily available. However, as Cochrane made clear in "Effectiveness and Efficiency",[11] reliable evidence about the effects of specific elements of health care, although essential for improving decisions about health care and research, is only part of what is needed for better decision making.

If better decisions are to lead to improved health, then effective mechanisms are needed for implementing them efficiently. Forms of care that have been shown to do more good than harm should be encouraged, while those that do more harm than good need to be discarded. Some forms of care will require weighing benefits and harms within patients individual circumstances, given their classification as trade off or close call decisions. The many forms of care which have unknown effects should, as far as possible, be used in the context of a research program to find out whether they help or do harm.

In addition, if people are to receive care which is appropriate, then policy makers and decision makers – ranging from ministers of health to individual clinicians and patients – must consider people's needs, the availability of resources, and priorities.

In making decisions about the care of individual patients, the results of the reviews must be integrated with the clinician's expertise, which has been acquired through experience and practice. The results must also be integrated with the patient's expertise, which derives from their knowledge of their condition (particularly if it is a chronic or recurrent health problem), the treatments on offer, and the receptivity of both the clinician and patient to shared decision making.

If operating in synchrony, these complementary forms of expertise are reflected in more efficient diagnosis and in more thoughtful identification and compassionate use of the predicaments, rights, and preferences of individual patients in making decisions about their care.

Despite the opposition of some, the popularity of EBHC continues to grow. Many practitioners recognise that ethical patient care should be based on the best possible evidence. In addition, increasing numbers of patients are demanding the right to participate in health decisions and requesting the evidence for available options. For these and other reasons, the fundamental concept behind evidence-based medicine and the use of the scientific method in the practice of clinical medicine – has been widely endorsed by medical opinion leaders, patients, and governments.

Rationale for this book

Generalist and specialist physicians and surgeons, nurses, occupational therapists, physiotherapists, and the other professionals caring for patients with musculoskeletal diseases are fortunate to have many excellent textbooks that provide a wealth of information regarding rheumatologic diseases. Such traditional textbooks concentrate on the pathophysiology of disease and are comprehensive in their scope. *Evidence-based Rheumatology* is not intended to replace these texts, since its focus is on clinical evidence.

Excellent electronic databases are available, and many traditional publications contain relevant research evidence and important summaries and reviews to support evidence-based practice. However, Cumbers and Donald[14] have found that physicians in clinical practice find the acquisition of data from these sources time-consuming. Their study revealed that even locating relevant articles required, on average, three days for practitioners with an onsite library and a week for those without such a facility. This book has been written for the purpose of saving valuable time for busy practitioners caring for patients with rheumatic disease.

The book cannot claim to be comprehensive; for example, the reader will not find chapters on some rare conditions. While we would have preferred to provide our readers with a more complete coverage of the topics, we had to establish a list of priority areas where we felt there was important evidence to be reviewed and summarised on one hand and available authors with the required expertise on the other. We hope that future editions will expand the number of topics that are included.

A limitation of any textbook is the timeliness of the information that it is possible to provide in print form. New evidence accumulates rapidly in clinical medicine and it is impossible to include the most up-to-date information in a textbook because of the time required for production. To meet the needs of our readers for the timeliest information it is planned to produce electronic updates of chapters at regular intervals. These updates, like those for the companion *Evidence-based* books, will appear on the book website http://www.evidbasedrheum.com

Special features

This text aims to do more than just summarise the best evidence for therapy. There has been an additional focus on the dissemination and integration of quality evidence into health and healthcare decisions, sometimes referred to as "knowledge translation". A feature of this text is the attempt to make the evidence more "usable" for both clinicians and consumers in five ways: web availability, simple quality grading, use of percentages, visual aids for Number Needed to Treat (NNT), and patient handouts.

Firstly, the clinician and consumer materials for each topic are available on the CD Rom (free with the book), and also on the free access book website http://www.evidbasedrheum.com. These sections will be organised for clinicians and consumers to easily print off for use as handouts for the clinic and the classroom. For instructions, please follow this Introduction.

Secondly, given the importance of an appreciation of the quality of the study, we have decided to use a scale that can be easily understood by all categories and levels of "users" – using the categories of Platinum, Gold, Silver, Bronze. Based on our previous experience and the challenges to numerative scales posed by Juni *et* al,[15] we have decided to focus on requiring a few validated criteria to decide which studies warrant the highest levels of Gold and Platinum; namely adequate sample size, completeness of follow-up, blindingz of outcome assessors and patients and concealment of allocation.

Levels of evidence used in this book

Methods for grading the scientific evidence have evolved over the past decade as EBHC has become increasingly important in clinical practice. There are a number of different grading systems available and some are very complex since they incorporate both the type of study and the quality of evidence.

We decided to use a common system of grading throughout the book to rank the strength of scientific evidence for each therapeutic agent. We reviewed multiple grading systems, including that recommended by the US Preventive Services Task Force Guidelines 2001,[16] the summary of systems rating strength of evidence by the Agency for Healthcare Research and Quality (ARHQ),[17] and the Oxford Centre for EBM 2001.[18] These grading systems were reviewed and by consensus process we derived a simplified grading system that included an assessment of quality and could be used by clinicians and patients as previously alluded. We chose four categories to rank the evidence from research studies: Platinum, Gold, Silver, and Bronze. These same levels of evidence are used to present consumer summaries throughout the book.

Grading for Evidence-based Rheumatology

Platinum level

The Platinum ranking is given to evidence that meets the following criteria, as reported: is a published systematic review that has at least two individual randomised controlled trials each satisfying the following:

- Sample sizes of at least 50 per group. If they do not find a statistically significant difference, they are adequately powered for a 20% relative difference in the relevant outcome.
- Blinding of patients and assessors for outcomes.
- Handling of withdrawals >80% follow up (imputations based on methods such as Last Observation Carried Forward (LOCF) acceptable).
- Concealment of treatment allocation.[19]

Gold level

The Gold ranking is given to evidence if at least one randomised controlled trial meets all of the following criteria for the major outcome(s), as reported:

- Sample sizes of at least 50 per group. If they do not find a statistically significant difference, they are adequately powered for a 20% relative difference in the relevant outcome.
- Blinding of patients and assessors for outcomes.
- Handling of withdrawals > 80% follow up (imputations based on methods such as Last Observation Carried Forward (LOCF) acceptable).
- Concealment of treatment allocation.[19]

Silver level

The Silver ranking is given to evidence if a systematic review or randomised trial that does not meet the above criteria. Silver ranking would also include evidence from at least one study of non-randomised cohorts who did and did not receive the therapy or evidence from at least one case-control study. A randomised trial with a "head-to-head" comparison of agents is considered Silver level ranking unless a reference is provided to a comparison of one of the agents to placebo showing at least a 20% relative difference.

Bronze level

The bronze ranking is given to evidence if at least one case series without controls (including simple before/after studies in which the patient acts as their own control) or is derived from expert opinion based on clinical experience without reference to any of the foregoing (for example, argument from physiology, bench research or first principles).

Evidence grades appear in shaded boxes.

The third item to aid "knowledge translation" is the provision of the information in tables in a clinically useful format. Where possible, the following data are provided: (a) if a scale, the range; (b) baseline rates; (c) relative effects; (d) NNT (number needed to treat), NNH (number needed to harm). The example table shown here is taken from Chapter 8 of the book (see end of Introduction for description).

Table 8.3 NNT for five year (high risk woman) and lifetime risk of fracture, with alendronate compared with no treatment (Cranney *et al*, 2002)[31]

Outcome	5 year and lifetime risk of fracture in untreated population	5 year and lifetime risk in a treated population	Relative risk with treatment (95% CI)	NNT
Vertebral fracture	5 year: 7·1%	5 year: 4%	0·52	5 year: 29
	Lifetime: 9·6%	Lifetime: 5%	(0·43–0·65)	Lifetime: 22
Non-vertebral	5 year: 19·8%	5 year: 10%	0·51	5 year: 10
fracture	Lifetime: 42·1%	Lifetime: 21%	(0·38–0·69)	LIfetime: 5

Fourthly, "face figures" are also included for a number of the outcomes. They use the transformation of the NNT (or NNH) data to "face tables". Visual Rx, a software program that was developed by Peter and Chris Cates[22] was used to calculate and convert the data to the face tables. The tables for the five year and lifetime risk of vertebral fractures for 100 high risk women comparing no treatment versus treatment with alendronate are presented on p xix.

Each display represents a total of 100 faces that are divided into three categories. The pale green faces are those patients who have a good outcome on both the control treatment and the active treatment. The red faces are those who suffer a bad outcome, whichever treatment they receive. The dark green faces are those patients that change their category of outcome depending on whether they are given the active

NNT for high risk women for 5 year prevention of vertebral fractures

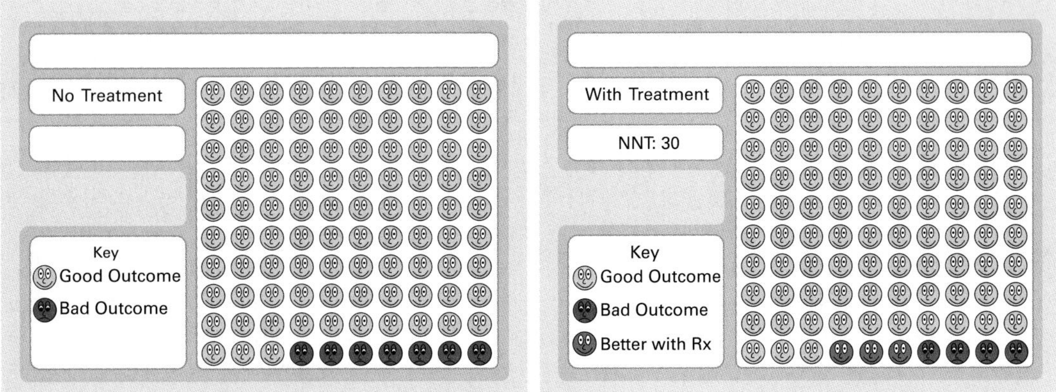

NNT for high risk women for lifetime prevention of vertebral fractures.

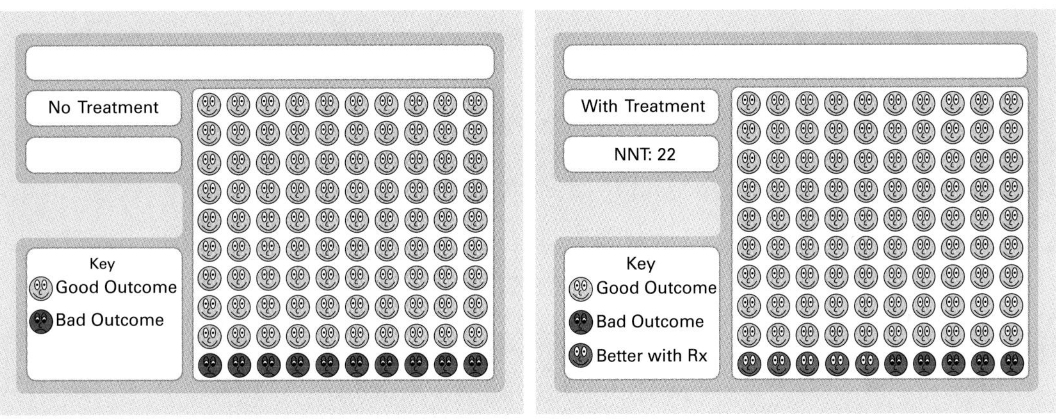

treatment or not. If the treatment is beneficial, as a consequence of being given the active treatment, the faces will appear as dark green. However, since it is not possible to tell who these patients are, all 100 have to be given active treatment for this group to benefit.

The above example of a face table displays the 5 year risk of vertebral fractures of 100 high risk women treated with or without alendronate. The first table, No Treatment, illustrates that 7 out of 100 women will have vertebral fractures if left untreated (red faces), while 93 out of 100 women left untreated will not have a vertebral fracture (pale green faces) with or without treatment. The second table, With Treatment, illustrates that if the 100 high risk women were treated with alendronate, then 4 out of 100 women will have vertebral fractures (red faces), while 3 out of 100 women will not have vertebral fractures due to alendronate – benefiting from treatment (dark green faces).

Fifthly, we have translated the evidence-based information about a number of treatments into a set of handouts for patients. These are reproduced in the book and are also available on the book website at http://www.evidbasedrheum.com to provide to patients and to use in consultation and for teaching and will also be made available on the Arthritis Society website at http://www.arthritis.ca.

The information about a treatment is presented as a consumer package in two parts: as a series of consumer summaries (1, 5, 15 minute handouts) and as a decision aid (45 minute handout). The series of consumer summaries consist of short consumer summaries and a long consumer summary that describe the disease and treatment at three different levels of detail. The different versions address the varying needs of the different patients who want varying quantities of detail about a treatment.

The "1 minute" consumer summary consists of a brief "bottom line" statement about the treatment. The "5 minute" summary includes some additional general information about the condition and treatment and a brief description of the results from studies regarding benefits and harms. The "15 minute" consumer summary provides more details about the evidence than the shorter summaries. It also provides more information about the condition and treatment, details about the types of studies analysed in the review of the literature, numerical data from the studies depicting the benefits and harms of the treatment and the "bottom line". The numerical data is presented as the number of patients out of 100 who improved with placebo or as the number of patients out of 100 who benefited from a treatment.

The second part of the consumer package, the Decision Aid, is a tool that incorporates the information from the consumer summaries together with the values and preferences identified by the patient; it guides patients in the decision making process, and enhances physician–patient interaction. Patients might take 45 minutes to use the decision aid and can use it in consultation with their physician. (See Chapter 4 for more details about decision aids.)

1 MINUTE CONSUMER SUMMARY
(bottom line)

How well does alendronate (Fosamax) work to treat and prevent osteoporosis in women after menopause?

What is the bottom line?

There is "Platinum" level evidence that women after menopause with osteoporosis, have fewer spine fractures when taking alendronate at 5 to 40 mg daily for 2 to 3 years. Women after menopause with osteoporosis have fewer hip and non-spinal fractures with 10 to 40 mg of alendronate for 2 to 3 years.

Alendronate for 2 to 3 years, increases bone mineral density.

Side effects such as heartburn or ulcers in the oesophagus or gullet may occur.

From Cranney A, Simon LS, Tugwell P, Adachi R, Ottawa Methods Group. Osteoporosis. In: *Evidence-based Rheumatology.* London: BMJ Books, 2003.

5 MINUTE CONSUMER SUMMARY

How well does alendronate (Fosamax) work to treat and prevent osteoporosis in women after menopause?

To answer this question, scientists found and analysed 11 studies testing alendronate in over 12 500 women after menopause. Women received 5 to 40 mg of alendronate as a pill daily for 1 to 4 years. These studies provide the best evidence we have today.

What is osteoporosis and how can alendronate help?
Osteoporosis is a condition of weak brittle bones that break easily. Breaks or fractures of the spine and hip or wrist (non-spinal fractures) may occur and often without a fall. Alendronate is a bisphosphonate and "antiresorptive agent" used to decrease fractures by slowing bone loss. There is some debate about whether alendronate decreases fractures, in women with normal or near normal bone density.

How well did alendronate decrease fractures and increase bone density?
In women after menopause who have osteoporosis, alendronate decreased the number of **spine** fractures more than a placebo or sugar pill. 10 to 40 mg of alendronate daily decreased the number of **non-spinal fractures** (such as wrist and hip) more than a placebo or sugar pill in women with osteoporosis, but not in women who have normal to near normal bone density.

Bone mineral density increased in the spine, hip and somewhat in the forearm.

Were there any side effects?
Heartburn or ulcers in the oesophagus or gullet may occur. But the number of women who stopped taking alendronate due to side effects was no different than the number of women who stopped taking a placebo.

1 minute summary →

What is the bottom line?
There is "Platinum" level evidence that women after menopause with osteoporosis, have fewer spine fractures when taking alendronate at 5 to 40 mg daily for 2 to 3 years. Women after menopause with osteoporosis have fewer hip and non-spinal fractures with 10 to 40 mg of alendronate for 2 to 3 years.

Alendronate for 2 to 3 years, increases bone mineral density.

Side effects such as heartburn or ulcers in the oesophagus or gullet may occur.

From Cranney A, Simon LS, Tugwell P, Adachi R, Ottawa Methods Group. Osteoporosis. In: *Evidence-based Rheumatology*. London: BMJ Books, 2003.

15 MINUTE CONSUMER SUMMARY

PAGE 1

How well does alendronate (Fosamax) work to treat and prevent osteoporosis in women after menopause?

What is osteoporosis and how can alendronate help?
Osteoporosis is a condition of weak brittle bones that break easily. In osteoporosis, breaks or fractures of the spine and hip, wrist or forearm (non-spinal fractures) may occur and often without a fall. Osteoporosis is detected using a bone density test that measures the amount of bone loss. A result that is at least 2·5 "standard deviations" below normal confirms the diagnosis. This means people have lost at least 25 per cent of their bone mass or density. Drugs have been developed to slow the bone loss.

Alendronate is a bisphosphonate drug and an "antiresorptive agent" that was developed for women after menopause to decrease fractures. Alendronate works by slowing bone loss or "resorption" and does not interfere with bone building or mineralisation. There is some debate about whether alendronate increases bone density in women after menopause who have normal to near normal bone density or who already have bone loss (as in osteoporosis) and whether it decrease all types of fractures, such as spine and non-spinal fractures.

How did the scientists find the information and analyse it?
To find out just how well alendronate works, the scientists searched for studies testing alendronate. Unfortunately, not all studies found were of a high quality and so only those studies that met high standards were examined in this summary.

Studies had to be randomised controlled trials – where a group of women after menopause (post menopausal) received alendronate and was compared to postmenopausal women who received a placebo (or sugar pill) for at least one year.
Studies had to show how well alendronate works by measuring bone mineral density (BMD) and the number of fractures (or breaks).

Which high quality studies were examined in the summary?
Eleven high quality studies were examined. The studies included 12 855 women after menopause (postmenopausal women) receiving 5 to 40 mg of alendronate daily for 1 to 4 years. Two studies provided alendronate to women with normal to near normal bone density to prevent bone loss and fractures and 9 studies provided alendronate to women who already had bone losses (or low bone mineral density – BMD). Some studies included women who already had a spine fracture.

How well did alendronate decrease fractures and increase bone density?
Spine fractures: Over a lifetime, in women who have normal to near normal bone density or osteoporosis:

5 out of 100 women receiving 5 to 40 mg of alendronate daily will have a spine fracture
10 out of 100 women receiving no treatment or a placebo (sugar pill) will have a spine fracture.

15 MINUTE CONSUMER SUMMARY

PAGE 2

- results from Cochrane Review and included trials

Hip and non-spinal fractures (wrist, etc.): Over a lifetime, in women who have **osteoporosis**:

21 out of 100 women receiving 10 to 40 mg of alendronate daily will have a hip fracture or other non-spinal fracture
42 out of 100 women receiving no treatment or a placebo (sugar pill) will have a hip fracture or other non-spinal fracture.

This means that 21 out of 100 more women benefited from taking alendronate than a placebo.

In women who have **normal to near normal** bone density:

the benefit of taking alendronate to prevent hip fracture or other non-spinal fractures is still in question since most of these women are at a lower risk of having a fracture.

The number of women taking 10 to 40 mg of alendronate daily over 2 to 3 years who will have a hip fracture is no different than the number of women taking a placebo (2 out of 100 compared to 4 out of 100 women). These numbers may also be due to chance and not to treatment with alendronate.

Bone mineral density (BMD): Bone mineral density increased in the lower spine and in the hip in **postmenopausal women** who had normal to near normal bone density and in women with osteoporosis who received 5 to 40 mg of alendronate. The increase in the bone density of the forearm was also increased but not as much as in the lower spine and hip.

Despite the fact that bone density increased after each year, the amount of the increase was less after each year.

Were there any side effects?
Side effects such as heartburn or ulcers in the oesophagus (or gullet) may occur. But the number of women who stopped taking alendronate due to side effects was no different than the number of women who stopped taking a placebo.

In the biggest study, 7 out of 100 women taking 5 to 40 mg of alendronate and 6 out of 100 women taking a placebo stopped their medication.

It will be long before we can assess what the rare and late side effects of alendronate.

15 MINUTE CONSUMER SUMMARY

PAGE 3

Bottom line

What is the bottom line?
There is "Platinum" level of evidence that women after menopause with normal to near normal bone density or osteoporosis, have fewer spine fractures when taking alendronate at 5 to 40 mg daily for 2 to 3 years.

Women after menopause with osteoporosis have fewer hip fractures and other non-spinal fractures with 10 to 40 mg of alendronate for 2 to 3 years. It is unclear whether women with normal or near normal bone density have fewer non-spinal fractures with alendronate.

Alendronate, at 10 to 40 mg daily for 2 to 3 years, increases bone mineral density in women after menopause with normal to near normal bone density or osteoporosis. This effect appeared to increase with larger doses of alendronate over longer periods of treatment.

Side effects such as heartburn or ulcers in the oesophagus (or gullet) may occur . However after 2 to 3 years of taking the pills, women after menopause do not appear to experience side effects that would cause them to stop taking alendronate. It is not certain yet what are the rare side effects of alendronate.

From Cranney A, Simon LS, Tugwell P, Adachi R, Ottawa Methods Group. Osteoporosis. In: *Evidence-based Rheumatology*. London: BMJ Books, 2003.

45 MINUTE DECISION AID

PAGE 1

Information about osteoporosis and treatment

What is osteoporosis?
Osteoporosis is a condition of weak, brittle bones that break easily. The most common breaks or fractures are in the spine, hip, wrist or forearm, and these may occur without a fall. Osteoporosis is detected using a bone density test that measures the amount of bone loss. A result that is at least 2·5 "standard deviations" below normal confirms the diagnosis. This means people have lost at least 25 per cent of their bone mass or density.

Hip fractures can cause severe disability or death.

Among 100 women with normal bone density, about **15** may break a hip in their lifetime.
Among 100 women with low bone density, about **35 to 75** may break a hip in their lifetime.

This number depends on *amount of bone loss, age*, and other risk factors, such as:

major bone-related risks: previous broken bones since age 50 (not from trauma); family history of fracture (e.g. mother who broke a hip, wrist, spine)
major fall-related risks: poor health; unable to rise from a chair without help; use of sleeping pills.

Spine fractures are more common, disabling, and painful. They can cause stooped posture and loss of height of up to 6 inches.

To find out your personal risk of broken bones, ask your doctor.

What can I do on my own to manage my disease?
Calcium and vitamin D   Regular impact exercises (e.g. walking)

What treatments are used for osteoporosis?
Three kinds of treatment may be used alone or together. The common (generic) names of treatment are shown below.

1. *Bone-specific drugs*
   Alendronate   Calcitonin   Etidronate   Risedronate
2. *Hormones that affect bones and other organs*
   Parathyroid hormone   Raloxifene   Hormone replacement therapy (oestrogen and progestin)
3. *Other*
   Hip protector pads

What about other treatments I have heard about?
There is not enough evidence about the effects of some treatments. Other treatments do not work. For example:

Calcitonin for non-spinal fractures
Etidronate for non-spinal fractures
Raloxifene for non-spinal fractures

What are my choices? How can I decide?
Treatment for your disease will depend on your condition. You need to know the good points (pros) and bad points (cons) about each treatment before you can decide.

45 MINUTE DECISION AID

PAGE 2

Osteoporosis decision aid

Should I take alendronate?

This guide can help you make decisions about the treatment your doctor is asking you to consider.

It will help you to:

1. Clarify what you need to decide.
2. Consider the pros and cons of different choices.
3. Decide what role you want to have in choosing your treatment.
4. Identify what you need to help you make the decision.
5. Plan the next steps.
6. Share your thinking with your doctor.

Step 1: Clarify what you need to decide
What is the decision?
Should I take alendronate to slow bone loss or prevent breaks?

Alendronate may be taken as a pill daily or once a week.

When does this decision have to be made? Check one

☐ within days   ☐ within weeks   ☐ within months

How far along are you with this decision? Check one

☐ I have not thought about it yet

☐ I am considering the choices

☐ I am close to making a choice

☐ I have already made a choice

45 MINUTE DECISION AID

PAGE 3

Step 2: Consider the pros and cons of different choices

What does the research show?
Alendronate is classified as: **Beneficial**

There is "Platinum" level evidence from 11 studies of 12 855 women after menopause that tested alendronate and lasted up to 4 years. The women had osteoporosis (low bone density) or normal to near normal bone density. These studies found pros and cons that are listed in the chart below.

What do I think of the pros and cons of alendronate?

1. Review the common pros and cons that are shown below.
2. Add any other pros and cons that are important to you.
3. Show how important each pro and con is to you by circling from one (*) star if it is a little important to you, to up to five (*****) stars if it is very important to you.

PROS AND CONS OF ALENDRONATE TREATMENT

PROS (number of people affected)	How important is it to you?	CONS (number of people affected)	How important is it to you?
Fewer broken bones in the spine 5 less women out of 100 have breaks in their spine over a lifetime with alendronate	* * * * *	**Side effects: heartburn, stomach irritation**	* * * * *
Fewer broken bones in the hip or wrist 21 less women out of 100 with **osteoporosis** have breaks in their hip or wrist over a lifetime	* * * * *	**Increases chance of developing ulcers in the oesophagus or gullet**	* * * * *
Increases bone density	* * * * *	**Must be taken in morning 1 hour before eating and sit or stand after taking the pill**	* * * * *
Flexible dosing may be taken once a week	* * * * *	**Personal cost of medicine**	* * * * *
Other pros	* * * * *	**Other cons**	* * * * *

What do you think about taking alendronate? Check ✓ one

☐ Willing to consider this treatment — Pros are more important to me than the Cons

☐ Unsure

☐ Not willing to consider this treatment — Cons are more important to me than the Pros

45 MINUTE DECISION AID

PAGE 4

Step 3: Choose the role you want to have in choosing your treatment

Check one

☐ I prefer to decide on my own after listening to the opinions of others

☐ I prefer to share the decision with: ____________________

☐ I prefer someone else to decide for me, namely: ______________

Step 4: Identify what you need to help you make the decision

What I know	Do you know enough about your condition to make a choice?	☐ Yes ☐ No ☐ Unsure
	Do you know which options are available to you?	☐ Yes ☐ No ☐ Unsure
	Do you know the good points (pros) of each option?	☐ Yes ☐ No ☐ Unsure
	Do you know the bad points (cons) of each option?	☐ Yes ☐ No ☐ Unsure
What's important	Are you clear about which **pros** are most *important to you?*	☐ Yes ☐ No ☐ Unsure
	Are you clear about which **cons** are most *important to you?*	☐ Yes ☐ No ☐ Unsure
How others help	Do you have enough support from others to make a choice?	☐ Yes ☐ No ☐ Unsure
	Are you choosing without pressure from others?	☐ Yes ☐ No ☐ Unsure
	Do you have enough advice to make a choice?	☐ Yes ☐ No ☐ Unsure
How sure I feel	Are you clear about the best choice for you?	☐ Yes ☐ No ☐ Unsure
	Do you feel sure about what to choose?	☐ Yes ☐ No ☐ Unsure

If you answered No or Unsure to many of these questions, you should talk to your doctor.

Step 5: Plan the next steps

What do you need to do before you make this decision?
For example: talk to your doctor, read more about this treatment or other treatments for osteoporosis.

Step 6: Share the information on this form with your doctor

It will help your doctor understand what you think about this treatment.

Structure of the book

Chapters 1–4 are methodology chapters relevant to an evidence-based approach to rheumatology. Chapter 1 reviews the important area of literature searching. A pivotal feature of a systematic review is the use of an unbiased comprehensive search strategy. Healthcare professionals have access to many resources through the internet. However, the process of searching for information is not simply a matter of plugging in a few keywords to one's favourite search engine. This chapter describes searching for evidence-based literature in the field of rheumatology.

Chapter 2 reviews work in rheumatology on outcomes, combining the results of studies and comparing the effects of different interventions while requiring that the endpoint of the study be comparable. In 1989 a review showed that there were still many problems with the endpoints employed in rheumatoid arthritis (RA) clinical trials;[21] the endpoints were not comprehensive and yet showed considerable overlap, and were insensitive to change. The stalemate was impeding progress and hampering the development of new treatments. This led to the establishment of a series of consensus conferences to develop an agenda to establish minimum core sets of outcomes that meet the OMERACT Methods "Filter" of validity, responsiveness, and feasibility.

Chapter 3, for example, reviews the issues relevant to incorporating the economic perspective in making decisions around therapy in rheumatologic conditions, while Chapter 2 addresses the concepts and issues relevant to the effective communication of the evidence to enable the patient or consumer and clinician to make an informed choice.

Chapters 5–13 are related to the clinical content areas. Each one presents in a similar perspective the best available evidence for helping to make choices about healthcare decisions. The published methodology for conducting a systematic review was applied.[19] All languages were included in the literature searches and when necessary translations were conducted. Authors for the clinical chapters included reviewers from North America (Canada and USA), Europe (France, Romania and the Netherlands), Australia, and Thailand. A description of the statistical methodology used for the NNT and NNH is provided.

The clinical chapters each report the results of the systematic review, RCT or observational studies, which are then presented in a clinically relevant manner using a statistical approach. Clinical case presentations within each chapter demonstrate how the evidence would be applied in making healthcare choices in practice. As new studies are completed, new evidence will be added to the data.

Number needed to treat (NNT)

When comparing a new treatment with a control (standard) treatment, the number needed to treat (NNT) is the number of patients who need to be treated with the new treatment rather than the control treatment in order for one additional patient to benefit. The NNT was calculated using one of several different methods depending on the clinical and research setting. More specifically, three methods were considered:

1. If a single study is available and the event rates in the treatment group (P_t) and the control group (P_c) are provided, then the NNT is the reciprocal of the risk difference (absolute risk reduction or ARR) given by $1/(P_c-P_t)$ or, if the outcome is beneficial, by $1/(P_t-P_c)$. Note, when there is no treatment effect the confidence limit of the risk difference includes 0 and NNT is infinite. The methods used for confidence interval calculations are outlined in Chapter 11 of *Statistics with Confidence*, 2nd edition.[22] If the ARR was significant, the confidence interval for NNT was calculated based on the reciprocals of the confidence limits of the ARR. The CIA software was used for the actual calculation.[22]
2. If several studies are available and a meta-analysis has been conducted yielding an overall weighted average estimate of relative risk (RR), then the NNT estimates are obtained by substituting the RR, along with an estimate of the prevalence of the condition in the population of interest, into the NNT formulation based on RR: NNT [1/(event rate*(1–RR)].[22] The Cates software,[21] Visual Rx 1.6, was used for the actual calculation. Visual Rx (available at http://www.nntonline.net/ebm/visualrx/try.asp) is designed to calculate numbers needed to treat (NNT) from the pooled results of a meta-analysis and produce a graphical display of the result.

   The original concept of presenting NNT graphically using faces was published by Laupacis *et al.*[23] The idea was reinforced by empirical work that was presented at the Seventh Annual Cochrane Colloquium in Rome in October 1999. There are many different statistical methods which can be used in calculating a summary estimate from the results of individual clinical trials and the NNT can be derived in different ways from each of these. Since the results are not always identical, Visual Rx accommodates a variety of methods using relative risk, Peto odds ratio, odds ratio, and event rates. In order to make the concept of NNT understandable to clinicians and patients, Visual Rx produces a graphical display representing the likely outcomes for a theoretical group of 100 patients who are given a particular treatment.

   Visual Rx is particularly useful in relation to the results of Cochrane Systematic Reviews, which are available electronically on the Cochrane Library at http://www.update-software.com/Cochrane. Visual Rx can only be used to display the results for dichotomous outcomes.
3. For continuous outcomes, the procedure by Altman was used to determine the estimate of NNT.[22] This procedure requires the identification of an effect size as a minimal important difference (MID) and the default value suggested was 0·5. The Wells software was used for the actual calculation.[24]

Number needed to harm (NNH) is similar to the NNT in the context of the mathematical calculation but differs in that the experimental treatment increases the probability of a harmful outcome compared to placebo[24,25,26]. This is to be considered when an adverse event is caused by the active treatment. The NNH is defined as the number of patients who receive the active therapy that will lead to one additional patient being harmed compared to those who receive placebo. The calculated NNH is usually accompanied by a 95% CI as that of the NNT. The NNH should be considered together with the NNT since an experimental treatment may help decrease the probability of one event, but may increase the probability of another adverse event, which might exceed the beneficial effect of the active therapy.

References

1 British Medical Research Council Investigation. Streptomycin treatment of pulmonary tuberculosis. *BMJ* 1948:770–82.

2 Empire Rheumatism Council: Multi-centre controlled trial comparing cortisone acetate and acetyl salicylic acid in the long-term treatment of rheumatoid arthritis. *Ann Rheum Dis* 1955;**14**:353.

3 Anon. How to read clinical journals V. To distinguish useful from useless or even harmful therapy. *Can Med Assoc J* 1981;**124**:1156–62.

4 *Evidence-based Healthcare* (quarterly journal 1997) (see http://www.harcourt-international.com/journals/ebhc/)

5 *Getting Research into Policy and Practice.* http://www.jsiuk-gripp-resources.net/gripp/do/viewPages?pageID=1.

6 Chalmers, I. The role of consumers in directing research. What do I want from health research and researchers when I am a patient? *BMJ* 1995;**310**:1315–18.

7 Moynihan R, Bero L, Ross-Dehnan D *et al.* Coverage by the news media of the benefits and risks of medications. *N Engl J Med* 2000;**342**(22):1645–50.

8 Rosenberg W, Donald A. Evidence-based medicine: an approach to clinical problem-solving. *BMJ* 1995;**310**:1122–6.

9 Boers M, Brooks P, Strand V, Tugwell P. The OMERACT filter for outcomes measures in rheumatology. *J Rheumatol* 1998;**25**(2):198–9.

10 Beckenhaugh RD, Instrup DM: Total hip arthroplasty: A review of 333 cases with long follow up. *J Bone Joint Surg (Am)* 1978;**60A**:306–13.

11 Cochrane AL. *Effectiveness and efficiency. Random reflections on health services.* London: Royal Society of Medicine, 1999.

12 Cochrane AL. 1931–1971: a critical review, with particular reference to the medical profession. In: *Medicines for the year 2000.* London: Office of Health Economics, 1979:1–11.

13 Cochrane Collaboration. *Cochrane Library.* Oxford: Update Software.

14 Cumbers BJ, Donald A. Evidence-based practice. Data day. *Health Serv J* 1999; April,**109**(5650):30–1.

15 Juni P, Witschi A, Bloch R, Egger M. The hazards of scoring the quality of clinical trials for meta-analysis. *JAMA* 1999;**282**:1054–60.

16 Harris RP, Helfnad M, Woolf SH et al. Current methods of the US Preventitive Services Task Force: a review of the process. *Am J Prev Med* 2001;**20**:21–35.

17 West S, King V, Carey TS *et al.* Systems to rate the strength of scientific evidence. http://www.ahcpr.gov/clinic/strevinv.htm.

18 Oxford Centre for EBM. http://www.latexresourcecenter.com/methodology.asp#tools.

19 Clarke M, Oxman AD, eds. *Cochrane Reviewer's Handbook 4.2* (updated March 2003). In: The Cochrane Library, Issue 2.Oxford: Update Software (updated quarterly), 2003.

20 Anderson JJ, Felson DT, Meenan RF, Williams HJ. Which traditional measures should be used in rheumatoid arthritis clinical trials? *Arthritis Rheum* 1989;**32**:1093–9.

21 Chris Cates. Visual Rx. http://www.nntonline.net/ebm/visualrx/try.asp

22 Altman DG, Machin D, Bryant TN, Gardner MJ. *Statistics with Confidence*, 2nd edn. London: BMJ Books, 2000.

23 Laupacis A, Sackett DL, Roberts RS. An assessment of clinically useful measures of the consequences of treatment. *N Engl J Med* 1988;**318**(26):1728–33.

24 Matthew J Wells. Wells Software. http://www.medicine.uottawa.ca/epid/eng/

25 Sackett DL, Haynes RB. Summarising the effects of therapy: a new table and some more terms (EBM Notebook). Evidence-Based *Medicine* 1997;July-August:103–4.

26 Glasziou P, Guyatt GH, Dans AL, Dans LF, Straus S, Sackett DL. Applying the results of trials and systematic reviews to individual patients (EBM Notebook). *Evidence-Based Medicine* 1998;November-December:165–6.

For additional information:

Evidence-based Healthcare (quarterly journal). http://www.harcourt-international.com/journals/ebhc/

Lavis, John *et al.* Program in policy decision-making (useful Bibliography). http://www.researchtopolicy.ca/

Alliance for Health Policy and Systems Research (for a more global angle). http://www2.alliance-hpsr.org/jahia/Jahia/cache/off

Abbreviations

ACE	angiotensin-converting enzyme
ACR	American College for Rheumatology
ACTH	adrenocorticotropic hormone
ANCA	antineutrophil cytoplasmic antibodies
Anti-dsDNA	anti-double stranded DNA (antibodies)
APL	anti-phospholipid antibodies
ARR	absolute risk reduction
AS	ankylosing spondylitis
AZA	azathioprine
BASDAI	Bath Ankylosing Spondylitis Disease Activity Index
BASFI	Bath Ankylosing Spondylitis Functional Index
BASMI	Bath Ankylosing Spondylitis Disease Metrology Index
BMD	bone mineral density
BVAS	Birmingham Vasculitis Activity Score
CCB	calcium channel blockers
CHD	coronary heart disease
CQ	chloroquine
CsA	ciclosporin
CSS	Churg Strauss syndrome
CTX	cyclophosphamide
CYC	cyclophosphamide
DAS	Disease Activity Score
DCART	disease controlling antirheumatic (drug) therapy
DMARDs	disease modifying antirheumatic drugs
DPGN	diffuse proliferative glomerulonephritis
ESR	erythrocyte sedimentation rate
ESRD	end stage renal disease
ESWT	extracorporeal shock wave therapy
EULAR	European League for Rheumatology
HCQ	hydroxycholoroquine
HRT	hormone replacement therapy
IBD	inflammatory bowel disease
ICER	incremental cost-effectiveness ratio
ILAR	International League for Rheumatology
ITT	intention to treat
IV Ig	intravenous gammaglobulin
JSW	joint space width
LOS	longitudinal observational studies
MA	meta-analysis
MCID	minimally clinically important differences
MMF	mycophenolate mofetil

6MP	6-mercaptopurine
MP	methylprednisolone
MPA	microscopic polyangiitis
MSU	monosodium urate
MTX	methotrexate
NNH	number needed to harm
NNT	number needed to treat
OA	osteoarthritis
OMERACT	Outcome Measures in Rheumatology (formerly Outcome Measures in Rheumatoid Arthritis Clinical Trials)
OP	osteoporosis
PDN	prednisone
PAN	polyarteritis nodosa
PCP	pneumocystis carinii
PP	plasmapheresis
QALY	quality adjusted life years
RA	rheumatoid arthritis
RCT	randomised controlled trial
ReA	reactive arthritis
RR	relative risk
RS	Reiter's syndrome
SERMs	selective (o)estrogen receptor modulators
SF	synovial fluid
SLAM	Systemic Lupus Activity Measure
SLE	systemic lupus erythematosus
SLEDAI	Systemic Lupus Erythematosus Disease Activity Index
SMD	standardised mean difference
SRC	scleroderma renal crisis
SSc	systemic sclerosis
SSZ	sulphasalzine
SUA	serum uric acid
THA	total hip arthroplasty
TKR	total knee replacement
US	ultrasound
VAS	visual analogue scale
WG	Wegener's granulomatosis
WHI	Women's Health Initiative
WMD	weighted mean difference
WOMAC	Western Ontario and McMaster University (Osteoarthritis Index)

Evidence-based Rheumatology CD Rom

Features

Evidence-based Rheumatology PDF eBook

- Bookmarked and hyperlinked for instant access to all headings and topics
- Fully indexed and searchable text – just click the "Search Text" button
- Free printable downloads of all consumer sections in the book
- Free printable downloads of all faces figures in the book
- Free printable download of the book Introduction

PDA edition sample chapter

- A chapter from Evidence-based Rheumatology, adapted for use on handheld devices such as Palm and Pocket PC
- Uses Mobipocket Reader technology, compatible with all PDA devices and also available for Windows
- Follow the on-screen instructions on the relevant part of the CD Rom to install Mobipocket for your device
- Full title available for purchase as a download from http://www.pda.bmjbooks.com

BMJ Books catalogue

- Instant access to BMJ Books full catalogue, including an order form

Evidence-based Rheumatology update website

- Direct link to free access book website (http://www.evidbasedrheum.com) which includes further information, printable clinical and consumer sections, faces figures and Introduction, and will also include regular updates for the book.

Instructions for use

The CD Rom should start automatically upon insertion, on all Windows systems. The menu screen will appear and you can then navigate by clicking on the headings. If the CD Rom does not start automatically upon insertion, please browse using "Windows Explorer" and double-click the file "BMJ_Books.exe".

Readers are encouraged to print off the clinical and consumer materials and faces figures and tables, along with the Introduction which explains their use, to share with patients and trainees. Simply click on "view/print consumer sections" to access the printable versions of these sections.

Tips

The viewable area of the PDF ebook can be expanded to fill the full screen width, by hiding the bookmarks. To do this, click and hold on the divider in between the bookmark window and the main window, then drag it to the left as required.

By clicking once on a page in the PDF ebook window, you "activate" the window. You can now scroll through pages uses the scroll-wheel on your mouse, or by using the cursor keys on your keyboard.

Note: the Evidence-based Rheumatology PDF eBook is for search and reference only and cannot be printed. A printable PDF version as well as the full PDA edition can be purchased from http://www.bmjbookshop.com

Troubleshooting

If any problems are experienced with use of the CD Rom, we can give you access to all content via the internet. Please send your CD Rom with proof of purchase to the following address, with a letter advising your email address and the problem you have encountered:

Evidence-based Rheumatology eBook access

BMJ Bookshop
BMA House
Tavistock Square
London
WC1H 9JR

Part I: Methodology in rheumatology

1
Literature searching

Jessie McGowan

Introduction

This chapter discusses how to locate and gather evidence. Performing a literature search is a vital step in the evidence-based process.[1] Healthcare professionals access the internet to search many resources, such as databases and website pages. Some of these databases, such as PubMed and CINAHL are available at no fee. Other databases, such as the Cochrane Library and Clinical Evidence, require a licensing agreement. Some countries have arranged for national licensing of certain products. For example, Australia, England, Wales, Ireland, Finland, Norway and South Africa have arranged national provisions to the Cochrane Library.

The process of searching for information is not simply a matter of plugging in a few keywords into one's favourite search engine. Very unfortunate outcomes can result from a search that does not locate all the appropriate literature. This is highlighted by an incident in which a healthy volunteer in an asthma and allergy related investigation died after inhaling the drug hexamethonium.[2,3] This chapter will focus on searching for evidence-based literature in the field of rheumatology.

Currently, there are no published standards or guidelines for literature searching in medicine or the health sciences. However, the Canadian Health Libraries Association/Association des bibliothèques de la santé, and the Medical Library Association of the United States have recommended that national guidelines or standards for literature searching be developed.[4] A protocol in the context of literature searching for health technology assessment has been developed. Steps to take in the course of the search are detailed so that another researcher should be able to duplicate the search strategy and retrieve comparable results.[5] The following chapter is based on the best available evidence from the current health and library literature.

It is important to remember that literature searching and information retrieval is a skill. Health librarians are professionals (with a master degree in library and information science) who specialise in this area. They should be consulted if training on using information resources or databases is required. They can be involved with the design and implementation of the literature search process either from a collaborative or from a consultative approach. It is a good idea to find out where to access health librarians in your location. One can start by contacting a local medical school, hospital, or professional association to ask if library services are available.

Healthcare professionals who want to take care of their patients in an evidence-based manner will need to know where and how to search the literature to locate the best available evidence. This chapter will outline the basics of identifying appropriate sources to locate health information and how to develop searching strategies.

The first step in the evidence-based process is to identify a clinical question or questions arising from a clinical scenario. Clinically, questions usually fall into one of four broad categories that include treatment/prevention, diagnosis, prognosis or aetiology/harm.

The literature search is the second step in the evidence-based process which is discussed in detail in the introductory portion of this book. Searching is completely dependent on the formation of a clear clinical question. The components of the clinical question (the patient/ population, the intervention/exposure, the comparison and the outcome) also form the components of the search strategy.

When searching for information, the following steps are suggested.

1. Form a clinical question.
2. Select sources to search.
3. Develop search strategies for the information sources based on the components of the clinical question.
4. Evaluate and appraise your search retrieval.
5. Consult with a librarian, as necessary.

The intellectual process of selecting information sources and developing search strategies will be presented using the following case presentation as an example.

Case presentation
A 62-year-old woman presents to your office with a recent history of lower back pain, which occurred after she slipped on the ice outside her house. Her family doctor ordered spinal x-rays that revealed a T12 compression fracture with a 50% loss of height. The family doctor also documented that the patient had risk factors for osteoporosis including low calcium intake, a maternal history of hip fracture, and a previous wrist fracture at age 55. She never took hormone replacement therapy after menopause, which occurred at age 47. Her family physician has heard about the drug etidronate at a recent conference (a first generation bisphosphonate). He wonders if this would be an appropriate treatment to prevent osteoporosis.

Several clinical questions can be derived from the above scenario, including the following therapy-related question:

Would taking the drug etidronate reduce this postmenopausal 62-year-old woman's risk of osteoporosis?

Patient: postmenopausal 62-year-old woman
Intervention: etidronate
Outcome: reduced risk of osteoporosis

Keep this question in mind as different information sources are discussed.

Selecting sources for locating evidence

Many different sources are available to locate information. However, not all of these sources are of equal value. Below is a description of the major sources of information that are used to locate information.

Expert opinion

Expert opinion refers to the consultation process, whether with a respected colleague, a specialist in the field or a supervisor. Expert opinion differs from the other sources of information in that it incorporates clinical experience. It is very convenient to ask a colleague about their experience in prescribing etidronate to patients. This can be advantageous because it allows for a focused response to the problem, which is something often not possible with the results of clinical trials. However, a disadvantage to using advice from colleagues is the susceptibility of the opinion to bias, as their responses may not be based on systematically collected information.

World Wide Web (WWW)

The World Wide Web (WWW) is part of the internet, a worldwide system of computer networks. The WWW is the most accessed part of the internet. Many healthcare professionals find it convenient to use the WWW to answer their questions because of its immediacy.

There are various types of health-related information found on the WWW, such as databases, full-text books and reference products, journals, and grey literature. Each of these information types is discussed separately in this chapter. Regardless of whether the book or journal formats are electronic or printed, the guidelines for the use and quality of the information is the same.

This section will focus on the textual content contained in websites. When looking for information on the internet, most users start by using one of the standard search engines (such as Google or AltaVista). Unfortunately, the information on the WWW is not well organised or consistently catalogued or indexed like the books in a library. There has been some effort to create an indexing system. Some web masters will use meta-tags. The meta-tags are imbedded in the coding of the website and are used to describe the content of the website. Search engines to locate websites also use meta-tags.

Unfortunately, much of the text that is located on a website is very difficult to validate and generalise. It can include expert opinion or incorrect and false information by non-experts. Therefore, searching the text of websites may only retrieve information that is based on opinion and not based on rigorous methodology.

In reviewing websites a healthcare professional needs to take into consideration information such as currency, authorship, ownership, and accuracy.[6] However, for standards relating to the content, healthcare professionals can use traditional measurements such as the levels of evidence and strength of recommendations. For example, in this scale the highest level of evidence for therapy is a systematic review of randomised controlled trials (RCTs). This scale ranks information based on the published research literature.[7] High quality, peer reviewed studies are most commonly found in the journal literature. They are not typically published on websites alone.

In a study on the examination of measurements that rate the quality on health information on the internet, the researchers were able to identify 51 rating instruments. Of these, only five had enough information to be evaluated. Of these remaining five, none was validated.[8]

To search the WWW for information about using etidronate to prevent osteoporosis we can begin by using a search engine.

Using Google, one of the standard search engines, searching the term *etidronate* retrieved many thousands of hits (links to websites that contain the information from the search question). However, searching the key words *etidronate, postmenopause* and *osteoporosis* retrieved four hits. The sources of the hits were located in journal articles.[9–12] The same search in AltaVista retrieved no hits. It is always advisable to use more than one search engine for a question. To execute a complete journal search, see the section on journals and bibliographic databases.

Textbooks/reference products

In the past, textbooks were the main repositories of information and knowledge. Textbooks are still important for locating established knowledge or information that is not rapidly changing. For example, human anatomical atlases do not need to be updated on a regular basis, we as humans are not continually changing. Textbooks are still needed for physicians to acquire comprehensive information from basic areas of knowledge.

One main criticism of books is that the information is often one or two years out of date by the time it is published, due to the long timelines required to publish books.[13] However, thanks to electronic media, some books can now be found on CD-ROM or updated regularly on the internet. For example, Harrison's Internal Medicine is not only available online, but it also has a version available for hand-held devices or personal digital assistants (PDA).

A second example, *Clinical Evidence* is a reference produced by the BMJ Publishing Group (http://www.clinicalevidence.com). It is a database driven by questions rather than by the availability of research evidence to help clinicians in making evidence-based decisions. It contains topics that are either common or important and then summarises the best available evidence to answer them. It identifies but does not try to fill important gaps in the evidence.

For our search to find a textbook with information about the use of etidronate in preventing osteoporosis, we would begin by searching library catalogues to locate textbooks. However, searching for textbooks can be difficult. For example, the healthcare professional will need to search not only for books about etidronate and osteoporosis, but review general textbooks on rheumatology, in which a chapter on the topic may be included.

The following is a small, selected list of national web catalogues:

- AMICUS – National Library of Canada (http://amicus.nlcbnc.ca/aaweb/amilogine.htm)
- Australian National Library (http://www.nla.gov.au/catalogue/)
- British Library (http://www.bl.uk/)
- National Library of Medicine's LOCATORplus (http://locatorplus.gov/)
- National Technical Information Services (http://www.ntis.gov/)
- Canadian Institute of Scientific and Technical Information (CISTI) (http://cat.cisti.nrc.ca/).

Cochrane Library

Healthcare professionals need to be aware of the Cochrane Library, an essential collection of databases to search. The Cochrane Library records the work of the Cochrane Collaboration – an international network that is committed to preparing, maintaining, and disseminating systematic reviews on the effects of health care. The Cochrane Collaboration has evolved rapidly since it was inaugurated, but its basic objectives and principles have remained the same as they were at its inception. It is an international organisation that aims to help people make well-informed decisions about health care by preparing, maintaining and ensuring the accessibility of systematic reviews of the effects of health care interventions. The Collaboration is built on ten principles:

- collaboration
- building on the enthusiasm of individuals
- avoiding duplication
- minimising bias
- keeping up to date
- striving for relevance
- promoting access
- ensuring quality
- continuity
- enabling wide participation.

The database collection is published quarterly and is designed to provide evidence for healthcare decision making.

The process to search the Cochrane Library is similar to the process used to search the US National Library of Medicine database MEDLINE. This searching process which will be discussed later in this chapter. A search of the Cochrane Library reveals a meta-analysis from the Cochrane Database of Systematic Reviews database entitled "Etidronate for treating and preventing postmenopausal osteoporosis". The data suggested a reduction in vertebral fractures.[14]

Synthesis journals

Healthcare professionals should be aware of secondary publications that were created to focus on evidence-based philosophies. These journals provide abstracts and commentaries of previously published clinically applicable research. Articles in these journals are selected based on strict quality criteria. These evidence-based journals include *ACP Journal Club, Evidence Based Medicine, Evidence Based Mental Health,* and *Evidence Based Nursing.*

A search of *ACP Journal Club* looking for the keywords "osteoporosis" and "etidronate" retrieved the citation "Etidronate for treating and preventing postmenopausal osteoporosis", the same citation already retrieved from the Cochrane Library.[15]

Evaluation of information sources

Journals are an important information tool for healthcare professionals to use to keep up-to-date with new research as well as professional news. Many healthcare professionals like to keep current by reading certain journals each month. This is very good for general knowledge. However, to understand a specific patient or problem, it is best to do a search for an article, regardless of what journal it is in, rather than just reviewing articles that are only in a few journals.

The most efficient way to locate articles is to search a bibliographic database. A record in a bibliographic database contains descriptive information such as a citation and subject heading (see Figure 1.1). Many bibliographic databases can be used to search for medical and health information. The best known of these databases is MEDLINE, which is produced by the US National Library of Medicine (NLM). This database currently contains over 11 million citations to articles published in international journals. MEDLINE is available from a number of different vendors. It is also available directly from NLM and this version of the database is called PubMed.

There are many important databases. For example, Embase is considered the European equivalent to MEDLINE. It is very important to consider searching all databases that may contain information relevant to a topic. For example, in our search on etidronate, MEDLINE (PubMed), Embase and Current Contents should be searched. A selected list of databases is available in Appendix 2 to this chapter.

An example of a MEDLINE record is shown in Figure 1.1.

Grey literature

Grey literature can also be an important source for locating quality information. Grey literature has been defined as: that which is produced on all levels of government, academics, business, and industry in print and electronic formats, but which is not controlled by commercial publishers.[16] Examples of grey literature include web pages, archives from email groups on the internet, eprints, technical reports, meetings, conference proceedings, newsletters, and theses.

Healthcare professionals conducting research for patients may find relevant information to answer clinical questions. In a study reviewing meta-analyses, it was concluded that physicians and researchers should make an effort to locate grey literature for inclusion to minimise bias.[17]

Accessing grey literature is difficult because it tends not to be recorded in standard bibliographic databases that primarily index journal articles (such as MEDLINE). However, a number of databases are now available to search grey literature. Other access points to grey literature include web search engines to search web pages (i.e., Google, AltaVista etc), online library catalogues (see above) and governmental websites. Examples of online grey literature databases include:

- NYAM Grey literature page (http://www.nyam.org/library/greylit/index.shtml)
- Sigle (http://www.kb.nl/infoler/eagle/frames.htm)
- Gray LIT Network (http://www.osti.gov/graylit/)
- National Technical Information Service (NTIS) (http://www.ntis.gov/)

In our scenario in searching for studies on etidronate for treating and preventing postmenopausal osteoporosis, a database that could be searched is the CRD Database (http://nhscrd.york.ac.uk/) from the NHS Centre for Reviews and Dissemination at the University of York, England. This database includes both published and grey literature. Results from a search of this database included 15 documents, 14 of which were already included in bibliographic databases. The one citation that was not published was a NHS report entitled: "Bisphosphonates (alendronate and etidronate) in the management of osteoporosis".[18]

Developing and executing search strategies in bibliographic databases

The best way to locate high level evidence is by searching bibliographic databases. A bibliographic database contains descriptive information (including the title, author name(s), source information, subject headings, sometimes an abstract) for publications. The following section describes how to search bibliographic databases. Other training manuals are available. For PubMed see the PubMed home page (http://pubmed.gov). As well, the US medical libraries that are part of the National Network of Libraries of Medicine have also created training materials on MEDLINE, PubMed, the NLM Gateway, and other databases at http://nnlm.gov/nnlm/online/pubmed/. Figure 1.2 outlines the steps involved in developing a search strategy.

Compose a clinical question

Let's consider our question again.

Would taking the drug etidronate reduce this postmenopausal 62-year-old woman's risk of osteoporosis?

Patient: postmenopausal 62-year-old woman
Intervention: etidronate
Outcome: reduced risk of osteoporosis

Identify relevant sources to search in

The following example will be for MEDLINE using the Ovid interface. However, other databases including Embase and Current Contents are also relevant.

Define the search strategy

Content searching

Next, the search question is reviewed and then split into concepts or elements that can be

Unique Identifier 11687195
Medline Identifier 21546913
Record Owner NLM

Authors Cranney A. Welch V. Adachi JD. Guyatt G. Krolicki N. Griffith L. Shea B. Tugwell P. Wells G.

Institution Medicine – Rheumatology, Ottawa Hospital, Civic Campus, 461, 737 Parkdale Ave, Ottawa, Ontario, Canada, K1Y 1J8. acranney@ottawahospital.on.ca

Title Etidronate for treating and preventing postmenopausal osteoporosis. [Review] [49 refs]

Source Cochrane Database of Systematic Reviews. (4):CD003376, 2001.
Abbreviated Source Cochrane Database Syst Rev. (4):CD003376, 2001.
NLM Journal Code 100909747
Journal Subset IM
Country of Publication England
MeSH Subject Headings Bone Density / de [Drug Effects]
*Etidronic Acid / tu [Therapeutic Use]
Female
Human
*Osteoporosis, Postmenopausal / dt [Drug Therapy]
Osteoporosis, Postmenopausal / pc [Prevention & Control]
Spinal Fractures / et [Etiology]

Abstract OBJECTIVES: To systematically review the efficacy of **etidronate** on bone density, fractures and toxicity in postmenopausal women. **SEARCH STRATEGY:** We searched MEDLINE from 1966 to December 1998, examined citations of relevant articles, and the proceedings of international osteoporosis meetings. We contacted osteoporosis investigators to identify additional studies, primary authors, and pharmaceutical industry sources for unpublished data. **SELECTION CRITERIA:** We included thirteen trials (with 1010 participants) that randomized women to **etidronate** or an alternative (placebo or calcium and/or vitamin D) and measured bone density for at least one year. **DATA COLLECTION AND ANALYSIS:** For each trial, three independent reviewers assessed the methodological quality and abstracted data. **MAIN RESULTS:** The data suggested a reduction in vertebral fractures with a pooled relative risk of 0·60% (95% CI 0·41 to 0·88). There was no effect on non-vertebral fractures (pooled relative risk 1·00, (95% CI 0·68 to 1·42)). **Etidronate** , relative to control, increased bone density after three years of treatment in the lumbar spine by 4·27% (95% CI 2·66 to 5·88), in the femoral neck by 2·19% (95% CI 0·43, 3·95) and in the total body by 0·97% (95% CI 0·39, 1·55). Effects were larger at 4 years, though the number of patients followed was much smaller. **REVIEWER'S CONCLUSIONS:** **Etidronate** increases bone density in the lumbar spine and femoral neck. The pooled estimates of fracture reduction with **etidronate** are consistent with a reduction in vertebral fractures, but no effect on non-vertebral fractures. [References: 49]

CAS Registry/EC Number 2809-21-4 (Etidronic Acid).
ISSN 1469-493X
Publication Type Journal Article. Review. Review, Academic.
Language English
Entry Date 20020419
Update Date 20020422

Figure 1.1 Example of a MEDLINE record.

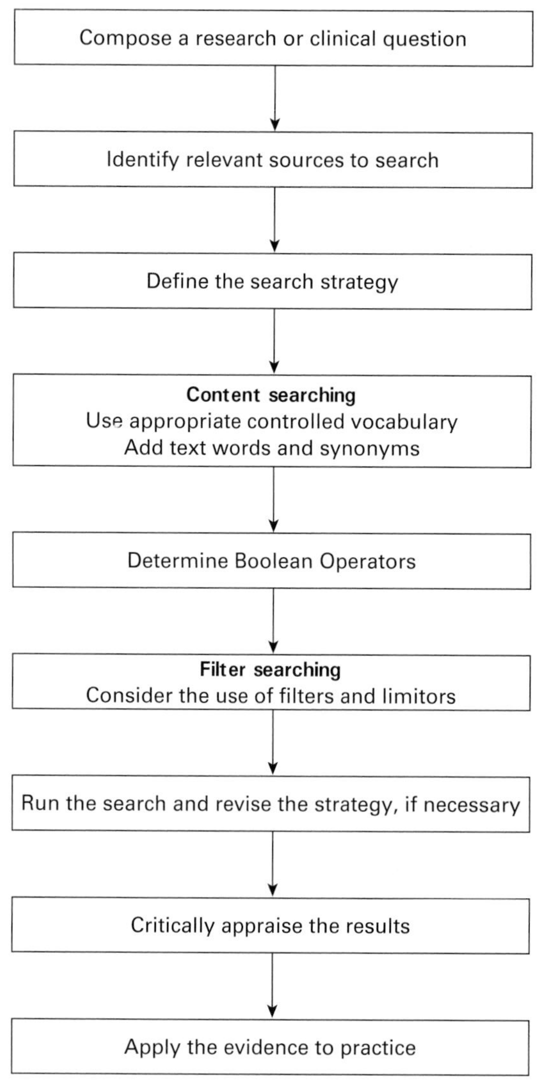
Compose a research or clinical question
Identify relevant sources to search
Define the search strategy
Content searching
Use appropriate controlled vocabulary
Add text words and synonyms
Determine Boolean Operators
Filter searching
Consider the use of filters and limitors
Run the search and revise the strategy, if necessary
Critically appraise the results
Apply the evidence to practice
Keep in mind: 1) the patient, 2) the intervention/ exposure, and 3) the outcome.
This can include databases like MEDLINE and Embase, or the Cochrane Library.
Break the question into concepts or elements that can be searched separately, and later combined. Define the content and filter searches.
Use the appropriate controlled vocabulary of the database you are searching. For example, in MEDLINE use MeSH (Medical Subject Headings). Use textwords and synonyms to search in non-indexed fields such as the title and abstract fields.
Use AND to retrieve records which contain both terms, use OR to retrieve records which contain either term, and use NOT to eliminate records with certain terms.
Filters can be added to retrieve specific search results. Some databases will allow limiting of searches to certain publication types (like RCTs), language, sex, age, etc.
Consult a librarian for assistance or to validate the search strategy.

Figure 1.2 Steps in developing an electronic search strategy.

searched separately. In the above search question, there are three main concepts:

- postmenopause
- osteoporosis
- etidronate.

When searching in any database, it is important to understand the controlled vocabulary of that database. In MEDLINE, MeSH (Medical Subject Headings) is the controlled vocabulary thesaurus. It consists of sets of terms that name subject headings in a hierarchical structure. This allows searching at various levels of specificity and relevancy.

The most common way to locate the appropriate MeSH in MEDLINE, is to use the *MeSH – Annotated Alphabetic List.* Online MeSH "scope notes" are available through some providers of MEDLINE. The scope notes provide useful information, such as the definition, year of entry, search notes, see-related and used-for terms. Some scope notes have more information than others. Another useful index is the *Permuted MeSH*, which consists of a listing of each significant word or root appearing in any MeSH heading or printed cross-reference. Because this index can be used to locate any word, regardless of word order, it is a useful way to locate the correct MeSH. Note: to use this index on line, type "ptx" before the one word you are searching (ptx will only work for one-word searching). For example: "ptx myocardial" will list every MeSH that has the word "myocardial" in it, such as myocardial infarction, myocardial ischaemia, myocardial depressant factor, etc. The *MeSH Tree Structures* arranges all MeSH in hierarchical order. This tool can be useful in locating broader and narrower terms for MeSH. Note: to use this index on line, type "tree" before the one word you are searching for, for example: "tree myocardial infarction". This will display the terms that are broader and narrower than this term.

The following MeSH are identified for the above search question:

- exp osteoporosis
- bone density
- exp menopause
- etidronic acid.

Using "exp" before a MeSH term, such as "exp osteoporosis" will allow the inclusion of all narrower terms under that heading. This is called exploding MeSH. This will search the main heading "osteoporosis" plus the narrower heading "osteoporosis, postmenopausal".

Occasionally in the MEDLINE database words are misspelled. Some of these originate in the printed manuscript and some through data entry at NLM. As well, depending on the number of index terms applied to an article, index terms may be omitted from articles.[19] Sometimes it may happen that a MeSH term has not been assigned to a new drug, or subject. In order to increase the sensitivity (i.e., to ensure that no relevant articles are missed), additional words may be added to search strategy. The Textword function searches for the occurrence of a word or phrase in the title (TI) and abstract (AB) fields. You can search these fields individually, or together by using the textword (TW). Some searchers will incorporate textwords (TW) and MeSH terms into their strategies. Be careful when you are textword searching, to account for variations in spelling, and synonyms, by using truncation.

- Post-menopause
  - post-menopaus$.tw.
  - postmenopaus$.tw.
  - Osteoporosis.tw.
  - osteoporosis.tw.
  - bone loss$.tw.
  - (bone adj2 densit$).tw.
- Etidronate
  - etidronate.tw.
  - (xidifon or xidiphon$).tw.
  - (ehdp or ethanehydroxydiphosphonate). tw.

The use of the "$" is for truncation. When searching for textwords where the suffix needs to be taken into account, you may truncate the term you are searching by adding the truncation symbol "$". For example, adenoma$.tw. will retrieve references in which the terms adenoma, adenomas, adenomatoid, adenomatous, and adenomatosis appear either in the titles or the abstracts. Remember to use the longest root of the term you are searching. For example: all$.tw. will retrieve "allergy", "allergies" as well as "alligators"!

Determine Boolean Operators

Boolean logic employs use of the terms "and," "or," and "not." These are called Boolean Operators, and are used to indicate the relationship between search terms (see Figure 1.3)

We have identified three concepts from our search strategy: post-menopause, osteoporosis, and etidronate. Within each of these concepts, we have different terms used for textwords, MeSH, and registry numbers. These are all terms about the same concept or like terms.

For our search strategy, we will want to combine our three concepts with AND. This will only retrieve articles that discuss all three concepts.

> Post-menopause AND Osteoporosis AND Etidronate

The resulting content searching section will be searched as follows:

1. exp osteoporosis/(note: includes osteoporosis, postmenopausal)
2. osteoporosis.tw.
3. bone density/
4. bone loss$.tw.
5. (bone adj2 densit$).tw.
6. or/2–5
7. exp menopause/
8. post-menopaus$.tw.
9. postmenopaus$.tw.
10. or/7–9
11. 6 and 10
12. 1 or 11
13. etidronic acid/
14. etidronate.tw,rn.
15. (xidifon or xidiphon$).tw.
16. (ehdp or ethanehydroxydiphosphonate).tw.
17. or/13–16
18. 12 and 17

Filter the search strategy

Filtering the literature search strategy for information of clinical significance will assist in the retrieval of relevant articles. The filters can be used depending on the type of clinical or research question being addressed. Some examples include limiting articles to publication types (i.e., meta-analysis, randomised controlled trials etc), articles on diagnosis, therapy, aetiology, prognosis, clinical practice guidelines, economic analysis, animal types, language etc.

The following search filters are based on informatics research.[20,21] The latter of these articles also includes a filter for searching for articles on prognosis, harm, and diagnosis.

Meta-analyses search filter (Hunt et al)[20]

This filter is designed to locate meta-analyses and systematic reviews.

1. meta-analysis.pt,sh.
2. (meta-anal: or metaanal:).tw.
3. (quantitativ: review: or quantitativ: overview:).tw.
4. (methodologic: review: or methodologic: overview:).tw.
5. (systematic: review: or systematic: overview).tw.
6. review.pt. and medline.tw.
7. or/1–7

RCT search filter (Haynes et al)[21]

This filter is designed to locate RCTs.

1. clinical trial.pt.
2. randomised controlled trial.pt.
3. tu.fs.
4. dt.fs.
5. random$.tw.
6. (double adj blind$).tw.
7. placebo$.tw.
8. or/1–8

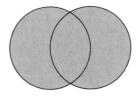

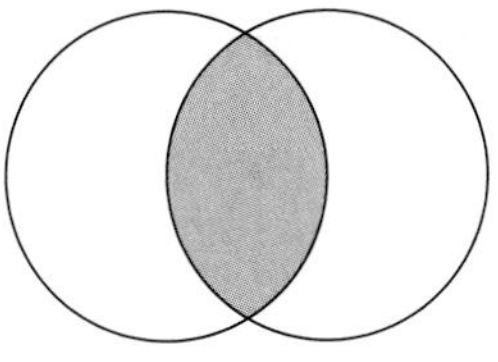
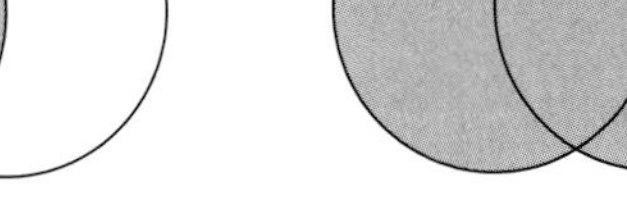
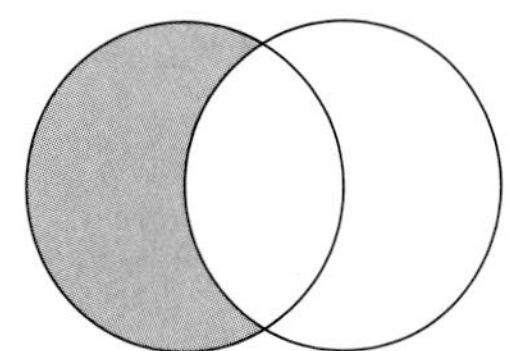

Figure 1.3

The combination of the content searching section and the filter sections are searched as follows:

1. exp osteoporosis/
2. osteoporosis.tw.
3. bone density/
4. bone loss$.tw.
5. (bone adj2 densit$).tw.
6. or/2–5
7. exp menopause/
8. post-menopaus$.tw.
9. postmenopaus$.tw.
10. or/7–9
11. 6 and 10
12. 1 or 11
13. etidronic acid/
14. etidronate.tw,rn.
15. (xidifon or xidiphon$).tw.
16. (ehdp or ethanehydroxydiphosphonate).tw.
17. or/13–16
18. 12 and 17
19. meta-analysis.pt,sh.
20. (meta-anal: or metaanal:).tw.
21. (quantitativ: review: or quantitativ: overview:). tw.
22. (methodologic: review: or methodologic: overview:).tw.
23. (systematic: review: or systematic: overview). tw.
24. review.pt. and medline.tw.
25. or/19–24
26. 18 and 25
27. clinical trial.pt.
28. randomised controlled trial.pt.
29. tu.fs.
30. dt.fs.
31. random$.tw.
32. (double adj blind$).tw.
33. placebo$.tw.
34. or/27–33
35. 18 and 34

Evaluating search strategies

In order to evaluate search strategies, the retrieval is measured in terms of precision (or specificity) and recall (or sensitivity). Precision refers to the proportion of citations that the search retrieves that are relevant to the question (i.e., the ability of the search to exclude irrelevant citations). Recall refers the proportion of all relevant citations in the database that the search retrieves (i.e., the ability to retrieve all relevant citations).

The goal of a good search strategy is to retrieve all the citations that are relevant to the question. One does not want to retrieve irrelevant citations or miss any relevant citations. Therefore, it is most important to consider recall in order not to miss relevant citations. While having low precision and reviewing irrelevant citations can be tedious, it is better to have a lower precision rate than to miss relevant citations. Unfortunately, searching will rarely, if ever, only retrieve relevant citations. However, there are techniques that can be used to improve both precision and recall.

If the search retrieves too many articles that are out of scope, then the precision is poor. To increase the precision of the search strategy, the following strategies are suggested:

- Use specific subject headings
- Use specific textwords
- Combine terms of different concepts using AND
- Limit or filter to relevant publication types
- Limit to age ranges or sex, if appropriate

If the search misses many relevant articles, then the recall is poor. To increase the recall of the search strategy, the following strategies are suggested:

- Include all subheadings
- Explode subject heading
- Do not use the "limit to focus" feature
- Add all relevant textwords
- Combine terms of related concepts using OR
- Exclude irrelevant concepts using NOT
- Use truncation
- Expand the time period of the search
- Search several databases

Library resources and services

This section briefly discusses the valuable resources and services that libraries provide. In an evidence-based environment, knowing who can help you to access materials quickly will save you time.

Libraries, like most services, are made up of different types of professionals. They can include librarians, library technicians, library assistants, and volunteers. Librarians have a postgraduate degree in library and information science. Library technicians have diplomas and are graduates of college training programmes in library and information science. Library assistants perform clerical functions in the library. Volunteers can perform duties such as shelving and photocopying. Together, they work to provide you with the best possible service.

Library staff can answer your questions, from simple enquiries, such as finding names and addresses or titles of books, to more complex enquiries, such as providing assistance and guidance regarding literature searches and collaboration on research projects. They can provide training sessions on different databases and using the internet.

Libraries can help you keep up-to-date on any subject in which you are interested. Current awareness services encompass a variety of services including photocopies of tables-of-contents, lists of new library acquisitions or recent publications, and SDI (selective dissemination of information) services. The SDI service is a monthly database update service to find relevant information on any subject from a number of databases.

Once you have found references or citations to materials you need, how do you actually get a copy? First, check your library to see if they have it. If they do not have the item you want, then you can request an interlibrary loan (ILL). Your library has access to many libraries throughout the country. The amount of time to receive your ILL will depend on a variety of factors, but libraries always try to get the document as fast as possible. Let your library know when you need to receive the item.

If you are not affiliated with a hospital, professional association or health sciences library, you may be able to access a fee-based service from one of these types of libraries, or you may be able to access a national library.

Appendices

Appendix 1: Additional MEDLINE Information

Exploding a MeSH heading will allow the inclusion of all narrower terms under that heading. For example, exploding the MeSH heading "myocardial infarction" ("exp myocardial infarction") will include the narrower MeSH headings: "myocardial stunning" and "shock, cardiogenic".

Subheadings (or qualifiers) are terms that are used in combination with MeSH. These terms can be used to help focus or narrow a search. For example: diabetes/dt,su - describes the term either with drug therapy (dt) or surgery (su), or with both.

The *floating subheading* looks for any MeSH term that uses that subheading. For example: dt.fs. retrieves aids/dt as well as asthma/dt or arthritis/dt.

The *exploded subheading* retrieves all occurrences of the subheading and related subheadings. For example the exploded therapy (th.xs.) includes many types of therapies including: diet, drug, nursing, prevention and control, rehabilitation, radiotherapy, surgery, and transplantation.

Field searching: each citation, or record in MEDLINE contains different *fields*. When you are searching using MeSH terms, you are searching the MeSH field. The following is a list of common MEDLINE fields.

Label/field	*Example*
UI Unique identifier	95262413.ui.
AU Author	tugwell p$.au.
IN Institution	Ottawa Health Research Institute.in.
TI Title	evidence-based.ti.
JN Journal	bmj.jn.
JW Journal Word	psychiatry.jw.
YR Year	1995.yr. or 95.yr
CP Country of Publication	canada.cp.
SH Medical Subject Headings	eye.sh. or eye/
FS Floating Subheading	dt.fs.
XS Exploded Subheading	th.xs.
AB Abstract	Evidence-based.ab.
RN Registry Number	tamoxifen.rn.
IS ISSN	0234-0009.is.
PT Publication Type	clinical trials.pt.
LG Language	eng.lg.
EM Entry Month	9501.em.
TW Textword	evidence-based.tw.

To search using the fields or labels, type the appropriate word or phrase, followed by the label inside dots (note: if you do not use the dots, you will receive an error message). For example if you want to search an author, type: tugwell p.au. or, if you want to find a journal, type: bmj.jn.

You may use an asterisk (*) before a MeSH term to restrict to focus. This means you will only retrieve documents in which the MeSH is considered a major focus in the article. This may be useful if you are interested in only a few citations on a general subject. This feature is not recommended for use when conducting research.

Textword searching: Sometimes it may happen that a MeSH term has not been assigned to a new drug, or subject, or sometimes you may have difficulty locating a MeSH term. The Textword function searches for the occurrence of a word or phrase in the title (TI) and abstract (AB) fields. You can search these fields individually, or together by using the textword (TW). Some searchers will incorporate textwords (TW) and MeSH terms into their strategies. Be careful when you are textword searching, by using truncation to account for variations in spelling, and synonyms.

How to limit (when the search retrieves too much): use "and" in other concepts, apply some limits (see below), remove any truncation, use more specific MeSH terms or use subheadings.

How to expand (when the search retrieval is too small): use "or" in additional synonyms or textwords, do not use limits, include all subheadings, use broader terms, "exp" MeSH terms, or truncate textwords.

In MEDLINE you may limit your search to citations on the following:

Abstracts (citations with)
Human
English language
Review
Language
Latest Update
Animal
Male
Female
Age Groups
Publication Year
Publication Type
Animal Types
Journal Subsets

Appendix 2: Selected list of databases

AMED (Allied and Complementary Medicine Database) – is produced by the British Library's Medical Information Centre in the United Kingdom. This database contains references from journals on alternative and complementary medicine going back to 1985. The thesaurus combines MeSH terms and additional AMED keywords. For more information, go to http://www.bl.uk/services/ information/amed.html.

Biological Abstracts – is produced in the US by BIOSIS and is reputed to be the world's most comprehensive reference database in the Life Sciences. Coverage includes original research reports and reviews in both the biological and biomedical areas. For more information, go to http://www.biosis.org/products_services/ba.html.

CINAHL (Cumulative Index to Nursing and Allied Health Literature) – is produced by CINAHL Information Systems. It covers the major English language literature in the areas of nursing, occupational and physical therapy and other allied health fields. For more information, go to http://www.cinahl.com/.

The Cochrane Library – is produced by Update Software for the Cochrane Collaboration and the NHS Centre for Reviews and Dissemination. The Cochrane Library is updated quarterly and contains several databases. The Cochrane Library includes the following databases:

- *The Cochrane Database of Systematic Reviews (CDSR)*: full text of completed reviews carried out by the Cochrane Collaboration, plus protocols for reviews currently in preparation.
- *The Database of Abstracts of Reviews of Effectiveness (DARE):* abstracts of other systematic reviews; comment on the quality of the methodology of reviews published in the medical literature.
- *The Cochrane Central Register of Controlled Trials (CENTRAL):* references to randomised controlled trials (RCTs) identified through hand searching of journals and searching of other databases.
- *The Cochrane Database of Methodology Reviews*: references to articles, etc dealing with the science/methods of systematic reviews, RCTs, etc.
- *The Cochrane Methodology Register:* is a bibliography intended to help those who are new to the science of reviewing to find additional material of interest and for those

who are already immersed in it to find something new.

- *The Health Technology Assessment Database (HTAD):* contains information on healthcare technology assessments.
- *The NHS Economic Evaluation Database (NHS EED):* abstracts of economic evaluations of healthcare interventions.

For more information, go to http://www.update-software.com/cochrane/.

Current Contents – is produced by the Institute for Scientific Information. This database allows the searching of up-to-date information by providing access to the tables-of-contents of over 7500 leading periodicals from around the world. For more information, go to http://www.isinet.com/isi/products/cc/.

Embase – is produced by Elsevier Science BV. It covers biomedicine and basic clinical sciences. Emphasis is given to covering the literature of drugs and pharmacology, including the biological effects of chemical compounds. The coverage of EMBASE includes a high proportion of European literature. For more information, go to http://www.embase.com/.

MEDLINE – is produced by the US National Library of Medicine. MEDLINE is the world's largest biomedical database. It encompasses information from Index Medicus, Index to Dental Literature, and International Nursing. The primary focus is on English language journals, although the scope is international. It also includes records formally indexed in the HealthSTAR, Bioethicsline and AIDSLINE databases. This database is available through the NLM gateway at http://gateway.nlm.nih.gov/, via PubMed at http://pubmed.gov and through a variety of database vendors.

OLDMEDLINE – is produced by the US National Library of Medicine. It provides access to the citations published in the *Cumulated Index Medicus* from 1960 through 1965 and the *Current List of Medical Literature* from 1957 through 1959. Unlike MEDLINE, this file contains no abstracts or MeSH heading data from NLM's current controlled vocabulary. It is searchable at http://gateway.nlm.nih.gov/.

PubMed – is produced by the US National Library of Medicine. It includes the MEDLINE database plus out-of-scope references from some MEDLINE journals (primarily general science and chemistry journals), for which the life sciences articles are indexed for MEDLINE. PubMed also includes articles that precede 1966 as well as some additional life science journals that submit full text to PubMedCentral. It is searchable at http://pubmed.gov.

PsycINFO – is produced by the American Psychological Association. This database indexes publications in psychology and related disciplines such as management, education, social work, psychiatry, medicine, and nursing. For more information, go to http://www.apa.org/psycinfo/products/psycinfo.html.

Web of Knowledge – is produced by Thomson ISI. It contains the electronic version of the Science Citation Index (as well as the Social Sciences Citation Index and Arts and Humanities Citation Index). It lists where a citation has been subsequently cited. Using this database to identify studies for a review requires that at least *one key citation exist* on a topic and that those reporting subsequent research cite the key article(s). For more information, go to http://www.isinet.com

References

1 Sackett DL, Straus SE, Richardson WS, Rosenberg W, Haynes RB. *Evidence-based medicine: how to practice and teach EBM.* Edinburgh: Churchill Livingstone, 2000.

2 Ramsey S. Johns Hopkins takes responsibility for volunteer's death. *Lancet* 2001;**358**(9277):213.

3 McLellan F. 1966 and all that: When is a literature search done? *Lancet* 2001;**358**(9282):646.

4 McGowan J. For expert literature searching, call a librarian. *CMAJ* 2001;**165**(10):301–2.

5 Bidwell S, Jensen MF. Chapter 3: Using a Search Protocol to Identify Sources of Information: the COSI Model. E-text on Health Technology Assessment (HTA) Information Resources. http://www.hlm.nih.gov/nichsr/ehta/chapter3.html (accessed June 24, 2002).

6 Silberg WM, Lundberg GD, Musacchio RA. Assessing, controlling, and assuring the quality of medical information on the internet: Let the reader and viewer beware. *JAMA* 1997;**277**(15):1244–5.

7 Oxford Centre for Evidence-based Medicine. *Levels of evidence and grades of recommendations*, 2001. http://163.1.96.10/docs/levels.html (accessed February 2002).

8 Gagliardi A, Jadad AR. Examination of instruments used to rate quality of health information on the internet: chronicle of a voyage with an unclear destination. *BMJ* 2002;**324**:569–73.

9 Wood AJJ. Treatment of postmenopausal osteoporosis. *NEJM* 1998;**338**(11):736–746. http://views.vcu.edu/womenshealth/polf/ostee-3.pdf (Accessed August 16, 2002).

10 Adachi JD, Bensen WG, Brown J, Hanley D, Hodsman A, Josse R, Kendler DL, Lentle B, Olszynski W, Ste-Marie LG, Tenenhouse A, Chines AA. Intermittent etidronate therapy to prevent corticosteroid-induced osteoporosis. *NEJM* 1997;**337**(6):382–7 (accessed August 16, 2002). (note: RCT)

11 Bisphosphonates in renal osteodystrophy. *MedFacts* 2002; **4**(1):1. http://www.nephrologypharmacy.com/downloads/medfacts4-1.pdf (accessed August 16, 2002).

12 Sambrook PN, Seeman E, Phillips SR, Ebeling PR. Preventing osteoporosis: outcomes of the Australian Fracture Prevention Summit. MJA 2002;176(8 Suppl):1–16. http://www.mja.com.au/public/issues/176_08_150402/s1-s16_fm.html (accessed August 16, 2002).

13 McKibbon A, Eady A, Marks S. *PDQ Evidence-based principles and practices*. BC Decker: Hamilton, 1999.

14 Cranney A, Welch V, Adachi JD, Guyatt G, Krolicki N, Griffith L, Shea B, Tugwell P, Wells G. Etidronate for treating and preventing postmenopausal osteoporosis. *Cochrane Database Syst Rev* (4):CD003376, 2001.

15 Cranney A, Welch V, Adachi JD *et al.* Etidronate for treating and preventing postmenopausal osteoporosis. *ACP Journal Club* 2002; May–June;136:98. Cochrane Database Syst Rev 2001;(4):CD003376.

16 GL'99 Conference Program. Fourth International Conference on Grey Literature: New Frontiers in Grey Literature.GreyNet, Grey Literature Network Service. Washington, DC, USA, 4–5 October 1999.

17 McAuley L, Pham B, Tugwell P, Moher D. Does the inclusion of grey literature influence estimates of intervention effectiveness reported in meta-analyses? *Lancet* 2000;**356**(9237):1228–31.

18 Best L, Milne R. Wessex Institute for Health Research and Development. Bisphosphonates (alendronate and etidronate) in the management of osteoporosis. DEC Report No. 79, 1998.

19 Coletti MH, Bleich HL. Medical Subject Heading used to search the biomedical literature. *JAMA* 2001;**8**(4):317–23.

20 Hunt DL, McKibbon KA. Locating and appraising systematic reviews. *Ann Intern Med* 1997;**126**(7):532–8.

21 Haynes RB, Wilczynski N, McKibbon KA, Walker CJ, Sinclair JC. Developing optimal search strategies for detecting clinically sound studies in MEDLINE. *JAMA* 1994;**1**(6):447–58.

2
OMERACT: an ongoing evidence-based initiative to improve the quality of outcome measures in rheumatology

Maarten Boers, Lee S Simon,
Vibeke Strand, Peter Brooks, Peter Tugwell

The OMERACT initiative

OMERACT (initially "Outcome MEasures in Rheumatoid Arthritis Clinical Trials", now "Outcome Measures in Rheumatology") is an informal gathering of professionals interested in outcome measurement in rheumatology. OMERACT organises conferences and manages a discussion list and a website on the internet (http://www.omeract.org). It has continuing endorsement of International League for Rheumatology (ILAR); most conferences have also been endorsed by the World Health Organisation (WHO).

OMERACT conferences

- **OMERACT 1:** Core set of measures to be included in all RA clinical trials ratified by World Health Organisation and International League of Associations for Rheumatology (WHO/ILAR).
- **OMERACT 2:** Cost-effectiveness, including both economic and safety considerations.
- **OMERACT 3:** Core sets for osteoarthritis, osteoporosis; psychosocial measures.
- **OMERACT 4:** RA (response criteria, imaging); ankylosing spondylitis and systemic lupus erythematosus (both: core set and response); longitudinal/ observational studies (measures and methods).
- **OMERACT 5:** Minimally clinically important differences; imaging; economic evaluation; toxicity.
- **OMERACT 6:** Consensus on health economics reference case for RA; provisional MRI scoring system for RA in hands. Workshops on: patient perspective; systemic sclerosis; osteoarthritis response; low disease activity state in RA; healing phenomena on radiographs in RA.

How does OMERACT work?

To reach consensus over what should be measured, and how, i.e. what measures are *applicable* in trials for each clinical indication, OMERACT works as follows. First, the organising committee polls experts and opinion leaders to generate interest in the topic at hand. These individuals then form a committee to guide the subsequent process. From the general domains of health status defined by the "D's" (Discomfort,

Disability, Dollar Cost, Death), specific domains are formulated for the topic in question. In each domain, measures are collected and tested for their applicability (see below). The domains and the applicable measures form the basis for the consensus guidelines.

The process is data-driven. Literature reviews and validation studies are usually performed by small groups. The formulation and selection of the domains are made by larger committees, and the presentation of evidence (both from literature and from targeted studies) and final selection occurs at the conference. Here, plenary presentations alternate with small group sessions where participants express their views and preferences. These views are brought back to the plenary session, where a final consensus is formulated, often with the help of interactive voting. Consensus does not always imply agreement on measures or domains; it can also mean the formulation of a research agenda in areas where data-driven decisions cannot be made. The process is iterative, in that guidelines are forever "preliminary" based on the assumption that future data (sometimes a direct result of the research agenda) will serve to refine or modify them.

The selection of applicable domains and measures based on the guidelines for validity formulated by Tugwell and Bombardier, based on their study of measurement methodology in psychology, but focused towards trials (see Related reading). OMERACT proposes a "Filter" for applicability of measures in a certain setting (see Related reading). The word "applicable" is intended to include all aspects necessary for proper selection of a measure.

The OMERACT Filter can easily be summarised in only three words: Truth, Discrimination, and Feasibility. Each word represents a question to be answered of the measure, in each of its intended settings:

Truth: is the measure truthful, does it measure what it intends to measure? Is the result unbiased and relevant? The word captures the issues of face, content, construct and criterion validity.

Discrimination: does the measure discriminate between situations that are of interest? The situations can be states at one time (for classification or prognosis) or states at different times (to measure change). The word captures the issues of reliability and sensitivity to change.

Feasibility: can the measure be applied easily, given constraints of time, money, and interpretability? The word captures an essential element in the selection of measures, one that in the end may be decisive in determining a measure's success.

OMERACT conferences in more detail

The idea for OMERACT was born in 1989 during Maarten Boers' training as a clinical epidemiologist in Canada (with Professor P. Tugwell, then at McMaster University, Hamilton). It became clear that despite several conferences and meetings held between 1980 and 1992, there were still many problems with the endpoints employed in rheumatoid arthritis (RA) clinical trials. The endpoints were not comprehensive and yet showed considerable overlap, and were insensitive to change. Opinions on the solution varied widely, and there was a considerable professional but also personal "transatlantic" divide (between Europe and the US/Canada). The stalemate was impeding progress and hampering the development of new treatments. Maarten Boers returned to The Netherlands in 1990 to take up his new position as a rheumatologist at the University of Maastricht (Department of Internal Medicine/ Rheumatology; head Professor Sj van der Linden). With Peter Tugwell, he decided to try to bring together in Maastricht all experts in the field, both clinicians and methodologists, to forge a consensus based on the available literature. Under the auspices of ILAR they contacted the European League for Rheumatology (EULAR), the American College for Rheumatology (ACR), and many other organisations actively working in this area. Other topics to be discussed were the utility of pooling endpoints, and response criteria.

In preparation for the conference, relevant literature was reviewed, summarised, and distributed to the participants, as well as a pre-conference questionnaire to poll opinions. At the conference, participants received plenary introductions but most of the work was done in small groups. These groups discussed patient and trial summaries ("profiles") based on real data to experience the relative importance of endpoints in the assessment of important improvements. The groups then discussed several propositions on the constitution of a core set of endpoints that should be included as a minimum in all RA clinical trials. The groups were run by the nominal group consensus technique aimed at bringing out all opinions and discussions in a balanced way. Final sessions were plenary and aided by an interactive voting system.

The end result was a core set that reflected scientific evidence, but also compromise in that it ended strife on endpoints on which, at that time, no decisive data were available. WHO and ILAR later ratified this core set at a conference in Geneva (see Boers *et al* (1994) in Related reading). To date, it remains the solid anchor on which all RA trials are now based. A more intangible result was the creation of a network of health professionals that has remained active to this day, as evidenced by the successful series of subsequent conferences, and a sharp increase in interest and publication of papers on related subjects. For instance, the OMERACT methodology was adopted by paediatrician-rheumatologists to develop a core set for juvenile chronic arthritis, and by other rheumatologists to develop a core set for ankylosing spondylitis (the "ASAS" group). An internet distribution list was set up to facilitate communication. Proceedings of OMERACT 1 were published in the *Journal of Rheumatology* (see OMERACT Bibliography).

The OMERACT committee was broadened by the inclusion of Professor Peter Brooks (then Professor of Medicine, University of Sydney; now Dean, Faculty of Health Science, University of Queensland). In June 1994 OMERACT 2 was held in Ottawa, Canada; it focused on the balance between efficacy and costs in the broad sense, including both economic and safety considerations. The conference led to the installation by ILAR of three Task Forces: one focuses on improvement of reporting and analysis of toxicity data (Chairman: Professor P. Brooks), the second focuses on the use of generic quality of life instruments (Chairman: Professor M. Boers), and the third on economic evaluations in rheumatology (Chairwoman Dr S. Gabriel). Proceedings of OMERACT 2 were published in the *Journal of Rheumatology* (see OMERACT Bibliography).

The third OMERACT conference took place in Cairns, Australia in 1996. It resulted in preliminary core sets of outcome measures for osteoarthritis and osteoporosis clinical trials, and started discussions on psychosocial measures in rheumatology (see OMERACT Bibliography).

The OMERACT committee was broadened by the inclusion of Professor Vibeke Strand (Division of Immunology, University of Stanford, Palo Alto, USA). In 1995 the development of two competing criteria to define improvement in a patient with RA ("ACR improvement" and "EULAR response") threatened to undermine the consensus that had been so successful in the definition of the first core set. Starting immediately after the third conference, the OMERACT committee decided to focus their efforts to resolve this problem. Happily it proved possible to convince the two principal scientists to cooperate in a joint effort to validate both criteria sets. Both scientists examined both core sets in predefined data sets, using their favourite methodology. This exercise proved that both criteria were of equal validity and equally applicable in practice. The results were presented and discussed at OMERACT 4, and appeared as a jointly authored paper in the proceedings of this conference (see OMERACT Bibliography). Other topics discussed at this conference included RA imaging, methods and measures in longitudinal/observational studies. Moreover, the ASAS group decided to present and receive feedback on their results on core set and response criteria in ankylosing spondylitis. For systemic lupus erythematosus agreement was reached on a core set of domains to be included in clinical trials and longitudinal studies. Further work was deferred until more data became available from randomised controlled trials. Finally, the progress of Task Forces instituted at previous meetings was presented.

The OMERACT committee was broadened by the inclusion of Associate Professor Lee S. Simon (then Harvard Medical School, Boston, USA; now Division Director, Analgesic, Anti-inflammatory, Ophthalmologic Drug Products (DAAODP), ODEV, Food and Drug Administration (FDA), Washington, DC). Toulouse, France hosted OMERACT 5 in 2000, just prior to the EULAR meeting in Nice. This conference was recognised as Euro-expert conference (European Community: Fifth Framework), with a special programme to train young European scientists in this field. Ten young European researchers (joined by several other young researchers from around the world) active in the field of outcome measurement in rheumatology were invited. They submitted an abstract, came to OMERACT, and participated in a pre-conference training session. This one-day session involved a primer on the OMERACT Filter and a critical appraisal of the candidate's current research by the OMERACT Faculty. The young researchers gave an oral presentation about their current research. All attendees subsequently fully participated in the OMERACT 5 conference.

At the conference four topics were discussed: minimally clinically important differences (MCID); imaging; economic evaluation; drug safety. The proceedings were published in the *Journal of Rheumatology* (see OMERACT Bibliography). Discussions in the MCID module included the concept of "major" (as opposed to "minimum") differences, new criteria for osteoarthritis, and a research agenda for osteoporosis and back pain. The economic module discussed key issues in the development of a reference case, the topic of consensus in OMERACT 6 (see below). In the imaging module, the concept of smallest detectable difference in radiographs was further explored in relation to expert-based or evidence-based MCID. Also, MRI, with RA hands as an example, was taken up as a key area for development of a validated scoring system. Like economics, this topic returned as a consensus module in OMERACT 6 (see below). Finally, the module on drug safety discussed a proposal to develop a large patient population cohort for long term safety monitoring in rheumatoid arthritis. This would consist of a combination of product-specific registries to follow a cohort of RA patients who receive a newly approved therapy, and the development of a much larger cohort of RA patients treated with multiple second line agents. The initiative to standardise the assessment of adverse effects in rheumatology clinical trials has resulted in a new instrument, an adaptation of an existing toxicity vocabulary and scoring system (see OMERACT 6 in OMERACT Bibliography). Those developing new studies are encouraged to incorporate this instrument so that experience can be obtained on how well it performs.

OMERACT 6 took place in Brisbane, Australia in April 2002. Just like previous OMERACT conferences, the format consisted of small group workshops alternating with plenary meetings. To accommodate the expanding number of topics that are timely and of interest, the executive committee decided to include only two full modules to formulate consensus guidelines. The remaining time was devoted to five workshops – some running in parallel. Workshops focused discussion and formulated a research agenda that will enable a full (consensus) module to be developed for a future conference.

The two consensus modules covered:

- Health economics: reference case for RA (minimum core format for presentation and analysis of economic studies in RA) The reference case developed previously was felt to be an appropriate example and it was decided that measures of pain, function, inflammation, quality of life, structural damage, and toxicity and comorbidity should be included in determining the "responder state" as an effective measure for estimation of cost effectiveness.
- Imaging: MRI in RA. Consensus on minimum assessment and evaluation protocol for the hands. This scoring system, known as the OMERACT-MRI score, involves scoring changes in the hands and wrist. It will be further developed by the expert group.

The five workshop topics discussed were as follows.

- Patient perspective: In the presence of a delegation of RA patients, this workshop discussed the input of patients into current measures in RA studies. This workshop identified the disparities between patient and health professional expectations of treatment and how these might influence outcome measurement. There was a strong feeling to continue patient input in the OMERACT process.
- Systemic sclerosis: Development of a research agenda towards a core set for use in clinical trials. This workshop reviewed current outcome measures across a wide range of organ systems in systemic sclerosis. Few had been validated according to the OMERACT filter, but a research agenda was developed to focus particularly on four areas – cardiopulmonary, quality of life, renal, and skin – in the first instance.
- Osteoarthritis: Further validation of the osteoarthritis research society international (OARSI) responder index. The OARSI (osteoarthritis research society international) response criteria were discussed and accepted for non-NSAID trials. Domains such as biochemical markers and MRI needed further development and would be discussed at future meetings.
- Low disease activity RA: Research agenda/ development of methodology to define a state of low disease activity in RA It was considered that pain, function, inflammation, quality of life, and structure/damage, toxicity (safety), and co-morbidity were useful in defining a low activity state and, along with sleep and energy/fatigue, should be part of the research agenda.
- Imaging: Research agenda to define healing/repair phenomena in radiographs of RA. It was accepted that repair (which was considered a better term than healing) did occur in some patients and that assessment by MRI should be pursued. Correlations with clinical and synovial biopsy data should also be pursued in a research agenda.

OMERACT 7 will take place in Asilomar, California USA in May 2004. It will revisit many of the topics previously discussed, but also take on new diseases such as psoriatic arthritis, gout and vasculitis, and new topics such as synovial biopsies and ultrasound. The website offers more detail (http://www.omeract.org).

In conclusion, OMERACT strives to improve outcome measurement in rheumatology through a data-driven, iterative consensus process. If nothing else, it has made the selection of applicable outcome measures more explicit.

OMERACT Bibliography

OMERACT 1. Maastricht, Netherlands, 1992

J Rheumatol 1993;20:526–91.

Outcome measures in rheumatoid arthritis clinical trials.

OMERACT 2. Ottawa, Canada, 1994

J Rheumatol 1995; 22:

979–99: Toxicity of antirheumatic drugs

1185–207: Health status benefit/utilities

1399–433: Health economics.

OMERACT 3. Cairns, Australia 1996

J Rheumatol 1997; 24:

763–802: Outcome measures in osteoarthritis

979–1011: Psychosocial function in musculoskeletal trials

1206–37 Outcome measures in osteoporosis.

OMERACT 4. Cancun, Mexico,1998

J Rheumatol 1999; 26:

199–228: Module updates

459–89: Measures and methods in longitudinal/observational studies

490–507: Lupus erythematosus: core set and response

705–51: Rheumatoid arthritis: response and imaging

945–1006: Ankylosing spondylitis.

OMERACT 5. Toulouse, France, 2000

J Rheumatol 2001; 28:

395–454: Minimum clinically important differences

640–73: Cost effectiveness

880–917: Imaging I. radiography

1113–61: Imaging II. MRI

1162–94: Drug safety.

OMERACT 6. Brisbane, Australia, 2002

J Rheumatol 2003; 30:

868–85: Patient perspective

886–96: economics reference case for RA

1102–9: imaging (repair)

1110–18: minimum clinically important difference/low disease activity state

1364–92: RA-magnetic resonance imaging

1630–47: Systemic sclerosis

1648–54: OARSI responder index in osteoarthritis

Related reading

Tugwell P, Bombardier C. A methodologic framework for developing and selecting endpoints in clinical trials. *J Rheumatol* 1982;**9**:752–62.

Boers M, Tugwell P, Felson DT, *et al.* World health organisation and international league of associations for rheumatology core endpoints for symptom modifying antirheumatic drugs in rheumatoid arthritis clinical trials. *J Rheumatol* 1994;**41**:86–9.

Tugwell P, Boers M, Baker P, Snider J. Endpoints in rheumatoid arthritis. *J Rheumatol* 1994;**21**:2–8.

Boers M, van Riel PLCM, Felson D, Tugwell P. Measuring activity of rheumatoid arthritis. *Baillière's Clin Rheumatol* 1995;**9**:305–17.

Boers M, Brooks P, Strand V, Tugwell P. The OMERACT Filter for outcome measures in rheumatology. *J Rheumatol* 1998;**25**:198–9.

Molenaar E, Boers M, Brooks P, Simon L, Strand V, Tugwell P. Recent developments for optimal endpoints in rheumatoid arthritis clinical studies. *Dis Management Hlth Outc* 2000;**8**:87–97.

Molenaar E, van der Heijde D, Boers M. Update on outcome assessment in rheumatic disorders. *Curr Opin Rheumatol* 2000;**12**:91–8.

Brooks P, Hochberg M. Outcome measures and classification criteria for the rheumatic diseases. A compilation of data from OMERACT (Outcome Measures for Arthritis Clinical Trials), ILAR (International League of Associations for Rheumatology), regional leagues and other groups. *Rheumatology (Oxford)* 2001;**40**:896–906.

3 Economics

Hilal Maradit Kremers, Sherine E Gabriel

Introduction

Even in the most affluent countries in the world, there are inadequate resources to provide all the medical care that is scientifically and theoretically available. Instead, choices must be made among alternatives. These choices must consider both cost and outcome.[1] Though these trade-offs are usually viewed as financial, they can also be viewed from a humanistic standpoint. In healthcare assessments it is imperative that outcomes and resource allocation be considered from these two standpoints.

In the case of investments in medical care, the return is measured not in dollars, but in improvements in health. An economic evaluation in health care must facilitate rational choices among complex alternatives by enumerating, quantifying, and comparing the various consequences. The humanistic outcomes include late complications and future effects and should include the importance as assessed by the patients. The financial outcomes are measured by costs and include the collective burden of insurance payments and taxes, as well as individual costs.

Economic evaluation has three dimensions (Figure 3.1).

- First: type of costs and benefits
  - Direct medical costs (for example, hospital stay)
  - Indirect medical costs (for example, lost wages)
  - Direct non-medical costs (for example, home care)
  - Intangible costs (for example, pain, suffering)
- Second: point of view
  - Provider
  - Payer
  - Patient
  - Society

This is important because the same item may be a cost from one point of view and a benefit from another.

- Third: methodological approach (Table 3.1)[2,3]
  - Cost–benefit: costs and benefits expressed in dollar terms
  - Cost minimization: compares two equivalent interventions with respect to financial costs only.
  - Cost–effectiveness: costs are expressed in terms of natural units (for example, years of life saved, number of attacks avoided, etc)
  - Cost utility: costs are expressed in terms of a measure of utility or patient preference (for example, quality adjusted life years (QALY))

In addition, there are cost-of-illness studies, which simply describe the impact of the disease and its consumption of resources as a result of the condition. These are used as a baseline for comparison prior to the discovery of new interventions.

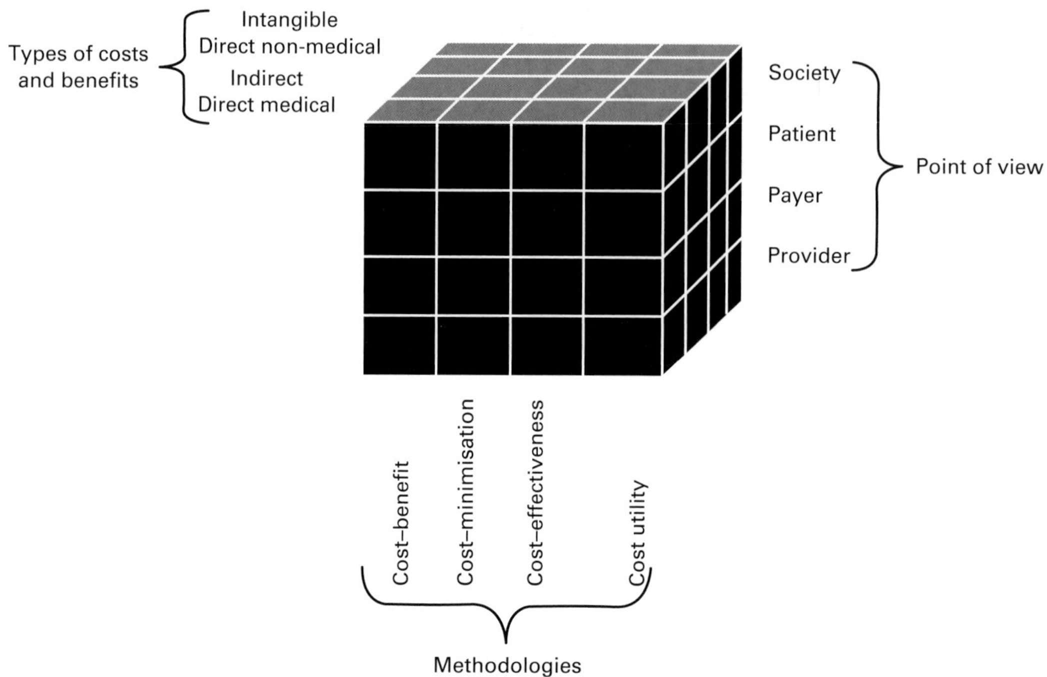

Figure 3.1 The three dimensions of economic evaluation (adapted from Beaton DE, *et al. J Clin Epidemiol* 2001;**54**:1204–17).

Table 3.1 Economic evaluation methodologies (from Bootman *et al*)[2,3]

Methodology	Cost measurement unit	Outcome unit
Cost–benefit	Dollars	Dollars
Cost-effectiveness	Dollars	Natural units (life-years gained, HAQ score, adverse GI effects averted)
Cost-minimisation	Dollars	Assume to be equivalent in comparative groups
Cost utility	Dollars	QALY or other utilities

Three principles of economic evaluation bear mention here.

- **Discounting:** The value of costs or effects occurring in the future must be adjusted downward to reflect their reduced importance compared with immediate consequences. This process of downward adjustment of future costs and effects, referred to as time discounting, is particularly important for chronic disease interventions in which the benefits may be immediate but adverse effects may occur far into the future (for example, liver toxicity with methotrexate), or in which the adverse effects may be immediate and the benefits delayed (for example, drug rash with hydroxychloroquine, sulphasalazine, or gold therapy). There is a danger that long term benefits and risks of a treatment will be missed in studies of short duration.
- **QALY:** Although one could enumerate and quantify medical outcomes along a variety of

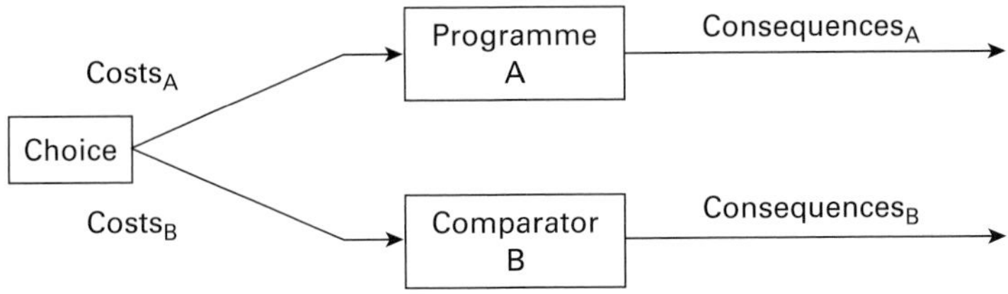

Figure 3.2 Formulation of an economic evaluation (Figure adapted from Drummond M, *et al. Methods for the economic evaluation of health care programmes 2nd ed.* Oxford: Oxford University Press, 1997).

dimensions, valuing one kind of outcome against another is essential if broad comparisons among alternatives are to be made. Thus, summary measures that combine the effects of an intervention on both the quality and length of life are optimal. The quality-adjusted life year (QALY) is a summary measure of effectiveness that allows comparison among interventions with different kinds of effects. The QALY aims to capture patients' relative preferences for different health effects, ranging from pain, to disability, to death. Does a patient prefer a reduced quality of life, if it provides them with a longer life expectancy or vice versa? However, methods for estimating QALY are still evolving.[4]

- **Sensitivity analysis:** Economic evaluation invariably involves identification of outcomes whose magnitude may be uncertain or unmeasured. These uncertain outcomes are often measured by suggestive evidence, consensus opinion or investigators' judgments being converted into explicit assumptions. Regardless of the source, analysis of the sensitivity of the findings to possible errors in assumptions is a necessary component of all economic evaluations.[5]

In an economic evaluation a choice often has to be made between competing alternatives (Figure 3.2). The general rule is that the difference in costs is compared with the difference in consequences in an incremental analysis. This determines whether the additional costs incurred by the new drug or intervention are worth the additional benefits derived from it.

$$\text{ICER} = \frac{\text{Costs}_A - \text{Costs}_B}{\text{Consequences}_A - \text{Consequences}_B}$$

The incremental cost-effectiveness ratio (ICER) is a method for comparing one choice alternative to another.

Development of drug-related interventions is often paralleled by a series of economic evaluations,[4] as summarised in Table 3.2.

Economic evaluation in rheumatology: the need for methodological standards

The past decade has witnessed remarkable advances in the field of rheumatology, with the introduction of several novel treatments for rheumatoid arthritis (RA) and other rheumatic diseases. Although many of these agents are quite costly, they may have major long term benefits, such as slowing disease progression and preventing disability. For new agents, such as these, to become introduced into our current healthcare environment, proof of benefit alone is not sufficient; it is necessary to demonstrate that the expected benefits of a new agent are worth the costs associated with its use. This can only

Table 3.2 Economic evaluation runs parallel to drug development[6]

Phase of drug development	Economic evaluation performed
Phase I and II	Cost-of-illness studies in order to help determine the potential market
Phase III Large, multicentre randomised controlled trials (RCT) to determine efficacy	Pharmacoeconomic evaluation to determine the cost-effectiveness of the intervention/drug in clinical trials
Phase IV Post marketing, data gathered to support the use of the drug in the community	Pharmacoeconomic evaluation to determine the cost-effectiveness of the intervention/drug in the community

be shown by formal economic evaluation that allows us to quantify and compare the benefits (such as prevented disability, improved quality of life, etc.) and the costs of medical interventions. Unfortunately, the science of economic evaluation and its application in rheumatology is not adequately developed to convincingly demonstrate the cost-efficiency of such therapies. A comprehensive literature review of all published economic evaluations in rheumatology identified only two studies that have been conducted according to internationally agreed upon criteria for economic evaluation.[7] In addition, literature reviews conducted by members of the OMERACT Health Economics Working Group show wide variation in the selection of measures of clinical efficacy and whether/how the costs of adverse events are incorporated into economic analyses.[8–10] This lack of agreement on methods is a threat to the validity, usability, and comparability of such research and has major implications on regulatory decisions since policy makers must allocate resources on the basis of economic efficiency.

Several reasons justify the need to achieve consensus on economic evaluation methods in rheumatology.

First, the recent explosion in the number of published economic analyses makes it important to identify key methodological standards so that studies can be appropriately compared and critically appraised.

Second, economic evaluations are meant, among other things, to inform choices about resource allocation. Methodology must exist, otherwise apparent differences in the relative cost-effectiveness of treatments may be attributable to differences in study methodology rather than true differences in the cost-effectiveness of the therapies/interventions.

Third, since the field of economic evaluation is still evolving, the discussion of standardization of methods is an essential first step on the path towards identifying research priorities in the field of economic evaluation.

Fourth, several jurisdictions are now requiring economic evaluations as part of the decision making process for reimbursement of health treatments and technologies. Indeed, methodological guidelines for performing such studies have already been developed in several countries.[11–14]

Finally, the emergence of innovative, highly effective, but costly new treatments for RA has created a need to more fully understand the economic implications of RA treatments.

In 1993, the Panel on Cost-effectiveness in Health and Medicine addressed the need for methodological standards by outlining an explicit set of minimum recommendations for use in a "reference case analysis". A reference case analysis is intended to provide decision makers with reassurance that the results of different cost-effectiveness analyses can be meaningfully compared to one another.[5]

Three notes of caution bear mention here. First, improvements in the quality and comparability of economic analyses do not in themselves provide the answer to how resources should be allocated in the pursuit of health. Economic analyses provide information that can help locate the trade-offs associated with different decisions, but these studies do not in themselves make decisions. Stronger methodology assures only that the information is more reliable[5]. Second, a reference case is intended to define a minimum set of standards for economic analysis that will enable comparisons across studies. A reference case is not intended to provide a "cookie-cutter" approach to economic analysis research. Instead, investigators are encouraged to go beyond these minimum methodological criteria to study novel methodological approaches that might be particularly informative in their individual studies. Third, a reference case is an evolving, not a static, concept. Reference cases need to be periodically evaluated as new methodological approaches are developed.

Literature review

Economic evaluations in rheumatic diseases, especially in RA and osteoarthritis (OA), have grown exponentially in recent years. A total of 57 published economic evaluations were identified during the 25 year period between 1970 and 1995. In contrast, 78 evaluations were published during the 5 years from 1996 to 2001 (Table 3.3). This trend is expected to continue along with advances in treatment of rheumatic diseases and the growing need for objective cost-effectiveness evaluations to inform allocation of healthcare resources.

Some of the published economic evaluations have been critically reviewed.[7–9,15–17] Herein, we provide a brief overview of published economic evaluations. We do not provide a comprehensive assessment of the quality of these evaluations. The evaluations vary considerably in their methodology. In addition, there are probably at least as many unpublished economic evaluations that were prepared as part of the registration of drugs in individual countries. Therefore, we encourage the reader to refer to the original documents for more detail. The citations of the studies reviewed in this section are listed in the Appendix to this chapter by disease area.

The majority of the published economic evaluations were conducted in the USA, United Kingdom, and Canada (Table 3.3). More than half the published evaluations were on OA and RA. The most common intervention studied was prevention of non-steroidal anti-inflammatory drug-induced gastropathy (including the cost-effectiveness of COX-2 inhibitors), followed by the value of total hip or knee arthroplasty and the cost-effectiveness of various preventive or primary care-based interventions. More recent evaluations focused on demonstrating the cost-effectiveness of new biologic therapies in RA.

Osteoporosis was another disease area where most evaluations focused on the value of hormone replacement therapy for prevention of osteoporotic fractures and the cost-effectiveness of screening strategies for different risk populations. Other disease areas were rarely studied (Table 3.3).

The majority of the economic evaluations were cost-effectiveness or cost-utility analyses.

Table 3.3 Summary of 135 published economic evaluations is rheumatology since 1970 (citations listed in the Appendix)

	Number (%)
Publication year	
1970–1979	2 (1)
1980–1989	10 (7)
1990–1995	45 (33)
1996–2001	78 (58)
Country	
United States	59 (44)
Canada	12 (9)
United Kingdom	16 (12)
Nordic countries	22 (16)
Others	26 (19)
Disease area	
Osteoarthritis and/or rheumatoid arthritis	74 (55)
Prevention of NSAID-induced gastropathy	25
Total hip or knee arthroplasty	16
Evaluation of treatment with new DMARDs	7
Others	26
Osteoporosis	34 (25)
Hormone replacement therapy	18
Low back pain	13 (10)
Lyme disease	3 (2)
Others	11 (8)
Analysis type	
Cost-minimisation or cost–benefit analysis	6 (4)
Cost-effectiveness analysis	83 (61)
Cost-utility analysis	31 (23)
More than 1 type of analysis	15 (11)
Viewpoint	
Society	38 (28)
Third party payer	34 (25)
Other	19 (14)
Not stated	44 (33)
Costs considered	
Direct costs only	99 (73)
Direct and indirect costs	32 (24)
Not stated	4 (3)
Time horizon	
≤ 1 year	59 (44)
>1–10 years	36 (27)
> 10 years	25 (19)
Not stated	15 (11)
Sensitivity analysis	
Yes	78 (58)
No	57 (42)

Clinical outcomes were expressed mainly as the cost per clinical event avoided or years of life saved. Cost-utility analyses evaluated costs per QALY gained or costs per unit change on certain quality of life scales. For valuation of health states (for example, QALY), only a few studies used directly elicited preferences from patients and general public. Instead, these were mostly derived either from the published literature or from expert opinions.

Most of the studies adopted the societal or the third-party payer perspective. While all studies examined direct medical costs, only a few also examined direct non-medical or productivity costs. The analysis timeframe was mostly one year or less. Only 19% of the evaluations considered a timeframe longer than 10 years.

Almost all of the evaluations used data from a variety of different sources. The data sources for clinical outcome measures included randomised controlled clinical trials, published observational studies, and administrative databases. Very few studies modelled beyond the duration of therapy or extrapolated long term outcomes using evidence from observational studies. Estimates of resource utilisation were obtained through observational data sources, randomised controlled trials, and expert judgement. Evaluation of financial costs was mainly based on administrative data sources or market prices (for example fee schedules, Medicare diagnosis-related group reimbursement rates). Few studies estimated opportunity costs and few reported cost items and quantities separately. Finally, sensitivity analyses were done only in approximately half of the studies and even these were not consistently reported. As the need for economic evaluations in rheumatology continues to grow, methodological standards will be increasingly required to ensure the validity, usability, and comparability of the findings.

OMERACT economics and the development of an RA reference case

One limitation of current methodological standards is that they are, of necessity, fairly general and tend to neglect the unique circumstances that surround particular clinical contexts. Recognising this problem, and the unique challenges surrounding economic analysis of RA and other rheumatic diseases, the Outcomes Measures in Rheumatology (OMERACT) Economics Working Group, a team of experts with methodological and clinical expertise, set out in 1994 to develop rheumatic disease specific reference cases for economic evaluation. The overall goal of this effort is to produce guidance documents to help standardise economic evaluations in rheumatological disorders.[18–37] These recommendations are intended to supplement (rather than replace) the generally accepted methodological standards and to facilitate their application in rheumatology.

When the OMERACT Economics Working Group first assembled in 1994, they reviewed the literature on the principles and application of economic analyses in the rheumatic diseases.[18] By 1997, the group had identified key elements of a reference case for RA and defined a preliminary methodological research agenda. The results of this work were presented in 1998 and published shortly thereafter.[22] In April 2000, the members of the Economics Group presented the results of original research that was aimed at addressing the methodological gaps identified in the previous report. These findings were synthesised into a document that summarised the methodological elements of consensus and of debate in economic evaluation of RA.[26] In February 2001, the group proposed preliminary reference case recommendations according to 13 previously identified methodological elements across three common rheumatological disorders, i.e., RA, OA, and osteoporosis.[30] A survey was

Table 3.4 Reference case recommendations for economic evaluations in RA[31]

Methodological element	Recommendation
1. Study horizon	Trial-based analysis, minimum 1 year Model-based analyses, minimum 5–10 years
2. Duration of therapy	Continuous
3. Extrapolation beyond trial duration	Report clinical trial data alone and extrapolate (model) using a synthesis of evidence from observational studies, trials, and other sources with sensitivity analysis (minimise use of expert opinion)
4. Modelling beyond therapy	No additional benefit or harm after therapy is stopped
5. Synthesis of comparisons where head-to-head trials do not exist	Synthetic comparisons by using relative effects from controlled trials
6. Clinical outcome measures	• Joint count • Pain by visual analogue scale • Physical measure of function (e.g. HAQ) • Measure of inflammation (CRP/ESR) • Health-related quality of life • Toxicity (report adverse effects with patients as the unit of analysis)
7. Mortality	Hazard rates for mortality from observational studies
8. Valuation of health states (e.g. QALY)	Patients' values for clinical choices, general population's values for health policy decisions
9. Resource utilisation	Include all associated direct medical and non-medical costs in the analysis, but report indirect costs (productivity losses) separately. When estimating mean costs in the presence of censoring due to discontinuation of therapy, adjust using appropriate statistical methods to allow for unequal exposure to risk of resource use
10. Discontinuation of therapy	Use discontinuation rates from trials, adjusted using observational data
11. Therapeutic sequence	Include modelling of most commonly used therapeutic sequence with sensitivity analysis to consider other strategies
12. Population risk stratification	Include clear definition of underlying population including low and high risk groups

developed to obtain feedback regarding these recommendations. The survey was circulated to 290 relevant experts. Excellent comments were obtained and revisions were suggested and made. The results of the survey demonstrated that there was no substantive disagreement on any of the recommendations. Following additional input and further discussions, reference case recommendations for RA resulting from the entire eight-year process were summarised and reported according to 12 central methodological elements and include:

study horizon; duration of therapy; extrapolation beyond trial duration; modelling beyond therapy; synthesis of comparisons where head-to-head trials do not exist; clinical outcome measures; mortality; valuation of health states (for example, QALY); resource utilisation; discontinuation of therapy; therapeutic sequence; and population risk stratification (see Table 3.4).[31]

The OMERACT Health Economics Working Group is an active, engaged methodological team that has developed the first disease-specific reference case recommendations for economic evaluation.[31] The goal of this initiative is to stimulate the transfer of the results of economic analyses into policy and practice through the use of rigorous, consensus-based methodological standards. In addition, this work aims to expedite and enhance the conduct of methodological research in economic analysis in rheumatology and to encourage networking among clinicians, policy makers, pharmaceutical industry scientists, health economists, and statisticians. Through these efforts, we hope to continue to work towards achieving the ultimate goal of not only creating common standards for economic evaluation in rheumatology, but also improving the scientific underpinnings of economic evaluation, particularly as these pertain to the rheumatic diseases.

Appendix

Rheumatoid arthritis (21 publications)

Pätiälä H, Niemelä P, Laurinkari J. Cost-benefit analysis of synovectomy of the knee. *Scan J Rheumatol* 1976;**5**: 227–32.

Anderson RB, Needleman RD, Gatter RA, Andrews RP, Scarola JA: Patient outcome following inpatient vs outpatient treatment of rheumatoid arthritis. *J Rheumatol* 1988;**15**:556–60.

Thompson MS, Read JL, Hutchings HC, Paterson M, Harris ED jr. The cost-effectiveness of auranofin: results of a randomised clinical trial. *J Rheumatol* 1988;**15**:35–42.

Helewa A, Bombardier C, Goldsmith CH, Menchions B, Smythe HA: Cost-effectiveness of inpatient and intensive outpatient treatment of rheumatoid arthritis: a randomised, controlled trial. *Arthritis Rheum* 1989;**32**:1505–14.

Gabriel SE, Jaakkimainen RL, Bombardier C: The cost-effectiveness of misoprostol for nonsteroidal antiinflammatory drug-associated adverse gastrointestinal events. Arthritis Rheum 1993;**36**:447–459.

Lambert CM, Hurst NP, Lochhead A, McGregor K, Hunter M, Forbes J: A pilot study of the economic cost and clinical outcome of day patient vs inpatient management of active rheumatoid arthritis. *Br J Rheumatol* 1994;**33**:383–8.

Bergquist SR, Felson DT, Prashker MJ, Freedberg KA. The cost-effectiveness of liver biopsy in rheumatoid arthritis patients treated with methotrexate. *Arthritis Rheum* 1995;**38**:326–33.

Erickson AR, Reddy V, Vogelgesang SA, West SG. Usefulness of the American College of Rheumatology recommendations for liver biopsy in methotrexate-treated rheumatoid arthritis patients. *Arthritis Rheum* 1995;38: 1115–19.

Al MJ, Michel BC, Rutten FF. The cost-effectiveness of diclofenac plus misoprostol compared with diclofenac monotherapy in patients with rheumatoid arthritis. *Pharmacoeconomics* 1996;**10**:141–51.

Anis AH, Tugwell PX, Wells GA, Stewart DG. A cost-effectiveness analysis of cyclosporine in rheumatoid arthritis. *J Rheumatol* 1996;**23**:609–16.

Criswell LA, Such CL. Cost-effectiveness analysis of drug therapies for rheumatoid arthritis. *J Rheumatol* Suppl 1996;**44**:52–5.

Kavanaugh A, Heudebert G, Cush J, Jain R. Cost evaluation of novel therapeutics in rheumatoid arthritis (CENTRA): a decision analysis model. *Semin Arthritis Rheum* 1996;**25**: 297–307.

Nordstrom DCE, Konttinen YT, Solovieva S, Friman C, Santavirta S. In- and out-patient rehabilitation in rheumatoid arthritis: a controlled open, longitudinal, cost-effectiveness study. *Scand J Rheumatol* 1996;**25**:200–6.

Lambert CM, Hurst NP, Forbes JF, Lochhead A, Macleod M, Nuki G. Is day care equivalent to inpatient care for active rheumatoid arthritis? Randomised controlled clinical and economic evaluation. *BMJ* 1998;**316**:965–9.

Verhoeven AC, Bibo JC, Boers M, Engel GL, van der Linden S. Cost-effectiveness and cost-utility of combination therapy in early rheumatoid arthritis: randomised comparison of combined step-down prednisolone, methotrexate and sulphasalazine with sulphasalazine alone. COBRA Trial Group. Combinatietherapie Bij Reumatoide Artritis. *Br J Rheumatol* 1998;**37**:1102–9.

Kobelt G, Eberhardt K, Jonsson L, Jonsson B. Economic consequences of the progression of rheumatoid arthritis in Sweden. *Arthritis Rheum* 1999;**42**:347–56.

Kristiansen IS, Kvien TK, Nord E. Cost-effectiveness of replacing diclofenac with a fixed combination of misoprostol and diclofenac in patients with rheumatoid arthritis. *Arthritis Rheum* 1999;**42**:2293–302.

Slothuus U, Brooks RG. Willingness to pay in arthritis: a Danish contribution. *Rheumatology* (Oxford) 2000;**39**:791–9.

Albert DA, Aksentijevich S, Hurst S, Fries JF, Wolfe F. Modeling therapeutic strategies in rheumatoid arthritis: use of decision analysis and Markov models. *J Rheumatol* 2000;**27**:644–52.

Choi HK, Seeger JD, Kuntz KM. A cost-effectiveness analysis of treatment options for patients with methotrexate-resistant rheumatoid arthritis. *Arthritis Rheum* 2000;**43**: 2316–27.

Suarez-Almazor ME, Conner-Sady B. Rating of arthritis health states by patients, physicians, and the general public. Implications for cost-utility analyses. *J Rheumatol* 2001;**28**:648–56.

Osteoarthritis (35 publications)

Liang MH, Cullen KE, Larson MG, *et al.* Cost-effectiveness of total joint arthroplasty in osteoarthritis. *Arthritis Rheum* 1986;**29**:937–43.

Hillman AL, Bloom BS: Economic effects of prophylactic use of misoprostol to prevent gastric ulcer in patients taking nonsteroidal anti-inflammatory drugs. *Arch Intern Med* 1989;**49**:2061–5.

Carrin GJ, Torfs KE. Economic evaluation of prophylactic treatment with misoprostol in osteoarthritic patients treated with NSAIDs. The case of Belgium. *Rev Epidemiol Sante Publique* 1990;**38**:187–99.

Edelson JT, Tosteson AN, Sax P: Cost-effectiveness of misoprostol for prophylaxis against nonsteroidal anti-inflammatory drug induced gastrointestinal tract bleeding. *JAMA* 1990;**264**:41–7.

Knill-Jones R, Drummond M, Kohli H, Davies L: Economic evaluation of gastric ulcer prophylaxis in patients with arthritis receiving non-steroidal anti-inflammatory drugs. *Postgrad Med J* 1990;**66**:639–46.

De Pouvourville G, Bader JP: Cost-effectiveness of preventive treatment with misoprostol in non-steroidal anti-inflammatory agents related gastric ulcers. *Gastroenterol Clin Biol* 1991;**15**:399–404.

Jönsson B, Haglund U: Cost-effectiveness of misoprostol in Sweden. *Int J Technol Assess Health Care* 1992;8:234–44.

McInnes J, Larson MG, Daltroy LH, *et al.* A controlled evaluation of continuous passive motion in patients undergoing total knee arthroplasty. *JAMA* 1992;**268**: 1423–8.

Chang RW, Falconer J, Stulberg SD, Arnold WJ, Manheim LM, Dyer AR: A randomised, controlled trial of arthroscopic surgery versus closed-needle joint lavage for patients with osteoarthritis of the knee. *Arthritis Rheum* 1993;**36**:289–96.

Weinberger M, Tierney WM, Cowper PA, Katz BP, Booher PA: Cost-effectiveness of increased telephone contact for patients with osteoarthritis: a randomised, controlled trial. *Arthritis Rheum* 1993;**36**:243–6.

Bentkover JD, Baker AM, Kaplam H. Nabumetone in elderly patients with osteoarthritis: economic benefits versus ibuprofen alone or ibuprofen plus misoprostol. *Pharmacoeconomics* 1994;**54**:335–42.

Bourne RB, Rorabeck CH, Laupacis A, *et al.* A randomised clinical trial comparing cemented to cementless total hip replacement in 250 osteoarthritic patients: the impact on health related quality of life and cost-effectiveness. *Iowa Orthop J* 1994;**14**:108–14.

Gabriel SE, Campion ME, O'Fallon WM: A cost-utility analysis of misoprostol prophylaxis for rheumatoid arthritis patients receiving nonsteroidal antiinflammatory drugs. *Arthritis Rheum* 1994;**37**:333–41.

Rorabeck CH, Bourne RB, Laupacis A, *et al.* A double-blind study of 250 cases comparing cemented with cementless total hip arthroplasty: cost-effectiveness and its impact on health-related quality of life. *Clin Orthop* 1994;**298**:156–64.

Healy WL, Kirven FM, Iorio R, Patch DA, Pfeifer BA. Implant standardization for total hip arthroplasty: an implant selection and a cost reduction program. *J Arthroplasty* 1995;**10**:177–83.

Healy WL. Economic considerations in total hip arthroplasty and implant standardization. *Clin Orthop* 1995;311:102–8.

Smalley WE, Griffin MR, Fought RL, Sullivan L, Ray WA. Effect of a prior-authorisation requirement on the use of nonsteroidal anti-inflammatory drugs by Medicaid patients. *N Engl J Med* 1995;**332**:1612–17.

Chang RW, Pellisier JM, Hazen GB. A cost-effectiveness analysis of total hip arthroplasty for osteoarthritis of the hip. *JAMA* 1996;**275**:858–65.

Furnes A, Lie SA, Havelin LI, Engesaeter LB, Vollset SE. The economic impact of failures in total hip replacement surgery: 28,997 cases from the Norwegian Arthroplasty Register, 1987–1993. *Acta Orthopaedica Scand* 1996;**67**:115–21.

Holzer SS, Cuerdon T. Development of an economic model comparing acetaminophen to NSAIDs in the treatment of mild-to-moderate osteoarthritis. *Am J Manag Care* 1996;II Suppl:S15–S26.

Cronan TA, Groessl E, Kaplan RM. The effects of social support and education interventions on health care costs. *Arthritis Care Res* 1997;**10**(2):99–110.

Fisher DA, Trimble S, Clapp B, Dorsett K. Effect of a patient management system on outcomes of total hip and knee arthroplasty. *Clin Orthop* 1997;**345**:155–60.

Rissanen P, Aro S, Sintonen H, Asikainen K, Slatis P, Paavolainen P. Costs and cost-effectiveness in hip and knee replacements: a prospective study. *Int J Technol Assess Health Care* 1997;**13**:575–88.

Saleh KJ, Wood KC, Gafni A, Gross AE. Immediate surgery versus waiting list policy in revision total hip arthroplasty: an economic evaluation. *J Arthroplasty* 1997;**12**:1–10.

Allhoff P, Graf von der Schulenburg JM. Zur Kostenwirksamkeit einer konservativen Gonarthrose-Therapie. *Z Orthop Ihre Grenzgeb* 1998;**136**:288–92.

Cronan T A, Hay M, Groessl E, Bigatti S, Gallagher R, Tomita M. The effects of social support and education on health care costs after three years. *Arthritis Care Res* 1998;**11**:326–34.

Fagnani F, Bouvenot G, Valat JP, *et al.* Medico-economic analysis of diacerein with or without standard therapy in the treatment of osteoarthritis. *Pharmacoeconomics* 1998;**13**:135–46.

Givon U, Ginsberg GM, Horoszowski H, Shemer J. Cost-utility analysis of total hip arthroplasties: technology assessment of surgical procedures by mailed questionnaires. *Int J Technol Assess Health Care* 1998;**14**:735–42.

Liaropoulos L, Spinthouri M, Ignatiades T, Ifandi G, Katostaras F, Diamantopoulos E. Economic evaluation of nimesulide versus diclofenac in the treatment of osteoarthritis in Greece. *Pharmacoeconomics* 1998;**14**:575–88.

Wammack L, Mabrey JD. Outcomes assessment of total hip and total knee arthroplasty: critical pathways, variance analysis, and continuous quality improvement. *Clinical Nurse Specialist* 1998;**12**:122–9.

Lord J, Victor C, Littlejohns P, Ross FM, Axford JS. Economic evaluation of a primary care-based education programme for patients with osteoarthritis of the knee. *Health Technol Assess* 1999;**3**:1–55.

Sevick MA, Bradham DD, Muender M, *et al.* Cost-effectiveness of aerobic and resistance exercise in seniors with knee osteoarthritis. *Med Sci Sports Exerc* 2000;**32**:1534–40.

Kocher MS, Erens G, Thornhill TS, Ready JE. Cost and effectiveness of routine pathological examination of operative specimens obtained during primary total hip and knee replacement in patients with osteoarthritis. *J Bone Joint Surg Am* 2000;**82**–A:1531–5.

Martí-Valls J, Alonso J, Lamarca R, *et al.* Efectividad y costes de la intervención de prótesis total de cadera en siete hospitales de Cataluña. *Med Clin (Barc)* 2000;**114**(Suppl 2):34–9.

Patrick DL, Ramsey SD, Spencer AC, Kinne S, Belza B, Topolski TD. Economic evaluation of aquatic exercise for persons with osteoarthritis. *Med Care* 2001;**39**:413–24.

Rheumatoid arthritis and osteoarthritis (18 publications)

Lorig KR, Mazonson PD, Holman HR: Evidence suggesting that health education for self-management in patients with chronic arthritis has sustained health benefits while reducing health care costs. *Arthritis Rheum* 1993;**36**:439–46.

Schwarz B. Die Kosten-Effektivität der Misoprostoltherapie in der Prävention NSAR-Induzierter Magenulzera. *Wien Klin Wochenschr* 1995;**107**:366–72.

Goldstein JL, Larson LR, Yamashita BD, Boyd MS. Management of NSAID-induced gastropathy: an economic decision analysis. *Clin Ther* 1997;**196**:1496–509.

Lavernia CJ, Guzman JF, Gachupin-Garcia ABS. Cost-effectiveness and Quality of Life in Knee Arthroplasty. *Clin Orthop* 1997;**345**:134–9.

Allard P, Deligne J, Van Bockstael V, Duquesnoy B. Is spa therapy cost-effective in rheumatic disorders? *Rev Rhum* 1998;**65**:600–2.

Kruger JM, Helmick CG, Callahan LF, Haddix AC. Cost-effectiveness of the arthritis self-help course. *Arch Intern Med* 1998;**158**:1245–9.

Maetzel A, Ferraz MB, Bombardier C. The cost-effectiveness of misoprostol in preventing serious gastrointestinal events associated with the use of nonsteroidal antiinflammatory drugs. *Arthritis Rheum* 1998;**41**:16–25.

McCabe CJ, Akehurst RL, Kirsch J, *et al.* Choice of NSAID and management strategy in rheumatoid arthritis and osteoarthritis: the impact on costs and outcomes in the UK. *Pharmacoeconomics* 1998;**14**:191–9.

Lawrence T, Moskal JT, Diduch DR. Analysis of routine histological evaluation of tissues removed during primary hip and knee arthroplasty. *J Bone Joint Surg Am* 1999;**81**: 926–31.

Motheral BR, Bataoel JR. A strategy for evaluating the novel COX-2 inhibitors versus NSAIDs for arthritis. *Formulary* 1999;**34**:855–63.

Walan A, Wahlqvist P. Pharmacoeconomic aspects of non-steroidal anti-inflammatory drug gastropathy. *Ital J Gastroenterol Hepatol* 1999;**31**(Suppl 1):S79–88.

Alvares JS. Analisis coste-efectividad de diclofenaco/ misoprostol (artrotec) en el tratamiento de los procesos osteoarticulares. *Anales Med Interna* 2000;**17**:477–84.

Davey PJ, Meyer E. The cost-effectiveness of misoprostol prophylaxis alongside long-term nonsteroidal anti-inflammatory drugs. Implications of the MUCOSA trial. *Pharmacoeconomics* 2000;**17**:295–304.

Haglund U, Svarvar P. The Swedish ACCES model: predicting the health economic impact of celecoxib in patients with osteoarthritis or rheumatoid arthritis. *Rheumatology* 2000;**39**(Suppl 2):51–6.

Krijnen P, Kaandorp CJ, Steyerberg EW, van Schaardenburg D, Moens HJ, Habbema JD. Antibiotic prophylaxis for haematogenous bacterial arthritis in patients with joint disease: a cost-effectiveness analysis. *Ann Rheum Dis* 2001;**60**:359–66.

Svarvar P, Aly A. Use of the ACCES model to predict the health economic impact of celecoxib in patients with osteoarthritis or rheumatoid arthritis in Norway. *Rheumatology* 2000;**39**(suppl 2):43–50.

Chancellor JVM, Hunsche E, de Cruz E and Sarasin FP. Economic evaluation of celecoxib, a new cyclo-oxygenase 2 specific inhibitor in Switzerland. *Pharmacoeconomics* 2001;**19**(Suppl 1): 59–75.

Zabinski RA, Burke TA, Johnson J, Lavoie F, Fitzsimon C, Tretiak R, Chancellor JVM. An economic model for determining the costs and consequences of using various treatment alternatives for the management of arthritis in Canada. *Phamacoeconomics* 2001;**19**(Suppl 1):49–58.

Osteoporosis (34 publications)

Weinstein MC. Estrogen use in postmenopausal women: costs, risks, and benefits. *N Engl J Med* 1980;**303**:308–16.

Weinstein MC, Schiff I. Cost-effectiveness of hormone replacement therapy in the menopause. *Obstet Gynecol Surv* 1983;**38**:445–55.

Van der Loos M, Paccaud F, Gutzwiller F, Chrzanowski R. Impact of hormonal prevention on fractures of the proximal femur in postmenopausal women: a simulation study. *Soz Praventivmed* 1988;**33**:162–6.

Tosteson AN, Rosenthal DI, Melton LJ, Weinstein MC. Cost-effectiveness of screening perimenopausal white women for osteoporosis: bone densitometry and hormone replacement therapy. *Ann Intern Med* 1990;**113**:594–603.

Weinstein MC, Tosteson ANA. Cost-effectiveness of hormone replacement. *Ann NY Acad Sci* 1990;**592**:162–72.

Tosteson AN, Weinstein MC. Cost-effectiveness of hormone replacement therapy after menopause. *Baillieres Clin Obstet Gynaecol* 1991;**5**:943–59.

Cheung AP, Wren BG: A cost-effectiveness analysis of hormone replacement therapy in the menopause. *Med J Aust* 1992;**156**:312–16.

Daly E, Roche M, Barlow D, Gray A, McPherson K, Vessey M. HRT: an analysis of benefits, risks and costs. *Br Med Bull* 1992;**48**:368–400.

Garton MJ, Torgerson DJ, Donaldson C, Russell IT, Reid DM. Recruitment methods for screening programmes: trial of a new method within a regional osteoporosis study. *BMJ* 1992;**305**:82–4.

Torgerson DJ, Reid DM. Osteoporosis prevention through screening: will it be cost-effective? *Baillieres Clin Rheumatol* 1993;**7**:603–22.

Torgerson DJ, Garton MJ, Donaldson C, Russell IT, Reid DM. Recruitment methods for screening programmes: trial of an improved method within a regional osteoporosis study. *BMJ* 1993;**307**:99.

Geelhoed E, Harris A, Prince R: Cost-effectiveness analysis of hormone replacement therapy and lifestyle intervention for hip fracture. *Aust J Publ Hlth* 1994;**18**:153–60.

Bendich A, Leader S, Muhuri P. Supplemental calcium for the prevention of hip fracture: potential health-economic benefits. *Clin Ther* 1999;**21**:(6), 1058–72.

Francis RM, Anderson FH, Torgerson DJ. A comparison of the effectiveness and cost of treatment for vertebral fractures in women. *Br J Rheumatol* 1995;**34**:1167–71.

Jönsson B, Christiansen C, Johnell O, Hedbrandt J. Cost-effectiveness of fracture prevention in established osteoporosis. *Osteoporos Int* 1995;**5**:136–42.

U.S. Congress, Office of Technology Assessment, Effectiveness and Costs of Osteoporosis Screening and Hormone Replacement Therapy, Volume 1: Cost-Effectiveness Analysis, OTA-BP-H-160 (Washington, DC: US Government Printing Office, August 1995).

Torgerson DJ, Kanis JA. Cost-effectiveness of preventing hip-fractures in the elderly population using vitamin-D and calcium. *QJM – J Assoc Phys* 1995;**88**:135–9.

Ankjaer-Jensen A, Johnell O. Prevention of osteoporosis: Cost-effectiveness of different pharmaceutical treatments. *Osteoporos Int* 1996;**6**:265–75.

Daly E, Vessey MP, Barlow D, Gray A, McPherson K, Roche M. Hormone replacement therapy in a risk–benefit perspective. *Maturitas* 1996;**23**:247–59.

Norlund A. Prevention of osteoporosis: a cost-effectiveness analysis regarding fractures. *Scand J Rheumatol* Suppl 1996;103:42–6.

Torgerson D, Donaldson C, Reid D. Using economics to prioritize research: a case study of randomised trials for the prevention of hip fractures due to osteoporosis. *J Hlth Serv Res Policy* 1996;**1**:141–6.

Garton MJ, Cooper C, Reid D. Perimenopausal bone density screening: will it help prevent osteoporosis? *Maturitas* 1997;**26**:35–43.

Kristiansen IS, Falch JA, Andersen L, Aursnes I. Use of alendronate in osteoporosis – is it cost-effective? *Tidsskr Nor Laegeforen* 1997;**117**:2619–22.

Visentin P, Ciravegna R, Fabris F. Estimating the cost per avoided hip fracture by osteoporosis treatment in Italy. *Maturitas* 1997;**26**:185–92.

Epstein RS, Feng W, Hirsch LJ, Kelly M. Intervention thresholds for the treatment of osteoporosis. Comparison of different approaches to decision-making. *Osteoporos Int* 1998;**8**(suppl 1):S22–27.

Jönsson B. Targeting high-risk populations. *Osteoporos Int* 1998;**8**(suppl 1):S13–16.

National Osteoporosis Foundation. Osteoporosis: review of the evidence for prevention, diagnosis, and treatment and cost-effectiveness analysis, status report. *Osteoporos Int* 1998;**8**(Suppl 4):S1–88.

Rosner AJ, Grima DT, Torrance GW, *et al.* Cost-effectiveness of multi-therapy treatment strategies in the prevention of vertebral fractures in postmenopausal women with osteoporosis. *Pharmacoeconomics* 1998;**14**:559–73.

Visentin P, Ciravegna R, Corcelli F, Fabris F. Cost-effectiveness of hip fracture prevention. *Epidemiologia Prevenzione* 1998;**22**:44–8.

Zethraeus N, Johannesson M, Jonsson B. A computer model to analyse the cost-effectiveness of hormone replacement therapy. *Int J Technol Assess Health Care* 1999;**15**:352–65.

Aursnes I, Storvik G, Gåsemyr J, Natvig B. A bayesian analysis of bisphosphonate effects and cost-effectiveness in post-menopausal osteoporosis. *Pharmacoepidemiol Drug Saf* 2000;**9**:501–9.

Solomon DH, Kuntz KM. Should postmenopausal women with rheumatoid arthritis who are starting corticosteroid treatment be screened for osteoporosis? A cost-effectiveness analysis. *Arthritis Rheum* 2000;**43**:1967–75.

Coyle D, Cranney A, Lee KM, Welch V, Tugwell P. Cost-effectiveness of nasal calcitonin in postmenopausal women – use of Cochrane collaboration methods for meta-analysis within economic evaluation. *Pharmacoeconomics* 2001;**19**:565–75.

Willis M, Odegaard K, Persson U, Hedbrant J, Mellstrom D, Hammar M. A cost-effectiveness model of tibolone as treatment for the prevention of osteoporotic fractures in postmenopausal women in Sweden. *Clin Drug Invest* 2001;**21**:115–27.

Lower back and/or neck pain (13 publications)

Brown KC, Sirles AT, Hilyer JC, Thomas MJ: Cost-effectiveness of a back school intervention for municipal employees. *Spine* 1992;**17**:1224–8.

Versloot JM, Rozeman A, van Son AM, van Akkerveeken PF: The cost-effectiveness of a back school program in industry: a longitudinal controlled field study. *Spine* 1992;**17**:22–7.

Mitchell LV, Lawler FH, Bowen D, Mote W, Asundi P, Purswell J: Effectiveness and cost-effectiveness of employer-issued back belts in areas of high risk for back injury. *J Occup Med* 1994;**36**:90–4.

Carey TS, Garrett J, Jackman A, McLaughlin C, Fryer J, Smucker DR. The outcomes and costs of care for acute low back pain among patients seen by primary care practitioners, chiropractors, and orthopedic surgeons. *N Engl J Med* 1995;**333**(14):913–17.

Malmivaara A, Hakkinen U, Aro T, *et al.* The treatment of acute low back pain: bed rest, exercises, or ordinary activity? *N Engl J Med* 1995;**332**:351–5.

Tuchin PJ, Bonello R. Preliminary findings of analysis of chiropractic utilization and cost in the workers compensation system of New South Wales, Australia. *J Manip Physiol Ther* 1995;**18**:503–11.

Malter AD, Larson EB, Urban N, Deyo RA. Cost-effectiveness of lumbar discectomy for the treatment of herniated intervertebral disc. *Spine* 1996;**21**:1048–55.

Skargren EI, Oberg BE, Carlsson PG, Gade M. Cost and effectiveness analysis of chiropractic and physiotherapy treatment for low back and neck pain: six-month follow-up. *Spine* 1997;**22**:2167–77.

de Lissovoy G, Brown RE, Halpern M, Hassenbusch SJ, Ross E. Cost-effectiveness of long-term intrathecal morphine therapy for pain associated with failed back surgery syndrome. *Clin Ther* 1997;**19**:96–112.

Hacker RJ. Comparison of interbody fusion approaches for disabling low back pain. *Spine* 1997;**22**:660–6.

Skargren EI, Carlsson PG, Oberg BE. One-year follow-up comparison of the cost and effectiveness of chiropractic and physiotherapy as primary management for back pain: subgroup analysis, recurrence, and additional health care utilization. *Spine* 1998;**23**:1875–83.

Goossens MEJB, Rutten-van Molken MPMH, Kole-Snijders AMJ, *et al.* Health economic assessment of behavioural rehabilitation in chronic low back pain: a randomised clinical trial. *Health Econ* 1998;**7**:39–51.

Moffett JK, Torgerson D, Bell-Syer SB, *et al.* Randomised controlled trial of exercise for low back pain: clinical outcomes, costs, and preferences. *BMJ* 1999;**319**: 279–83.

Lyme disease

Lightfoot RW Jr, Luft BJ, Rahn DW, *et al.* Empiric parenteral antibiotic treatment of patients with fibromyalgia and fatigue and a positive serologic result for Lyme disease: a cost-effectiveness analysis. *Ann Intern Med* 1993;**119**: 503–9.

Eckman MH, Steere AC, Kalish RA, Pauker SG. Cost-effectiveness of oral as compared with intravenous antibiotic therapy for patients with early Lyme disease or Lyme arthritis. *N Engl J Med* 1997;**337**:357–63.

Nichol G, Dennis DT, Steere AC, *et al.* Test-treatment strategies for patients suspected of having Lyme disease: a cost-effectiveness analysis. *Ann Intern Med* 1998;**128**:37–48.

Others

Tompkins RK, Burnes DC, Cable WE: An analysis of the cost-effectiveness of pharyngitis management and acute rheumatic fever prevention. *Ann Intern Med* 1977;**86**: 481–92.

Coulehan JL, Baacke G, Welty TK, Goldtooth NL: Cost-benefit of a streptococcal surveillance program among Navajo Indians. *Publ Hlth Rep* 1982;**97**:73–7.

Tsevat J, Durand-Zaleski I, Pauker SG: Cost-effectiveness of antibiotic prophylaxis for dental procedures in patients with artificial joints. *Am J Publ Hlth* 1989;**79**:739–43.

Bakker C, Hidding A, van der Linden S, van Doorslaer E: Cost-effectiveness of group physical therapy compared to individualized therapy for ankylosing spondylitis: a randomised controlled trial. *J Rheumatol* 1994;**21**:264–8.

McInnes PM, Schuttinga J, Sanslone WR, Stark SP, Klippel JH. The economic impact of treatment of severe lupus nephritis with prednisone and intravenous cyclophosphamide. *Arthritis Rheum* 1994;**37**:1000–6.

Ferraz MB, O'Brien B. A cost-effectiveness analysis of urate lowering drugs in nontophaceous recurrent gouty arthritis. *J Rheumatol* 1995;**22**:908–14.

Goossens ME, Rultenvan Molkan MP, Leidl RM, Bos SG, Viaeyen JW, Teeken-Gruben NJ. Cognitive–educational treatment of fibromyalgia: a randomised clinical trial: II. Economic evaluation. *J Rheumatol* 1996;**23**:1246–54.

Helliwell PS. Comparison of a community clinic with a hospital out-patient clinic in rheumatology. *Br J Rheumatol* 1996;**35**:385–8.

Lafuma A, Fagnani F, Meunier PJ. An economic evaluation of tiludronic acid treatment in Paget's disease of bone. *Pharmacoeconomics* 1997;**12**:460–74.

Grzybicki DM, Callaghan EJ, Raab SS. Cost-benefit value of microscopic examination of intervertebral discs. *J Neurosurg* 1998;**89**:378–81.

Klein-Gitelman MS, Waters T, Pachman LM. The economic impact of intermittent high-dose intravenous versus oral corticosteroid treatment of juvenile dermatomyositis. *Arthritis Care Res* 2000;**13**:360–8.

References

1 Eisenberg JM. Clinical economics. A guide to the economic analysis of clinical practices. *JAMA* 1989;**262**(20):2879–86.

2 Bootman JL, Townsend RJ, McGhan WF. Introduction to pharmacoeconomics. In: Bootman JL, Townsend RJ, McGhan WF, eds. *Principles of pharmacoeconomics, 2nd ed.* Cincinnati, OH: Harvey Whitney Books Company, 1996:5–18.

3 Drummond MF. Basic types of economic evaluation. In: Drummond MF, O'Brien BJ, Stoddart GL, Torrance GW, eds. *Methods for the economic evlaution of health care programmes, 2nd ed.* New York: Oxford University Press; 1997:6–26.

4 Drummond MF, Davies L. Economic analysis alongside clinical trials: revisiting the methodological issues. *Intl J Technol Assess Health Care* 1991;**7**(4):561–73.

5 Gold MR, Siegel JE, Russell LB, Weinstein MC. *Cost-effectiveness in health and medicine,* Vol II. New York, NY: Oxford University Press, 1996.

6 Hanley JA. The robustness of the "binormal" assumptions used in fitting ROC curves. *Med Decis Making* 1988;**8**(3):197–203.

7 Chapman RH, Stone PW, Sandberg EA, Bell C, Neumann PJ. A comprehensive league table of cost-utility ratios and a subtable of "panel-worthy" studies. *Med Decis Making* 2000;**20**:451–67.

8 Cranney A, Coyle D, Welch V, Lee KM, Tugwell P. A review of economic evaluation in osteoporosis. *Arthritis Care Res* 1999;**12**(6):425–34.

9 Maetzel A, Ferraz MB, Bombardier C. A review of cost-effectiveness analyses in rheumatology and related disciplines. *Curr Opin Rheumatol* 1998;**10**(2):136–40.

10 Tugwell P. Economic evaluation of the management of pain in osteoarthritis. *Drugs* 1996;**52** Suppl 3:48–58.

11 National Institute for Clinical Excellence. Technical Guidance for Manufacturers and Sponsors on Making a Submission to a Technology Appraisal. www.nice.org.uk *(Technology Appraisals)* [World Wide Web]. March 2001. Available at: www.nice.org.uk (Technology Appraisals).

12 Canberra: Department of Health and Community Services. *Commonwealth of Australia Guidelines for the Pharmaceutical Industry on Preparation of Submissions to the Pharmaceutical Benefits Advisory Committee: Including Economic Analyses* 1995.

13 Canadian Coordinating Office for Health Technology Assessment (CCOHTA). *Guidelines for economic evaluation of pharmaceuticals, 2nd ed.* Ottawa, Canada, 1997.

14 Murray CJ, Evans DB, Acharya A, Baltussen RM. Development of WHO guidelines on generalized cost-effectiveness analysis. *Health Econ* 2000;**9**(3):235–51.

15 Ferraz MB, Maetzel A, Bombardier C. A summary of economic evaluations published in the field of rheumatology and related disciplines. *Arthritis Rheum* 1997;**40**(9):1587–93.

16 Rothfuss J, Mau W, Zeidler H, Brenner MH. Socioeconomic evaluation of rheumatoid arthritis and osteoarthritis: a literature review. *Semin Arthritis Rheum* 1997;**26**(5):771–79.

17 Ruchlin HS, Elkin EB, Paget SA. Assessing cost-effectiveness analyses in rheumatoid arthritis and osteoarthritis. *Arthritis Care Res* 1997;**10**(6):413–21.

18 O'Brien B. Principles of economic evaluation for health care programs. *J Rheumatol* 1995;**22**(7)1399–402.

19 Drummond M, O'Brien B. Economic analysis alongside clinical trials: practical considerations. The Economics Workgroup. *J Rheumatol* 1995;**22**(7):1418–19.

20 Drummond M, Ferraz MB, Mason J. Assessing the cost-effectiveness of NSAID: an international perspective. *J Rheumatol* 1995;**22**:1408–11.

21 Gabriel SE. Economic evaluation using mathematical models: the case of misoprostol prophylaxis. *J Rheumatol* 1995;**22**(7):1412–14.

22 Gabriel SE, Tugwell P, O'Brien B, *et al.* Report of the OMERACT Task Force on economic evaluation. *J Rheumatol* 1999;**26**(1):203–6.

23 Gabriel SE. OMERACT 5 economics working group report: Introduction. *J Rheumatol* 2001;**28**(3):640.

24 Gabriel SE, Drummond MF, Coyle D, *et al.* OMERACT 5 – Economics working group: summary, recommendations, and research agenda. *J Rheumatol* 2001;**28**(3):670–3.

25 Suarez-Almazor M, Connor-Spady B. Rating of arthritis health states by patients, physicians, and the general public. Implications for cost-utility analyses. *J Rheumatol* 2001;**28**(3):648–56.

26 Coyle D, Welch V, Shea B, Gabriel S, Drummond MF, Tugwell P. Issues of consensus and debate for economic evaluation in rheumatology. *J Rheumatol* 2001;**28**(3): 642–7.

27 Merkesdal S, Ruof J, Huelsemann JL, *et al.* Development of a matrix of cost domains in economic evaluation of rheumatoid arthritis. *J Rheumatol* 2001;**28**(8):657–61.

28 Ruof J, Merkesdal S, Hulsemann JL, *et al.* Cost assessment instruments in rheumatology: evaluation of applied isntrument characteristics. *J Rheumatol* 2001; **28**(3):662–5.

29 Ruff B. OMERACT: Economic evaluations and health policy. *J Rheumatol* 2001;**28**(3):666–9.

30 Gabriel SE, Tugwell P, Drummond M. Progress towards an OMERACT–ILAR guideline for economic evaluations in rheumatology. *Ann Rheum Dis* 2002;**61**:370–3.

31 Gabriel S, Drummond M, Maetzel A, *et al.* OMERACT 6 economics working group report: a proposal for a reference case for economic evaluation in rheumatoid arthritis. *J Rheumatol* 2003;**30**:886–90.

32 Maetzel A, Tugwell P, Boers M, et al. Economic evaluation of programs or interventions in the management of rheumatoid arthritis: defining a consensus-based reference case. *J Rheumatol* 2003;**30**:891–6.

33 Gabriel SE. Controversies in economic evaluation in the rheumatic diseases [editorial; comment]. *J Rheumatol* 1999;**26**(9):1859–60.

34 Guillemin F. The value of utility: assumptions underlying preferences and quality adjusted life years [editorial] [see comments]. *J Rheumatol* 1999;**26**(9):1861–3.

35 O'Brien B. Statistical analysis of cost-effectiveness data. *J Rheumatol* 1999;**26**(10):2078–80.

36 Maetzel A, Bombardier C. Give observational studies a chance: Better observational studies make better economic evaluations. *J Rheumatol* 1999;**26**(11):2298–9.

37 Cranney A, Coyle D, Welch V, Lee K, Tugwell P. Current controversies in cost-effectiveness analysis of osteoporosis therapies. *J Rheumatol* 1999;**26**(11): 2300–2.

4

Knowledge translation for patients: methods to support patients' participation in decision making about preference-sensitive treatment options in rheumatology

Annette M O'Connor, Dawn Stacey, France Légaré, Nancy Santesso

Case presentation Part I: Mrs C

Mrs C, a 51-year-old Caucasian woman, recently started on oestrogen and progestin for hot flashes that disturbed her sleep and affected her ability to function at work and at home. She was otherwise healthy, with no risk factors for heart disease, thromboembolic disease, or breast cancer. A recent mammogram and breast exam were normal. She has not had any fractures in the past, however, her mother suffered from an osteoporotic fracture. Other risk factors for osteoporosis were negative.

Results of her bone density test indicating osteoporosis (T-score = 2.5 standard deviations below normal) were reviewed today, along with long term treatment options for Mrs C to consider. However, she was not sure of her preference and requested information and help with deliberation.

Evidence-based medicine integrates clinical experience with patients' values using the best available evidence.[1] In the past, physicians took responsibility not only for being well informed about the benefits and harms of medical options but also for judging the value for their patients. Physicians acted as agents in the best interest of their patients.[2] However, patients are now asking to be involved and share the responsibility in making health-related decisions.[3–4] In response, a shared decision making approach is advocated in which patients are recognised as the best experts for judging "values" (also known as preferences). Preferences are an individual's desirability of an outcome either under conditions of certainty (values) or uncertainty (utilities). Evidence-based decision aids supplement physicians' counselling regarding preference-sensitive options so that patients can: (a) understand the probable consequences of options; (b) consider and clarify the value they place on the consequences; and (c) participate actively with their physician in selecting the best option for themselves.

This chapter discusses practical and effective methods that practitioners can use for providing patients with evidence-based information and guidance in decision making to facilitate their involvement as partners in making treatment decisions. Three issues are discussed. First, we explore the types of decisions in rheumatology and the clinician's role in providing decision support. Next, we describe the efficacy of practical tools, known as decision aids, to prepare patients to participate in decision making regarding preference-sensitive options. Finally, we introduce a library of simple, evidence-based rheumatology decision aids that can be supplemented with additional information and integrated into clinical, patient education, and health information services.

What are the classes of decisions in rheumatology?

The goal in decision making is to select options that increase the *likelihood* of *valued* health outcomes and minimise the chance of *undesired* consequences according to the best available scientific *evidence*.[1] In some cases, the best strategy is clear because the evidence of benefits and harms is known and the harms are minimal relative to the benefits. For these decisions, most clinicians would recommend an option and most informed patients, placing a greater value on benefits relative to harms, would agree to take it. Unfortunately, many decisions in health care do not have clear answers because the benefit/harm ratios are unknown or the decision depends on how people value benefits versus harms. For these more difficult decisions, clinicians do not routinely recommend the option but provide access to information about benefits, harms, and scientific uncertainties so that patients can consider their associated values.

To guide practitioners and patients in understanding which decisions have clear answers and which ones do not, treatment options are being classified not only according to the strength of scientific evidence but also the magnitude of benefit/harm ratios. Table 4.1 summarises the classification schemes of Chalmers[5] and the US Preventive Task Force.[6] The Chalmers' terminology is used in this textbook: beneficial; likely to be beneficial; trade-off between benefits and harms; unknown effectiveness; unlikely to be beneficial; and likely to be ineffective or harmful. Although the classification is useful in guiding decision making and counselling, there are some limitations to consider when using evidence-based texts:

> Fitting interventions into these categories is not always straightforward. For one thing, the categories represent a mix of several hierarchies: the level of benefit (or harm), the level of evidence (RCT or observational data), and the level of certainty around the finding (represented by the confidence interval). Another problem is that much of the evidence that is most relevant to clinical decisions relates to comparisons between different interventions rather than to comparison with placebo or no intervention. A third problem is that interventions may have been tested, or found to be effective, in only one group of people, such as those at high risk of an outcome. But perhaps most difficult of all has been trying to maintain consistency across different topics.[5]

What is the clinician's role in providing decision support by class of decisions?

There are both commonalities and differences in counselling according to the classifications for decisions. In general, the counsellor's role is to facilitate the patient's participation in ways that respect the patient's values, personal resources, and capacity for self-determination. Among the classes of decisions, the commonalities include providing patients with the opportunity to be actively involved in deliberation, planning, and implementing the chosen option. However, the goals, intensity of decision support, and rationale are different.

"Beneficial and likely beneficial": For beneficial and likely beneficial decisions, practitioners usually recommend a treatment and briefly

Table 4.1 Schemes for classifying medical options according to the strength of scientific evidence and magnitude of benefit/harm ratios

Chalmer's scheme used in clinical evidence[5]			
Rating	Evidence of Intervention effectiveness	Magnitude of benefit over harm	US Preventive Task Force Guidelines[6]
Beneficial	Clear evidence from RCTs	Expectation of harms is small compared to benefits.	A • Strongly recommend • good quality evidence • substantial magnitude of benefit over harm
Likely to be beneficial	Less well established than beneficial rating		B • Recommend in favour of routine provision • fair evidence • moderate benefit
Trade-off between benefits and harms	Clinicians and patients should weigh the beneficial and harmful effects according to individual circumstances and priorities		C • Close call, no recommendation either for or against routine provision • good or fair evidence • small magnitude of benefit or sensitive to patient values
Unknown effectiveness	Insufficient data		I • Insufficient evidence to recommend either for or against routine provision • poor quality evidence
Unlikely to be beneficial	Less well established than likely to be beneficial rating		D • Recommend against routine provision
Likely to be ineffective or harmful	Clear evidence	Harmfulness demonstrated	• good or fair evidence • zero or negative magnitude of benefit over harm

explain the rationale for treatment and its benefits and harms. Patients are asked if they agree to take it. With information provided in accordance with patients' beliefs, most patients will acknowledge the greater value of the benefits compared to the harms, and will be interested in trying the recommended option. Practitioners need to be aware of the beliefs, values, attitudes and intention held by the patients to support decision making in the most favourable direction.[7]

Once agreement is reached, the focus of support can move from decision making to the more challenging task of implementing the decision, which frequently requires changing behaviour and ensuring continuance of the chosen option. We know that over half of patients prescribed medications have difficulties with follow-though because: (a) they are not convinced of the need or they have personal attitudinal beliefs that do are not in accord with the benefits or risks associated with this medication; (b) someone important to them might not support this decision; or (c) there are too many barriers to making the changes necessary to take medications over the long term. Indeed, 15–25% do not fill their prescription and only 50% are taking treatment at one year following a prescription.[8] Involving patients in their care can address these issues. Indeed, doing so improves control of their disease and continuance of therapy.

For implementation of the decision, a motivational and tailored interviewing strategy is effective in identifying: (a) patients' beliefs, values, attitudes, priorities, motivations, and confidence in making the recommended change; and (b) personal barriers for uptake.[9] This counselling strategy reflects a change in emphasis from a passive "informed consent" process to a more active engagement, which has been called "evidence-informed patient choice", "collaborative care", "shared decision making" or "patient–physician concordance". There is coherence within these frameworks of "patient-centred care" for which the patient is considered as a unique human being with the interaction aimed at seeing the situation through the individual patient's eyes.[10–12] It includes sharing power and responsibility based on a therapeutic alliance in order to reach an agreement about the problem, the options, and the role in decision making.[13]

Case presentation Part II: Mrs C

Calcium and vitamin D are beneficial treatments that are usually recommended as part of the treatment for osteoporosis. Therefore, Mrs C's practitioner used a motivational and tailored counselling technique to negotiate the course of action for these beneficial options.

"As you know, you have osteoporosis, which is ....

For women with your level of bone density, we routinely recommend you take calcium and vitamin D every day to help prevent any further bone loss.

The scientific evidence is strong that the benefits are substantial and the harms are minimal.

But of course, your opinion counts in deciding whether you agree that the benefits outweigh the harms.

On the benefit side.......calcium and vitamin D reduce the chances of broken hips and spines... .....

On the harm side, side effects include...."

"What do you think about the benefits and harms?"

"Do you agree that this therapy is worth taking, or do you have concerns about it still...

"Do you have other questions or concerns?"

If the patient agrees to take it:

"Here are some common reasons people have difficulty taking their pills every day:"

- not convinced of the need
- worried about side effects
- don't believe in taking pills
- expense
- hassle
- hard to work into daily routine
- not ready, confident or motivated to change.

"Do any of these apply to you? What would help overcome these difficulties? Are there any other reasons it may be hard for you to take your pills every day."

Trade-off between benefits and harms" or "uncertain effectiveness": In contrast to beneficial options, counselling for these types of decisions is usually non-directive, because the best choice for an individual depends on how the patient values the benefits, harms, and scientific uncertainties (see Table 4.2). There is no evidence-based "right" decision. Moreover, there is a need to describe options, benefits, harms, and scientific uncertainties in more detail in order to create realistic expectations, clarify values, and enable participation in decision making. To streamline the process, evidence-based decision aids have been developed to prepare patients for discussions with their practitioners. These improvements will lead to enhanced accountability, informed consent, and, in some situations, have the potential to reduce litigation.[14]

Choices may or may not involve making a change in behaviour (for example if status quo is an option); in cases where it does, motivational and tailored interviewing described previously may be helpful to assist the individual with follow-through on their chosen option.

The criteria for judging the success of counselling with these types of decisions can be challenging to identify because the outcomes are unknown or involve making value trade-offs. For decisions requiring trade-offs, we can expect that patients will experience both benefits and harms. The key is to determine the option whose potential harms patients find least objectionable, and whose benefits they value most. In other words, success is the extent to which the choice is informed and matches the patients' values. With this approach, patients may be more likely to stick with their choice and to express less regret over the negative consequences of the choice.

Case presentation Part III: Mrs C

Mrs C's rheumatologist told her that in the short term, because she was pleased with the relief of hot flashes, she could continue on hormone therapy (HT) for both menopausal symptoms and osteoporosis. However, the osteoporosis therapy needed to be taken long term and she should consider other medication options (in addition to the calcuim, vitamin D, and physical activity) to prevent further bone loss and subsequent fractures. The rheumatologist arranged for her to review a decision aid outlining her options of staying on hormones for the year or switching to a bisphosphonate therapy now (see Appendix: Decision Aid on p. 57).

How do patient decision aids differ from usual patient education material?

Patient decision aids are standardised, evidence-based resources that facilitate the process of decision making and enhance practitioner–patient interaction. According to the Cochrane definition, they are "interventions designed to help people make specific and deliberative choices among options (including the status quo) by providing (at a minimum) information on the options and outcomes relevant to a person's health status".[15] Information is a necessary but not a sufficient element of decision aids.[16] Patients need to learn how to personalise the information and communicate their values to practitioners. Decision aids are designed to supplement rather than replace the patient–practitioner interaction.

Compared to conventional education materials, patient decision aids present the treatments as a choice of options and include personalised information about options, outcomes, probabilities, and uncertainties in sufficient detail for decision making. The decision aid then facilitates patients' clarifying their personal desirability of potential benefits relative to potential harms. Many aids include balanced examples of how others deliberate about options and also guide

Table 4.2 Practitioners' decisions support process for preference-sensitive decisions

Attribute	Preference-sensitive decision support description
Directiveness and focus	No routine recommendation; usually no right or wrong choice Non-directive counselling usually involving more detailed personalised information and values clarification Focus on decision making is usually longer than for beneficial options Choosing status quo (watchful waiting) is often a valid option; therefore, focus on implementing change depends on choice
Goals	Decision making process Participates in decision making and care according to preference Informed of available options, benefits, harms, probabilities, scientific uncertainties Values clarified related to benefits and harms More certain about best personal option (lower decisional conflict) Self-confidence and skill in decision making Progresses through stages of decision making Change process (only relevant if choice involves a change in the status quo) Self-confidence and skill in priority setting, identifying and addressing barriers, and implementing change. Progresses through stages of change Behavioural and clinical outcomes Choice matches patient values for benefits, harms, scientific uncertainties Continuance of chosen option (if choice changes status quo) Health outcomes may be variable due to: (a) scientific uncertainty; or (b) trade-offs in harm/benefit ratio Less decisional regret Future decisions Transfers learned skills in decision making and change processes to future decisions
Decision support process	1. Clarify decision and decisional support needs Explain condition stimulating need for a decision Summarise options, benefits, harms, scientific uncertainties Assess preferred role in decision making Screen for decisional conflict regarding best option and deficits in knowledge, values clarity, and support 2. Address decisional support needs Provide or refer patient for decision support (with information, decision aids, and/or referral to other team members as needed) to: o Guide patient in steps of decision making process o Provide information o Clarify values o Provide access to examples of others' decisions o Identify questions and leaning toward options Discuss understanding and questions, acknowledge values, and determine preferred option(s) 3. Facilitate progress in stage of decision making Obtain agreement regarding choice or commitment to take steps toward making a choice 4. Discuss implementation of choice (if choice involves change in status quo) Assess patient's motivation and confidence to implement choice Discuss barriers to implementation and potential solutions Negotiate arrangements for implementation and follow-up

people in the steps of collaborative decision making. Decision aids are delivered as self-administered or practitioner-administered tools within one-to-one or group situations. The mediums for delivery include decision boards, interactive computer programs, audio-guided workbooks, and pamphlets. Many developers use more than one medium and there is a shift toward internet-based delivery systems. The timing of delivering decision aids in the process of clinical care (for example, before, during, or after counselling) depends on practitioners' usual counselling practices and the availability of patient education and information services. Ideally, most decision aids are designed for use in preparation for counselling.[15]

General patient education resources are inadequate as a decision aid because they are not geared to a specific decision and they are frequently designed to obtain passive informed consent or to promote adherence to a specific recommended option. For example, 54 patient education resources in the United Kingdom that were reviewed by patients and practitioners were found to be inadequate for patient decision making.[17] These resources were rated as: being either too simple or too technical; excluding discussion of treatment options; offering inadequate information on treatment effectiveness, self-management or prevention; not necessarily having evidence-based quality information; and more likely to emphasize benefits while minimizing possible harms.

Several theoretical frameworks have guided the development of patient decision aids.[18–24] Most frameworks are based on decision theories from economics[25–26] and cognitive psychology[27] that describe how patients decide or ought to make decisions. Many frameworks broaden this cognitive perspective to include emotional, social, or environmental dimensions.[28–32]

The four key elements frequently found in decision aids are information, values clarification, examples of others, and guidance in the decision making process:

Information tailored to a patient's health status: Information is provided on: the condition, disease, or developmental transition stimulating the decision; the health care options available; the outcomes of options, including how they affect patient functioning; and the probabilities associated with outcomes. The information is clearly presented as a "choice situation". According to the Cochrane definition,[15] the minimum requirement to be classified as a decision aid is to include information on options and outcomes relevant to the patient's health status.

Values clarification: Information on treatment benefits and harms helps patients implicitly to form judgements of their value, especially if there are descriptions of physical, emotional, and social impacts on functioning. However, many decision aids also include values clarification exercises to explicitly consider and communicate the personal importance of each benefit or harm. There are several strategies, including balance scales, relevance charts, or trade-off techniques. For example, in balance scales, patients are asked to rate the degree of personal importance associated with each of the possible outcomes (see Appendix: Decision Aid on p 57). The familiar 'five star' rating system helps the practitioner understand which benefits and harms are most salient to the patient in decision making.

Examples of other patients: People are social learners and therefore, patients often like to learn from others who have faced the same situation. Some decision aids provide a balanced illustration of how others deliberate about options and arrive at decisions based on their personal situation.

When examples are used, it is important to ensure balanced representation of the choice made.

Guidance or coaching in shared decision making: Skills and confidence associated with participating in decision making are developed by guiding patients in the steps involved with decision making and coaching in communicating to others their preferences, values, and personal issues. Guidance and coaching are included in some decision aids.

Do patient decision aids work?

A Cochrane Collaboration Systematic Review of 35 randomised trials of decision aids provides clear answers about the efficacy of decision aids for improving the quality of decision making.[15] Decision aids improve patients' knowledge of options, create realistic perceptions of the probabilities of benefits and harms, reduce decisional conflict (uncertainty about the best course of action) increase the proportion of patients who make a choice, improve the match between what patients' value and what they choose, and enhance participation in decision making without affecting anxiety. One additional trial has shown improvement in agreement between patients and their providers about the decision making process.[33]

More research is needed on which decision aids work best with which decisions and which types of patients. As well, evaluation is needed on their acceptability to diverse groups of practitioners and patients, their impact on patient–practitioner communication, and their effects on continuance with chosen options, preference-linked health outcomes, practice variations, and use of resources. There continue to be questions about the essential elements in decision aids and whether or not information is enough, as a minimum requirement.

There is a need to examine ways to integrate patient decision aids into clinical practice. In a recent qualitative study of practitioner's attitudes to decision aids, response to open-ended questions suggested that there are four unique barriers/facilitators to implementing patient decision aids in general and specialty medical practices.[34] The first barrier was awareness that the decision aid exists. Another barrier was accessibility to decision aids with a recommendation from practitioners that this needs to be smooth, automatic, and timely. The third barrier was acceptability. Practitioners identified that decision aids, similar to the logistical barriers for implementing evidence in clinical practice,[35] need to be compatible with their practice and personal beliefs, up-to-date, attractive, easy to use, and not require additional cost, time, or equipment. Finally, practitioners identified needing to feel motivated to use it by factors such as time saving, avoidance of repetition, not requiring extra calls from patients, potential to decrease litigation, and improved rationing of health care with the possibility of reducing waiting-list pressures. For example, internet-based decision aids have many advantages that include increased availability, decreased expenses, ease of updating, and access either within patients' homes, practitioners' offices, or public libraries.[36] However, internet-based decision aids requiring internet connection may impede access to patients who lack computer resources and skills.

Current strategies under evaluation to improve patient and practitioner access to decision aids include the use of call centres staffed by nurses and imbedding decision aids in the routine process of care.

Which patient decision aids exist?

To improve access to decisions aids, the Cochrane Collaboration Systematic Review Team, examining the effectiveness of decision aids, established an Inventory of Patient Decision

Aids.[15] The inventory includes information on the topic, author, location, last update, delivery format, evaluation status, availability, and relevant publications. For decision aids that are available for use, there is a more detailed description of their contents and a quality rating; access to this information is available at a patient-friendly A to Z library on the web. In the most recent update, over 300 patient decision aids were identified, and the four relevant to rheumatology are listed in Table 4.3. Several of these decision aids are available on the internet. To obtain the most recent version of the inventory and access to the A to Z library of decision aids, visit the Ottawa Health Research Institute website http://www.ohri.ca and follow the links to patient decision aids.

Given the wide range of decision aids available and the diverse methodologies used in their development and evaluation, the Cochrane Collaboration Review Team of Patient Decision Aids developed a standardised quality assessment process,[15] whose acronym is "CREDIBLE": **C**ompetently developed and developers, **R**ecently updated, **E**vidence-based, **D**evoid of conflicts of **I**nterest, **B**a**L**anced, and **E**fficacious (see Box 4.1).

Expanding the library of evidence-based rheumatology decision aids

Given the evidence supporting the use of patient decision aids in facilitating the decision making process, the paucity of decision aids in rheumatology, and the labour-intensive nature of developing and updating decision aids, a starting point for developing a library of evidence-based rheumatology decision aids is proposed. The goal of these new rheumatology decision aids is to provide a user-friendly, direct to consumer, link with condition-oriented, evidence-based reviews using a structured process to facilitate shared decision making.

The first series in a library of evidence-based rheumatology decision aids is presented at the end of several chapters in this book. Their format is based on several sources: the Cochrane definition of decision aids;[15] a patient decision template for screening or treatment options;[37] the CREDIBLE quality indicators;[15] and a generic decision support tool known as the Ottawa Personal Decision Guide that was developed using the clinically based Ottawa Decision Support Framework.[38]

These rheumatology decision aids include two sections:

- an introduction to the specific rheumatology condition.
- systematic guidance in the 6 steps of deliberation, tailored to a specific option (see Appendix: Decision Aid on p 57).

Three of the four key elements for decision aids are included: information on options and outcomes, values clarification, and guidance in decision making. The only missing element is examples of how other patients made their decisions. These aids are to be publicly accessible on the book website (http://www.evidbasedrheum.com) as well as the Canadian Arthritis Society website (http://www.arthritis.ca). With ongoing online evaluations of these decision aids, the plan is to eventually develop a "People Like Me" series of balanced examples of different patients' deliberations about options or to refer patients to websites such as Database of Individual Patients' Experience (DIPEX) in Oxford (http://www.dipex. org/EXEC).[39] DIPEX has a current proposal to describe patients' experiences with arthritic conditions.

We will now look at each section of these rheumatology decision aids in turn.

Section I: Introduction to the rheumatology condition The first section of the simple decision aid provides information about the condition, possible outcomes and consequences

Table 4.3 Available up-to-date rheumatology-related patient decision aids

First author	Title	Delivery format	Content elements	Update status	Evaluation status	Access
Healthwise Knowledgebase (Boise, ID)	Making the decision about joint replacement surgery (hip/knee)	Internet	Information Discusses values Examples of others Coaching in decision steps	Updated May - 2001	Not evaluated	Check the following website for links to the complete inventory of decision aids, some online decision aids and detailed reviews. http://www.ohri.ca/decisionaid and follow links for Patient Decision Aids
Foundation for Informed Medical Decision Making (Hanover, NH)	Treatment choices for knee osteoarthritis	Video and booklet	Information Discusses values Examples of others Coaching decision steps	Reviewed Oct. 2002	Evaluation in progress	
Healthwise Knowledgebase Boise, ID	Deciding whether to get a dual-energy X-ray absorptiometry (DEXA) test to diagnose osteoporosis	Internet	Information Discusses values Examples of others Coaching in decision steps	Updated Sept. 2002	Not evaluated	
Cranney (Ottawa, CAN)	Making choices: Osteoporosis treatment options	Audio-guided booklet	Information Discusses values Exercise to weigh the pros and cons Examples of others Coaching in decision steps	Updated 2003	Pilot tested and randomised trial in progress	

without treatment, evidence-based self-care recommendations, and options for treating the condition. Practitioners can individualise the options by highlighting those that are most suitable for the individual patient to consider.

Section II: Decision Aid The second section provides specific information about the options and guides patients in assessing their decision support needs. It is designed to summarise the decision and process in preparation for counselling with the practitioners.

1. Identifying the decision, timing, and stage in decision making.
2. Summarising the specific option(s) being considered with pros and cons, and when available probabilities of outcomes.

   The option is classified using the Chalmers criteria. A values clarification exercise is included for patients to begin to focus on which outcomes are most important to them. Patients are invited to add additional pros and cons before rating the importance they attach to each using a "one to five" star rating system. As part of this step, patients are asked for their overall leaning for or against the option.
3. Communicating the patient's preferred role in decision making.
4. Assessing current decision making needs using the Decisional Conflict Scale.

   This Decisional Conflict Scale (see Appendix: Decision Aid on p 57), was developed to determine whether a patient is experiencing decisional conflict about the decision and to identify some of the key determinants contributing to decisional conflict (for example, feeling uninformed, unclear about values, unsupported in decision making).[40] Decisional conflict is a state of uncertainty about the course of action to take and is frequently characterised by difficulty

Box 4.1 CREDIBLE Cochrane criteria for evaluating the quality of patient decision aids[52]

C – Competently developed
Were the credentials of developers included in the decision aid?
Was the development process published or easily accessible?

R – Recently updated
Was the decision aid published or updated within the past 5 years?
Was an update policy or statement included or known?

E – Evidence-based
Is there a description of a link to an evidence review group or the process used to identify and appraise evidence?
Are scientific references to trials or systematic reviews used to support statements describing benefits/harms of treatment/screening?
Is there a description of the level of uncertainty regarding evidence?

DI – Devoid of conflicts of interest
Was sponsorship free from perceived conflict of interest?

BL – BaLanced presentation of options, benefits, and harms
Were all options presented (including, if appropriate watchful waiting)?
Are potential harms as well as potential benefits presented?
Does data regarding user responses indicate at least two-thirds of users find it balanced?

E – Efficacious at improving decision making
Did the evaluations show that the decision aid improved knowledge of options?
Did the evaluations show that the decision aid is acceptable to the users?
Did evaluations show other benefits?
Did evaluations show it was free from adverse effects?
Did the evaluation include a randomised controlled trial design?

in making a decision, vacillation between choices, procrastination, being preoccupied with the decision, and having signs and symptoms of distress or tension.

The Decisional Conflict Scale has good reliability and validity in a variety of clinical settings.[40–46] The scale can be used to assess baseline needs and to monitor progress following interventions such as decision aids. Greater decisional conflict occurs in those who (a) delay decisions compared to those who implement and stick with decisions; (b) score lower on knowledge tests; (c) are in the early phases of decision making compared to later phases; or (d) have not yet received decision support compared to those who have.[42–43,45–50] Those who have unresolved decisional conflict following counselling will be more likely to have downstream problems of failure to stick with chosen option, regret, and dissatisfaction, highlighting the need to resolve these issues at the time of decision making.

5. Planning next steps for taking action.
6. Encouraging patient to share the completed decision aid with their doctor to communicate knowledge and values associated with a health-related decision "at a glance". Alternatively, the guide can be completed together with the practitioner to structure the process of decision making. In addition, it provides a generic process that can be applied to future health-related decisions.

A similar guide is being used in nurse call centres and patient information services as part of the process of care. However, referrals to these types of services are intended to complement and streamline the decision making process rather than replace discussion with the patient's physician. Most patients have made it clear that individual consultation with their practitioner about options is extremely important.[3]

What are the advantages and disadvantages of using rheumatology decision aids?

These new rheumatology decision aids have five main advantages.

- They provide a direct link to *evidence-based healthcare practices* with the focus on translating the evidence into patient-friendly information that is suitable for decision making. This link to evidence improves the shelf-life of the tools and the credibility of the information provided. Further it permits a simple tool for communicating the evidence to patients.
- They can be *individualised*. Together with their practitioner, patients can discuss risk-based information, determine relevant options for consideration, and share their values associated with those options.
- The two-section approach permits *easy updating* of the individual sections and information provided.
- The explicit *values clarification* ensures that patients and their healthcare providers consider their values associated with the decision and facilitates sharing of these values.
- The guidance in steps for making any health-related decision may enhance the transferability of skills to subsequent decisions.

However, there are some limitations to consider. First, the expanded library of decision aids needs to be evaluated. Second, there is no information on how others have made similar decisions. This limitation can be addressed by referring patients to examples of others in existing decision aids found in the inventory and/or practitioners sharing their experiences with other patients or arranging for contact with other patients within the medical practice, support groups, or rheumatology volunteer organisations.

Another limitation is that these rheumatology decision aids do not address behaviour change following decision-making. Therefore, motivational and tailored interviewing or other techniques focused specifically on behaviour modification may need to be added for implementation of decisions.

Finally, the challenge of imbedding patient decision aids as part of the process of care is a limitation that is addressed in the next section.

How do clinicians integrate decision aids into their practice?

Practitioners are essential for clarifying the decision, identifying patients in decisional conflict or requiring decision support, referring patients to the appropriate resources including decision aids as part of the process of care, and following up on patients' responses in the decision aids to facilitate progress in decision making. Patients prefer face-to-face contact with a practitioner to individualise the information and guide them in decision making.[3,51] Patient decision aids are designed to enhance this interaction rather than replace it.

To use decision aids in practice, the following steps can be followed by your team:

1. **Clarify the decision** including specific options the patient needs to consider.
2. **Refer the patient to the decision aid.** Endorsement of patient information from one's personal practitioner is highly valued by patients.[3] Direct patients to the book website (http://www.evidbasedrheum.com or http://www.arthritis.ca) to access a decision aid or provide them with photocopies of the two sections of the rheumatology decision aids:
   - condition-specific introductory page
   - option specific decision aid
3. **Explain how the decision aid is used in your practice.** Instruct the patient to review the information and complete the decision aid in preparation for a follow up discussion.
4. **Refer to the decision aid at follow up discussion.** It is important that the practitioner acknowledges patients' responses to their decision aid. Use the decision aid as a communication tool to focus the patient–practitioner dialogue. At a glance, you can quickly learn how your patients see the decision. You can:
   - clarify their understanding of the benefits and harms,
   - acknowledge their values as revealed by the patient's rating of importance on the balance scale,
   - answer their questions, and
   - facilitate decision making according to the patient's preference for decision participation and leaning toward options. Knowing a patient's preference for participation and leaning can assist you to judge how quickly you can move from facilitating decision making to follow up planning.

These steps can be completed by the individual practitioner or shared among team members. When shared within a clinical team, it is better to determine who on the team will be responsible for each part of the process. In the absence of staff to help with this process, referral to call centres staffed by nurses or patient information services may be an option to prepare patients for a dialogue. This decision aid can also be used by patients when discussing their options and preferences with important others such as a spouse, family member, or friend.

Case presentation Part IV: Mrs C

Mrs C completed the decision aid while the rheumatologist saw other patients. The rheumatologist then reviewed with Mrs C her completed Osteoporosis alendronate specific Decision Aid (see Appendix: Decision Aid on p 57), acknowledging the importance she placed on preventing fractures and her concerns about the effects of taking alendronate. Mrs C's questions were answered.

Together Mrs C and her rheumatologist determined that alendronate was the "best" treatment option for her. Mrs C was motivated to take it and did not anticipate any barriers to taking it along with the calcium and vitamin D.

Evaluating the new rheumatology decision aids

Formal evaluations of these new decision aids are under way, including effective models for imbedding decision support as part of the process of care. Practitioners can evaluate their usefulness in practice by noting whether: patients are better prepared to discuss options; the need to repeat factual information is reduced; and ascertainment of patients' values is improved. Practitioners can also note whether, following counselling, patients resolve their decisional conflict (for example, by repeating the Decisional Conflict Scale) and progress through the stages of decision making. If the practice is linked to a larger patient information system, the effects of introducing decision aids on renewal of prescriptions, satisfaction with counselling, health outcomes, and use of health services can also be monitored.

Conclusions

Rheumatology patients are likely to experience some difficulty in making health-related decisions. Systematic reviews do not usually contain patient summaries adequate for patient participation in making preference-sensitive decisions or necessary for adaptation into decision aids. The rheumatology decision aids, found at the end of some chapters and on the free access book website http://www.evidbasedrheum.com as well as the http://www.arthritis.ca website, have the potential to improve the quality of patient decision making, facilitate the integration of patient values into evidence-based medical practice, and enhance the practitioner– patient interaction. A quality decision is informed, based on values, implemented, and results in satisfaction with the process of decision making. The challenge is developing best practices for implementing decision aids as part of the process of care.

References

1 Sackett DL, Straus SE, Richardson WS, Rosenberg W, Haynes RB. *Evidence-based medicine. How to practice and teach EBM, 2nd edn.* Edinburgh: Churchill Livingstone, 2000.

2 Gafni A, Charles C, Whelan T. The physician–patient encounter: the physician as a perfect agent for the patient versus the informed treatment decision-making model. *Soc Sci Med* 1998;**47**(3):347–54.

3 O'Connor AM, Drake ER, Wells GA, Tugwell P, Laupacis A, Elmslie T. A survey of the decision-making needs of Canadians faced with complex health decisions. *Health Expectations* 2003;**6**:97–101.

4 Martin S. "Shared responsibility" becoming the new medical buzz phrase. *CMAJ* 2002;**167**(3):295.

5 Chalmers I, *Clinical Evidence*, Volume 2, BMJ Publications, 1999. [http://www.clinicalevidence.com/lpBinCE/lpext.dll?f=templates&fn=main-h.htm&2·0]

6 Harris RP, Helfand M, Woolf SH *et al.* Current methods of the US preventive services Task Force: a review of the process. *Am J Prevent Med* 2001;**20**: (3 suppl) 21–35.

7 Rutter D, Quine L *et al.* Social cognition models and changing health behaviours. In: Rutter D, Quine L, eds. *Changing health behaviour. Intervention and research with social cognition models.* Buckingham: Open University Press, 2002:1–27.

8 Vermeire E, Hearnshaw H, ValRoyen P, Denekens J. Patient adherence to treatment: three decades of research. A comprehensive review. *J Clin Pharm Ther* 2001;**26**(5): 331–42.

9 Orbell S, Sheeran P. Changing health behaviours: the role of implementation intentions. In: Rutter D, Quine L,

eds. *Changing health behaviour. Intervention and research with social cognition models.* Buckingham: Open University Press, 2002:123–37.

10 Mead N, Bower P. Patient-centredness: a conceptual framework and review of the empirical literature. *Soc Sci Med* 2000;**51**(7):1087–110.

11 Stewart M. Towards a global definition of patient centred care. *BMJ* 2001;**322**(7284):444–5.

12 Weston WW, Brown JB, Stewart MA. Patient-centred interviewing Part I: Understanding patients' experiences. *Can Fam Phys* 1989;**35**(Jan):147–51.

13 Brown JB, Weston WW, Stewart MA. Patient-centred interviewing Part II: Finding common ground. *Can Fam Phys* 1989;**35**(January):153–57.

14 Lester G, Smith S, Listening and talking to patients. A remedy for malpractice suits? *West J Med* 1993;**158**: 268–72.

15 O'Connor AM, Stacey D, Entwistle V *et al. Decision aids for people facing health treatment or screening decisions* (Cochrane Review). In: Cochrane Collaboration. *Cochrane Library.* Issue 3. Oxford: Update Software, 2003.

16 O'Connor A. Using patient decision aids to promote evidence-based decision making. *Am Coll Phys Evidence-Based Med* 2001;**6**(4):101–2.

17 Coulter A, Entwistle V, Gilbert D. Sharing decisions with patients: Is the information good enough? *BMJ* 1999;**318**:318–22.

18 Charles C, Gafni A, Whelan T. Decision-making in the physician–patient encounter: Revisiting the shared treatment decision–making model. *Soc Sci Med* 1999;**49**:651–61.

19 Entwistle VA, Sheldon TA, Sowden A, Watt IS. Evidence-informed patient choice. Practical issues of involving patients in decisions about healthcare technologies. *Int J Technol Assess Hlth Care* 1998;**14**(2):212–25.

20 Hersey J, Matheson J, Lohr, K at the Research Triangle Institute. *Consumer health informatics and patient decision-making.* (AHCPR Pub. No. 98-N001). Rockville, MD: Agency for Health Care Policy and Research, 1997.

21 Llewellyn-Thomas H. Presidential Address. *Med Decision Making* 1995;**15**(2):101–6.

22 Mulley A. Outcomes research: implications for policy and practice. In: Smith R, Delamother T eds. *Outcomes in clinical practice.* London: BMJ Books, 1995.

23 O'Connor AM, Tugwell P, Wells GA *et al.* A decision aid for women considering hormone therapy after menopause: Decision support framework and evaluation. *Patient Educ Counselling* 1998;**33**(3);267–79.

24 Rothert M, Talarcyzk GJ. Patient compliance and the decision making process of clinicians and patients. *J Compliance Health Care* 1987;**2**,55–71.

25 Fischhoff B. Clinical decision analysis. *Operations Res* 1980;**28**(1):28–43.

26 Keeney RL. Decision analysis: An overview. *Operations Res* 1982;**30**:803–38.

27 Tversky A, Kahneman D. The framing of decisions and the psychology of choice. *Science* 1981:**211**:453–8.

28 Ajzen I, Fishbein M. *Understanding attitudes and predicting social behaviour.* Englewood Cliffs: Prentice Hall, 1980.

29 Bandura A. Self-efficacy mechanism in human agency. *Am Psychol* 1982;**37**:122–47.

30 Janis IL, Mann L. *Decision making.* New York: The Free Press, 1977.

31 Norbeck JS. Social support. *Ann Rev Nurs Res* 1988;**6**:85–109.

32 Orem DE. *Nursing: Concepts of practice, 5th edn.* Toronto: Mosby, 1995.

33 Légaré F, O'Connor AM, Graham I *et al.* The effect of decision aids on the agreement between women's and physician's decisional conflict about hormone replacement therapy. *Patient Educ Counseling* 2003; **50**:211–221.

34 Graham ID, Logan J, O'Connor A, Weeks K, *et al.* A qualitative study of physicians' perceptions of three decision aids. *Patient Educ Counseling* 2003;**2055**:1–5.

35 Freeman AC, Sweeney K. Why general practitioners do not implement evidence: qualitative study. *BMJ* 2001;**323**:1100–4.

36 Deyo RA. A key medical decision maker: the patient. *BMJ* 2001;**323**(7311):466–7.

37 Holmes-Rovner M, Llewellyn-Thomas H, Entwistle V *et al.* Patient choice modules for summaries of clinical effectiveness: A proposal. *BMJ* 2001;**322**:664–7.

38 O'Connor AM, Jacobsen MJ, Stacey D. An evidence-based approach to managing women's decisional conflict. *JOGNN* 2002;**31**(5):570–81.

39 See website: http://www.dipex.org/EXEC

40 O'Connor AM. Validation of a decisional conflict scale. *Med Decision Making* 1995;**15**(1):25–30.

41 Bunn H, O'Connor AM. Validation of client decision making instruments in the context of psychiatry. *Canad J Nursing Res* 1996;**28**(3):13–27.

42 Drake E, Engler-Todd L, O'Connor AM, Surh L, Hunter A. Development and evaluation of a decision aid about prenatal testing for women of advanced maternal age. *J Genet Counseling* 1999;**8**(4):217–33.

43 Fiset V, O'Connor AM, Evans WK, Graham I, DeGrasse C, Logan J. The development and evaluation of a decision aid for patients with stage IV non-small cell lung cancer. *Health Expectations* 2000;**3**(2):125–36.

44 O'Connor A, Jacobsen MJ, Elmslie T *et al.* Simple versus complex patient decision aids: Is more necessarily better? *Med Decision Making* 2000;**20**(4):496(Abstract).

45 O'Connor AM, Tugwell P, Wells G *et al.* Randomised trial of a portable, self-administered decision aid for post-menopausal women considering long-term preventive hormone therapy. *Med Decision Making* 1998;**18**(3): 295–303.

46 Cranney A, Jacobsen MJ, O'Connor AM, Tugwell P, Adachi JD. A decision aid presenting multiple therapeutic options for women with osteoporosis: Development and evaluation. *Med Decision Making* 2001;**21**(6):547 (Abstract).

47 Stacey D, O'Connor A, DeGrasse C, Verma S. Development and evaluation of a breast cancer prevention decision aid for higher risk women. *Health Expectations* 2003;**6**(1):3–18.

48 Grant FC, Laupacis A, O'Connor AM, Rubens F, Robblee J. Evaluation of a decision aid for autologous predonation for patients before open-heart surgery. *CMAJ* 2001;**164**(8):1139–44.

49 Comeau, C. Evaluation of a decision aid for family members considering long-term care options for their relative with dementia. Unpublished Master's thesis, University of Ottawa, Ottawa, Ontario, Canada, 2001.

50 Mitchell SL, Tetroe J, O'Connor AM. A decision aid for long-term tube feeding in cognitively impaired older persons. *J Am Geriatr Soc* 2001;**49**:1–4.

51 Nair K, Dolovich L, Cassels A *et al.* What patients want to know about their medications. Focus group study of patient and clinician perspectives. *Can Fam Physician* 2002;**48**:104–10.

52 Stacey D, O'Connor AM, Rovner D *et al.* Cochrane Inventory and evaluation of patient decision aids. *Med Decision Making* 2001;**21**(6):527 (Abstract).

53 Brown JP, Josse RG. 2002 clinical practice guidelines for the diagnosis and management of osteoporosis in Canada. *CMAJ* 2002;**167**:S1–S34.

Evidence-based Osteoporosis Decision Aid for Mrs C

Information about osteoporosis and treatment

What is osteoporosis?

Osteoporosis is a condition of weak brittle bones that break easily. The most common breaks or fractures are in the spine, hip or wrist and these may occur without a fall. Osteoporosis is detected using a bone density test that measures the amount of bone loss. A result that is at least 2·5 "standard deviations" below normal confirms the diagnosis. This means people have lost at least 25 per cent of their bone mass or density.

Hip fractures can cause severe disability or death.

- Among 100 women with normal bone density, about **15** may break a hip in their lifetime.
- Among 100 women with low bone density, about **35 to 75** may break a hip in their lifetime.

This number depends on *amount of bone loss, age*, and other risk factors such as:

- *Major bone related risks:* previous broken bones since age 50 (not from trauma); family history of fracture (e.g. mother who broke a hip, wrist, spine)
- *Major fall related risks:* poor health; unable to rise from a chair without help; use of sleeping pills.

Spine fractures are more common, disabling, and painful. They can cause stooped posture and loss of height of up to 6 inches.

To find out your personal risk of broken bones, ask your doctor.

What can I do on my own to manage my disease?

✓ Calcium and Vitamin D

✓ Regular impact exercises (e.g. walking)

What treatments are used for osteoporosis?

Three kinds of treatment may be used alone or together. The common (generic) names of treatment are shown below.

1. Bone specific drugs
   - Alendronate
   - Calcitonin
   - Etidronate
   - Risedronate
2. Hormones that affect bones and other organs
   - Parathyroid hormone
   - Raloxifene
   - Hormone replacement therapy (oestrogen and progestin)
3. Other
   - Hip protector pads

What about other treatments I have heard about?

There is not enough evidence about the effects of some treatments. Other treatments do not work or may not work to stop all types of fractures. For example:

- Calcitonin for non-spinal fractures
- Etidronate for non-spinal fractures
- Raloxifene for non-spinal fractures

What are my choices? How can I decide?

Treatment for your disease will depend on your condition. You need to know the good points (pros) and bad points (cons) about each treatment before you can decide.

Osteoporosis decision aid

Should I take alendronate?

This guide can help you make decisions about the treatment your doctor is asking you to consider.

It will help you to:

1. Clarify what you need to decide.
2. Consider the pros and cons of different choices.
3. Decide what role you want to have in choosing your treatment.
4. Identify what you need to help you make the decision.
5. Plan the next steps.
6. Share your thinking with your doctor.

Step 1: Mrs C clarifies what she needs to decide

What is the decision?

Should I take alendronate to slow bone loss or prevent breaks?

Alendronate may be taken as a pill daily or once a week.

When does this decision have to be made? Check ✓ one

☐ within days ☑ within weeks ☐ within months

How far along are you with this decision? Check ✓ one

☐ I have not thought about it yet

☑ I am considering the choices

☐ I am close to making a choice

☐ I have already made a choice

Step 2: Mrs C considers the pros and cons of different choices

What does the research show?

Alendronate is classified as: Beneficial

There is 'Platinum' level evidence from 11 studies of 12 855 women after menopause that tested alendronate and lasted up to 4 years. The women had osteoporosis (low bone density) or normal to near normal bone density. These studies found pros and cons that are listed in the chart below.

What do I think of the pros and cons of alendronate?

1. Review the common pros and cons that are shown below.
2. Add any other pros and cons that are important to you.
3. Show how important each pro and con is to you by circling from one (*) star if it is a little important to you, to up to five (*****) stars, if it is very important to you.

PROS AND CONS OF ALENDRONATE TREATMENT

PROS (number of people affected)	How important is it to you?	CONS (number of people affected)	How important is it to you?
Fewer broken bones in the spine 5 less women out of 100 have breaks in their spine over a lifetime with alendronate	(* * * *) *	**Adverse effects: heartburn stomach irritation**	(*) * * * *
Fewer broken bones in the hip or wrist 21 less women out of 100 with osteoporosis have breaks in their hip or wrist over a lifetime	(* * * *) *	**Increases chance of developing ulcers in the oesophagus or gullet**	(* *) * * *
Increases bone density	(* *) * * *	**Must be taken in morning 1 hour before eating and sit or stand after taking the pill**	(*) * * * *
Flexible dosing May be taken once a week	(*) * * * *	**Personal cost of medicine**	(*) * * * *
Other pros: *I will be doing something about my osteoporosis*	(* *) * * *	**Other cons:** *I may forget to take the medicine*	(* *) * * *

Mrs C checks what she thinks about alendronate:

☑ Willing to consider this treatment — Pros are more important to me than the cons

☐ Unsure

☐ Not willing to consider this treatment — Cons are more important to me than the pros

Step 3: Mrs C chooses what role she wants to have in choosing her treatment

☐ I prefer to decide on my own after listening to the opinions of others

☑ I prefer to share the decision with: My Rheumatologist

☐ I prefer someone else to decide for me, namely: ________________

Step 4. Mrs C identifies what she needs to help her make the decision

		Yes	No	Unsure
What I Know	Do you know enough about your condition to make a choice?	☑	☐	☐
	Do you know which options are available to you?	☑	☐	☐
	Do you know the good points (pros) of each option?	☑	☐	☐
	Do you know the bad points (cons) of each option?	☑	☐	☐
What's important	Are you clear about which **pros** are most *important to you?*	☑	☐	☐
	Are you clear about which **cons** are most *important to you?*	☑	☐	☐
How others help	Do you have enough support from others to make a choice?	☑	☐	☐
	Are you choosing without pressure from others?	☑	☐	☐
	Do you have enough advice to make a choice?	☐	☑	☐
How sure I feel	Are you clear about the best choice for you?	☐	☑	☐
	Do you feel sure about what to choose?	☐	☑	☐

If you answered No or Unsure to many of these questions, you should talk to your doctor.

Step 5: Mrs C plans the next steps

Mrs C decided to talk to her rheumatologist and to someone who has taken alendronate. She also wants to find out about tapering hormone therapy if she decides to take alendronate.

Step 6: Mrs C shares this information with her doctor

Part 2: Finding, evaluating, and applying the evidence of rheumatological disorders

5
Gout

Naomi Schlesinger Ralph Schumacher, Ottawa Methods Group

Introduction

Gout is a condition in which uric acid, a waste product that occurs naturally within the body, rises above normal levels. Rather than being flushed by the kidneys and through the urine, as it normally is, it forms crystals and deposits in the joints. These deposits give rise to inflammation of the joints, causing pain, swelling, redness, and tenderness. Most typically the joint affected is that of the big toe, but gout can also affect the ankle, knee, foot, hand, wrist, and elbow. Monosodium urate (MSU) crystals may also form deposits in other areas, such as under the skin or in other soft tissues, and in the kidney or urinary tract.

Methodology and literature search (see Introduction p xiii)

Literature searches were used in order to retrieve all relevant material, for both acute and chronic gout.

In general the approach used was to restrict searches in Medline and Embase to RCTs or randomised longitudinal series, as well as systematic reviews of gout treatment.

Gout – acute

1. exp anti-inflammatory agents, non-steroidal/
2. anti-inflammatory agents, non-steroidal.rn.
3. (nsaid or nsaids).tw.
4. meclofenamic acid.tw,rn.
5. (sulindac or tolmetin or naproxen).tw,rn.
6. (phenylbutazone or ketoprofen).tw,rn.
7. (indomethacin or ibuprofen or curcumin).tw,rn.
8. (flurbiprofen or diclofenac or clofazimine).tw,rn.
9. (aspirin or antipyrine or aminopyrine).tw,rn.
10. nonsteroidal anti-inflammatory.tw.
11. non-steroidal anti-inflammatory.tw.
12. or/1–11
13. (corticoid$ or corticosteroid$).tw.
14. exp Adrenal Cortex Hormones/
15. Glucocorticoid$.tw,sh,rn.
16. or/13–15
17. colchicine.tw,sh.
18. 12 or 16 or 17
19. gout.tw,sh.
20. acute.tw. or acute diseases/
21. 19 and 20
22. 18 and 21
23. tu.fs.
24. dt.fs.
25. random$.tw.
26. (double adj blind$).tw.
27. placebo$.tw.
28. or/23–27
29. 22 and 28
30. meta-analysis.pt,sh.
31. (meta-anal: or metaanal:).tw.
32. (quantitativ: review: or quantitativ: overview:).tw.
33. (methodologic: review: or methodologic: overview:).tw.
34. (systematic: review: or systematic: overview).tw.

35. review.pt. and medline.tw.
36. or/30–35
37. 22 and 36

Gout – chronic

1. allopurinol.tw,sh,rn.
2. (cellidrin or lopurin or milurit$ or zyloprim).tw.
3. 1 or 2
4. probenecid.tw,sh,rn.
5. (benemid or probecid).tw.
6. 4 or 5
7. 3 or 6
8. chronic.tw. or chronic diseases/
9. gout$.tw,sh.
10. 8 and 9
11. 7 and 10
12. tu.fs.
13. dt.fs.
14. random$.tw.
15. (double adj blind$).tw.
16. placebo$.tw.
17. or/12–16
18. 11 and 17
19. meta-analysis.pt,sh.
20. (meta-anal: or metaanal:).tw.
21. (quantitativ: review: or quantitativ overview:).tw.
22. (methodologic: review: or methodologic: overview:).tw.
23. (systematic: review: or systematic: overview).tw.
24. review.pt. and medline.tw.
25. or/19–24
26. 11 and 25

Case presentation

A 55-year-old male has a ten year history of arthritis. He has had multiple attacks of arthritis involving his left wrist, left knee, both ankles, and first toes. He never had a joint aspiration. He was placed on allopurinol 300 mg daily and was given no other medications for his arthritis. He is complaining of a one-day history of right ankle and first toe pain. The pain woke the patient from sleep. There is associated redness and swelling. He has a temperature of 100·7 °F. He denies any trauma and feels okay otherwise. He does not watch his diet and drinks beer on a regular basis, mostly during the weekends, although he was advised to stop drinking. He takes a daily 80 mg aspirin. His father suffers from renal stones. There is no history of gout in the family. Physical examination is remarkable for a swollen, red right ankle and first toe. There is warmth, tenderness, and reduced range of motion of his right ankle and toe. Apparent tophi are appreciated in the helix of his right ear. There is a large tophus in his right olecranon bursa and on two fingers in his left hand. His serum creatinine is 1·2 mg/dl. His uric acid is 7·7 mg/dl.

Question 1

Do we need to aspirate the joint to determine the diagnosis?

During the 1960s, McCarty and Hollander[1] described the currently accepted method for establishing a definite diagnosis of gout: needle aspiration of the acutely inflamed joint or suspected tophus. In some asymptomatic patients, MSU crystals are also detected in joints in which there is no inflammation,[2,3] and this is also felt to confirm the diagnosis. Wallace *et al* published preliminary criteria for the diagnosis of gout in 1977.[4] Thirty-eight rheumatologists in different centres collected data on 706 patients. An analysis of over 200 variables for five groups was performed. Patient groups included: patients with gout, pseudogout, rheumatoid arthritis less than 2 years or more than 2 years, and septic arthritis. Thirteen criteria for the diagnosis of acute gout were described. These include: more than one attack of acute arthritis; maximum inflammation developed within a day;

monarthritis; redness over joints; first metatarsal phalangeal painful/swollen; unilateral first metatarsal phalangeal attack; unilateral tarsal joint attack; tophus; hyperuricaemia; symptomatic swelling within a joint on radiography; subcortical cysts without erosions on radiography; MSU crystals in synovial fluid (SF) during attack; and SF culture negative for organism during attack. One needs 6 out of 13 minor criteria or one major criterion (MSU crystals in SF or tophus) to make the diagnosis of gout by these criteria.

Evidence summary: Bronze

No RCTs of influence on therapy affecting patient outcomes. Although intuitively crystal proven diagnosis is ideal, no studies have compared cost and outcome of attempted crystal proven diagnosis versus clinical diagnosis in determining outcome of care. Quality control of crystal identification has been a concern. While the number of crystals is diagnostically irrelevant, false negative results increase when crystals are scarce;[5] inter-laboratory reliability is very poor.[6–8] When synovial fluid samples containing a variety of crystals are sent to different laboratories every type of error has commonly occurred: false negatives, false positives and misclassification. This leads to the concern that the technique as currently used lacks both sensitivity and specificity.[9]

Case presentation

When the clinical appearance suggests gout then do a SF aspiration on at least one occasion from the acutely involved joint. Aspiration of the joint could also rule out infection, although this seems unlikely in this case.

Question 2

Should the serum uric acid measurement change our thoughts as to what the diagnosis is?

Serum uric acid (SUA) measurement is by definition the method of detecting hyperuricaemia. When reviewing SUA levels, it is important to remember, that despite the fact that SUA levels less than 8 mg/dl are considered to be normal in many hospitals, levels greater than 6·8 mg/dl are above saturation level and may allow deposition of gouty crystals. As many as 39–42% of patients may have normal SUA levels during bouts of acute gouty arthritis,[10,11] so that this is not a reliable method for diagnosis of gout. Serum uric acid levels can also be elevated in other situations such as psoriasis and myeloproliferative disorders or renal insufficiency without gout.

Campion *et al*[12] examined the rates of occurrence of a first episode of gouty arthritis based on 30–147 human years of prospective observation. A cohort of 2046 initially healthy men in the Normative Aging study was followed for 14·9 years with serial examinations of SUA. This study found an incidence rate of gouty arthritis was 4·9% per year for the group with a prior SUA of 9 mg/dl or greater. The incidence rate of gouty arthritis was 0·5% per year for the group with a prior SUA of 7–8·9 mg/dl and 0·1% for SUA levels below 7 mg/dl. Serum uric acid may be normal during attacks, possibly in part due to uricosuric effects of inflammatory cytokines.

Evidence summary: Bronze

No studies have addressed the impact of basing initial therapeutic decisions on serum urate levels.

Case presentation

The serum uric acid would not influence our diagnosis but if it is still elevated it will help direct the increase in the patient's allopurinol dose or be certain about the patient's compliance. SUA level would not change the management of acute gout.

Question 3

Should we check a 24 hour urine collection for uric acid. Is it a valuable test?

This is controversial. A recent review of gout treatment,[13] advocates beginning urate-lowering therapy with allopurinol without measuring the uric acid excretion in most patients, as allopurinol is effective whether the hyperuricaemia is due to overproduction or underexcretion. Others[14,15] find the 24 hour urine collection for uric acid valuable in assessing risk of stones, elucidating underlying factors, and determining which urate-lowering agent to use (allopurinol or a uricosuric drug). If patients are not overexcreting uric acid and have normal renal function then a uricosuric can be used, although there is no specific evidence to support this. There is evidence supporting the fact that uricosuric is less effective in patients with renal insufficiency.

In patients with gout the incidence of uric acid stones was 23% in those with urinary uric acid levels less than 600 mg per day compared with 50% in those with uric acid levels greater than 1000 mg per day.[16] In another study, 11% of patients with uric acid excretion less than 300 mg per day had uric acid stones.[17]

When 24 hour values were first used for clinical purposes, subjects were maintained on a purine-free diet for at least a week, and collections were done on three successive days. The individual 24 hour urine collection for uric acid is such that any single 24 hour value is only a mediocre predictor of what a repeat collection might show.[18] There is great individual variation.[19] Excretion rates vary due to the fact that up to one-third of specimens are not a full 24 hour specimen, uric acid crystals are missed at the bottom of the urine jug, dietary intake of purines in the daily diet fluctuates, and there is variation of fractional intestinal uricolysis.[20]

Evidence summary: Bronze

No RCTs of influence on therapy affecting patient outcomes.

Case presentation

A 24 hour urine for uric acid is not necessary, since it would not influence the treatment at this point.

Question 4

How should we treat this patient whom we suspect has acute gouty arthritis?
What are the non-pharmacological ways of treating gout?

Joint motion may increase inflammation due to experimental gouty arthritis whereas rest of an affected joint may aid in its resolution.[21] Less medication may be needed if the patient can rest the afflicted joint for 1–2 days.[22]

Avoiding factors important in the development of gout among asymptomatic hyperuricaemic patients may reduce gouty attacks. Avoiding diuretics, weight gain, and alcohol consumption may lead to a decrease in gouty arthritis. In a population survey conducted 1991–2 in Kin Hu Kinmen, Taiwan,[23] alcohol consumption, OR 2·31 (1·04, 5·54) and central obesity, OR 2·43 (1·14, 5·29), were found to be independent predictors of gout among hyperuricaemic patients irrespective of serum uric acid (SUA) level. In a prospective study of 233 asymptomatic hyperuricaemics[24] the SUA level, OR 1·84 (1·24, 2·72), alcohol consumption, OR 3·45 (1·58, 7·56), use of diuretics, OR 6·55 (92·98, 14·35), and excessive weight gain OR 1·91 (0·98, 4·01) were independent factors affecting the onset of gout among hyperuricaemic men.

Cold applications may be a useful adjunct to treatment of acute gouty arthritis (Table 5.1).[25] In

Table 5.1 **Number needed to treat for patients undergoing treatment with ice in conjunction with prednisone and colchicine (Schlesinger *et al*, 2002)[25]**

Outcome	Standardised mean difference (95% CI)	% benefiting (95% CI)	NNT (95% CI)
Pain	1·15 (0·16, 2·41)	48% (8, 67)	3 (2, 13)

a very small prospective randomised trial acute gouty arthritis patients treated with topical ice had a greater reduction in pain ($p = 0{\cdot}021$), joint circumference, and synovial fluid volume compared to the control group. There were 10 patients in the ice group and 9 controls. The changes in joint circumference and synovial fluid were not statistically significant.

Heat application to an inflamed joint can exacerbate experimental urate crystal-induced inflammation.[26]

Evidence summary: Silver

One small RCT (less than 10 patients per group) suggests benefit of ice applied to the inflamed joint.

Case presentation

Topical ice treatment can be used at the onset of the acute gouty attack since it reduces severity and length of attack and serves as an analgesic. This treatment may not be needed in this patient since his attack has been caught very early.

Question 5

Should the patient be on a reduced purine or other diet?

A case series of 15 patients found that a strict purine-free diet will reduce serum uric acid by 15–20%.[27] In yet another case series[28] Dessein and colleagues followed a group of 13 gouty men with a diet moderately decreased in calories and carbohydrates, increased in protein, and with replacement of saturated fat with unsaturated fat since this enhances insulin sensitivity and therefore may promote a reduction in SUA. The mean SUA decreased by 18% in gouty patients after 4 months of dietary intervention. This was accompanied by a 67% reduction in monthly gouty attack frequency. They suggest that a lowered insulin resistance results in increased uric acid clearance from the renal tubule, as a result of the stimulation by insulin of tubular ion exchange. Thus these case series found benefit from re-evaluation of the current dietary recommendations for patients with gout, with limitation of carbohydrate intake, an increased proportional intake of protein, and the use of unsaturated fat in all patients.

Evidence summary: Bronze

No RCTs. Two observational studies found that a low purine diet will reduce serum uric and one of these reported a lower frequency of gouty attacks.

Case presentation

For this patient the allopurinol should be optimised. The patient should avoid foods that have very high purine content such as hearts, herring, sardines, and mussels. Once the allopurinol dose is adjusted to the SUA the content of the food that the patient eats is less important. He should be encouraged to reduce his alcohol use as alcohol can increase uric acid production and decrease clearance.

Question 6

Does aspirin treatment affect the SUA?

Aspirin is known to have a bimodal effect on renal handling of uric acid. High doses (>3 g/day are uricosuric, while low doses (1–2 g/day) cause uric acid retention.[29] The role of low dose aspirin in uric acid handling was examined in two recent studies. In a prospective study by Caspi *et al*[30] the effect of mini-dose aspirin (75–325 mg/day) on renal function and uric acid handling in elderly patients was assessed. Within one week minor decreases in renal function and uric acid excretion were seen in elderly patients (without known renal disease, hyperuricaemia or gout) hospitalised for a variety of reasons. These effects were gradually reduced despite administering increasing dosages of aspirin. (Uric acid excretion gradually returned to near baseline levels after doses were increased to 150 mg/day and 325 mg/day.) Concomitant diuretic therapy and low serum albumin seemed to increase the susceptibility to these adverse effects. In another study no change in SUA or in 24 hour urinary excretion of uric acid was seen when 325 mg of daily aspirin was administered to patients with gouty arthritis taking a stable dose of probenecid.[31]

Evidence summary: Bronze

Case series found mixed results, but no major concerns.

Case presentation

The effects of low dose aspirin, if they occur, should be considered, but the use of aspirin should not be discouraged if it is needed for other medical reasons. In this patient it would be fine to continue low dose aspirin, but important to ensure that he has adequate reason to be taking it.

Question 7

What pharmacological treatment should we give this patient for his acute gouty attack?

Colchicine

Colchicine is effective in the treatment of acute gout but has a high frequency of gastrointestinal adverse effects.

A review by Ben-Chetrit and Levy[32] found that only one placebo-controlled trial of colchicine treatment in acute gout was ever done and that all other data reported were accumulated by review rather than by prospective experimentation. Ahern *et al*[33] studied 43 patients (40 men, 3 women); 22 patients were put on colchicine 1 mg then 0·5 mg every 2 hours until complete response or toxicity. Twenty-one patients were in the placebo group. No NSAIDs were used during the study. All had crystals in the synovial fluid. In this placebo-controlled study, two-thirds of the colchicine treated patients improved after 48 hours but only one-third of the patients receiving placebo demonstrated similar improvement (Table 5.2). The colchicine-treated patients responded earlier. Colchicine was more effective when used within 24 hours of an acute attack. In all patients taking colchicine, diarrhoea and/or vomiting occurred at a median time of 24 hours (range 12–36 hours) or after a mean dose of 6·7 mg of colchicine after oral administration and before full clinical improvement[33] (Table 5.3). Gastrointestinal adverse effects are not uncommon in patients either initiating or on long term colchicine therapy. This narrow benefit to toxicity ratio has limited the use of colchicine. Colchicine has the smallest benefit to toxicity ratio of the drugs that are used in the management of gout.[34]

Evidence summary: Silver

One RCT found benefit from colchicines but a very high frequency of adverse effects.

Table 5.2 Number needed to treat for patients receiving oral colchicine (Ahern *et al*, 1987)[33]

Outcome	Improved with placebo	Improved with colchicine	Relative risk of improvement with colchicine (95% CI)	Absolute benefit increase (95% CI)	NNT (95% CI)
Improved in 48 hours (50% decrease in baseline measures)	7/21 (33%)	15/22 (68%)	2·05 (1·05,3·99)	35% (5, 58)	3 (2, 20)

Table 5.3 Number needed to harm for patients receiving oral colchicine (Ahern *et al*, 1987)[33]

Outcome	Placebo	Colchicine	Relative risk adverse effect colchicine (95% CI)	Absolute Risk increase	NNH (95% CI)
Diarrhoea and/or vomiting	0/21 (0%) (however 5 did experience nausea)	22/22 (100%)	Not calculated	100% (79, 100)	1 (1, 1)

Table 5.4 Treatment of acute gouty arthritis with placebo alone

Reference	Study	No.	Days of treatment/ regimen	Qualifiers/diagnosis	Outcomes
Bellamy[35]	Placebo only	11	7 days no treatment	Acute podagra (1–5 days) with prior attacks and hyperuricaemia. No treatment	Day 4: 2/11 withdrew due to severe persistent pain By day 5: all remaining patients showed some improvement in pain By day 7: all remaining patients showed some improvement in swelling. Tenderness improved in 7/9 patients. Resolution of pain occurred in only 3/9 patients

NSAIDs

There are no RCTs directly comparing colchicines to NSAIDs (Table 5.4). A number of head to head studies show equivalence between many NSAIDs (Table 5.5).

Despite this lack of rigorous evidence and the unlikeliness that more placebo controlled trials will be done, two recent reviews of gout treatment written by American physicians state that NSAIDs are the preferred treatment for acute gouty arthritis.[14,15] Harris *et al* suggest that determination of therapeutic success is not which NSAID is chosen but rather how soon NSAID therapy is initiated.[14]

As can be seen in the table below, many clinicians use NSAIDS alone or in combination with colchicine; however, there is no evidence to support combined use (Table 5.6).

Evidence summary: Silver

No RCT of NSAIDs with placebo or colchicine-control. The majority of seven head-to-head RCTs showed faster recovery than a previous series of untreated patients.

Table 5.5 Treatment of acute gouty arthritis with NSAIDs

Reference	Study	No.	Days of treatment/ regimen	Qualifiers/ diagnosis	Outcomes
Smythe[36]	Double blind, indomethacin (I) *v* phenylbutazone (P)	28 (31 attacks)	*n* = 16 I: 200 mg 1st 24 hr, followed by 150 mg per 24 hr, then 100 mg per 24 hr. *n* = 15 P: 800 mg 1st 24 hr, followed by 600 mg per 24 hr then 400 mg per 24 hr	Generally accepted clinical grounds	Number of days (range) to resolution for clinical outcomes: Complete subjective relief: P = 5 (2–17); I = 5 (2–13) Rest pain: P = 4 (1–11); I = 3(1–6) Tenderness: P = 6 (2–17); I = 4 (1–7) Heat: P = 3 (1–8); I = 2 (1–4) Erythema: P = 3 (1–8); I = 2 (1–4) Swelling: P = 6 (1–17); I = 3 (1–6) Number of recurrences within 14 days: P = 1; I = 3 Toxicity: P = 1 (pitting oedema); I = 1 (drowsiness)
Rousti[37]	Double blind, indomethacin (I) *v* proquazone (P)	18	10 days of P 300 mg TID BID *n* = 9 *v* I:50 mg TID BID *n* = 9	SUA crystals in some *x*-ray films	Improvement appeared in 2–3 days for both groups. Complete remission: P = 6/9; I = 4/9 Good result: P = 1/9; I = 4/9 Slight improvement: P = 1/9; I = 1/9 No response: P = 1; I =1 Significant decrease in SUA values was noted in proquazone group. As well, 2 patients in this group experienced mild GI symptoms
Altman[38]	Double blind ketoprofen (K) *v* indomethacin (I)	59	*n* = 29 100 mg K *v* *n* = 30 I 50 mg TID	MSU crystals or clinical criteria	More than 90% in each group reported pain relief within 1st day of treatment. Discontinuation of treatment due to complete or substantial pain relief by day 5/29: K = 7/29; I = 6/30. Withdrawal due to drug-related GI disorder: K = 3; I = 3

(Continued)

Table 5.5 *(Continued)*

Reference	Study	No.	Days of treatment/ regimen	Qualifiers/ diagnosis	Outcomes
Weiner 1979[39]	Double blind fenoprofen (F) *v* phenylbutazone (P)	30	4 days *n* = 15 F: 3·6 g first day then 3 g qd *n* = 15 P:700 mg first day then 400 mg qd	MSU crystals	Both equally effective. Reduction in pain, heat, swelling, redness Day 4: F = 77%; P = 81%
Shresta[40]	Double blind IM ketorolac (K) *v* indomethacin (I) PO	20	*n* = 10 60 mg K IM and oral placebo *v* *n* = 10 50 mg I TID for 2 days then 50 mg BID for 5 days and IM placebo	Wallace criteria	At 2 hr, mean pain score for K had decreased from 4·5 ± 0·71 to 1·4 ± 1·43. For I decrease from 4·4 ± 0·70 to 1·5 ± 1·18. At 6 hours, some rebound pain was noted with K. Thereafter, K pain scores returned to 2 hour level and did not differ from I
Macagno[41]	Double blind etodolac (E) *v* naproxen (N)	61	7 days *n* = 31 E 300 mg BID v *n* = 30 N 500 mg BID		Significant improvement from baseline in pain, swelling, tenderness, erythema, joint heat, range of motion, and global assessment for both groups at all time points. Day 2 overall improvement: E = 81%; N = 53% Day 7 overall improvement: E = 97%; N = 93%
Schumacher[42]	Double blind etoricoxib (E) *v* indomethacin (I)	150	14 days *n* = 75 E 120 mg *v* *n* = 75 I 50 mg TID	Wallace criteria	Proportion of clinically meaningful responses: 4 hr: I = 25%; E = 35% Day 2: I = 60%; E = 55% Day 5: I = 85%; E = 78% Day 8; I = 93%; E = 95% Drug-related adverse effects: I = 46·7%; E = 22·7%

Case presentation

How the patient has previously been treated and responded should be reviewed. If there is no reason to do otherwise, the patient should be given full dose NSAID and colchicine should be avoided if possible because of its high frequency of adverse effects.

Question 8

Should we give this patient IV colchicine?

Two recent published letters[48,49] support use of intravenous (IV) colchicine for acute gout. On the other hand, inappropriate use of the drug happens not uncommonly and therefore many clinicians have advocated restriction or outright ban of IV colchicine therapy.[50–52] The American

Table 5.6 Survey studies of treatment of acute gouty arthritis

Reference	Country	No. of rheum	Colchicine as primary agent	Colchicine plus NSAIDs	NSAIDs alone
Bellamy[43]	Canada	71	6%		
Stuart[44]	New Zealand	26	12%	25%	Indomethacin used in 73%
Ferraz[45]	Brazil		57%		
Rozenberg[46]	France	750	63%	32%	5%
Schlensinger[47]	USA	100		69%	33%

Association of Poison Control Centers toxic exposure surveillance system recorded 33 colchicine-related deaths from 1985 to 1997.[53]

The role of intravenous (IV) colchicine is also limited by its small benefit to risk ratio. Serious systemic reactions can occur with IV colchicine administration. These include: bone marrow suppression, renal failure, alopecia, disseminated intravascular coagulation, hepatic necrosis, diarrhoea, seizures, and death.[50] Guidelines for the administration of IV colchicine have been published.[50]

Evidence summary: Bronze

Clinical opinions are mixed. There are no RCTs of IV colchicine. Toxicity is a major concern.

Case presentation

It is our opinion that IV colchicine should not be used in acute gout because of its toxicities, with the possible exception of its use in patients who are not able to take anything by mouth.

Question 9

Are steroids useful in the treatment of acute gout?

Other treatments for acute gout need further evaluation. These include intra-articular corticosteroids once infection is excluded; adrenocorticosteroids inpatients in whom NSAIDs are contraindicated, and adrenocorticotropic hormone (ACTH) intramuscularly or subcutaneously.

Intra-articular corticosteroids are currently accepted as beneficial when only one or two joints are actively inflamed.[54] Patients with polyarticular gout who demonstrate suboptimal or delayed response to oral NSAIDs or who have contraindications to usual NSAIDs may also benefit from adjunctive corticosteroid injections into joints with persistent synovitis.[55] In a recent case series,[56] small intra-articular doses of triamcinolone acetonide (10 mg in knees and 8 mg in small joints) were felt to have helped resolve 20 attacks of gout in 19 men. Joints involved were 11 knees, 4 metatarsophalangeal joints, 3 ankles, and 2 wrists. All had MSU crystals identified in the joints. After intra-articular injection of triamcinolone acetonide in 11 joints (55%) the attack had resolved at 24 hours and in 9 joints (45%) at 48 hours. All the attacks were fully resolved at 48 hours.

In a prospective case series using either IV methylprednisolone or oral prednisone corticosteroid treatment for acute gout inpatients who had contraindications to use of NSAIDs, Groff *et al*[57] noted improvement within 12–48 hours. Thirteen consecutive patients with 15 episodes of acute gout were treated with systemic corticosteroids. Sufficient records were available on 12 patients and 13 attacks: mean age 65 years; 7 men and 5 women; 8 of the 12 had MSU proven gout. In 11 of 13 attacks complete resolution of the signs and symptoms occurred within 7 days and within 10 days in the remainder. Patients with more than five involved joints required longer courses of therapy (mean: 17 days). Nine patients received an initial dose of 20–50 mg/day with a tapering dose over a mean time of 10·5 days (4–20 days). Three patients with greater than five joints involved, longer duration of symptoms, and one with multiple myeloma received either IV prednisolone or a prolonged prednisone tapered over a mean of 17 days. Comparison of different dosing regimens has not been done.

Alloway *et al*[58] reported 23 patients presenting within 5 days of onset of an acute gouty attack. They noted that resolution of all symptoms occurred at an average of 8 days for indomethacin (50 mg TID PO) treated patients and 7 days for patients treated with triamcinolone (60 mg IM). Despite the fact that the triamcinolone acetonide patients tended to have a longer duration of symptoms before the onset of therapy and a greater number of joints involved, resolution of all symptoms occurred on average 1 day quicker. However, the difference was not statistically significant.

The exact mechanism of action of ACTH is largely unknown. Ritter *et al*[59] conducted a retrospective review of 33 patients with acute gout (38 episodes) and 5 patients with acute pseudogout (5 episodes) who received ACTH. These patients had multiple medical problems. Eleven patients had a crystal diagnosis. The most commonly documented indications for ACTH were: congestive heart failure (CHF) (n = 18), chronic renal failure (CRF) (n = 20), history of gastrointestinal (GI) bleeding (n = 10), and lack of response to NSAIDs or colchicine (n = 6). Mean age 66 years (43–93). Patients were treated with ACTH IV (n = 27), IM (n = 6) or SC (n = 5). Thirty-four episodes of gout were treated with 40 IU of ACTH q 8 hours and four episodes were treated with 80 IU every 8 hours. Doses were tapered each day according to clinical improvement (decrease in synovitis, improved ROM). The most common regimen (90%) was 40 IU every 8 hours then 40 IU every 12 hours and then 40 IU once a day. Duration of therapy was 1–14 days. Prophylactic colchicine was given in 79% of patients (n = 30) as the ACTH was tapered. A 97% resolution rate was reported (Table 5.7). In some resolution was within the first day. Mean time to complete resolution was 5·5 days. A relapse rate of 11% (n = 4) was noted. The authors concluded that ACTH is effective in patients with multiple medical problems such as CHF, CRF, and GI bleeding.

In a prospective quasi-randomised (patients alternately assigned) study involving 76 patients who presented within 24 hours of onset of an acute gouty attack, Axelrod and Preston[60] compared parental ACTH (a single dose of 40 IU administered intramuscularly) with oral indomethacin 50 mg four times daily with food until pain subsided (Table 5.7). For subsequent attacks patients continued treatment with the assigned study medication and were followed for one year. During each treatment course the patients were treated and observed for 5 hours until released. Patients reported for follow-up 5–7 days after each attack and were assessed for time to pain relief, ability to walk, and occurrence of adverse effects. Diagnosis was confirmed by MSU crystals in all patients. The mean pain interval from administration of the study drug to complete pain relief was 3 ± 1 hour with corticotropin and 24 ± 10 hours with indomethacin ($p < 0{\cdot}0001$). Pain resolved within 4 hours and no adverse effects were noted in 36 patients who received ACTH IM for their gouty attack. They concluded that the patients who received ACTH experienced a quicker onset of pain relief than those who received oral indomethacin. However,

Table 5.7 Treatment of acute gouty arthritis with ACTH

Reference	Study	No.	Days of treatment/ regimen	Qualifiers/ diagnosis	Assessment criteria
Ritter[59]	Retrospective ACTH IM, IV, SC 40 IU *v* 80 IU	33 patients; 38 attacks	1–14 days; IV ($n = 27$), IM ($n = 6$), SC ($n = 5$) 34: 40 IU ACTH q8hr–q12hr-qd; 4: 80 IU ACTH q8hr Prophylactic colchicine in 79% ($n = 30$)	MSU ($n = 11$)	97% had complete resolution. Mean time to resolution: 5·5 days Relapse: $n = 4$ (11%)
Axelrod[60]	Single blind prospective ACTH *v* indomethacin	76	ACTH 40 IU IM *v* indomethacin 50 mg q6hr	MSU in all Within 24 hr of attack No tophi No CRF No probenecid/ allopurinol/ colchicine	Hours to complete pain relief: ACTH = 3 (SD1); indomethacin = 24 (SD 10). % of patient visits in follow up year attributable to relapse: ACTH 5%; indomethacin 7·5%
Seigel[61]	Prospective ACTH *v* triamcinolone	31	ACTH 40 IU IM *v* triamcinolone 60 mg IM	Crystal proven gout of <5 days' duration	Resolution of all symptoms occurred at an average of 8 days for both groups. Fewer repeat injections in triamcinolone group (5/16) *v* (11/15) 2 patients from ACTH arm transferred to acetonide due to rebound arthritis

their studied patients had to present within 24 hours of the onset of an acute gouty attack, could not have tophaceous gout or renal insufficiency, and could not be taking colchicine, allopurinol or probenecid. Their results, therefore, may not be reproducible in a more complicated patient population. In addition their study was not blinded and no adverse effects with ACTH were recorded.

In a small RCT Siegel *et al*[61] compared patients receiving a single dose of 40 IU intramuscular ACTH ($n = 16$) with patients receiving intramuscular 60 mg triamcinolone acetonide ($n = 15$) in acute gout (Table 5.7).

Both groups had similar mean times to complete resolution (7·9 and 7·6 days, respectively). The triamcinolone group required fewer repeat injections compared with the ACTH group. Repeat injection was needed in 5 of 16 patients receiving ACTH but only 11 of 15 receiving triamcinolone and many ACTH patients required a third injection to treat rebound attacks. This could have been related to a lack of equivalent doses between the two medications. Thus, there are no convincing data that such therapy is superior to corticosteroids.

Future studies are needed to directly compare ACTH treatment with other regimens in the management of acute gout.

Evidence summary: Silver

One RCT showed a faster response with ACTH compared with indomethacin.

Case presentation

An NSAID should be used. Corticosteroids and ACTH are often reserved for more severe cases or people with contraindications to colchicine and NSAIDs. We would not use it in this patient unless his attacks have been hard to control or his serum creatinine level rises.

Question 10

How should we treat this patient in the long term?
Should we give colchicine prophylactically and if so, for how long?

Wortmann, as one expert, states that colchicine prevents acute gouty attacks in 85% of patients initiating commencing treatment with urate lowering drugs and should be discontinued after the serum urate has been "controlled" and the patient has not had an acute attack for 1–3 months.[13] The basis for this recommendation is not given. Emmerson[62] recommended continuing colchicine intake for at least a year, again without supporting data. Ben Chetrit and Levy in an update on colchicine[32] recommend a daily prophylactic dose of approximately 1 mg and state the drug is effective in preventing attacks and diminishing their severity. Others[63,64] emphasise the risks of routine colchicine treatment in all patients being treated with urate lowering drugs and state that the actual risk of precipitating an attack of gout is at the most 24%.

The practice of using colchicine as prophylaxis against acute gouty attacks was introduced by Cohen over 50 years ago.[65] In 1961, Yu and Gutman analysed the use of colchicine prophylaxis in gout over a mean period of 5 years in 208 patients. They compared colchicine alone in 119 patients with a combination of colchicine with probenecid in 89 patients. The doses ranged from 0·5 mg to 2 mg a day for a duration of 2 to more than 10 years. Before institution of prophylaxis the course of attacks was classified as severe in 76 (37%) and moderately severe in 24 (11%). Patients with mild or rare attacks were excluded from the study. After prophylaxis the courses were considered severe in 2 (1%), moderately severe in 24 (11%), mild in 72 (35%), and virtually attack-free in 110 (53%) of patients. They conclude that both colchicine alone or in combination with probenecid was effective in preventing acute gout.[66] However, the authors reported the outcome of only 208 of their 614 patients. Patients who were excluded were also prescribed colchicine but their outcomes were not reported. The patients were instructed to abort attacks by immediately taking extra doses of colchicine (2 or 3 mg for 1–2 days). They were instructed not to drink and some were on a low purine diet. In addition, they were all put on uricosuric drugs from the start of the prophylactic colchicine regimen or shortly after. In 1982[67] Yu published a report on the efficacy of colchicine prophylaxis in articular gout; this was a reappraisal after 20 years of the outcome in 540 patients. This further uncontrolled study showed that colchicine diminishes recurrence of gouty attacks. Again many patients were prescribed hypouricemic agents. Li-Yu *et al*,[68] in a study of urate lowering, showed that the frequency of attacks was reduced in the patients given colchicine prophylaxis compared with those who stopped taking colchicine, even among those with urate levels lowered for one year. In 1974, Paulus *et al*[34] published the results of a randomised controlled trial that evaluated prophylactic colchicine therapy in patients treated with probenecid. In this 6 month double blind study of 51 patients with recurrent tophaceous and non-tophaceous gout patients were randomly allocated to receive probenecid 1·5 g/day and colchicine 1·5 mg/day or probenecid

1·5 g/day with placebo. In the event of an acute attack, patients were to record the attack and take additional colchicine, indomethacin, or phenylbutazone until the attack subsided. Only attacks judged as moderate or severe by the investigators were incorporated in the analysis. The authors analysed only the patients (n = 38) who showed a sustained reduction in serum uric acid. They assumed that these were the compliant patients. There were 35 attacks of acute gout during the 94 patient-months of therapy in patients taking placebo–probenecid and 23 attacks during 109 patient-months of therapy in the patients taking colchicine–probenecid. The authors concluded that treatment with 1·5 mg/day of colchicine in divided doses significantly reduced the frequency of attacks of acute gout in patients whose hyperuricaemia was controlled by probenecid.

No randomised controlled trial has examined prescription of colchicine as a single drug therapy for the prophylaxis of acute gouty arthritis. The effectiveness of colchicine prophylaxis as an isolated therapy is still to be confirmed by placebo controlled trials. Another issue is prophylaxis with NSAIDs. There are no comparative studies with colchicines.

Evidence summary: Silver

There is limited evidence in one RCT where colchicine was used in combination with probenecid for a reduction in recurrent gouty attacks in patients with a sustained reduction in serum uric acid.

Case presentation

Prophylactic colchicine should be used when initiating hyparicemic therapy or when increasing the dose of the hypouricaemic agent. This patient should take colchicines as he has persistent tophi and is at risk of acute attacks. This treatment should be continued until his SUA is <6·0 and the tophi have been depleted.

Question 11

When should we start urate lowering drugs?

This is a controversial point. Expert opinion varies; some advocate that only patients who suffer more than four episodes per year should be treated.[63] Importantly, cost-effectiveness of urate lowering therapy has been studied, with the conclusion that therapy is cost-saving in patients who have two or more attacks a year.[69] Patients with tophi should receive urate lowering agents, as they can resolve tophi.

Evidence summary: Bronze

There are no RCTs. Experts recommend that urate lowering drugs should be started after repeated attacks. In this patient allopurinol should be continued.

Question 12

Does the frequency of acute gout increase during the first months of treatment intended to normalise SUA?

It is postulated that a major change in SUA induced by initiating or stopping urate lowering drugs may precipitate an attack or even prolong an attack in progress. Data to support this is limited. Case reports of acute episodes of gout after starting allopurinol were documented as far back as 1964.[70] In a case series, 11 of 45 patients given allopurinol developed an acute gouty attack.[71] Most of these patients developed the attack while on a low purine diet, 1 mg PO of oral colchicine and 2 litres of water a day to induce diuresis. In another case series,[72] of 64 patients taking a variety of uricosuric agents while taking colchicine treatment, 15 developed acute gout. In two, this was severe enough to stop uricosuric treatment.

Evidence summary: Bronze

Only case reports are available.

Question 13

Should we be using uricosuric drugs or xanthine oxidase inhibitors?

The two main classes of drugs used to treat chronic gout are the uricosuric drugs and the xanthine oxidase blockers. In a survey of prescribing practices in Ontario, Canada, 99% of rheumatologists elected to start allopurinol as their urate lowering drug therapy.[43] In another study, 66% of rheumatologists prescribed allopurinol as their initial urate lowering drug[73] while in yet another study 30% of French rheumatologists were reported as never using uricosurics.[74] No studies have evaluated these differences in approach.

In a much needed prospective open study, 86 male patients with chronic gout who fulfilled the 1977 ARA preliminary criteria for the classification of gout,[4] the efficacy of allopurinol and benzbromarone was compared in reducing serum urate.[75] Patients were randomised into two groups. One group received a daily allopurinol dose of 300 mg and the other received a daily benzbromarone dose of 100 mg. Both groups included underexcretors and normal execretors of uric acid. Patients receiving allopurinol showed a mean reduction of serum urate of 2·75 mg/dl while patients receiving 100 mg of benzbromarone had a 5·04 mg/dl reduction in their serum urate. Fifty-three per cent of patients receiving allopurinol and 100% of patients receiving benzbromarone achieved optimal serum urate levels at such doses. Renal function improved and no renal stones were observed among the benzbromarone-treated group. Benzbromarone was found to be effective (including underexcretors of urate) in controlling serum urate levels in doses ranging from 50 to 100 mg per day. Allopurinol was not tested at higher doses, which may be needed in some patients.

In a comparative study (randomisation unclear) comparing allopurinol treatment with uricosuric drug treatment in 183 gouty patients by Weinberger *et al*,[76] patients treated by allopurinol for a prolonged period of time had disappearance of attacks after 4 years of treatment while uricosuric therapy did not cause the same decrease in appearance of attacks. This is compatible with other studies, indicating that allopurinol is more effective in reducing the frequency of arthritis (that is, gouty attacks).[77,78]

In a quasi-randomised (even/odd hospital numbers) prospective study by Scott comparing long term effects of allopurinol with those of uricosuric treatment in uncomplicated gout, it is concluded that there is no clear advantage to the use of allopurinol versus probenecid.[79] In this study, 37 men were allocated to receive either allopurinol (n = 20) or uricosuric drugs (n = 17). Mean follow up was 18·6 months for the allopurinol group and 19·6 months for patients taking uricosuric drugs. It is important to note the doses of allopurinol 300 mg a day (n = 12), 400 mg (n = 6) and 600 mg (n = 2). Dosage was decided dependent on SUA. The goal was a "normal" SUA (6 mg/100ml in men and postmenopausal women and 5 mg/100dl in premenopausal women). Probenecid, on the other hand, was started at 1 g daily and upped to 2 g daily in all patients in the group after 2 weeks in order to achieve an adequate uricosuric response. Five patients on probenecid were changed to sulphinpyrazone 400 mg daily because of adverse effects (flatulence, pruritus, difficulty swallowing or bad taste). All patients received daily colchicine (0·5 mg twice to three times). Colchicine was withdrawn after several months in patients who became free of symptoms. Despite the difference in dosing, the mean serum uric acid was lower in the group receiving allopurinol 4·7 (range: 2·6–5·5) versus the mean SUA in the group receiving uricosuric drugs 5·2 (range: 3·8–7·3). Half of the patients of both groups had no further attacks at the last assessment.

Evidence summary: Silver

Two RCTs found that uricosuric drugs or xanthine oxidase inhibitors both reduce serum uric acid. One RCT showed no difference in frequency of clinical gouty attacks.

Case presentation

In this patient the use of allopurinol in a dose that would achieve a SUA of ≤ 6 mg/dl is an advisable treatment. Therefore, the patient should stick with the allopurinol.

Question 14

How low should the plasma urate be lowered to deplete urate stores and to prevent acute gouty attacks?

Maintaining SUA level at less than 6 mg/dl and not just within the "normal range" has been proposed to help assure resolution of tophi and eventual cessation of acute gouty attacks. Bomalaski *et al*[3] showed that monosodium urate crystals persisted in 58% of asymptomatic knees of patients with non-tophaceous gout despite lowering of SUA to less than 7·1 mg/dl for varying periods. In a prospective (divided according to SUA level but not randomised) study by Li-Yu *et al*,[68] 57 patients were divided into two groups: one that had a SUA >6 mg/dl and one that had SUA successfully lowered to ≤6 mg/dl for at least one year. Knee joint aspirates were performed in 32 patients. Fifty-six per cent of patients who maintained their SUA at less than 6 mg/dl had MSU crystals depleted from their knee joints and seemed to do better. A cohort study found that attacks diminished once allopurinol was started, even before SUA was normal.[78] Longer follow ups on crystal disappearance and tophi depletion are needed.

Evidence summary: Silver

One cohort study found that patients who maintained their SUA at less than 6 mg/dl had MSU crystals depleted from their knee joints and seemed to do better.

Case presentation

In this patient it is advisable to aim for SUA ≤ 5–6mg/dl and measure tophi in order to ensure that there is a decrease.

Question 15

How long should we be treating patients with urate lowering drugs?

Uric acid lowering upon treatment with allopurinol treatment is dose-dependent. Many patients are maintained on a fixed dose of allopurinol, usually 100 mg or 300 mg per day and dose is not adjusted to SUA level. Most believe that patients with chronic gout need SUA concentrations to be kept low to prevent further attacks. There are no studies on this. Allopurinol "holidays" have been studied. Urate levels rise when allopurinol is stopped and tophi and attacks can recur.[80] In a prospective RCT by Bull *et al*,[81] intermittent administration of allopurinol was found to be less effective in controlling gouty attacks than continuous treatment. In the continuously treated group (n = 20) SUA levels were controlled and no further attacks of gout occurred after 2 years (Table 5.8).

In the group treated intermittently (n = 20) SUA levels fell during administration of the drug but rose rapidly afterwards. In 7 of the 20 patients, attacks of gouty arthritis persisted.

Evidence summary: Silver

In one RCT intermittent administration of allopurinol resulted in more frequent gouty attacks than continuous administration.

Case presentation

Continuous treatment in order to maintain SUA ≤ 6 mg/dl would be the appropriate treatment.

Table 5.8 Number needed to treat for patients receiving continuous (300 mg/day) versus intermittent (8 weeks in 12 months) administration of allopurinol (Bull and Scott, 1989)[81]

Outcome	Intermittent allopurinol	Continuous allopurinol	Relative risk or improvement allopurinol (95% CI)	ARR	NNT (95% CI)
Patients with gouty attacks after 2 years	7/20 (35%)	0/20 (0%)	Unable to calculate	35% (11, 57)	3 (2, 9)

Question 16
When do we use surgical treatment?

Surgical treatment may be required for refractory cases of tophaceous gout. A recent case report[82] described a patient with chronic tophaceous gout who presented with a progressively enlarging painful mass on the plantar aspect of the first metatarsophalangeal joint measuring 4·8 cm by 2·5 cm, which caused difficulty wearing shoes and walking. The patient was allergic to allopurinol and failed a course of probenecid treatment. The patient underwent extirpation of a tophaceous mass and is now able to walk without discomfort. Large tophi have been excised for mechanical and cosmetic reasons but healing can be difficult if overlying skin is compromised. It is proposed that removal of tophi can decrease the urate load that has to be removed by drugs.

Evidence summary: Bronze

A case report found benefit from surgical removal of tophaceous masses.

Case presentation

Medical management would be advised in this patient before moving on to surgical intervention.

References

1 McCarty DJ, Hollander JL. Identification of urate crystals in gouty synovial fluid. *Ann Intern Med* 1961:**54**:452–602.

2 Weinberger A. Schumacher HR, Agudelo CA. Urate crystals in asymptomatic metatarsophalangeal joints. *Ann Intern Med* 1979;**92**:56–7.

3 Bomalaski JS, Lluberas G, Schumacher HR, Jr. Monosodium urate crystals in the knee joints of patients with asymptomatic nontophaceous gout. *Arthritis Rheum* 1986;**29**:1480–4.

4 Wallace SL, Robinson H, Masi AT, Decker JL, McCarty DJ, Yu TF. Preliminary criteria for the classification of the acute arthritis of primary gout. *Arthritis Rheum* 1977;**20**:895–900.

5 Von Essen R, Holtta AMH, Pikkarainen R. Quality control of synovial fluid crystal identification. *Ann Rheum Dis* 1998;**57**:107–9.

6 Hasselbacher P. Variation in synovial fluid analyses by hospital laboratories. *Arthritis Rheum* 1987;**30**:637–42.

7 Schumacher HR, Sieck MS, Rothfuss C, Clayburne GM, Baumgarten DF, Mochan BS. Reproducibility of synovial fluid analyses; a study among four laboratories. *Arthritis Rheum* 1986;**29**:770–4.

8 McGill NW, York H. Reproducibility of synovial fluid examination for crystals. *Aust NZ J Med* 1991;**34**:710–13.

9 Dieppe P, Swan A. Identification of crystals in synovial fluid. *Ann Rheum Dis* 1999;**58**:261–3.

10 Schlesinger N, Baker DG, Schumacher HR, Jr. Serum uric acid during bouts of acute gouty arthritis. *J Rheum* 1997;**24**(11):2265–6.

11 Logan JA, Morrison E, McGill PE. Serum uric acid in acute gout. *Ann Rheum Dis* 1997;**56**:696–7.

12 Campion EW, Glynn RJ, DeLabry LO. Asymtomatic hyperuricemia. Risks and consequences in the Normative Aging study. *Am J Med*;1986;**82**:421–6.

13 Wortmann RL. Effective treatment of gout: An analogy. *Am J Med* 1998;**105**(6):513–14.

14 Harris MD, Siegel LB, Alloway JA. Gout and hyperuricemia. *Am Fam Physician* 1999;**59**(4):925–34.

15 McDonald E, Marino C. Stopping progression to tophaceous gout. When and how to use urate-lowering therapy. *Postgrad Med* 1998;**104**(6):117–27.

16 Yu TF, Gutman AB. Uric acid nephrolithiasis in gout: predisposing factors. *Ann Intern Med* 1967;**67**:1133.

17 Hall AP, Barry PE, Dawber TR, McNamara PM. Epidemiology of gout and hyperuricemia. A long-term population study. *Am J Med* 1967;**42**:27.

18 Pak CYC, Peterson R, Poindexter JR. Adequacy of a single stone risk analysis in the medical evaluation of urolithasis. *J Urol* 2001;**165**:378–81.

19 Ricos C, Jimenez CV, Hernandez A *et al.* Biological variation in urine samples used for analyte measurements. *Clin Chem* 1994;**40**:472–7.

20 Simkin PA. When, why, and how should we quantify the excretion rate of urinary uric acid. *J Rheumatol* 2001;**281**:207–10.

21 Agudelo CA, Schumacher, HR Jr, Phelps P. Effect of exercise on urate crystal-induced inflammation in canine joints. *Arthritis Rheum* 1972;**15**:609–16.

22 Schumacher, HR Jr. Crystal induced arthritis: An overview. *Am J Med* 1996;**100**(Suppl 2A):46–52.

23 Lin KC, Lin HY, Chou P Community based epidemiological study on hyperuricemia and gout in Kin-Hu, Kimmen. *J Rheumatol* 2000;**27**:1045–50.

24 Lin KC, Lin HY, Chou P. The interaction between SUA level and other risk factors on the development of gout among asymptomatic hyperuricemic men in a prospective study. *J Rheumatol* 2000;**27**:1501–23.

25 Schlesinger N, Baker DG, Beutler AM, Hoffman BI, Schumacher HR, Jr. Local ice therapy during bouts of acute gouty arthritis. *J Rheumatol* 2002;**29**:331–4.

26 Dorwart BB, Hansell JR, Schumacher HR, Jr. Effects of cold and heat on urate-induced synovitis in dog. *Arthritis Rheum* 1974;**17**:563–71.

27 Nicholas A, Scott JT. Effect of weight loss on plasma and urinary levels of uric acid. *Lancet* 1972;**2**:1223–4.

28 Dessein PH, Shipton AE, Stanwix AE, Joffe BI, Ramokgadi J. Beneficial effects of weight loss associated with moderate calorie/carbohydrate restriction, and increased proportional intake of protein and unsaturated fat on serum and lipoprotein levels in gout: a pilot study. *Ann Rheum Dis* 2000;**59**:539–43.

29 Yu TF, Gutman AB. Study of the paradoxical effects of salicylate in low, intermediate and high dosage on the renal mechanisms of excretion of urate in man. *J Clin Invest* 1959;**38**:1298–313.

30 Caspi D, Lubart E, Graff E, Habot B, Yaron M, Segal R. The effect of mini-dose aspirin on renal function and uric acid handling in elderly patients. *Arthritis Rheum* 2000;**43**:103–8.

31 Harris M, Bryant R, Danaher P, Alloway J. Effect of low dose daily aspirin on serum urate levels and urinary excretion in patients receiving probenecid for gouty arthritis. *J Rheumatol* 2000;**27**:2873–6.

32 Ben-Chetrit E, Levy M. Colchicine: 1998 update. *Semin Arthritis Rheum* 1998;**28**:48–59.

33 Ahern MJ, Reid C, Gordon TP. Does colchicine work? Results of the first controlled study in gout. *Aust NZ J Med* 1987;**17**:301–4.

34 Paulos HE, Schlosstein LH, Godfrey RC, *et al.* Prophylactic colchicine therapy in intercritical gout. *Arthritis Rheum* 1987;**17**:609–14.

35 Bellamy N, Downie WW, Buchanan WW. Observations on spontaneous improvement in patients with podagra: implications for therapeutic trials of non-steroidal anti-inflammatory drugs. *Br Clin Pharm* 1987;**24**(1):33–6.

36 Smythe CJ, Percy Js. Comparison of indomethacin and phenylbutazone in acute gout. *Ann Rheum Dis* 1973;**32**(4):351–3.

37 Rousti A, Vainio U. Treatment of acute gouty arthritis with proquazone and indomethacin. A comparative double-blind trial. *Scand J Rheumatol* 1978;Suppl 21,15–17.

38 Altman RD, Honig S, Levin JM, Lightfoot RW. Ketoprofen versus indomethacin in patients with acute gouty arthritis: A multicenter, double blind comparative study. *J Rheumatol* 1988;**15**:1422–6.

39 Weiner GI, White SR, Weitzner RI, Rubenstein HM. Double blind study of phenoprofen versus phenylbutazone in acute gouty arthritis. *Arthritis Rheum* 1979;**22**:425–6.

40 Shresta M, Morgan DL, Moreden JM, Singh R, Nelson M, Hayes JE. Randomised double-blind comparison of the analgesic efficacy of intramuscular ketorolac and oral indomethacin in the treatment of acute gouty arthritis. *Ann Emerg Med* 1995;**26**:682–6.

41 Macagno A, Di Giorgio E, Romanowicz A. Effectiveness of etodolac (Lodine) compared with naproxen in patients with acute gout. *Curr Med Res Opin* 1991:**12**:423–9.

42 Schumacher HR, Boice J, Dahikh DI, *et al.* Randomised double blind trial of etoricoxib and indomethacin in treatment of acute gouty arthritis. *BMJ* 2002;**324**: 1488–92.

43 Bellamy N, Gilbert JR, Brooks PM, Emmerson BT, Campbell J. A survey of current prescribing practices of anti-inflammatory and urate lowering drugs in gouty arthritis in the Province of Ontario. *J Rheumatol* 1988;**15**:1841–71.

44 Stuart RA, Gow PJ, Bellamy N, Campbell J, Grigor R. A survey of current prescribing practices of anti-inflammatory and urate lowering drugs in gouty arthritis *NZ Med J* 1991;**104**:118–21.

45 Ferraz MB, Sato EI, Nishie IA, Visioni RA. A survey of current prescribing practices in gouty arthritis and symptomatic hyperuricemia in San Paulo, Brazil. *J Rheumatol* 1994;**21**(2):374–5.

46 Rozenberg S, Lang T, Laatar A, Koeger AC, Orcel P, Bourgerois P. Diversity of opinions on the management of gout in France. A survey of 750 rheumatologists. *Rev Rhum (Engl Ed)* 1996,**63**:255–61.

47 Schlesinger N, Johanson WG, Jr, Jyoti Rao, Jayanti Rao, Schumacher HR, Jr. A survey of current evaluation and treatment of gout. *Arthritis Rheum* 1999;**42**(9, Supplement):S536.

48 Guazzo E. Use of intravenous colchicine for podagra. *Am Fam Physician* 1999;**60**:2504–5.

49 Stephan WH. Use of intravenous colchicine in patients with acute gout. *Am Fam Physician* 2000;**61**:2343–4.

50 Wallace SL, Singer JZ. Review: systemic toxicity associated with the intravenous administration of colchicine – guidelines for use. *J Rheumtol* 1988;**15**:495–9.

51 Evans IT, Wheeler MT, Small RE, *et al.* A comprehensive investigation of inpatient colchicine use shows more education is needed. *J Rheumatol* 1996;**23**:143.

52 Roberts WN, Liang MH, Stern SH. Colchicine and acute gout. Reassessment of risks and benefits. *JAMA* 1987;**257**:1920–2.

53 Mullins ME, Carrico EA. Horowitz Z. Fatal cardiovascular collapse following acute colchicine ingestion. *Clin Toxicol* 200;**38**:51–4.

54. Gordon GV, Schumacher HR. Management of gout. *Am Fam Physician* 1969;**10**:62–6.

55 Gray RG, Tenenbaum J, Gottlieb NL. Local corticosteroid injection treatment in rheumatic disorders. *Semin Arthritis Rheum* 1979;**10**:231–54.

56 Fernandez C, Noguera R, Gonzalez JA, Pasquel E. Treatment of acute attacks of gout with small doses of intraarticular triamcinolone acetonide. *J Rheumatol* 1999;**26**:2285–6.

57 Groff GD, Franck WA, Raddatz DA. Systemic steroid therapy for acute gout: A clinical trial and review of the literature. *Semin Arthritis Rheum* 1990;**19**:329–36.

58 Alloway JA, Moriarty MJ, Hoogland YT, Nashel D. Comparison of triamcinolone acetonide with indomethacin in the treatment of acute gouty arthritis *J Rheumatol* 1993;**20**:111–13.

59 Ritter J, Kerr LD, Valeriano-Marcet J, Spiera H. ACTH revisited: effective treatment for acute crystal induced synovitis in patients with multiple medical problems. *J Rheumatol* 1994;**21**:696–9.

60 Axelrod D, Preston S. Comparison of parenteral adrenocorticotropic hormone with oral indomethacin in the treatment of acute gout. *Arthritis Rheum* 1988;**31**:803–5.

61 Seigel LB, Alloway JA, Nashel DJ. Comparison of adrenocorticotropic hormone and triamcinolone acetonide in the treatment of gouty arthritis. *J Rheumatol* 1994;**21**:1325–7.

62 Emmerson BT. The management of gout. *N Engl J Med* 1996:**334**:455–51.

63 Fam AG. Should patients with interval gout be treated with urate lowering drugs? (editorial) *J Rheumatol* 1995;**22**:1621–3.

64 Ferraz MB. An evidence based appraisal of the management of tophaceous interval gout. *J Rheumatol* 1995;**22**:1618–20.

65 Cohen A. Gout. *Am J Med Sci* 1936;**192**:448–93.

66 Yu TF, Gutman AB. Efficacy of colchicine prophylaxis in gout. *Ann Intern Med* 1961;**55**:179–192.

67 Yu TF The efficacy of colchicine prophylaxis in articular gout – a reappraisal after 20 years. *Semin Arthritis Rheum* 1982;**12**:258–64.

68 Li-Yu J, Clayburne G, Sieck M, *et al.* Treatment of chronic gout. Can we determine when stores are depleted enough to prevent attacks of gout? *J Rheumatol* 2001:**28**:577–80.

69 Ferraz MB, O'Brien B. A cost effectiveness analysis of urate lowering drugs in nontophaceous recurrent gouty arthritis. *J Rheumatol* 1995;**22**:908–14.

70 Yu TF, Gutman AB. Effect of allopurinol (4-hydroxypyrazolo(3,4-d)pyrimidine) on serum and urinary uric acid in primary and secondary gout. *Am J Med* 1964;**37**:885–98.

71 Delbarre F, Amor B, Auscher C, DeGery A. Treatment of gout with allopurinol. *Ann Rheum Dis.* 1966;**25**:627–33.

72 Thompson GR, Duff IF, Robinson WD, Mikklesen WM, Galindez H. Long term uricosuric therapy in gout. *Arthritis Rheum* 1962;**5**:384–96.

73 Medellin MV, Erickson AR, Enzenauer RJ. Variability of treatment for gouty arthritis between rheumatologists and primary care physicians. *J Clin Rheumatol* 1997;**3**:24–7.

74 Pawlotsky Y. What is the optimal treatment for acute crystal induced arthritis? *Rev Rheum [Engl Ed]* 1996;**63**:231–3.

75 Perez-Ruiz F, Alonso-Ruiz A, Calaabozo M, Herrero-Beites A, Garcia-Erauskin G, Ruiz-Lucea E. Efficacy of allopurinol and benzbromarone for the control of hyperuricemia. A pathogenic approach to the treatment of primary chronic gout. *Ann Rheum Dis* 1998;**57**(9):545–9.

76 Weinberger A, Schreiber M, Sperling O, DeVeris A. Comparative evaluation of uricosuric and allopurinol treatment in a series of 183 patients gouty patients. *Intern Rev Rheum* 1975;**5**:681.

77 Rundles RW, Metz EN, Silberman HR. Allopurinol in the treatment of gout. *Ann Intern Med* 1966;**64**:229–58

78 Beutler Am, Rull M, Schlesinger N, Baker DG, Hoffman BI, Schumacher HR, Jr. Treatment with allopurinol decreases the number of acute gout attacks despite persistently elevated serum uric acid. *Clin Exp Rheumatol* 2001;**19**:595.

79 Scott JT. Comparison of allopurinol to probenecid. *Ann Rheum Dis* 1966;**25**:623–6.

80 Levinson DJ, Becker MA. Clinical gout and the pathogenesis of hyperuricemia. In: McCarty DJ, Koopman WJ, eds. *Arthritis and allied conditions, 12th edn.* Philadelphia: Lea and Febriger, 1993:1773–818.

81 Bull PW, Scott JT. Intermittent control of hyperuricemia in the treatment of gout. *J Rheumatol* 1989;**16**:1246–8.

82 Nass JE, Sanders LJ. Chronic tophaceous gout in a patient with a history of allopurinol toxicity. *Cutis* 1998;**62**(5):239–41.

Gout
Summaries and decision aids

Gout and NSAIDs
Summaries and decision aid

How well do non-steroidal anti-inflammatory drugs (NSAIDs) work to treat gout and is one better than the other?

To answer this question, scientists found and analysed 8 studies testing NSAIDs in 366 people with gout. People received either pills or injections of NSAIDs. These studies provide the best evidence we have today.

What is gout and how can it be treated?

Gout is a type of arthritis in which there is a build up of crystals from uric acid in the joints of the body. In gout, the body either makes too much uric acid or it is not able to flush out excess uric acid from the body fast enough. When it builds up, the uric acid forms into crystals and deposits in joints (especially in the big toe). It can also deposit under the skin and in the kidneys. In the joint, the deposits can cause pain, swelling, and tenderness. An attack of gout may occur suddenly and go away on its own after 7 to 10 days or the pain and swelling can come on slowly and last for long periods. Non-steroidal anti-inflammatory drugs (NSAIDs), such as indomethacin, naproxen, etodolac or etoricoxib, are often used to decrease the pain and swelling. In people who cannot take NSAIDs because of side effects or when NSAIDs are not working, there are other treatments such as corticosteroids or colchicine.

How well did NSAIDs work?

A study of people who **did not receive treatment for gout** showed that gout will not likely improve before 7 days without using NSAIDs.

Seven studies that compared different NSAIDs to each other all showed that people improved when receiving NSAIDs. But the studies have not shown which NSAID works better.

What side effects occurred with NSAIDs?

Side effects that occurred were stomach and intestinal problems, such as ulcers and bleeding (3 out of 100 people had these side effects), vomiting, headache, dizziness, and sleepiness. NSAIDs may not be safe in people with kidney disease, ulcers, high blood pressure, bleeding problems, and heart failure.

What is the bottom line?

There is "Silver" level evidence that non-steroidal anti-inflammatory drugs (NSAIDs) decrease pain and swelling in gout. NSAIDs also decrease the length of the attack.

It is not clear which NSAID works better.

Based on Schumaucher R, Schlesinger N, Baker D, Ottawa Methods Group. Gout. In: *Evidence-based Rheumatology*, London: BMJ Books, 2003.

How well do non-steroidal anti-inflammatory drugs (NSAIDs) work to treat gout and is one better than the other?

What is gout and how can it be treated?

Gout is a type of arthritis in which there is a build up of crystals from uric acid in the joints of the body. Normally, the body makes uric acid and flushes out the excess in the urine. But in gout, the body either makes too much uric acid or it is not able to flush out the excess fast enough. When it builds up, the uric acid forms into crystals and deposits in the joints, especially in the big toe. It can also deposit under the skin and in the kidneys. In the joint, the deposits can cause pain, swelling and tenderness.

An attack of gout may occur suddenly and go away on its own after 7 to 10 days or the pain and swelling can come on slowly and last for long periods. Non-steroidal anti-inflammatory drugs (NSAIDs), such as indomethacin, naproxen, etodolac or etoricoxib, are often used to decrease the pain and swelling. But, it is unclear if one NSAID works better than the other and which NSAIDs may cause more side effects. In people who can't take NSAIDs because of side effects or when NSAIDs are not working, there are other treatments such as corticosteroids or colchicine

How did the scientists find the information and analyse it?

The scientists searched for studies and reviews of the literature that examined the treatment of gout with NSAIDs. Not all studies found were of a high quality and so only those studies that met high standards were selected.

Which high quality studies and reviews were examined in this summary?

Eight studies were examined in this summary.

One study examined 11 patients with gout who did not receive any treatment. The seven other studies tested 366 patients who received an NSAID. NSAIDs tested were indomethacin, phenylbutazone, proquazone, ketoprofen, fenoprofen, ketorolac (IV), etodolac, naproxen or etoricoxib. One of these studies tested 75 patients receiving indomethacin and 75 patients receiving etoricoxib for 8 days.

How well did NSAIDs work?

The study with patients who **did not receive any treatment** for gout showed that gout will not likely improve before 7 days without using NSAIDs. This was because

- 18 out of 100 patients needed treatment because the pain did not improve after 4 days
- 81 out of 100 patients had **some** improvement in pain after 5 days
- 27 out of 100 patients had complete improvement after 7 days.

The 7 studies that compared different NSAIDs to each other all showed that patients improved when receiving NSAIDs. Some of the results from the studies are shown:

- all patients improved with indomethacin or phenylbutazone after 2 to 3 days
- 90 out of 100 patients had some pain relief after 1 day and 22 out of 100 had complete relief from pain after 5 days with indomethacin or proquazone
- 79 out of 100 patients improved after 4 days with fenoprofen or phenylbutazone
- 80 out of 100 patients had half the pain after 2 hours with ketorolac or indomethacin
- 28 out of 100 patients had no pain or mild pain after 4 hours with etoricoxib or indomethacin.

Specifically, one study testing indomethacin showed that:

- about 20 out of 100 patients had no pain or mild pain after 4 hours
- about 60 out of 100 patients had no pain or mild pain after 2 days
- about 83 out of 100 patients had no pain or mild pain after 5 days.

The studies have not shown which NSAID works better.

What side effects occurred with NSAIDs?

Side effects that occurred in these short studies were stomach and intestinal problems, vomiting, headache, dizziness and sleepiness.

Specifically, one study showed that

- 60 out of 100 patients had these side effects with an NSAID (indomethacin)
- 11 out of 100 patients stopped taking the NSAID (indomethacin) because of these side effects.

NSAIDs may not be safe in people with kidney disease, ulcers, high blood pressure, bleeding problems, and heart failure.

Serious side effects: Very large studies need to be done to test serious side effects of NSAIDs. But very large studies have not been done for gout. Studies of NSAIDs in other conditions have shown that bleeding stomach ulcers or holes in the lining of the gut occur more often with NSAIDs. Normally, these side effects occur in 1 to 5 out of 100 patients. But, some studies testing NSAIDs show that these serious side effects may occur more often than normal. For patients that have more chances of stomach problems, a type of NSAID called a coxib or Cox-2 inhibitor is safer on the stomach and intestines.

What is the bottom line?

There is "Silver" level evidence that non-steroidal anti-inflammatory drugs (NSAIDs) decrease pain and swelling in gout. NSAIDs also decrease the length of the attack.

It is not clear which NSAID works better.

Based on Schumaucher R, Schlesinger N, Baker D, Ottawa Methods Group. Gout. In: *Evidence-based Rheumatology.* London: BMJ Books, 2003.

Information about gout and treatment

What is gout?

Gout is a type of arthritis in which there is a build up of uric acid in the joints of the body. Normally, the body makes uric acid and flushes out the excess in the urine. But in gout the body either makes too much uric acid or is unable to flush out the excess fast enough. When it builds up, the uric acid forms into crystals and deposits in the joints, especially in the big toe. It can deposit under the skin and in the kidneys. This causes pain, swelling, and tenderness in that area of the body. Attacks of gout may occur suddenly or the pain and swelling can come on slowly and last for long periods.

If left untreated, the attack may end after 7 to 10 days, but can last weeks. However, attacks will still occur with pain and swelling, and uric acid may build up and lead to

- tophi (uric acid deposits under the skin and elsewhere)
- limited ability to do daily activities
- kidney stones
- permanent damage to joints.

What can I do on my own to manage my disease?

✓ rest during attack
✓ put less stress on joints
✓ cold packs
✓ maintain a healthy weight
✓ relax
✓ avoid excess carbohydrates and purines
✓ avoid alcohol

What treatments are used for gout?

Five kinds of treatment may be used alone or together. The common (generic) names of treatment are shown below.

1. *Pain medicines and non-steroidal anti-inflammatory drugs (NSAIDs) for attacks*
   - Acetylsalicylic acid
   - Celecoxib
   - Diclofenac
   - Etodolac
   - Etoricoxib
   - Indomethacin
   - Ketoprofen
   - Meloxicam
   - Naproxen
   - Rofecoxib
   - Tolmetin
   - Valdecoxib
2. *Colchicine for attacks or to prevent gout*
   - Allopurinol
   - Benzbromarone
   - Probenecid
3. *Uric acid lowering drugs to prevent gout*
4. *Corticosteroid injections for attacks*
   - Adrenocorticosteroids
   - Adrenocorticotropic hormone (ACTH)
5. *Diet therapy*
   - Low purine diet
   - Low carbohydrate

What are my choices? How can I decide?

Treatment for your disease will depend on your condition. You need to know the good points (pros) and bad points (cons) about each treatment before you can decide.

Gout decision aid

Should I take non-steroidal anti-inflammatory drugs (NSAIDs)?

This guide can help you make decisions about the treatment your doctor is asking you to consider.

It will help you to

1 Clarify what you need to decide.
2 Consider the pros and cons of different choices.
3 Decide what role you want to have in choosing your treatment.
4 Identify what you need to help you make the decision.
5 Plan the next steps.
6 Share your thinking with your doctor.

Step 1: Clarify what you need to decide

What is the decision?

Should I take non-steroidal anti-inflammatory drugs to decrease the pain and swelling in gout?

NSAIDs may be taken as a pill daily.

When does this decision have to be made? Check ✓ one

☐ within days ☐ within weeks ☐ within months

How far along are you with this decision? Check ✓ one

☐ I have not thought about it yet

☐ I am considering the choices

☐ I am close to making a choice

☐ I have already made a choice

Step 2: Consider the pros and cons of different choices
What does the research show?

NSAIDs are classified as: **Likely benefical**

There is 'Silver' level evidence from 8 studies of 366 people that tested NSAIDs. The studies lasted up to 2 weeks. These studies found pros and cons that are listed in the chart below.

What do I think of the pros and cons of non-steroidal anti-inflammatory drugs (NSAIDs)?

1 Review the common pros and cons.
2 Add any other pros and cons that are important to you.
3 Show how important each pro and con is to you by circling from one (*) star if it is a little important to you, to up to five (*****) stars if it is very important to you.

PROS AND CONS OF NON-STEROIDAL ANTI-INFLAMMATORY DRUGS (NSAIDS)

PROS (number of people affected)	How important is it to you?	CONS (number of people affected)	How important is it to you?
Improves pain and swelling 83 out of 100 people had no pain or mild pain after 5 days of taking indomethacin	* * * * *	Gout may improve on its own without treatment after 7 to 10 days	* * * * *
Decreases length of attack	* * * * *	Side effects: stomach and intestinal side effects, vomiting, headache, dizziness and tiredness 60 out of 100 people had side effects with indomethacin 11 out of 100 people stopped taking indomethacin because of side effects	* * * * *
Other pros:	* * * * *	May make high blood pressure worse and may not be safe in people with kidney disease	* * * * *
		Rare serious harms 1 to 5 more people out of 100 will get a bleeding stomach ulcer or a hole in the lining of their gut when taking NSAIDs	* * * * *
		Personal cost of medicine	* * * * *
		Other cons:	* * * * *

What do you think of NSAIDs? Check ✓ one

☐ Willing to consider this treatment — Pros are more important to me than the cons

☐ Unsure

☐ Not willing to consider this treatment — Cons are more important to me than the pros

Step 3: Choose the role you want to have in choosing your treatment
Check ✓ one

☐ I prefer to decide on my own after listening to the opinions of others

☐ I prefer to share the decision with: ____________________

☐ I prefer someone else to decide for me, namely: ____________

Step 4: Identify what you need to help you make the decision

What I know	Do you know enough about your condition to make a choice?	☐ Yes	☐ No	☐ Unsure
	Do you know which options are available to you?	☐ Yes	☐ No	☐ Unsure
	Do you know the good points (pros) of each option?	☐ Yes	☐ No	☐ Unsure
	Do you know the bad points (cons) of each option?	☐ Yes	☐ No	☐ Unsure
What's important	Are you clear about which **pros** are most *important to you?*	☐ Yes	☐ No	☐ Unsure
	Are you clear about which **cons** are most *important to you?*	☐ Yes	☐ No	☐ Unsure
How others help	Do you have enough support from others to make a choice?	☐ Yes	☐ No	☐ Unsure
	Are you choosing without pressure from others?	☐ Yes	☐ No	☐ Unsure
	Do you have enough advice to make a choice?	☐ Yes	☐ No	☐ Unsure
How sure I feel	Are you clear about the best choice for you?	☐ Yes	☐ No	☐ Unsure
	Do you feel sure about what to choose?	☐ Yes	☐ No	☐ Unsure

If you answered No or Unsure to many of these questions, you should talk to your doctor.

Step 5: Plan the next steps
What do you need to do before you make this decision?

For example: talk to your doctor, read more about this treatment or other treatments for gout.

Step 6: Share the information on this form with your doctor

It will help your doctor understand what you think about this treatment.

6

Systemic lupus erythematosus

Joel Schiffenbauer, Eliza Chakravarty, Vibeke Strand

Introduction

Systemic lupus erythematosus (SLE) is an autoimmune disease affecting multiple organ systems. Its clinical course is typically characterised by remissions and relapses, although some patients have prolonged periods of continuous disease activity. Manifestations of active disease or its treatment may result in permanent end organ dysfunction. The protean nature of organ system involvement in SLE requires that events as diverse as renal failure, thrombosis, seizures, cerebrovascular accident (CVA), and cognitive dysfunction must be considered when identifying goals for treatment. Chronic use of glucocorticoids may result in osteonecrosis, osteoporosis, muscle atrophy, and/or infections. Use of immunosuppressive agents may lead to infections, bone marrow suppression, and lymphoproliferative disorders. Both high dose glucocorticoids and cytotoxic agents may adversely affect health-related quality of life. As these therapies have significant risk/benefit profiles, it is important that treatment interventions in SLE be directed at reversible processes.

Mortality from SLE has improved considerably over the past several decades. In 1955, 5 year survival rates were reported to be only 50–60%; in the 1980s the 5 year survival was about 90%.[1] Recent reports indicate ≥ 90% survival over 10 years, in part attributed to earlier diagnoses and improvements in treatment, including use of low dose immunosuppressive agents as steroid sparing therapy.[2,3] However, death rates for patients with SLE remain three to five times higher than in the general population, and are related both to disease activity and its treatment. Prognostic factors also include age of onset, gender, race, and socioeconomic status.[2–4]

SLE is associated with significant morbidity, including organic brain dysfunction, Sjögren's syndrome, as well as organ involvement described above. Osteoporosis, hypertension, cataracts, hyperlipidaemia, obesity, and diabetes are well recognised complications of chronic glucocorticoid use. An important problem gaining attention is the increased risk of arteriosclerotic cardiovascular disease and myocardial infarctions in patients with SLE. In one study, women with SLE aged 35–44 years were more than 50 times more likely to have a myocardial infarction than women of similar age in the Framingham Offspring study.[5] The causes are likely multifactorial, resulting not only from the disease itself (even when attempting controls for known risk factors), but also its treatment, as well as anti-phospholipid antibodies (APL).

It is of the utmost importance to choose therapies demonstrated to have a potential impact on the morbidity and mortality associated with active SLE. The questions and responses that follow attempt to provide the best evidence available supporting treatment of various manifestations of SLE, relying on data from randomised controlled

The opinions and assertions expressed in this chapter are the private views of the authors. No endorsement by the Food and Drug Administration is intended or should be inferred.

trials (RCTs). Where RCTs are unavailable, data from longitudinal observational studies or continuation series following randomised assignment to treatment group will be discussed, recognising that conclusions from this type of evidence are more limited.

Methodology (see Introduction, p xiii)

In general the approach used was to restrict searches in Medline, Embase and CCTR to RCTs or randomised longitudinal series, as well as systematic reviews of SLE treatment. Open label, long term follow up from RCTs is provided where applicable. We also conducted hand searches of bibliographic references and contacted content experts for additional studies.

Outcomes

RCTs designed to study treatments in SLE need to utilise outcome measures that capture clinically important endpoints, and identify those which represent important benefits to the patient.

Most clinical trial data in SLE have been collected in patients with SLE nephritis, where "objective" measures of renal function including 24 hour urines for creatinine clearances and quantification of proteinuria, defined changes in microscopic urinalyses, doubling of serum creatinine, and end stage renal disease have been utilised as primary outcomes. Other than in nephritis, there are a limited number of RCTs and longitudinal observational studies (LOS) in SLE as few other organ system manifestations have been considered as easily evaluated using similar "objective" outcome measures. Certainly haematological disease including thrombocytopenia, haemolytic anaemia, and autoimmune leucopenia may be objectively measured in similar fashion – but these manifestations are not as common, and are typically associated with a variety of other organ system involvement in SLE. It remains difficult to perform RCTs in SLE, for a number of reasons, not least of which includes the length of time necessary to demonstrate significant clinical benefit.

Therefore, the goal of the SLE module at the "Outcome Measures in Rheumatology Clinical Trials" (OMERACT) 4 meeting was to begin to address this issue. Rather than attempting to define a core set of outcome measures, it was elected to define a core group of outcome domains to be evaluated in RCTs or LOS in SLE. Each of six breakout groups considered a variety of outcome domains (and applicable instruments for each domain) and reached a consensus that, in RCTs and LOS in SLE, five domains should be included as a minimum: disease activity, damage, health status/HRQOL as well as adverse effects and health utilities/economic measures, both already ratified by previous OMERACT conferences.[6]

As reviewed in this chapter, none of the RCTs or LOS in SLE included all recommended domains. None the less we have sought to cite reported outcome measures in the context of recommended domains, although development of most disease activity indices and the American College of Rheumatology/Systemic Lupus International Cooperating Clinics: SLICC damage index occurred after completion of many RCTs discussed here. The outcome measures reported in the cited studies considered to address these domains are shown in the Box on the next page.

Evaluating the evidence

Literature search

A broad search was conducted from SLE to determine all high quality relevant studies in the area. All of the evidence needed to answer the questions in this chapter can be identified from the search.

1. exp Lupus Erythematosus, Systemic/
2. Lupus Erythematosus.tw.
3. (lupus adj2 (systemic or nephritis or vasculitis)).tw.

4. or/1–3
5. clinical trial.pt.
6. randomised controlled trial.pt.
7. random$.tw.
8. (double adj blind$).tw.
9. placebo$.tw.
10. case report/or exp case-control studies/
11. exp cohort studies/
12. Controlled Clinical Trials/
13. Or/5–12
14. 4 and 13

The treatment of SLE remains unproven. Definitions utilised in analysed RCTs and LOS are shown in the Box below. We have endeavoured to group outcome measures reflecting similar domains together.

Outcome domains as recommended by OMERACT

Disease activity:
- Disease Activity Scores: SLEDAI, SLAM, BILAG, ECLAM, SELENA SLEDAI, SLAM-R
- Definitions of active nephritis by U/A, 24 hour CCr, proteinuria, renal flare

Damage:
- ACR/SLICC Damage Index
- Deterioration of renal function:
- End stage renal disease [ESRD]
- Doubling of serum creatinine
- Chronicity index on biopsy

Health status/HRQOL: SF-36
Should also include:
- Economic costs including health utilities
- Adverse effects

Definitions of outcomes utilised in this review

I. Deterioration of renal function
Steinberg *et al*[9]: degree of change from baseline required to denote deterioration: creatinine clearance to 10 ml/min; urinary sediment: 2x increase in RBCs or RBC casts from baseline; 24 hour urine protein: 20% change (at least 1 g/day); serum complement: 20 mg/100 ml; anti-dsDNA antibodies: 2x increase; extrarenal disease: double blind clinical evaluation

II. Severe lupus nephritis
Sesso *et al*[25]: defined as "nephritic urine sediment" *[not further defined]* or urinary protein >3·0 g/day and impaired renal function (creatinine clearance <80 ml/min or a recent reduction of at least 30% from baseline); if creatinine clearance remained stable then histology consistent with diffuse proliferative GN had to be present.

III. Renal flare
Donadio *et al*[57]: development of one of the following: decrease in renal function (reduction in creatinine clearance by ≥ 25% within 3–6 months; nephrotic syndrome (either relapse or new manifestation *[not further defined]*) or increased proteinuria of 2 g per 24 hours from baseline or within 3–6 months.

Illei *et al*[12]: an episode of increased activity of SLE nephritis; classified as either proteinuric (defined as an increase in proteinuria > 2 g/day with a stable serum creatinine level and inactive urinary sediment-no cellular casts and <10 RBCs/hpf) or nephritic (defined as mild or severe; mild: defined as reappearance of cellular casts or >10 RBCs/hpf with an increase in proteinuria <2 g/day and with a stable serum creatinine level; severe: defined as reappearance of cellular casts or >10 RBCs/hpf with an increase in serum creatinine 30% over the level at the time of complete response regardless of the level of proteinuria).

Alarcon-Segovia *et al*[23]: that it be attributed to SLE by the treating physician and/or medical monitor and one or more of the following three criteria were met:

1 a reproducible increase from baseline in 24 hour urine proteinuria;

2 a reproducible increase from baseline in serum creatinine of greater than 20% or at least 0·3 mg/dl, whichever was greater, accompanied by proteinuria (>1000 mg/24 hours), haematuria (>4 RBC/HPF) and/or red cell casts; or
3 new reproducible haematuria (>11–20 RBC/HPF) or a reproducible increase in haematuria by two grades compared to baseline associated with greater than 25% dysmorphic red blood cells of glomerular origin, exclusive of menses, accompanied by either ≥ 800 mg increase in 24 hour protein or new appearance of RBC casts

IV. Treatment failure
Gourley *et al*[11]; Illei *et al*[12]: composite of any of the following events: need for immunosuppressive therapy not dictated by protocol treatment, doubling of serum creatinine or death.

Houssiau *et al*[17]: defined as one of the following three features:

1 Absence of a primary response;
— (a) for patients with baseline serum creatinine levels ≥1·3 mg/dl and <2·6 mg/dl: serum creatinine levels ≥1·3 at 6 months;
— (b) for patients with baseline serum creatinine > 2·6 mg/dl: serum creatinine levels which did not improve by 50% at 6 months;
— (c) for patients with nephrotic syndrome but without renal impairment at baseline: persistence of nephrotic syndrome at 6 months.

2 Glucocorticoid resistant flare. Doubling of serum creatinine over the lowest value reached at any time during follow up and confirmed on two consecutive visits ≥1 month apart.

Chan *et al*[13]: defined as one of the following: 24 urine protein levels ≥3 g/24 hours, 0·3–2·9 g/24 hours, and serum albumin levels <3·9 g/dl; increase in serum Cr ≥0·6 mg/dl; creatinine clearance >15% above baseline; discontinuation of treatment due to adverse effects.

V. Non-responders
Gourley *et al*[11]: defined as >10 RBC/hpf or cellular casts on urinalysis, proteinuria >1 g/day and doubling of serum creatinine.

VI. High risk group
Steinberg *et al*[9]: patients with active nephritis who have, in addition, chronic sclerotic atrophic and/or fibrotic changes on kidney biopsy.

VII. Renal remission
Gourley *et al*[11]: defined <10 dysmorphic RBC/hpf absence of cellular casts and <1 g/day proteinuria.

Sesso *et al*[25]: after 6 months: "trend of improvement" in serum creatinine, urinary sediment or proteinuria.

VIII. Complete response
Illei *et al*[12]: presence of three criteria ≥6 months: serum creatinine <130% of the lowest level during treatment, proteinuria <1 g/day, absence of cellular casts and <10 RBC/hpf. Patients had to be off all immunosuppressive therapy, hydroxychloroquine, and prednisone (≥10 mg/day or equivalent).

IX. Complete renal remission
Chan *et al*[13]: proteinuria < 0·3 g/24 hours, with normal urinary sediment, normal serum albumin, and serum creatinine and creatinine clearance values within 15% of baseline values.

X. Partial response/stabilisation of renal function **Illei *et al*[12]:** stable values of serum creatinine (<150% of the lowest level during treatment) for at least 6 months without immunosuppressive therapy regardless of levels of urinary protein sediment.

XI. Partial remission

Chan *et al*[13]: 24 hour proteinuria between 0·3 and 2·9 g with serum albumin levels ≥3·0 g/dl and stable renal function.

XII. Number needed to treat

Bansal *et al*[8]: reciprocal of the absolute risk difference; number of patients needed to treat to prevent one occurrence of a specific outcome (such as death or renal failure).

Case presentation: Patient 1

A 25-year-old African American female with known systemic lupus erythematosus on prednisone 5 mg for previous arthritis presents with fatigue and swelling of her feet. She is found to have haematuria and proteinuria on urine dipstick. On further evaluation she has RBC casts along with 1 g of proteinuria. Serum creatinine is 2·2 mg/dl. A renal biopsy demonstrates diffuse proliferative glomerulonephritis. She is concerned about the use of cyclophosphamide after the potential adverse effects are explained to her.

Case presentation: Patient 2

A 27-year-old female school teacher has been diagnosed with systemic lupus erythematosus based on a 9 month history of fatigue, mild non-deforming arthritis of the hands, malar rash, oral ulcers, and intermittent mild pleuritic chest pain. Laboratory evaluation is significant for an ANA (antinuclear antibody) titre of 1:640, mildly decreased serum complements, and a mild anaemia of chronic disease. She has no evidence of renal or other internal organ involvement, no other medical problems, and is currently taking only over-the-counter analgesics with minimal relief. She wants to avoid oral steroids because of concerns of weight gain, osteoporosis, and high cholesterol that had occurred in her mother during chronic steroid treatment for lupus.

Question 1

In a patient with active manifestations of SLE nephritis does the use of CTX improve survival (including mortality and ESRD) compared with steroids alone?

Question 2

Does combination treatment with steroids and CTX improve survival over steroids or CTX alone?

Two meta-analyses address the treatment of SLE nephritis. A meta-analysis by Felson and Anderson published in 1984[7] examined data from eight RCTs in which patients were randomly assigned to receive either prednisone alone or prednisone plus immunosuppressive agents: CTX or AZA (n = 250). This analysis concluded that patients receiving treatment with immunosuppressive agents and prednisone had less deterioration in renal function (p = 0·006), were less likely to develop end stage renal disease (p = 0·023) or die from renal disease (p = 0·024) than patients receiving steroids alone. Subjects with biopsy proven diffuse proliferative glomerulonephritis (DPGN) showed the most significant improvement with combination treatment compared with prednisone alone (deterioration in renal function: p = 0·008; ESRD: p = 0·012; nephritis-related death: p = 0·017) compared with those without DPGN (deterioration in renal function: p = 0·416; ESRD: p = 0·986; nephritis-related death: p = 0·642). Use of either immunosuppressive agent alone (AZA or CTX) failed to show significant improvement compared with steroids alone for any outcome.

A second, more recent meta-analysis by Bansal and Beto published in 1997[8] examined 19 trials in SLE nephritis (n = 440), comparing treatment with oral prednisone alone, AZA alone, AZA with prednisone, oral CTX with prednisone, and IV CTX with prednisone. Primary outcomes included ESRD and mortality. When compared to oral prednisone alone, pooled data comparing

Table 6.1 Adverse effects (Gourley *et al*, 1996)[11]

Adverse effect	MP alone	CTX alone	MP+ CTX
Avascular necrosis	6 (22%)	3 (11%)	5 (18%)
Amenorrhoea	2 (10%)	11 (52%)	12 (57%)
One or more infections	2 (7·4%)	7 (26%)	9 (32%)
Neutropenic fever	0	1 (3·7%)	1 (3·6%)
Herpes zoster infection	1 (3·7%)	4 (15%)	6 (21%)
Cervical dysplasia	0	3 (11%)	2 (7·1%)
Death	0	2 (7·4%)	1 (3·6%)

immunosuppressive agents plus prednisone with oral prednisone alone demonstrated greater efficacy for both outcomes with immunosuppressive use (absolute risk differences 12·9% for ESRD and 13·2% for mortality). When comparing outcomes by treatment group, statistically significant differences favoured IV CTX for ESRD (absolute risk difference 16·2%), oral prednisone plus either immunosuppressive agent (oral AZA or CTX) for ESRD (absolute risk difference 16·9%), and IV CTX for mortality (absolute risk difference 19·9%). Neither immunosuppressive agent was shown more effective than the other, either for ESRD or mortality. A number needed to treat analysis indicated that treating 7 patients with IV CTX prevented one case of ESRD and treating 5 patients averted one death. Using either immunosuppressive agent the numbers needed to treat were 7·8 and 7·6 patients, for ESRD and total mortality, respectively.

Together, these 2 meta-analyses indicate that combined use of immunosuppressive agents with prednisone can improve outcomes in SLE nephritis. They do not distinguish between use of either oral CTX or AZA, but do favour treatment with IV CTX. The meta-analyses do not address the morbidities associated with the use of either of these immunosuppressive agents, especially oral or IV CTX. Based on the patient populations studied, this approach should be reserved for patients with proliferative class III–V lesions on renal biopsy.

Two particular studies included in the meta-analysis described above deserve special mention here for containing the elements of rigorously designed trials. The first is the study by Steinberg *et al.*[9] in which patients with SLE nephritis were randomly assigned to receive placebo or cyclophosphamide. The trial was double blind and treatment allocation was concealed by providing numbered envelopes with random assignments to the hospital pharmacy. "Therapist physicians" adjusted doses of medication while "observer physicians" reported clinical changes without knowledge of laboratory data. However, the study was 10 weeks in duration and included 13 patients, with biopsies performed in only 8. The results showed no differences in creatinine clearance, although patients receiving CTX showed greater improvement in more assessments (creatinine clearance, urinary sediment, 24 hour urine protein, serum complement, anti-DNA antibodies, extrarenal manifestations of SLE) than those treated with placebo ($p < 0{\cdot}005$ by Spearman rank correlation). Overall the difference between the placebo and cyclophosphamide treatment groups was significant ($p < 0{\cdot}001$).

The second study, also by Steinberg *et al*,[10] used a similar design to examine the effects of cyclophosphamide or AZA versus placebo in SLE nephritis. This RCT was only 10 weeks in duration: 10 patients were assigned to

Table 6.2 Adverse effects (Illei *et al*, 2001)[12]

Adverse effect	Methylprednisolone group	Cyclophosphamide group	Combination group
Avascular necrosis	6/20 (30%)	7/19 (36%)	8/21 (31%)
Osteoporosis	3/24 (13%)	5/21 (23%)	5/24 (21%)
Premature amenorrhoea	7/21 (30%)	12/20 (60%)	12/23 (52%)
Infection	2/27 (8%)	7/27 (26%)	9/28 (32%)
Herpes zoster	2/27 (7%)	7/27 (26%)	9/28 (32%)
Death	1/27	5/27	5/28

cyclophosphamide, 13 to azathioprine, and 15 to placebo. All 38 patients had renal biopsies. Renal function, urine sediment, proteinuria, anti-DNA, C3, and symptoms were assessed. Cyclophosphamide was significantly superior to both azathioprine ($p < 0.02$) and placebo ($p < 0.001$) for all six measures and for the three renal measures alone (creatinine clearance, urine sediment, proteinuria; cyclophosphamide versus azathioprine $p < 0.005$; cyclophosphamide versus placebo, $p < 0.005$).

Although these studies were relatively small and of short duration, they are two of the most rigorously designed studies that support use of cyclophosphamide in SLE nephritis, the results of which are further supported by additional studies described below.

The results of these meta-analyses are supported by two recent publications that provide cumulative data on additional patients not included in the meta-analyses. Gourley *et al*[11] reported results in 82 patients from the National Institutes of Health (NIH]) RCT in patients with active SLE nephritis (defined as >10 RBC/hpf and cellular casts on urinalysis, proteinuria > 1 g/day and a renal biopsy with proliferative nephritis: biopsy class III–V). They compared three different interventions over at least 1 year: (1) bolus methylprednisolone (MP) (1 g/m^2) monthly; (2) bolus CTX (0·5–1 g/m^2) monthly for 6 months and then quarterly; (3) bolus MP and CTX. Primary outcomes included: patients who achieved renal remission, number of non-responders (patients with persistent nephritis as defined above: >10 RBC/hpf and cellular casts on urinalysis, proteinuria >1 g/day, and doubling of serum creatinine); and adverse effects. Patients were randomly assigned to one of the three treatment regimens by drawing from a masked card sequence derived from a random numbers table. There was no discussion of blinding.

Of 82 patients, 17 were censored during the study for: pregnancy ($n = 4$), failure to return for follow up ($n = 5$), protocol violations ($n = 2$), excessive nausea and vomiting ($n = 1$), allergy to MP ($n = 2$), and 3 deaths. Of 27 patients in the MP alone group, 7 achieved remission compared with 13/27 receiving CTX ($p = 0.038$) and 17/28 combination MP + CTX ($p < 0.001$); remission rates in the CTX group were not statistically different from combination treatment ($p = 0.16$). Inclusion of all censored patients coding them as non-responders demonstrated that renal remission was statistically significant in the combination MP + CTX treatment group ($p = 0.02$): responders: MP alone 10/27; CTX 19/27; combination 25/28. Adverse effects included: avascular necrosis, amenorrhoea, infections (pulmonary, gastrointestinal, cardiovascular, herpes zoster), neutropenic fever, cervical dysplasia, and death (see Table 6.1). Together, they included: MP alone: 12 events, 7·4% patients; CTX alone: 35 events, 41% patients; combination MP + CTX: 40 events, 43% patients.

Table 6.3 Adverse effects (% patients at risk) (Austin *et al*, 1986)[14]

Adverse effect	Prednisone	AZA	Oral CTX	Oral AZA + CTX	IV CTX
Major infection	25	11	17	14	10
Herpes zoster	7	11	33	32	25
Haemorrhagic cystitis	0	0	17	14	0
Cancer	0	11	17	0	0
Premature ovarian failure	8	18	71	53	45

In a second publication, Illei *et al*[12] reported an extended follow up of 82 patients (median 11 years) from the Gourley study. Primary outcomes were treatment failure (defined above) and adverse effects. Patients receiving CTX or combination therapy were significantly less likely to develop treatment failure ($p = 0{\cdot}002$ MP versus combination; $p = 0{\cdot}24$ for combination versus CTX; $p = 0{\cdot}04$ for MP versus CTX). However, in an intent to treat analysis, including all patients entered into the series, there were no significant differences between treatments in the risk for death or ESRD.

Adverse effects included avascular necrosis, osteoporosis, premature amenorrhoea, infection, herpes zoster, and death (Table 6.2).

These two reports support the conclusions of both meta-analyses, that combination treatment with immunosuppressive agents and glucocorticoids is more efficacious than glucocorticoids alone. With the benefit of longer term follow up, the Illei report indicates that pulse MP added to IV CTX may improve long term renal outcomes without additive toxicity. However, these studies illustrate the risks associated with use of immunosuppressive agents, including infections and amenorrhoea. Reports of skin cancer and myeloproliferative disorders are increased with use of both CTX and AZA, and bladder cancer with CTX. Interestingly, only one death due to malignancy in the two series was secondary to acute myelogenous leukaemia (AML), in an individual who never received alkylating agents. However, cervical dysplasia was more common in the group receiving CTX. Nevertheless, total deaths were lower in the groups receiving immunosuppressive agents. The benefits of CTX therapy therefore must be weighed against its potential risks, over short and long term use.

Evidence summary: Silver

Two systematic reviews and two subsequent trials of various approaches show that the optimal approach is the addition of an immunosuppressive agent to prednisone. This combination improves survival in patients with SLE nephritis.

Silver level evidence studies suggest that CTX plus prednisone appears to offer better outcomes than immunosuppressive agents such as AZA, but this has not been definitively proven.

Based on the weight of evidence, it is possible that future studies in SLE nephritis will be required to use CTX plus prednisone as the gold standard against which new therapies will be compared. These RCTs will likely be add-on trials (all patients receive glucocorticoids and CTX upon which the new therapy or placebo are superimposed), or will be "head to head" comparisons with CTX (see the study by Chan *et al* using MMF for an example.[13]

Case presentation

For Patient 1, cyclophosphamide and steroids would be appropriate therapy, although the patient remains concerned about potential toxicity.

Table 6.4 Cause of death (numbers of patients) (Steinberg and Steinberg)[15]

Cause of death	Prednisone (n = 30)	AZA (n = 20)	Oral CTX (n = 18)	Oral AZA + CTX (n = 23)	IV CTX (n = 20)	Total
CRF	5	3	2	1	0	11
Infection	3	2	2	1	2	10
Cerebral haemorrhage	2	1	0	1	1	5
Other haemorrhage	1	0	1	0	0	2
Other CVA	0	0	1	1	0	2
CNS-SLE/suicide	1	1	0	0	0	2
Cardiac	0	0	1	0	1	2
TTP	0	0	0	1	0	1
Total	12	7	7	5	4	35

Question 3

In a patient with severe manifestations of active SLE, is pulse intravenous CTX as effective and less toxic than daily oral CTX therapy?

Two reports have directly compared the efficacy and safety of IV versus oral CTX. In the first RCT, by Austin *et al*,[14] 107 patients with SLE nephritis were randomly assigned to receive high dose oral prednisone (1 mg/kg), oral AZA (up to 4 mg/kg/day), oral CTX (up to 4 mg/kg/day), combined oral AZA and CTX (up to 1 mg/kg/day of each) or intravenous CTX (0·5–1 g/m^2) every 3 months. Patients received oral prednisone as needed for control of extrarenal disease in all groups except those receiving high dose prednisone treatment. Patients were randomly assigned by drawing from a masked card sequence based on a table of random numbers; no mention of blinding was made. Outcomes included renal failure, death, and adverse effects. A total of 111 patients were entered; 4 were excluded because they did not complete a minimum 3 months of protocol treatment, leaving 107 patients with follow up data.

The probability of no renal failure across treatment groups was statistically better in those receiving IV CTX versus prednisone ($p = 0·027$). In the high risk group the probability of no renal failure favoured treatment with IV CTX over prednisone ($p = 0·014$); and was statistically significant compared with low risk patients ($p = 0·005$). In each case, results with IV were better than using oral CTX.

Comparing treatment groups, overall adverse effects were significantly less with prednisone and AZA than with oral CTX ($p < 0·05$); combined AZA and CTX versus IV CTX ($p < 0·05$); prednisone, AZA, and IV CTX versus oral CTX or combined AZA plus CTX ($p < 0·01$); and prednisone and AZA versus AZA plus CTX and IV CTX ($p < 0·010$). For each reported complication there were fewer with IV than oral CTX (Table 6.3).

In a follow up of the Austin study, Steinberg and Steinberg[15] reported long term preservation of renal function in 111 patients with SLE nephritis. Treatment regimens between oral prednisone (1 mg/kg); oral AZA (1–4 mg/kg/day); oral CTX (1–4 mg/kg/day); combined oral AZA and CTX (1 mg/kg/day each), and intravenous CTX (0·5–1 g/m^2) were compared. Patients in the groups other than high dose prednisone received a maintenance regimen of prednisone 10–20 mg every other day. Endpoints were progression to ESRD or death in all 111 patients (ITT population). Progression to ESRD was not statistically different between prednisone alone or AZA (p = 0·09); but was with IV CTX (p = 0·0025); AZA plus CTX (p = 0·001); and oral CTX (p = 0·032). Deaths were not statistically different between treatment groups, combining all four immunosuppressive treatment groups compared to prednisone (p = 0·24) or comparing all CTX treatment groups with prednisone (p = 0·20). In the high risk group patients receiving prednisone alone demonstrated most rapid progression to renal failure: IV CTX versus prednisone (p = 0·004); AZA plus CTX (p = 0·04); oral CTX (p = 0·04). In all analyses the IV CTX treatment group fared better than the oral CTX group.

Patients receiving IV CTX had equal or fewer complications than those receiving oral CTX.

Evidence summary: Silver

IV CTX appears to be more effective in delaying ESRD and preventing death than oral CTX with fewer complications, although these results do not become apparent until a minimum of 5 years follow up. There is mainly Silver level evidence to support the use of IV CTX and this appears to be the preferred approach to the treatment of SLE nephritis. However, the optimal dosing regimen and number of treatment courses remain to be identified.

Case presentation

For Patient 1 IV cyclophosphamide is the preferred route of treatment, especially since the patient has expressed reservations about the use of cyclophosphamide in general.

Question 4

In a patient with active manifestations of SLE are there any treatment regimens using CTX which are associated with less toxicity and similar relapse rates?

A single RCT directly addressed the most appropriate timing of CTX use. Boumpas *et al*[16] reported on 65 patients randomly assigned to one of three treatments: monthly IV infusions of methylprednisolone (1 g/m^2), IV CTX (0·5–1 g/m^2) monthly for 6 months, IV CTX monthly for 6 months followed by quarterly infusions for a further 2 years; all patients received prednisone. Randomisation was performed by drawing from a set of masked cards. Blinding was not discussed. The primary outcome was renal insufficiency defined by sustained doubling of serum creatinine; exacerbations of nephritis were also evaluated. No randomised patients were lost to follow up.

The probability of renal insufficiency occurring was statistically less in the continued CTX treatment group than methylprednisolone alone (p = 0·037) over a 5 year period of follow up. End stage renal disease occurred in 6/25 (24%) methylprednisolone, 5/20 (25%) 6 month CTX treatment, and 2/20 (10%) continued CTX treatment groups; for doubling in serum creatinine: methylprednisolone 12/25 (48%), 6 month CTX 7/20 (35%), continued CTX 3/20 (15%). In the methylprednisolone treatment group 13/25 (52%) had stable renal function, 13/20 (65%) in the 6 month CTX group, and 17/20 (85%) receiving continued CTX treatment. The probability of no exacerbation in renal disease in the continued CTX group was statistically significant compared with methylprednisolone (p = 0·006).

In a recent RCT, Houssiau *et al*[17] compared the efficacy of two different treatment regimens of CTX. Ninety patients were randomised by minimisation to receive either high dose IV CTX (6 monthly pulses, initially 0·5 g/m^2, then titrated to WBC counts, followed by two quarterly pulses) or low dose IV CTX regimen (six fortnightly pulses at a fixed dose of 500 mg) each of which was followed by AZA (2 mg/kg/day). Blinding was not discussed. In an intent to treat analysis, with median follow up of 41 months), there were no statistically significant differences between treatment groups for treatment failures (Kaplan Meier analysis, p = 0·64), remission of renal disease (p = 0·36), renal flare (p = 0·80) or severe infection (p = 0·20). It was concluded that a remission-inducing regimen of low dose IV CTX was as effective as a high dose regimen, provided each regimen was followed by long term AZA administration.

Evidence summary: Silver

An extended course of pulse IV CTX including the addition of quarterly maintenance doses was more effective than 6 months of pulse CTX only in preserving renal function and reducing the number of renal flares. However, low doses of IV CTX followed by continued AZA may be equally effective. Oral CTX and AZA may be less effective, but superior to corticosteroid therapy alone.

It is challenging to provide recommendations for any specific treatment regimen as differences in baseline characteristics between study populations, protocol design, treatments used, duration of trials etc make comparisons difficult. Although the Houssiau study begins to address this question, additional studies to identify a more optimal dosing regimen of CTX are necessary.

Case presentation

It was explained to Patient 1 that the optimal dosing regimen for cyclophosphamide was not known, but that tolerability issues support the use of IV dosing. Her treating physician recommended a dose of 0·5 g/m^2.

Question 5

Are there alternatives to CTX that improve survival compared to glucocorticoids alone? In a patient who refuses CTX, is resistant to CTX, or has toxicity from CTX are there alternative therapies that improve survival and/or maintain renal function?

It would be useful to know that a number of alternative therapies were demonstrated to improve mortality, reduce the development of ESRD in SLE nephritis, and were better tolerated than CTX. Although there are several studies that have examined the use of alternative therapies in SLE nephritis, none has specifically examined efficacy in patients who have failed CTX. To illustrate the lack of consensus as to what to use in this situation, Houssiau *et al*[17] listed immunosuppressive agents used after initial failure of treatment. These included additional IV or oral CTX (after the use either the low or high dose IV CTX regimen), mycophenolate mofetil (MMF), ciclosporin (CsA), or 6-mercaptopurine (6-MP). Published reports examining alternative therapies to CTX have addressed the issue in "head to head" comparisons of immunosuppressive agents and will be discussed below.

Both meta-analyses cited in the response to Question 1 assessed renal outcomes with use of AZA. In the Felson meta-analysis,[7] pooled analyses indicated that both AZA as well as CTX were associated with a 40% reduction in the rates of adverse renal outcomes in comparison to steroids alone. In the Bansal meta-analysis, rates of total mortality and ESRD were not significantly different between CTX and AZA, nor for AZA and prednisone. Point estimates for absolute risk differences always favoured AZA, although the confidence intervals for the comparison of AZA versus prednisone included 0 for both outcomes and was therefore not statistically significant.

Ginzler *et al*[18] published a double blind crossover trial in 1976 comparing AZA alone to AZA plus CTX. No specific discussion of the method of blinding or method of randomisation was provided. Therapeutic success was defined as patients with normal or stable serum creatinine, complement, and urine protein and RBCs were absent from urinalysis while receiving

Table 6.5 Adverse effects (number observed/number at risk) (Boumpas *et al*, 1992)[16]

Adverse effect	Methylprednisolone	Short course CTX	Long course CTX
Major infection	0/25	1/20	1/20
Herpes zoster	3/25	2/20	1/20
Malignancy	0/25	0/20	1/20
Haemorrhagic cystitis	0/25	0/20	0/20
Premature ovarian failure	0/15	3/16	5/13
Osteonecrosis	3/17	3/16	4/14
Cataracts	6/17	5/15	3/14

≤ 20 mg of prednisone. Patients who were therapeutic failures on one regimen (AZA 2·5 mg/kg/day versus AZA plus CTX each at 1·25 mg/kg/day, randomly assigned) were crossed over to the other regimen. Two patients in the AZA group and 3 in the combined AZA plus CTX group crossed over to the opposite regimen. The alternate regimen was successful in 1 of 2 patients switching to AZA plus CTX and 2 of 3 to AZA alone.

Although definitive proof awaits additional data, the meta-analyses and above report indicate that AZA is efficacious in the treatment of SLE nephritis.

Several alternative therapies have been examined for the treatment of lupus nephritis. Each therapy will be discussed in turn. Plasmapheresis will be discussed below (see Question 10).

Chan *et al*[13] published an RCT comparing combination treatment with MMF and prednisolone to oral CTX and prednisolone. Forty-two patients with diffuse proliferative glomerulonephritis were randomly assigned (no discussion of method of randomisation was provided) to receive either: oral MMF (started at 1 g twice a day) plus oral prednisolone or oral CTX (2·5 mg/kg/day) plus oral prednisolone; after 6 months the dose of MMF was halved and CTX was replaced by AZA (1·5 mg/kg/day); after 12 months MMF was replaced by AZA at 1·5 mg/kg/day. There was no discussion of blinding. The incidence of complete remission (defined as urinary protein < 0·3 g per 24 hours, with normal sediment, normal serum albumin, values for both serum creatinine and creatinine clearance that were 15% or less above the baseline value) was the primary endpoint; secondary endpoints included partial remission, adverse effects, and doubling of serum creatinine, relapse of SLE, and death. Outcomes in all 42 patients were reported. There was no discussion of equivalence margins or whether the study was powered to detect a difference between treatment effects.

There were no statistical differences between groups in complete remissions or partial remissions, treatment failures, relapses or discontinuations of treatment (all outcomes, $p = 1·00$) and deaths ($p = 0·49$). Times to complete remission ($p = 0·15$), partial remission ($p = 0·81$), and relapse ($p = 0·70$) were not different between groups. There were significant improvements from baseline in serum C3, albumin, serum creatinine ($p = 0·02$ for MMF and $p = 0·01$ for CTX) and urinary protein excretion but not for creatinine clearance ($p = 0·15$ in MMF and $p = 0·18$ in CTX groups).

There were no statistical differences in adverse effects, including: infections ($p = 0·45$), herpes zoster ($p = 0·60$), leucopenia, alopecia,

Table 6.6 Adverse effects (Houssiau *et al*, 2002)[17]

Adverse effect	All patients ($n = 89$)	High dose IV CTX ($n = 45$)	Low dose IV CTX ($n = 44$)
Death	2	0	2
ESRD	3	2	1
Doubling of serum creatinine	4	1	3
Severe infection (total)	24	17	7
Leucopenia (<4000/microlitre)	10	5	5
Menopause	4	2	2
Avascular necrosis	1	1	0

amenorrhoea (p = 0·09) or diarrhoea, as well as deaths (p = 0·49).

This single RCT demonstrated that MMF and prednisolone appeared to be as effective as CTX and prednisolone, both followed by AZA and prednisolone, in patients with SLE nephritis. Patients in this study had little evidence of chronic glomerular changes; those with serum creatinine >3·4 mg/dl were excluded and only 3/42 were men, indicating few individuals with poor prognostic indicators were included in the trial.

In a small study Boletis *et al*[19] randomised 14 patients with proliferative SLE nephritis who had received prednisone and monthly IV CTX (1 g/m^2) for 6 months to receive monthly intravenous immunoglobulin (IVIG) (400 mg/kg monthly) for 18 months or IV CTX every 2 months for 6 months and quarterly for one year. There was no discussion of methods of randomisation or blinding. All 14 patients completed the study and results from all enrolled patients were presented. There were no substantial changes in serum creatinine (p = 0·83) or creatinine clearance (p = 0·80) in both groups; mean changes in proteinuria were similar (p = 0·71). No patient withdrew due to adverse effects or deterioration of renal function.

Therefore, IVIG may be useful in maintaining remission in those who have responded to CTX therapy.

Fu *et al*[20] reported a trial in 40 children with SLE nephritis class III–IV and normal creatinine clearances previously treated with IV methylprednisolone followed by oral prednisolone. With persistent heavy proteinuria, they were randomised to receive either ciclosporin (CsA) (started at 5 mg/kg/day every 12 hours and adjusted to trough levels between 75 and 150 ng/ml) or CTX (2 mg/kg/day) plus prednisolone (2 mg/kg/day). The treatment code was contained in sealed completely opaque envelopes numbered in sequence according to a table of random numbers. No mention of blinding was made. Results in 38 of 40 patients were analysed; 2 in the CsA group withdrew due to acute exacerbations of SLE nephritis. Proteinuria improved significantly in both groups – CsA $p < 0·05$; CTX plus prednisolone $p < 0·01$ – without significant changes in creatinine clearance in either group. In the CsA group, anti-ds DNA antibodies, CH50, and C3 levels significantly improved ($p < 0·05$ for all); anti-dsDNA antibody levels only improved in the CTX plus prednisolone group ($p < 0·01$). Growth rate increased significantly after one year with CsA treatment, and remained unchanged in the CTX plus prednisolone group ($p < 0·01$). Adverse effects including hypertension, diabetes, paraesthesias and tremor were not reported during treatment.

There are no other RCTs examining CsA in the treatment of SLE nephritis.

Evidence summary: Silver

In summary, the preferred alternative to CTX appears to be AZA and there is RCT evidence that AZA is effective in reducing adverse renal outcomes and mortality for treatment of SLE nephritis . Other RCTs showed benefit with MMF and CsA on some outcomes , although longer term studies with other outcomes including development of ESRD and doubling of serum creatinine etc are required before any of these regimens can be recommended with confidence.

Case presentation

Patient 1 remained undecided about therapy. The patient seemed interested in MMF and the results of the study using MMF were further discussed. She was reminded that this was a single RCT supporting its use. Azathioprine might also be an option for this patient. Ultimately the patient chose MMF because of safety concerns with the use of cyclophosphamide.

Question 6

What are effective approaches to the treatment of a flare or relapse of SLE nephritis?

There are no RCTs specifically examining treatment of relapses or flares in SLE nephritis after either response to or failure of initial therapy. Various approaches to the treatment of relapses in RCTs to date will be presented.

In the NIH case series reported by Gourley *et al*[11] patients who were no longer receiving monthly therapy but who had evidence of reactivation of glomerular disease after the first year of treatment (defined as new active nephritis with an increase of at least 50% of two of the following: number of dysmorphic RBC, number of cellular casts, proteinuria, or serum creatinine) received their originally assigned regimen (IV methylprednisolone, IV CTX or combination).

In a systematic follow up of the Gourley study, Illei *et al*[12,21] identified the outcomes of all 82 patients. Additional immunosuppressive therapy after the protocol completion was required in 34 patients: high dose corticosteroids ($n = 2$), IV CTX ($n = 26$) or combination ($n = 6$). Reasons for additional therapy included persistent nephritis ($n = 24$), renal flare ($n = 9$), or major extrarenal flare ($n = 1$). The specific outcomes in each group were not provided.

Means of handling treatment failures in the reported RCTs may provide some insight as to how to treat relapses. Illei *et al*[21] examined the prevalence of renal flares in the cohort of patients who had originally participated in two RCTs at the NIH.[11,16] Of 82 patients, 73 had an initial complete response, and 19 a partial response/stabilisation. There were a total of 29 flares (6 were proteinuric and 23 nephritic) in the complete response group and 12 flares (2 proteinuric and 10 nephritic) in the partial responders. In patients with initial complete responses who subsequently flared, treatment included IV CTX with or without IV methylprednisolone in 12 of 29 flares; 5 received other immunosuppressive agents including pulse methylprednisolone, AZA, or cladribine; 4 received prednisone alone and 8 of 29 received no therapy. Three patients progressed to ESRD. In the partial response group 6/12 were treated with IV CTX with or without pulse methylprednisolone, 4 received other immunosuppressive agents, and one each received prednisone or no therapy. Eight patients progressed to ESRD.

Houssiau *et al*[17] summarised the immunosuppressive regimens prescribed to patients after failure of the initial treatment regimen in the EU RCT comparing low to continuous dose CTX. Patients failing either low or high dose IV CTX were given additional doses of IV CTX as well as CsA, MMF, 6-MP, and oral CTX. No dose or

Table 6.7 Adverse effects (Chan *et al*, 2000)[13]

Adverse effect	MMF ($n = 21$) n	%	CTX ($n = 21$) n	%
Infection				
Herpes zoster	2	33	2	20
Tuberculosis	0		1	10
Other				
Amenorrhoea	0		2	23
Death	0		2	10

duration of treatment was provided. In the study by Fu *et al*[20] subjects with SLE nephritis initially unresponsive to oral prednisolone received pulse IV methylprednisolone. If patients continued to have active nephritis they were then randomised to receive either CsA or prednisolone plus CTX.

Evidence summary: Bronze

No specific recommendations can be made in terms of the optimal approach to treatment of relapse or flare of SLE nephritis. A number of alternative approaches have been used in clinical practice, but none has proven effective. Based purely on clinical grounds it appears that treatment of relapses depends at least to some extent on when the relapse occurs. Those occurring after the first 6 months of monthly IV CTX therapy during the initiation of quarterly treatment would likely necessitate the re-institution of monthly IV CTX therapy. Relapses that occur during the first 6 months of monthly IV CTX pulses may signify that therapy was ineffective, necessitating a complete change in immunosuppressive regimens.

Question 7

In a patient in whom remission has been successfully achieved with CTX, which drugs are the most effective (for example, AZA) maintenance treatments ? After remission, are there any therapies effective for long term maintenance?

There are no RCTs in which all patients are initially treated with the same regimen of CTX and then randomised to receive alternative therapies once a remission (or stabilisation) is achieved. There is an ongoing randomised controlled study in Europe examining the role of CsA versus AZA in preventing renal flares after remission is initially induced with CTX plus steroids. Houssiau *et al*[17] used AZA maintenance therapy following a comparison of high with low dose IV CTX. Mok *et al*[22] prescribed AZA for at least another 18 months after comparing IV CTX with sequential oral CTX for 6 months. Chan *et al*[13]) used AZA (2 mg/kg/day) after comparing oral MMF with oral CTX. The studies discussed above illustrate various forms of maintenance therapy but no specific conclusions regarding their efficacy can be reached.

Alarcon-Segovia *et al*,[23] in a double blind placebo controlled study of 230 SLE patients, determined if LJP 394 delayed or prevented renal flares in SLE patients with a history of renal disease (patients not enrolled if they had evidence of active renal disease within 3 months of screening). In the intent to treat population, time to renal flare was not significantly different between treatment groups but LJP 394 treated patients had a longer time to institution of high dose corticosteroids and/or CTX (HDCC) ($p = 0{\cdot}033$) and required 41% fewer treatments with HDCC ($p = 0{\cdot}026$). In the high affinity population (patients with high affinity anti-dsDNA antibody binding to the nucleotide epitope on LJP 394), the active treatment group experienced a longer time to renal flare ($p = 0{\cdot}008$), 67% fewer flares ($p = 0{\cdot}008$), longer time to HDCC ($p = 0{\cdot}002$), and 62% fewer treatments with HDCC ($p = 0{\cdot}001$) compared with placebo.

Serious adverse effects were observed in 26/114 (23%) of LJP 394 treated patients and 34/116 (29%) placebo patients. Most were not considered related to treatment.

Evidence summary: Bronze

The use of maintenance therapy must be guided by the long term risk/benefit ratio and although AZA appears to be the most frequently used agent, there are no data to support its effectiveness when used in this fashion. Additional studies examining the use of LJP 394 in individuals with a history of SLE nephritis are awaited, to better answer this question.

Case presentation

Patient 1 remained on MMF and continues to do well.

Question 8

In a patient with active SLE do high dose (or pulse) steroids improve mortality or morbidity?

Several studies have attempted to address this issue. In a very small RCT Liebling *et al*[24] studied 9 patients with SLE nephritis who were randomly assigned to receive monthly IV methylprednisolone (1 g) on three consecutive days for 12 months or placebo. Daily oral prednisone doses (most individuals were on prednisone 60 mg just before entering the study) were aggressively tapered on an individual basis during the study by one of the investigators. The study was double blind; patients received identically packaged methylprednisolone or placebo; the method of randomisation was not mentioned.

Mean values for all creatinine clearances over the course of the study were significantly better in the active treatment group than placebo ($p < 0{\cdot}05$). At the end of treatment there were no differences between groups in serum creatinine, creatinine clearances or proteinuria. At the last reported follow up, 35 months in the active group and 26 months in placebo since last pulse treatment, serum creatinine and creatinine clearances were significantly different ($p < 0{\cdot}02$). During this follow up period the mean daily prednisone dose was 8·1 in the active and 17·5 mg in the placebo group ($p < 0{\cdot}025$). Two patients in placebo developed ESRD; one died while awaiting dialysis.

This small RCT indicates that pulse methylprednisolone is more effective than placebo in treating SLE nephritis, even with relatively short term follow up periods of less than 3 years. One patient developed aseptic necrosis of the hip one year and 4 months after the last pulse; one patient developed glucose intolerance; one patient developed arthralgias. There were significantly fewer infections in the methylprednisolone group ($p < 0{\cdot}05$ by Fisher exact test). There were no significant changes in laboratory testing.

In the Boumpas[16] RCT cited under Question 4 it was demonstrated that pulse CTX is more effective than pulse methylprednisolone in preserving renal function and that a continued course of CTX reduces the risk of renal flare, compared with only 6 months' treatment with CTX.

In a third study Sesso *et al*[25] randomly assigned 29 patients (the method of randomisation was not provided) to receive IV CTX (0·5–1 g/m^2) monthly for 4 months, bimonthly for 4 and then quarterly for 6 months, or IV methylprednisolone 10–20 mg/kg with maximal dose of 1 g) in three daily doses followed by three single monthly doses, bimonthly for 4 and quarterly for 6 months. There was no discussion of a method of blinding. Outcomes assessed included death, progression to ESRD (or doubling of serum creatinine over baseline), remission and exacerbation of nephritis, and complications of therapy. Follow up was up to 18 months. Outcomes were provided in all 29 patients. The probability of not developing ESRD or doubling serum creatinine were not significantly different ($p > 0{\cdot}20$) between treatment groups, nor the probability of survival without renal failure ($p > 0{\cdot}20$). There were 2 deaths in IV CTX and

3 in the methylprednisolone groups; and 8 and 9 remissions, respectively (both were not significantly different). One patient in each group died from pulmonary infection; one receiving CTX developed tuberculous meningitis and recovered. There were no malignancies, osteonecrosis, or haemorrhagic cystitis reported. In summary, these results suggest that pulse CTX is as effective as pulse methylprednisolone in preserving renal function.

In a fourth study, the report by Illei *et al* on the long term follow up of the NIH RCT, cited previously,[12] with benefit of longer term follow up, pulse methylprednisolone added to IV CTX appeared to improve long term renal outcome without additive toxicity.

Evidence summary: Silver

IV CTX appears to be superior to pulse methylprednisolone alone for treatment of SLE nephritis.

The combination of IV CTX and pulse methylprednisolone may provide additional benefit over CTX alone with little additional risk for adverse effects. However, this approach has not been shown to improve mortality or decrease the risk of developing ESRD.

Case presentation

The use of pulse corticosteroids would be appropriate and this was also discussed with Patient 1. Based on the above study results, the patient preferred not to use pulse corticosteroid therapy.

Question 9

Is the approach to therapy for membranous SLE nephritis different than for proliferative nephritis? Is CTX efficacious for membranous nephritis, for example does it improve survival or time to ESRD?

Unfortunately there are no prospective RCTs that specifically address treatment of membranous SLE nephritis. While several reported RCTs include a limited number of patients with membranous disease, there are either too few patients included, or renal outcomes are not segregated by histopathological type, to allow any specific conclusions. Reports of treatment that do separate out patients with membranous lesions in SLE have been either case reports or retrospective reviews. In the absence of data, clinicians have extrapolated from RCTs in proliferative idiopathic membranous nephritis. This is problematic because SLE membranous disease has several pathological characteristics which distinguish it from proliferative idiopathic membranous nephritis, and its natural history is unknown. Additional factors relating to the influence of other organ system disease on renal function make direct comparisons difficult.

Chan *et al*[26] reported a case series in which a cohort of 20 patients with nephrotic syndrome due to pure membranous SLE nephritis received oral prednisolone and oral CTX initially followed by AZA for maintenance treatment. This study was neither randomised nor controlled. This study demonstrated that renal function remained stable during follow up for 73 ± 49 months.

Based on the above discussion, no specific recommendations can be made for appropriate therapy for pure membranous nephritis in SLE. The reader is referred to a recent review of the topic[27] for more information and a bibliography. Further studies of the treatment of membranous nephritis in SLE are needed.

Evidence summary: Bronze

There is insufficient evidence on whether to treat these patients differently from patients with proliferative nephritis.

Question 10

Does plasmapheresis add to the efficacy of prednisone and CTX and improve morbidity or mortality in SLE nephritis?

Plasmapheresis (PP) theoretically can remove pathogenic autoantibodies which may ameliorate disease activity. Lewis *et al*[28] studied 86 patients with SLE nephritis randomised to receive prednisone and CTX (2 mg/kg orally; standard therapy) or standard therapy plus PP (three times weekly for 4 weeks). Randomisation sequences were generated by the Biostatistical Coordinating Center which issued treatment assignments by telephone. No discussion of blinding was presented. Outcomes included: time to death, ESRD (renal failure, initiation of dialysis, or renal transplant), length of time before a treatment stopping point (as defined in the article, examples included increase in serum creatinine, ESRD, major extrarenal manifestation etc) was reached, as well as changes in 24 hour urinary protein and serum creatinine, IgG anti-dsDNA antibody, cryoglobulin, and Complement 3 and 4 levels.

The study was terminated early (after 86 subjects entered) because results showed no significant differences between treatment groups in primary outcome measures ($n = 86$). P values for each of the endpoints are as follows: death ($p = 0{\cdot}39$); renal failure ($p = 0{\cdot}39$); renal failure or death ($p = 0{\cdot}26$), treatment stopping points ($p = 0{\cdot}35$). P values for other endpoints include: proportion surviving ($p = 0{\cdot}41$); proportion surviving without renal failure ($p = 0{\cdot}26$); proportion who had not reached treatment stopping points ($p = 0{\cdot}30$).

There were statistical differences only in laboratory parameters in the PP treatment group: serum IgG lower weeks 2–6 ($p < 0{\cdot}05$), anti-dsDNA antibody levels lower at weeks 2,3,5 ($p < 0{\cdot}05$), and cryoglobulins lower weeks 2–7 ($p < 0{\cdot}05$).

Results in the PP group were actually numerically worse in almost every endpoint although PP treatment did not appear to increase the risk for infections in these immunosuppressed patients with severe SLE nephritis.[29]

Derksen *et al*[30] examined the short term effects of PP versus cytotoxics in steroid resistant SLE nephritis. Twenty subjects who had an insufficient response to treatment with steroids alone for at least 3 weeks were randomly assigned to PP three times a week for 3 weeks (9 patients) or immunosuppressive agents (11; AZA in 7 and CTX in 4; dose of AZA and CTX was 2 mg/kg orally). Patients were assigned treatment by drawing lots from a card sequence derived from a random numbers table. No discussion of blinding was provided. At 3 weeks 5 patients were determined to have had a "sufficient" response, 3 in the PP and 2 in the immunosuppressive groups. Longer term follow up was confounded by changes in treatments within groups. In conclusion, this short study did not support the use of PP.

Because PP may lead to a rebound in antibody production thereby resulting in higher anti-dsDNA antibody levels that might obscure the positive effects of PP, coadministration of immunosuppressive agents has been advocated.to prevent this rebound. Wallace *et al*[31] studied 19 subjects who were randomised to receive six pulses of CTX (750 mg/m^2) alone or pulse CTX preceded in each cycle by three daily plasmaphereses; prednisone was used in both groups. The method of randomisation was not provided. No discussion of blinding was presented. Outcomes included: serum creatinine, anti-DNA, C3, 24 hour urine protein, serum albumin, and SLAM scores. All but one patient was analysed; the one dropout after 2 months protocol treatment was due to a femoral fracture following an injury. SLAM scores improved in both groups (change from study entry to 2 years significant at $p = 0{\cdot}02$ for CTX and $p = 0{\cdot}01$ for CTX/PP) without significant differences between groups. No patient died.

Three patients in each group were considered to be in renal remission (defined by serum creatinine <1·4, 24 hour urine protein < 500 mg, absence of urinary casts, normal blood pressure, serum albumin >4·0).There were no significant differences between groups in each of the parameters measured.

Evidence summary: Silver

Three RCTS found no benefit from plasmapheresis. It does not appear at this time that PP offers additional efficacy over and above a regimen of prednisone and CTX, although in the short term, PP does not appear to increase the risk of infection.

Case presentation

Patient 1 was not offered PP as an option at the time of presentation.

Question 11

Is there evidence that any therapies are effective in the treatment of neuropsychiatric SLE?

Neuropsychiatric SLE (NPSLE) includes a diverse set of clinical disorders with multiple manifestations ranging from headaches to seizures, strokes, psychosis, or transverse myelitis, and is likely to be caused by multiple mechanisms including autoantibodies (such as anti-phospholipid, anti-neuronal and anti-dsDNA antibodies etc), microvasculopathy, and inflammation (with local cytokine production). The key to diagnosis is identifying whether NPSLE manifestations are due to SLE, infection, adverse effects due to medications such as steroid psychosis, or metabolic abnormalities including uraemia. Unfortunately, there are no specific laboratory studies that can be used to confirm the diagnosis. Many clinical manifestations such as transverse myelitis are relatively rare, therefore attempts to define and rigorously study NPSLE in RCTs have been exceedingly difficult.

A recent Cochrane systematic review[32] attempted to assess the efficacy and safety of CTX and methylprednisolone in the treatment of NPSLE. However, the authors found no RCTs comparing the use of these therapies for the treatment of NPSLE. Of 16 studies cited, 11 referred only to renal disease and did not include information about other clinical manifestations of SLE. Of the remaining 5 studies, one was a protocol, one included only patients taking different regimens of CTX where only laboratory findings were analysed, and the last three included patients with systemic manifestations of SLE but did not include sufficient information. The authors concluded that there was "no evidence of effect" and not that there was "evidence of no effect".

It is worth mentioning two recent abstracts relating to therapy of NPSLE. In the first, Barile *et al*[33] randomised patients with NPSLE manifestations including refractory seizures, peripheral neuropathy, optic neuritis, transverse myelitis, coma, brainstem disease, and cranial neuropathy, to receive either IV CTX or IV methylprednisolone monthly. After a minimum of 4 months of follow up (up to 12 months) 12/20 patients on CTX improved compared with 7/11 on methylprednisolone ($p < 0·01$). There were 11 infections in CTX group and 7 in the methylprednisolone group.

In the second abstract, Van Vollenhoven *et al*[34] examined the effects of DHEA on cognitive function in lupus. Patients were randomised to either DHEA or placebo. Patients treated with DHEA showed a significant improvement in attention/concentration and memory/learning ($p < 0·02$ overall). The number of responders was greater in the DHEA versus placebo group for attention/concentration ($p < 0·05$) and

Table 6.8 Summary of RCts in the treatment of lupus nephritis with cytotoxic

Study	No.	Drugs	Level of evidence*	Outcomes	Comments; renal pathology
Felson[7]	250	P, I	Silver	Mortality and ESRD decrease with I	Meta-analysis of 8 studies
Bansal[8]	440	P, I	Silver	Mortality and ESRD decrease with I	Meta-analysis of 19 studies
Steinber[9]	38	P + C or A or placebo	Silver (double blind and placebo)	For renal measures (Cr clearance, urine sediment, proteinuria) C > A ($p < 0{\cdot}005$) or placebo ($p < 0{\cdot}005$)	3 with membranous, one with biopsy not available for review; remainder with DPGN
Steinberg[10]	13	Placebo or C + P	Silver	C>placebo for 5 indexes including anti-DNS, serum C, urine sediment, proteinuria, extra-renal disease ($p < 0{\cdot}001$)	No biopsies reported
Gourley[11]	82	IV MP, IV C, combo	Silver (not blinded)	Renal remission C>MP ($p = 0{\cdot}038$)	All with proliferative GN on biopsy
Illei[12]	82	IV MP, IV C, combo	Silver	Treatment failure lower in C ($p = 0{\cdot}04$) and combo ($p = 0{\cdot}002$) groups compared to M but no difference in death or ESRD	Follow up of Gourley[11] study
Chan[13]	42	Oral MMF + prednisolone, oral CTX + prednisolone	Silver	No statistical difference for complete remission ($p = 1{\cdot}0$), partial remission (1·0), treatment failure (1·0), relapse (1·0), death (0·49)	All with DPGN
Austin[14]	107	Oral P, oral A, C, combo, IV C	Silver	Prob. to no renal failure IV C>P ($p = 0{\cdot}027$)	60 with DPGN, 11 with membranoproliferative, 7 focal, 16 with membranous, 7 mesangial, 6 no biopsy
Steinberg[15]	111	P, oral A, C, IV C, combo	Silver	ESRD: IV C> P ($p = 0{\cdot}0025$) oral C>P ($p = 0{\cdot}032$)	Long term follow up of Austin[14] study
Boumpas[16]	65	MP, C (long and short course)	Silver	Renal insufficiency M *v* C ($p = 0{\cdot}037$)	56 with DPGN, 3 with membranous, 5 with focal
Houssiau[17]	90	High dose IV C, low dose IV C	Silver	No difference between groups for treatment failure, renal remission, renal flares	21 class III; 62 class IV; 7 class V

(Continued)

Table 6.8 (Continued)

Study	No.	Drugs	Level of evidence*	Outcomes	Comments; renal pathology
Ginzler[18]	14; cross over	A, low dose A plus C	Silver (blinded but no placebo)	No difference in changes in creatinine, proteinuria, C3	2 membranous; all others with DPGN
Boletis[19]	14	IV Ig, IV C	Silver	No difference in change in creatinine or Cr clearance ($p = 0{\cdot}80$)	11 with type III; 3 with type IV
Sesso[25]	29	IV C, IV M	Silver	Prob. not developing renal failure ($p > 0{\cdot}20$); prob. survival without renal failure ($p > 0{\cdot}20$)	23 with class IV renal biopsy; 1 with class III; 3 with class II; not available in 2
Lewis[28]	86	P + C, P + C + PP	Silver	No difference in primary outcomes including time to death, time to renal failure	Terminated after 86 subjects entered; 24 class III; 35 class IV; 26 class V; one non-qualifying biopsy
Wallace[31]	19	Pulse C, pulse C + PP	Silver	No differences between groups	12 with class IV and 6 with class III; one dropped out
Carette[54]	53	Oral A, C, P alone	Silver	Prob. stable renal function C>P ($p = 0{\cdot}03$) Prob. avoiding renal failure C>P ($p = 0{\cdot}07$)	40 with DPGN. 4 membranous, 2 focal, 5 mesangial
Dinant[55]	41	Oral P, oral C, A, IV C	Silver	No difference for renal outcomes, change serum creat. or Cr clearance	26 with DPGN; 5 membranous, 4 membranoproliferative, 3 focal, 2 mesangial
Decker[56]	38	P alone, P + oral C, P + oral A	Silver	No differences for Cr clearance	All with DPGN
Donadio[57]	50	P, oral C + P	Silver	Prob. stable renal course Oral C>P ($p \cong 0{\cdot}04$)	All with DPGN
Donadio[58]	19 entered (16 completed)	P alone, P + A	Silver	No difference in renal biopsies or Cr clearance at 6 months	Biopsies at start and at 6 months with scoring by activity
Donadio[59]	39	P, P + C	Silver	No differences in Cr clearance ($p = 0{\cdot}93$); proteinuria ($p = 0{\cdot}33$); prob. no further renal progression C>P ($p \cong 0{\cdot}03$)	Active GN on biopsy not otherwise specified; 22/39 biopsies with crescents
Donadio[60]	16	P alone, P + A	Silver	No difference in major renal flares	Extension of 1972 study
Balletta[61]	10	P alone, P + CsA	Silver	Proteinuria decreased in CsA group from baseline while in P group there was no change	2 DPGN; 1 membranous;1 focal; 1 mesangioproliferative; 1 membranoproliferative

(Continued)

Table 6.8 (*Continued*)

Study	No.	Drugs*	Level of evidence*	Outcomes	Comments; renal pathology
Hahn[62]	24	P alone, A + P	Silver	No differences in deaths, renal or extra-renal disease	Focal GN 8, membranous 3, membranoproliferative 9
Sztejnbok[63]	35	P alone, P + A	Silver	Decrease morbidity and mortality in A group	No biopsy
Cade[64]	50	P alone, A + P, A alone, A + heparin	Silver.	Combination of A + P or A + heparin improved survival compared to A or P alone	Biopsy results not provided

Abbreviations: P = prednisone; MP = methylprednisolone; C = cyclophosphamide; A = azathioprine; CsA = cyclosporin; IV = intravenous; PP = plasmapharesis; IV Ig = intravenous gammaglobulin; MMF = mycophenolate mofetil.

*Studies are designated Silver because they were in general not blinded. There was no discussion of allocation concealment.

memory/learning ($p < 0{\cdot}01$). Changes in cognitive scores did not correlate with changes in depression scores. The complete results of both of these abstracts are pending at the time of writing.

Evidence summary: Bronze

In clinical practice immunosuppressive agents as well as adjunctive therapy directed at the specific manifestation (such as treatment of seizures with anti-seizure medications) are used. Improved diagnostic techniques are needed to better define the multiple manifestations of NPSLE, as well as RCTs to examine treatment with immunosuppressive agents.

Question 12

Aside from steroids and NSAIDs, are there any medications that are effective in treating cutaneous and musculoskeletal manifestations of SLE? Is antimalarial therapy effective in the treatment of active SLE or the prevention of SLE flares?

Antimalarials have been used for the treatment of mild to moderate SLE since the 1940s.[35] Because of its efficacy and safety profile, hydroxychloroquine or chloroquine are now considered the main treatments for cutaneous and musculoskeletal manifestations of SLE. Despite widespread use there are relatively few RCTs assessing their efficacy in SLE.

The first placebo RCT with hydroxychloroquine enrolled 47 patients with stable SLE who were randomised to either continue their usual dose of medication or receive placebo (Canadian Hydroxychloroquine Study Group[36]). Outcome measures included SLE flares: defined as the development or worsening of specific clinical manifestations of SLE according to ARA criteria and an early version of the SLEDAI (Systemic Lupus Erythematosus Disease Activity Index), before it had been fully validated. During the 24-week study, 16/22 or 73% patients withdrawn from hydroxychloroquine experienced a flare, compared with 9/25 or 36% continuing treatment (time to flare $p = 0{\cdot}02$ versus placebo). Disease flares were characterised predominantly by cutaneous disease, nasopharyngeal ulcerations, arthritis, and constitutional symptoms. In 6 patients severe exacerbation of SLE required withdrawal from the study, 5/22 or 23% in placebo and 1/25 or 4% in active treatment. There was no statistical difference in the changes of prednisone dose between the groups.

This trial was not designed to address safety as all patients had been receiving hydroxychloroquine for 6 months prior to study entry. The authors concluded that hydroxychloroquine may contribute to continued control of active disease and its continued use may prevent mild to moderate SLE flares. These positive results prompted continued observation of these patients over a longer follow up period. Although treating physicians were allowed to make therapeutic choices after the 6 month RCT, patients were encouraged to continue their assigned therapy (hydroxychloroquine or not). Following 42 months of treatment, a retrospective report[37] indicated that major SLE flares occurred less frequently in patients taking hydroxychloroquine (28% *v* 50% placebo; relative risk reduction of 57%, which did not reach statistical significance. Adverse effects were not reported.

A single RCT addressed the efficacy of chloroquine diphosphate in the management of patients with mild to moderate manifestations of SLE: 24 patients were randomised to receive 250 mg chloroquine diphosphate or placebo daily.[38] Primary outcomes included the number of SLE flares and decrease in daily prednisone requirements. There was no discussion of randomisation or blinding other than the use of a placebo. There was a statistically significant reduction in number of flares in patients receiving active therapy (2/11 or 18% *v* 10/12 or 83% placebo, $p < 0{\cdot}01$); and a significant difference in the number of patients able to reduce their prednisone dose > 50% of baseline (82% *v* 25%, $p < 0{\cdot}01$). There were no significant differences in SLEDAI scores between treatment groups.

One episode of dyspepsia, in a patient receiving placebo, required withdrawal from the study. No other adverse effects, including retinal toxicity were reported.

The Cooperative Systemic Studies of the Rheumatic Diseases conducted a multicentre, double blind placebo RCT evaluating 200 mg hydroxychloroquine BID for the treatment of SLE associated arthralgias and/or non-erosive arthritis in 71 patients.[39] Patients with abnormal renal function or active manifestations of disease requiring >10 mg prednisone daily were excluded. There were no significant differences between treatment groups by joint tenderness and swelling scores, although patient-assessed joint pain was improved in the hydroxychloroquine group compared with placebo. Twenty-nine patients (41%) discontinued study participation early, the majority for lack of efficacy, further confounding interpretation of the results. Two patients (both in active treatment) withdrew due to adverse effects: one each for rash and dizziness. The benefit of hydroxychloroquine treatment for articular manifestations of SLE are modest at best, and are not well supported by this study.

Evidence summary: Silver

Three RCTs found mixed results to support the use of antimalarials to prevent flares of SLE. As these trials were of short duration and included only small sample sizes, it is not possible to assess the safety of antimalarials or their long term efficacy in the treatment of SLE, based on their results.

Case presentation

The use of antimalarials and the adverse effects were discussed with Patient 1. She elected to start an antimalarial.

Hydroxychloroquine at 200–400 mg/day were recommended to Patient 2 to treat her malar rash and arthritis. Its low adverse effect profile and possibility of reducing the frequency and severity of subsequent flares was appealing to the patient and she elected to start antimalarial therapy.

Question 13

Can hydroxychloroquine be continued if a patient with SLE becomes pregnant?

Antimalarials are known to cross the placenta,[40] although most data regarding their use during pregnancy are restricted to retrospective case series.[41–43] A placebo RCT examining the use of hydroxychloroquine during pregnancy was recently published.[44] Twenty patients at between 8 and 18 weeks of pregnancy were randomised to receive an unstated dose of hydroxychloroquine or identical placebo. Significant improvement in skin disease as well as decreases in prednisone doses at delivery were reported in patients taking hydroxychloroquine compared with placebo. There were no SLE flares in the active treatment group compared with 3 of 10 receiving placebo, but this did not reach statistical significance. There were no statistical differences in SLEDAI scores or fetal outcomes between the groups. Examination of all offspring between 1·5 and 3 years of age, including ophthalmological examination, did not reveal any abnormalities. However the sample size was small and composed of a heterogeneous mixture of patients with discoid and systemic manifestations, prior antimalarial use and naive patients. As patients were not randomised to treatment until later in pregnancy (8–18 weeks, average 11 weeks) important information about exposure early in pregnancy was not obtained.

Evidence summary: Silver

This is a small RCT suggesting that hydroxychloroquine use during pregnancy appears to be well tolerated without significant adverse effects to mother or fetus.

Case presentation

The issue of hydroxychloroquine use during pregnancy was discussed with Patient 2. She was uncomfortable continuing the medication in the event of a pregnancy because of the lack of adequate data based on a single trial involving few subjects. She plans to discontinue hydroxychloroquine prior to planning a pregnancy.

Question 14

What is the role for DHEA in the treatment of active SLE? Can it be used to achieve a sustained reduction in steroid dose? Are there any other benefits of DHEA for lupus patients?

Several lines of evidence have suggested administration of dehydroepiandrosterone (DHEA), a naturally occurring adrenal androgen, for the treatment of mild to moderate manifestations of SLE.[45]

The first RCT randomised 28 patients to receive 200 mg DHEA or identical placebo daily for 3 months.[46] Patients were allowed to continue baseline corticosteroids or hydroxychloroquine; changes in these medications were allowed at the discretion of the treating physician. Clinical outcomes included changes in SLEDAI score and prednisone doses at 3 months; there was no significant difference between treatment groups in either measure. The incidence of flares was evaluated retrospectively, defined as the use of the term "flare" by the primary treating physician. There were fewer "flares" in the DHEA (3/14) than the placebo group (8/14), which approached, but did not meet statistical significance ($p = 0{\cdot}053$).

Acneiform dermatitis was the most frequently reported adverse event (8/14 patients receiving active treatment versus 1/14 patients placebo). Hirsutism, weight gain, rash, menstrual irregularities, and emotional lability were reported with similar frequencies in both groups.

Following this trial, a large multicentre placebo RCT evaluated the steroid-sparing effects of

DHEA.[47] Patients with SLE, receiving 10–30 mg prednisone daily were randomised to receive placebo (*n* = 64), 100 mg (*n* = 63) or 200 mg (*n* = 64) DHEA daily for 7–9 months. Patients must have failed a steroid taper within the prior 6 months; stable doses of NSAIDs and hydroxychloroquine were allowed; immunosuppressants were excluded. Daily doses of prednisone were reduced by algorithm each month in patients with stable or improving SLEDAI scores. The primary outcome measure was the number of patients who were able to taper prednisone doses to less than or equal to ≤7·5 mg/day for 2 consecutive months, including the last two months of the trial. There was a dose-dependent effect of DHEA administration on the number of responders (200 mg prasterone 55%, 100 mg prasterone 44%, and placebo 41%), however, this did not meet statistical significance (p = 0·111, 200 mg DHEA *v* placebo). A subgroup analysis of patients with active disease at baseline, defined as a SLEDAI score >2, showed statistically more responders receiving 200 mg DHEA compared with placebo (51% *v* 29%, p = 0·031), and more patients with a mean number of days with prednisone doses ≤7·5 mg/day (93% *v* 60%, p = 0·015).

Two patients were reported with serious adverse effects: 1 patient each in the placebo and 200 mg DHEA groups with pneumonia. Of other adverse effects, only acne occurred with a significantly higher rate in patients receiving DHEA (41% in 200 mg and 100 mg combined versus 19% in placebo).

A second multicentre placebo RCT evaluated the effect of DHEA on disease activity and reduction of flares in female patients with mild to moderate SLE.[48] One hundred and twenty patients with active SLE were randomised to receive 200 mg DHEA or placebo daily for 24 weeks. Patients were required to have SLEDAI scores > 2 at entry and were maintained on stable doses of prednisone or other immunosuppressive agents. The primary outcome measure was mean change in Systemic Lupus Activity Measure (SLAM) score at 24 weeks. Secondary outcomes included time to first flare (defined as in ongoing SELENA study) and changes in SLEDAI scores. There were no statistically significant differences in mean changes in SLAM or SLEDAI scores between treatment groups. Flares were less common in patients receiving DHEA than placebo (11/60 (18·3%) versus 20/59 (33·9%), p value not stated) and there was a statistically significant difference between groups for time to first flare (p = 0·044).

Two of 60 patients receiving DHEA and 4/59 in placebo discontinued study participation early – reasons were not reported. Serious adverse effects were reported in 7/61 (11·5%) patients in active treatment compared with 18/59 (30·5%) in placebo (p = 0·010). The authors stated that most serious adverse effects were related to SLE flares, but specific data were not provided. There were insufficient data provided in the publication to analyse the safety of DHEA in this RCT.

One small RCT has been published evaluating DHEA for the treatment of serious manifestations of SLE.[49] Nineteen male and female SLE patients with severe renal, haematological, or serosal involvement were randomised to receive 200 mg DHEA or placebo daily in addition to stable doses of prednisone and immunosuppressive medications for 6 months. The clinical outcome was stabilisation of disease activity as well as bone densitometry and SLEDAI scores. There were no significant differences between patients achieving response criteria (defined specifically for each manifestation) between treatment groups (7/9 DHEA *v* 4/10 placebo, p = 0·10). Improvement in renal manifestations did not differ between the two groups. Treatment with DHEA was shown to have statistically significant benefit in preserving bone mineral density in the lumbar spine in patients taking DHEA (p < 0·05).

Three serious adverse effects were reported during this 6 month RCT; none was considered related to administration of the study drug. Acne, hirsutism, and menstrual irregularities were the most common non-serious adverse effects recorded.

Evidence summary: Silver

Two RCTs examining the efficacy of DHEA for the treatment of mild to moderate disease manifestations of SLE activity found mixed results, with the majority unable to show a statistically significant benefit. One RCT in more severe disease did not show clinical benefit. DHEA may, however, play a role in the prevention of steroid-induced osteoporosis in patients with SLE. DHEA does appear to be well tolerated, with adverse effects predominantly related to androgenic properties of the medication.

Case presentation

The use of DHEA was discussed with Patient 2. DHEA was not recommended for the treatment of her symptoms as it has not been consistently shown to treat active manifestations of disease. DHEA may have a role in preserving bone mineral density in this patient, however she decided against it because of concerns of acne and hirsutism.

Question 15

Are there any therapies that are steroid-sparing in mild to moderate SLE? Do these drugs improve survival or prevent organ damage? Do these drugs reduce the incidence of flares?

Several therapies have been studied for their use in the treatment of mild to moderate lupus. Hydroxychloroquine and DHEA are perhaps the best studied, and are discussed above. The published RCTs examining the efficacy of milder therapies are limited to single studies each for methotrexate and bromocriptine.

Based on its efficacy for the treatment of rheumatoid arthritis, low dose weekly methotrexate was studied in the treatment of mild to moderate lupus. A single RCT has been published to date.[50] Forty-one patients with active disease were enrolled in a 6 month double blind, placebo controlled study. Patients were not taking hydroxychloroquine or other immunosuppressive drugs and were on an average 16–17 mg prednisone daily. Method of randomisation was not discussed. Patients took 15–20 mg oral methotrexate or identical placebo each week. After the first month, treating physicians were permitted to adjust the dose of prednisone based on individual assessment of lupus activity. Main outcomes were SLEDAI scores and change in dose of prednisone during the study. Mean SLEDAI scores were significantly improved in the methotrexate group when compared to the placebo group at 3–6 months of follow up ($p < 0{\cdot}05$). In addition, 13/20 (72·2%) of patients receiving methotrexate were able to reduce their prednisone dose by >50% compared to 1/21 (5·0%) of patients receiving placebo ($p < 0{\cdot}001$). Cutaneous and musculoskeletal manifestations appeared to be the most responsive to methotrexate.

The safety of methotrexate was also examined in this study. The only reported adverse effects in patients receiving placebo were 3/21 patients with mild dyspepsia. No infections were noted. In contrast, numerous adverse effects were reported in patients taking methotrexate. Four patients developed infections: 2 urinary tract infections, 1 patient with lobar pneumonia, and 1 patient was withdrawn from the study after the development of pulmonary tuberculosis. Oral ulcers developed in 6 patients, and dyspepsia in 9. Ten patients (50%) in the methotrexate group had transaminitis during the study.

Four patients discontinued study treatment prematurely: 2 patients receiving placebo for lack of efficacy after hospitalisations due to increased SLE activity and 2 on methotrexate due to adverse effects: 1 pulmonary tuberculosis and 1 urticaria.

This single RCT in a small number of patients showed some benefit in cutaneous and articular symptoms with use of weekly methotrexate, demonstrating a steroid-sparing effect. However, the adverse effects including infections associated with use of methotrexate are of concern.

Bromocriptine, an inhibitor of prolactin secretion, was studied for the treatment of mild to moderate SLE in 66 patients randomised to receive 2·5 mg bromocriptine or placebo daily for12 months.[51] Clinical outcomes included changes in background prednisone doses and number of SLE flares, defined as onset of manifestations of active disease not present at baseline or increases in SLEDAI scores >3. There were no significant differences in SLEDAI scores, number of flares or average prednisone dose at the end of the study between the two groups.

Any conclusions from this RCT are limited by the large number of patients who did not complete the trial. In the bromocriptine group, 12/36 (33·3%) discontinued prematurely: 3 for pregnancy, 4 were lost to follow up, and 5 for adverse effects, including nausea and headaches. A similar number, 11/30 (36·7%), in the placebo group dropped out early: 5 patients for adverse effects of nausea and headache, 2 for pregnancy, and 3 were lost to follow up. There was one death. It is not stated whether these patients were included in the analysis. Based on these results, bromocriptine does not appear to have efficacy for the treatment of active SLE nor does it have any steroid-sparing effects.

Evidence summary: Silver

Methotrexate: One RCT found that methotrexate appears to have some efficacy as a steroid-sparing agent and for the treatment of cutaneous and articular manifestations of SLE. Use of weekly methotrexate was associated with a high rate of adverse effects, which may limit its use. These studies were designed to exclude patients with known severe organ damage, and are of too short a duration to evaluate progression to organ damage or effects on survival.

Bromocriptine: One RCT found no benefit.

Case presentation

For Patient 2, it was recommended that she begin therapy with hydroxychloroquine based on its efficacy and low risk of adverse effects. The use of methotrexate was not recommended as initial therapy, given a higher rate of adverse effects. It may be considered in the future if she has active cutaneous or articular manifestations that remain unresponsive to hydroxychloroquine alone.

Question 16

Can biological markers be used to predict flares and alter therapy?

It is believed that prevention of relapses of clinical SLE over time will lead to a reduction in irreversible organ damage and ultimately improve morbidity and mortality. The concept of prevention of relapses presupposes that clinical flares can be predicted either by changes in renal function or following biological markers such as anti-dsDNA antibodies or complement, or a number of cytokine or cytokine receptor levels in serum. Close monitoring of these markers and aggressive treatment prompted by changes in these markers have been advocated as an approach to prevent or reduce the severity of SLE flares. An uncontrolled prospective trial[52] demonstrated improved long term outcome in patients with SLE nephritis in whom normalisation of serum complement and anti-DNA antibody levels were maintained.

Bootsma *et al*[53] studied 156 patients with SLE. When increases in anti-dsDNA antibodies were observed, patients were randomised to receive either conventional treatment (treatment with prednisone and cytotoxic drugs were given only for clinical relapses) or conventional treatment including an additional 30 mg prednisone daily for a rise in anti-dsDNA antibody titres (to a maximum of 60 mg qd; and a defined tapering schedule). Increases in anti-dsDNA antibodies occurred in 46 patients, 24 of whom received conventional treatment only and 22 an additional increase in steroids.

During the RCT (mean follow up for the two groups was similar, 580 *v* 556 days) 2 of 22 patients in the steroid + conventional treatment group had a clinical relapse, compared with 20 of 24 receiving conventional therapy. The cumulative risk of a major SLE flare was not significantly different between the two groups ($p = 0{\cdot}12$) but the risk of any flare (major or minor) was less in the expectantly treated patients ($p < 0{\cdot}001$). Mean doses of prednisone were higher in the prednisone + conventional treatment group ($p = 0{\cdot}025$), although cumulative doses did not differ significantly ($p = 0{\cdot}068$). There were more proven infections in the conventional treatment group ($p = 0{\cdot}005$).

Early aggressive treatment of an increasing anti-DNA titre in patients without clinical evidence of changing disease activity may be appropriate in a subset of patients with SLE. Identifying these individuals may be worthwhile, although at this time further studies are needed to confirm these findings and demonstrate an improvement in long term morbidity and mortality.

Evidence summary: Silver

One RCT showed benefit from an additional 30 mg prednisone daily for a rise in anti-dsDNA antibody titres.

Discussion of intervention

Case presentation

Patient 1: It was explained to the patient that the medical literature supports the use of IV cyclophosphamide to treat the type of kidney disease that she has and that the use of IV monthly pulse cyclophosphamide, in general, is well tolerated. The patient remained concerned with the adverse effects of cyclophosphamide, and after further discussion it was elected to treat the patient with high dose (but not pulse) steroids in combination with mycophenolate mofetil. Hydroxychloroquine was also added to her regimen because of the severity of her presentation and the relative safety profile of the drug. She had no complication or adverse effects of therapy except for acne. The patient's haematuria gradually resolved and she continued to have only trace amount of proteinuria. Serum creatinine dropped to 1·3.

Patient 2: The patient presents with mild to moderate lupus and wants to avoid systemic steroid therapy. It was explained to her that the medical literature suggests that hydroxychloroquine has efficacy to treat cutaneous and articular manifestations of lupus without risks of serious adverse effects. Methotrexate has also been shown to have some efficacy. However, its safety profile would make it a second line therapy in her situation. There is no evidence to support the use of DHEA or bromocriptine for treatment of her symptoms although DHEA may help to prevent bone loss associated with lupus. The patient elected to take hydroxychloroquine with resolution of arthritis and rash over the next several months. She has flares of arthralgias which are managed by NSAIDs. She continues to be followed on a regular basis to monitor for signs of SLE flares and asymptomatic renal disease.

Future research needs

There is still a lack of controlled clinical trials evidence to guide therapy of SLE. Future randomised controlled trials need to include:

- studies to identify a valid renal responder index
- studies to identify the optimal dosing regimen (including dose, duration, mode of administration) for CTX for lupus nephritis
- studies to examine the role of other immunosuppressive agents either in induction or remission therapy
- studies to identify techniques to diagnose NPSLE
- studies to identify the appropriate therapies for the various manifestation of NPSLE
- studies to examine the potential role of biologics (for example cytokines) in SLE
- studies to examine the optimal role of additional therapies such as hydroxychloroquine, bromocriptine, DHEA, methotrexate, or azathioprine in lupus.

References

1 Uramoto KM, Michet CJ, Thumbo J, *et al.* Trends in the incidence and mortality of systemic lupus erythematosus, 1950–1992. *Arth Rheum* 1999;**42**:46–50.

2 Abu-Shakra M, Urowitz MB, Gladman DD, Gough J. Mortality studies in systemic lupus erythematosus. Results from a single center. *J Rheumatol* 1995;**22**:1259–64.

3 Abu-Shakra M, Urowitz MB, Gladman DD, Gough J. Mortality studies in systemic lupus erythematosus. Results from a single center. *J Rheumatol* 1995;**22**:1265–70.

4 Cervera R, Khamashita MA, Font J, *et al.* Morbidity and mortality in systemic lupus erythematosus during a 5-year period. *Medicine* 1990;**78**:167–75.

5 Manzi S, Meilahn EN, Rairie JE, *et al.* Age specific incidence rates of myocardial infarction and angina in women with systemic lupus erythematosus: comparison with the Framingham study. *Am J Epidemiol* 1997;**145**: 408–15.

6 Strand V, Gladman D, Isenberg D. Endpoints: consensus recommendations from OMERACT IV. *Lupus* 2000;**9**:322–7.

7 Felson DT, Anderson J. Evidence for the superiority of immunosuppressive drugs and prednisone over prednisone alone in lupus nephritis. *N Engl J Med* 1984;**311**:1528–33.

8 Bansal VK, Beto JA. Treatment of lupus nephritis: a meta-analysis of clinical trials. *Am J Kidney Dis* 1997;**29**:193–9.

9 Steinberg AD, Kaltreider HB, Staples PJ, *et al.* Cyclophosphamide in lupus nephritis: a controlled trial. *Ann Intern Med* 1971;**75**:165–171.

10 Steinberg AD, Decker JL. A double blind controlled trial comparing cyclophosphamide, azathioprine and placebo in the treatment of lupus glomerulonephritis. *Arth Rheum* 1974;**17**:923–37.

11 Gourley MF, Austin HA, Scott D, *et al.* Methylprednisolone and cyclophosphamide alone or in combination in patients with lupus nephritis. *Ann Intern Med* 1996;**125**:549–57.

12 Illei GG, Austin HA, Crane M, *et al.* Combination therapy with pulse cyclophosphamide plus pulse methylprednisolone improves long term renal outcome without adding toxicity in patients with lupus nephritis. *Ann Intern Med* 2001;**135**:248–57.

13 Chan TM, Li FK, Tang CSO, *et al.* Efficacy of mycophenolate mofetil in patients with diffuse proliferative lupus nephritis. *N Engl J Med* 2000;**343**: 1156–62.

14 Austin HA, Klippel JK, Balow JE, *et al.* Therapy of lupus nephritis. *N Engl J Med* 1986;**314**:614–19.

15 Steinberg AD, Steinberg SC. Long term preservation of renal function in patients with lupus nephritis receiving treatment that includes cyclophosphamide versus those treated with prednisone only. *Arth Rheum* 1991;**34**: 945–50.

16 Boumpas DT, Austin HA, Vaughn EM, *et al.* Controlled trial of pulse methylprednisolone versus two regimens of pulse cyclophosphamide in severe lupus nephritis. *Lancet* 1992;**340**:741–5.

17 Houssiau FA, Vasconcelos C, D'Cruz D, *et al.* Immunosuppressive therapy in lupus nephritis. *Arth Rheum* 2002;**46**:2121–31.

18 Ginzler E, Diamond H, Guttadauria M, Kaplan D. Prednisone and azathioprine compared to prednisone plus low dose azathioprine and cyclophosphamide in the treatment of diffuse lupus nephritis. *Arth Rheum* 1976;**19**:693–9.

19 Boletis JN, Ioannidis JPA, Boki KA, Moutsopoulos HM. Intravenous immunoglobulin compared with

cyclophosphamide for proliferative lupus nephritis. *Lancet* 1999;**354**:569–70.

20 Fu LW, Yang LY, Chen WP, Lin CY. Clinical efficacy of cyclosporin A neoral in the treatment of pediatric lupus nephritis with heavy proteinuria. *Br J Rheum* 1998;**37**:217–21.

21 Illei GG, Takada K, Parkin D, *et al.* Renal flares are common in patients with severe proliferative lupus nephritis treated with pulse immunosuppressive therapy. *Arth Rheum* 2002;**46**:995–1002.

22 Mok CC, Ho C, Siu YP, *et al.* Treatment of diffuse lupus glomerulonephritis: a comparison of two cyclophosphamide containing regimens. *Am J Kidney Dis* 2001;**38**:256–64.

23 Alarcon-Segovia D, Tumlin J, Furie RA, *et al.* LJP 394 for the prevention of renal flare in patients with systemic lupus erythematosus: Results from a randomised, double blind, placebo controlled study. *Arthritis Rheumatol* 2003;**48**(2):442–54.

24 Liebling MR, McLaughlin K, Boonsue S, *et al.* Monthly pulses of methylprednisolone in SLE nephritis. *J Rheumatol* 1982;**9**:543–8.

25 Sesso R, Monteiro M, Sato E, *et al.* A controlled trial of pulse cyclophosphamide versus pulse methylprednisolone in severe lupus nephritis. *Lupus* 1994;**3**:107–12.

26 Chan TM, Li FK, Hao WK, *et al.* Treatment of membranous lupus nephritis with nephrotic syndrome by sequential immunosuppression. *Lupus* 1999;**8**:545–51.

27 Kolasinski SL, Chung JB, Albert DA. What do we know about lupus membranous nephropathy? An analytic review. *Arth Care Res* 2002;**47**:450–5.

28 Lewis EJ, Hunsicker LG, Lan S, *et al.* A controlled trial of plasmapharesis therapy in severe lupus nephritis. *N Engl J Med* 1992;**326**:1373–9.

29 Pohl MA, Lan S, Berl T, *et al.* Plasmapharesis does not increase the risk for infection in immunosuppressed patients with severe lupus nephritis. *Ann Intern Med* 1991;**114**:924–9.

30 Derksen RHWM, Hene RJ, Kallenberg CGM, *et al.* Prospective multicenter trial on the short term effect of plasma exchange versus cytotoxic drugs in steroid resistant lupus nephritis. *Neth J Med* 1988;**33**:168–77.

31 Wallace DJ, Goldfinger D, Pepkowitz SH, *et al.* Randomised controlled trial of pulse/synchronization cyclophopsphamide apheresis for proliferative lupus nephritis. *J Clin Apheresis* 1998;**13**:163–6.

32 Trevisani VFM, Castro AA, Neto JF, *et al.* Cyclophosphamide versus methylprednisolone for treating neuropsychiatric involvement in systemic lupus erythematosus. *Cochrane Database Syst Rev* (2):CD00329, 2002.

33 Barile L, Olguin L, Ariza R, *et al.* Controlled clinical trial of cyclophosphamide vs methylprednisolone in severe neurologic manifestation in SLE. *Arth Rheum* (abstracts) 2001;88.

34 Van Vollenhoven RF, Elliott D, Powell M, *et al.* Dehydroepiandrosterone improves cognitive function in patients with systemic lupus erythematosus–results of double blind placebo controlled pilot study. *Arth Rheum* (abstracts) 2001;26.

35 D'Cruz D. Antimalarial therapy: a panacea for mild lupus? *Lupus* 2001;**10**:148–51.

36 The Canadian Hydroxychloroquine Study Group. A randomised study of the effect of withdrawing hydroxychloroquine sulfate in systemic lupus erythematosus. *N Engl J Med* 1991;**324**:150–4.

37 The Canadian Hydroxychloroquine Study Group. A long-term study of hydroxychloroquine withdrawal on exacerbations in systemic lupus erythematosus. *Lupus* 1998;**7**:80–5.

38 Meinao IM, Sato EI, Andrade LEC, *et al.* Controlled trial with chloroquine diphosphate in systemic lupus erythematosus. *Lupus* 1996;**5**:237–41.

39 Williams HJ, Egger MJ, Singer JZ, *et al.* Comparison of hydroxychloroquine and placebo in the treatment of the arthropathy of mild systemic lupus erythematosus. *J Rheumatol* 1994;**21**:1457–62.

40 Costedoat-Chalumeau N, Amoura Z, Aymard G, *et al.* Evidence of transplacental passage of hydroxychloroquine in humans. *Arthritis Rheum* 2002;**46**:1123–4.

41 Parke AL. Antimalarial drugs, systemic lupus erythermatosus and pregnancy. *J Rheumatol* 1988;**15**:607–10.

42 Parke AL, West B. Hydroxychloroquine in pregnant patients with systemic lupus erythematosus. *J Rheumatol* 1996;**23**:1715–18.

43 Buchanan NMM, Toubi E, Khamashta MA, *et al.* Hydroxychloroquine and lupus pregnancy: review of a series of 36 cases. *Ann Rheum Dis* 1996;**55**:486–8.

44 Levy RA, Vilela VS, Cataldo MJ, *et al.* Hydroxychloroquine (HCQ) in lupus pregnancy: double-blind and placebo-controlled study. *Lupus* 2001;**10**:401–4.

45 van Vollenhoven RF. Dehydroepiandrosterone in systemic lupus erythematosus. *Rheum Dis Clin North America* 2000;**26**:349–62.

46 van Vollenhoven R, Engleman EG, McGuire JL. Dehydroepiandrosterone in systemic lupus erythematosus: results of a double-blind, placebo-controlled, randomised clinical trial. *Arthritis Rheum* 1995;**38**:1826–31.

47 Petri MA, Lahita RG, van Vollenhoven RF, *et al.* Effects of prasterone on corticosteroid requirement of women with systemic lupus erythematosus: a double-blind, randomised, placebo-controlled trial. *Arthritis Rheum* 2002;**46**:1820–9.

48 Chang DM, Lan JL, Lin HY, Luo SF. Dehydroepiandrosterone treatment of women with mild-to-moderate systemic lupus erythematosus: a multicenter randomised, double-blind, placebo-controlled trial. *Arthritis Rheum* 2002;**46**:2942–7.

49 van Vollenhoven RF, Park JL, Genovese MC, West JP, McGuire JL. A double-blind, placebo-controlled, clinical trial of dehydroepiandrosterone in severe systemic lupus erythematosus. *Lupus* 1999;**8**:181–7.

50 Carneiro JRM, Sato EI. Double blind, randomised, placebo controlled clinical trial of methotrexate in systemic lupus erythematosus. *J Rheumatol* 1999;**26**: 1275–9.

51 Alvarez-Nemegyei J, Cobarrubias-Cobos A, Escalante-Triay F, Sosa-Muòoz J, Miranda JM, Jara LJ. Bromocriptine in systemic lupus erythematosus: a double-blind, randomised, placebo-controlled study. *Lupus* 1998;**7**:414–19.

52 Appel AE, Sablay LB, Golden RA, *et al.* The effect of normalization of serum complement and anti-DNA antibody on the course of lupus nephritis. *Am J Med* 1978;**64**:274–83.

53 Bootsma H, Spronik P, Derksen R, *et al.* Prevention of relapses in systemic lupus erythematosus. *Lancet* 1995;**345**:1595–9.

54 Carette S, Klippel JH, Decker JL, *et al.* Controlled studies of role immunosuppressive drugs in lupus nephritis. *Ann Intern Med* 1983;**99**:1–8.

55 Dinanat HJ, Decker JL, Klippel JH, *et al.* Alternative modes of cyclophosphamide and azathioprine therapy in lupus nephritis. *Ann Intern Med* 1982;**96**:728–36.

56 Decker JL, Klippel JH, Plotz PH, Steinberg AD. Cyclophosphmaide or azathioprine in lupus glomerulonephritis. *Ann Intern Med* 1975;**83**:606–15.

57 Donadio JV, Holley KE, Ferguson RH, Ilstrup DM. Treatment of diffuse proliferative lupus nephritis with prednisone and combined prednisone and cyclophosphamide. *N Engl J Med* 1978;**299**:1151–5.

58 Donadio JV, Holley KE, Wagoner RD, *et al.* Treatment of lupus nephritis with prednisone and combined prednisone and azathioprine. *Ann Intern Med* 1972;**77**:829–35.

59 Donadio JV, Holley KE, Ferguson RH, Ilstrup DM. Progressive lupus glomerulonephritis. *Mayo Clin Proc* 1976;**51**:484–94.

60 Donadio JV, Holley KE, Wagoner RD, *et al.* Further observation on the treatment of lupus nephritis with prednisone and combined prednisone and azathioprine. *Arth Rheum* 1974;**17**: 573–81.

61 Baletta M, Sabella D, Magri P, *et al.* Cyclosporin plus steroids versus steroids alone in the treatment of lupus nephritis. In: Sessa, Meroni, Battini, eds. *Contrib Nephrol* 1992;**99**:129–36.

62 Hahn BV, Kantor OS, Osterland CK. Azathioprine plus prednisone compared with prednisone alone in the treatment of systemic lupus erythematosus. *Ann Int Med* 1975;**83**:597–605.

63 Sztejnbok M, Stewart A, Diamond H, Kaplan D. Azathioprine in the treatment of systemic lupus erythematosus. *Arth Rheum* 1971;**14**:639–45.

64 Cade R, Spooner G, Schlein E, *et al.* Comparison of azathioprine, prednisone, and heparin alone or combined in treating lupus nephritis. *Nephron* 1973:**10**:37–56.

Systemic lupus erythematosus
Summaries and decision aids

Lupus kidney disease and immunosuppressive agents Summaries and decision aid

How well do immunosuppressive agents, such as cyclophosphamide plus steroids, work to treat lupus kidney disease (SLE nephritis) and how safe are they?

To answer this question, scientists found and analysed 2 reviews of the literature and 2 more studies testing medications in people with lupus kidney disease. People received either pills (by mouth, oral) or injections (IV) of medications for kidney lupus disease. These studies provide the best evidence today.

What is lupus kidney disease and how is it treated?

SLE (systemic lupus erythematosus) or simply "lupus" is a group of diseases in which the body's immune system fights or attacks itself. Lupus can cause swelling, pain, and damage to many organs of the body such as the skin, heart, lungs, brain and kidneys. When people with lupus have kidney problems or kidney disease, it is called SLE nephritis or lupus kidney disease. Drugs are prescribed to prevent kidney failure. Corticosteroids such as prednisone, are used with immunosuppressive agents or cytotoxics, such as cyclophosphamide (Cytoxan), azathioprine (Imuran) or mycophenolate mofetil (Cellcept).

How well did cyclophosphamide plus steroids work to treat lupus kidney disease?

The reviews and studies showed that people who in addition to prednisone, received cyclophosphamide or azathioprine had less of a decrease in kidney function, were less likely to develop kidney failure or die from kidney disease than people who received prednisone alone. Cyclophosphamide or azathioprine alone showed the same improvements seen with prednisone alone. One of the reviews also found that oral azathioprine and oral cyclophosphamide worked just as well as the other.

What were the side effects?

Side effects such as menstrual periods stopping in women (amenorrhoea), infections, death of bone tissue, bone loss, cervical dysplasia (precancerous change to cells in the cervix), and death due to complications from infections may occur when taking steroids and immunosuppressive agents.

What is the bottom line?

There is "Silver" level evidence that taking steroids (such as prednisone) with immunosuppressive agents (cyclophosphamide or azathioprine) is better than taking corticosteroids alone to improve kidney function and survival in patients with lupus kidney disease.

Side effects of cyclophosphamide and azathioprine, include infections, cancer, and death from complications of the drugs.

From Schiffenbauer J, Chakravarty E, Strand V. Systemic lupus erythematosus. In: *Evidence-based Rheumatology*, London, BMJ Books, 2003.

How well do immunosuppressive agents, such as cyclophosphamide, plus steroids, work to treat lupus kidney disease (SLE nephritis) and how safe are they?

What is lupus kidney disease and how is it treated?

SLE (systemic lupus erythematosus) or simply "lupus" is a group of diseases in which the body's immune system does not work properly. Normally, the body's immune system fights or attacks germs but in lupus the body starts to attack itself. Lupus can cause swelling and damage to many organs of the body such as the skin, heart, lungs, brain and kidneys. Lupus occurs in cycles, where there are periods of pain and illness or periods of little or no pain and illness (remission). When people with lupus have kidney problems or kidney disease, it is called SLE nephritis.

Drugs are prescribed to treat the kidney disease to prevent the kidneys from failing. The drugs can decrease swelling in the kidney and control the immune system. Corticosteroids such as prednisone are used with immunosuppressive agents or cytotoxics, such as cyclophosphamide (Cytoxan) and azathioprine (Imuran), or mycophenolate mofetil (Cellcept). Most of these drugs can be taken by mouth or by injection (IV) and sometimes alone or in combination. Unfortunately, these drugs can cause side effects that can cause damage in the body and therefore it is important to determine which medications taken alone or in combination work and which are safe.

How did the scientists find the information and analyse it?

The scientists searched for studies and reviews of the medical literature that examined the treatment of lupus kidney disease. Not all studies and reviews found were of a high quality and so only those studies that met high standards were selected.

Which high quality studies and reviews were examined in this summary?

There were two reviews of the literature and 2 more studies examined in this summary. Two high quality studies included in the one review of the literature are also described. All patients tested had lupus kidney disease.

- One review examined 8 studies that compared the effects of prednisone and a placebo to prednisone with an immunosuppressive agent such as cyclophosphamide or azathioprine.
- The other review examined 19 studies that compared the effects of prednisone to prednisone plus one immunosuppressive agent (cyclophosphamide or azathioprine) or to azathioprine alone.
- One study in the above review compared the effects of prednisone to prednisone and cyclophosphamide in 13 patients over 10 weeks. And the other study compared the effects of prednisone to prednisone plus cyclophosphamide or prednisone plus azathioprine in 38 patients over 10 weeks.
- The two recent studies compared 82 patients receiving methylprednisolone (MP) or cyclophosphamide; or MP plus cyclophosphamide over 1 year and over 11 years.

How well did cyclophosphamide plus steroids work to treat lupus kidney disease?

The first review showed that patients who received, in addition to prednisone, oral cyclophosphamide or azathioprine had less decrease in kidney function, were less likely to develop kidney failure or die from kidney disease than patients who received prednisone alone. Patients with "diffuse proliferative glomerulonephritis" (a form of damage in the kidney) had the most improvement with cyclophosphamide plus prednisone or azathioprine plus prednisone. Cyclophosphamide or azathioprine alone showed the same improvements seen with prednisone alone.

The second review showed that patients who received, in addition to prednisone, cyclophosphamide or azathioprine were less likely to develop kidney failure or die from kidney disease than patients who received prednisone alone. This review found the same results as the first review and also found that azathioprine and cyclophosphamide worked just as well as the other.

Specifically, two high quality Gold studies in the review showed that after 10 weeks of treatment:

- more patients improved on more tests for kidney function with prednisone plus cyclophosphamide than with prednisone plus a placebo
- other symptoms of lupus (for example: rashes, fever, arthritis, mouth sores, and swelling around the lungs and heart) went away (in 5 out of 9 patients) or did not occur in patients who received prednisone plus cyclophosphamide. But the symptoms stayed or did occur (6 out of 15 patients) in patients receiving prednisone alone.

The results of the best two most recent studies showed that after 1 year:

— Renal remission (period of little or no swelling in the kidney) occurred in

- 26 out of 100 patients receiving methylprednisone alone
- 48 out of 100 patients receiving cyclophosphamide alone
- 61 out of 100 patients receiving methylprednisone and cyclophosphamide together.

— Improved kidney function occurred in

- 37 out of 100 patients receiving methylprednisone alone
- 70 out of 100 patients receiving cyclophosphamide alone
- 89 out of 100 patients receiving methylprednisone and cyclophosphamide together.

What were the side effects?

Side effects such as menstrual periods stopping in women (amenorrhoea), infections, death of bone tissue (avascular necrosis), bone loss (osteoporosis), cervical dysplasia (precancerous change to cells in the cervix), and death due to complications from infections may occur when taking steroids and immunosuppressive agents.

After 1 year, more patients had side effects when taking methylprednisone and cyclophosphamide together compared to patients taking either drug on its own.

In the best study testing cyclophosphamide plus methylprednisone for 1 year, side effects occurred in:

- 7 out of 100 patients receiving methylprednisone alone
- 41 out of 100 patients receiving cyclophosphamide alone
- 43 out of 100 patients receiving methylprednisone and cyclophosphamide together.

What is the bottom line?

There is "Silver" level evidence that taking steroids (such as prednisone) with immunosuppressive agents (cyclophosphamide or azathioprine) is better than taking corticosteroids alone to improve kidney function and survival in patients with lupus kidney disease.

Side effects of cyclophosphamide and azathioprine, include infections, cancer, and death from complications of the drugs.

From Schiffenbauer J, Chakravarty E, Strand V. Systemic lupus erythematosus. In: *Evidence-based Rheumatology,* London: BMJ Books, 2003

Information for lupus kidney disease (SLE nephritis) and treatment

What is lupus kidney disease?

SLE (systemic lupus erythematosus) or simply "lupus" is a group of diseases in which the body's immune system does not work properly. Normally, the body's immune system fights or attacks germs but in lupus the body starts to attack itself. Lupus can cause swelling, pain and damage to many organs of the body such as the skin, heart, lungs, brain and kidneys. When people with lupus have kidney problems or kidney disease, it is called SLE nephritis.

Lupus usually occurs in cycles, where there are periods of pain and illness or periods of little or no pain and illness. If the swelling is not treated, it can cause permanent damage. In lupus kidney disease, pain and swelling in the kidney can cause permanent damage to the kidney that can lead to

- swollen feet and legs (water retention)
- kidneys stop working
- need for dialysis or kidney transplant
- death.

What can I do on my own to manage my disease?

✓ exercise ✓ avoid alcohol ✓ relaxation

What treatments are used for lupus kidney disease?

Three kinds of treatment may be used alone or together. The common (generic) names are shown below.

1. *Oral or IV corticosteroids*
   - Prednisone
   - Prednisolone
   - Methylprednisolone
2. *Immunosuppressive agents (cytotoxics)*
   - Azathioprine
   - Cyclophosphamide
   - Mycophenolate mofetil
3. *Alternative therapies*
   - Ciclosporin
   - IV immunoglobulins

What about other treatments I have heard about?

There is not enough evidence about the effects of some treatments. Other treatments may not work. For example:

- Plasmapheresis (may not work)
- LJP 394 (need more research)
- Dehydroepiandrosterone (DHEA) (need more research)

What are my choices? How can I decide?

Treatment for your disease will depend on your condition. You need to know the good points (pros) and bad points (cons) about each treatment before you can decide.

Lupus kidney disease (SLE nephritis) decision aid

Do I agree to take the recommended treatment of steroids (such as prednisone) plus cyclophosphamide?

This guide can help you make decisions about the treatment your doctor is asking you to consider.

It will help you to:

1. Clarify what you need to decide.
2. Consider the pros and cons of different choices.
3. Decide what role you want to have in choosing your treatment.
4. Identify what you need to help you make the decision.
5. Plan the next steps.
6. Share your thinking with your doctor.

Step 1: Clarify what you need to decide

What is the decision?

Do I agree to take the recommended treatment of steroids (such as prednisone) plus cyclophosphamide?

In addition to the dose of prednisone, cyclophosphamide may be taken as a pill daily or as an injection into the veins (IV).

When does this decision have to be made? Check ✓ one

☐ within days ☐ within weeks ☐ within months

How far along are you with this decision? Check ✓ one

☐ I have not thought about it yet

☐ I am considering the choices

☐ I am close to making a choice

☐ I have already made a choice

Step 2: Consider the pros and cons of different choices

What does the research show?

Cyclophosphamide plus steroids is classified as: Likely beneficial

There is "Silver" level evidence from 2 reviews and 2 studies of people with lupus kidney disease who took immunosuppressive agents plus corticosteroids. The studies lasted for up to 10 weeks to 11 years. These studies found pros and cons that are listed in the chart below.

What do I think of the pros and cons of cyclosphosphamide plus steroids?

1. Review the common pros and cons.
2. Add any other pros and cons that are important to you.
3. Show how important each pro and con is to you by circling from one (*) star if it is a little important to you, to up to five (*****) stars if it is very important to you.

PROS AND CONS OF CYCLOPHOSPHAMIDE PLUS STEROIDS

PROS (number of people affected)	How important is it to you?	CONS (number of people affected)	How important is it to you?
Improves symptoms of lupus kidney disease 61 out of 100 people had little or no symptoms	* * * * *	Side effects: serious infections, hair loss, sore bladder, blood in urine, bone loss, death of bone tissue in 43 out of 100 people	* * * * *
Improves other symptoms of lupus rashes, fever, mouth sores, and arthritis disappeared in 55 out of 100 people No one developed more symptoms of lupus while taking pills	* * * * *	Long term harms: cancer, diabetes, early menopause, bladder tumours, other cancers and death	* * * * *
Improves kidney function in 89 out of 100 people	* * * * *	Personal cost of medicine	* * * * *
Lowers chances of needing kidney dialysis or kidney transplantation	* * * * *	Extra clinic visits and blood tests needed	* * * * *
Other pros:	* * * * *	Other cons:	* * * * *

What do you think about taking cyclophosphamide plus steroids? Check ✓ one

☐ Willing to consider this treatment
Pros are more important to me than the Cons

☐ Unsure

☐ Not willing to consider this treatment
Cons are more important to me than the Pros

Step 3: Choose the role you want to have in choosing your treatment Check ✓ one

☐ I prefer to decide on my own after listening to the opinions of others

☐ I prefer to share the decision with: ______________________

☐ I prefer someone else to decide for me, namely: ______________

Step 4: Identify what you need to help you make the decision

What I know	Do you know enough about your condition to make a choice?	☐ Yes ☐ No ☐ Unsure
	Do you know which options are available to you?	☐ Yes ☐ No ☐ Unsure
	Do you know the good points (pros) of each option?	☐ Yes ☐ No ☐ Unsure
	Do you know the bad points (cons) of each option?	☐ Yes ☐ No ☐ Unsure
What's important	Are you clear about which **pros** are most *important to you?*	☐ Yes ☐ No ☐ Unsure
	Are you clear about which **cons** are most *important to you?*	☐ Yes ☐ No ☐ Unsure
How others help	Do you have enough support from others to make a choice?	☐ Yes ☐ No ☐ Unsure
	Are you choosing without pressure from others?	☐ Yes ☐ No ☐ Unsure
	Do you have enough advice to make a choice?	☐ Yes ☐ No ☐ Unsure
How sure I feel	Are you clear about the best choice for you?	☐ Yes ☐ No ☐ Unsure
	Do you feel sure about what to choose?	☐ Yes ☐ No ☐ Unsure

If you answered No or Unsure to many of these questions, you should talk to your doctor.

Step 5: Plan the next steps

What do you need to do before you make this decision?

For example: talk to your doctor, read more about this treatment or other treatments for lupus kidney disease.

Step 6: Share the information on this form with your doctor

It will help your doctor understand what you think about this treatment.

7
Osteoarthritis

Thao Pham, Marlene Fransen, Philippe Ravaud, Maxime Dougados, Ottawa Methods Group

Introduction

Osteoarthritis (OA) is often called "wear and tear" of the joints. OA causes certain parts of the joints to weaken and break down. Cartilage, the tough elastic material that cushions the ends of the bones, begins to crack and get holes in it. Bits of cartilage can break off into the joint space and irritate soft tissues, such as muscles, and cause problems with movement. Much of the pain of OA is a result of muscles and other tissues that help joints move (such as tendons and ligaments) being forced to work in ways for which they were not designed, as a result of damage to the cartilage. Cartilage itself does not have nerve cells, and therefore cannot sense pain, but muscles, tendons, ligaments, and bones do. After many years of cartilage erosion, bones may actually rub together, further increasing pain. Bones can also thicken and form growths, called spurs or osteophytes. Also, when cartilage is weak or damaged, extra stress is placed on the surrounding bones causing excessive blood flow (hyperaemia) that can cause pain, especially at night.

Case presentation

Mrs Smith, 64 years old, 81 kilos, 1·57 m, is complaining of mechanical (occurring after physical activities), chronic (more than 1 year) pain localised at the medial compartment of the right knee. The physical examination is normal.

The radiographs (anteroposterior view of both knees, standing position) performed 1 month ago showed a joint space narrowing of the tibiofemoral compartment joint space width (JSW): 5 mm at the left knee and 2 mm at the right knee), together with osteophytes of the tibial plateau.

Mrs Smith is wondering:

1. Which kind of painkillers she can take when the pain is no longer tolerable (Question 1).
2. Whether compounds such as glucosamine sulphate, chondroitin sulphate or diacerein can improve her condition (Questions 2 and 9).
3. Which kind of exercises might help her (Question 3).
4. Whether the use of sticks, specific shoes or insoles may slow the natural history of the disease (Question 7).

After a 6 month period of follow up, she returns because of an acute (less than 7 days) painful (at night and during the day) exacerbation of the knee pain. You are considering a knee aspiration together with an intra-articular injection of steroids (Questions 4, 5, and 6). You also try to convince her to lose weight, but she needs convincing (Question 8).

After a 5 year period, she returns again because she feels her condition has deteriorated.

The radiographs reveal the disappearance of joint space, pain is now interfering with most of her daily activities. She is 69 years old, without any concomitant disease except mild coronary disease and a moderate hypertension. Total knee arthroplasty has dramatically improved the condition of her brother-in-law and she is wondering whether such treatment might now be indicated to improve her condition (Question 10).

Literature search

General strategy

Start by searching for evidence syntheses with the Cochrane Library and with MEDLINE (Ovid, PubMed), looking specifically for meta-analyses. Both sources are rich in systematic reviews of numerous aspects of OA. When a systematic review is identified, then also search in MEDLINE (PubMed) to identify randomised controlled trials (RCTs) published after the publication date of the systematic review.

Searching for evidence syntheses: primary search strategy

Cochrane Library: osteoarthritis

MEDLINE (Ovid): Database: MEDLINE <1996 to September week 1 2002>: osteoarthritis AND (randomised controlled trials OR review literature OR decision making):

1. exp osteoarthritis/ or osteoarthritis.tw.
2. (meta-analysis or review).pt.
3. (meta-anal$ or metaanal$).tw.
4. (clinical trial or randomised controlled trial).pt.
5. (random$ or placebo).tw.
6. (double adj blind).tw.
7. 1 and (or/2–6)

Evaluating the evidence

Question 1

As first line symptomatic therapy, should we use NSAIDs or simple analgesics?

Additional literature search

Cochrane Library: osteoarthritis AND (non-steroidal anti-inflammatory drug OR analgesic)

MEDLINE (Ovid): Database: MEDLINE <1996 to April Week 3 2002>: osteoarthritis AND (randomised controlled trials OR review literature OR decision making) AND (non-steroidal anti-inflammatory drug OR analgesic OR acetamoniphen OR paracetamol):

1. osteoarthritis (all subheadings)
2. randomised controlled trials
3. review literature
4. decision making.
5. or/ 2–4
6. 1 and 5
7. anti-inflammatory agents, non-steroidal
8. analgesics
9. acetaminophen
10. paracetamol
11. or/ 7–10
12. 6 and 11

MEDLINE (PubMed): osteoarthritis, randomised controlled trials, review, NSAIDs, acetaminophen (4).

NSAIDS

In the Cochrane Library there are two systematic reviews of non-aspirin, non-steroidal anti-inflammatory drugs (NSAIDS) in the treatment of clinical and/or radiological confirmed OA of the knee and hip.[1,2] The outcome measures included validated measures of pain, physical function, patient global assessment, number of withdrawals due to lack of efficacy. Sample size calculation were assessed for the detection of clinically relevant changes in outcome measures. In spite of the large number of publications, there are few RCTs (16 trials have been identified for knee OA and 44 for hip OA). These trials appear to be weakened by the lack of standardisation of outcome assessments and of NSAID doses. No clear recommendations for the choice of specific NSAID therapy can be offered on this analysis.

Table 7.1 Number needed to treat for acetaminophen versus placebo (Amadio, 1983)[3]

Outcome	Improved with placebo	Improved with acetaminophen	Relative risk of improvement with acetaminophen (95% CI)	Absolute Benefit Increase (95% CI)	NNT(95% CI)
Rest pain	1/22 (5%)	16/22 (73%)	16·00 (2·32, 110·45)	68% (41, 83)	2 (2, 3)
Pain on motion	2/22 (9%)	15/22 (68%)	7·50 (1·94, 28·99)	59% (31,76)	2 (2, 4)
Physician global assessment	1/21 (5%)	20/21 (95%)	20·00 (2·95, 135·76)	90% (65, 96)	2 (2, 2)
Patient global	1/19 (5%)	18/19 (95%)	18·00 (2·66, 121·26)	89% (62, 96)	2 (2, 2)

Simple analgesics

There is some evidence that simple and narcotic analgesics, with little or no anti-inflammatory effect are comparably effective in the treatment of OA of the hip and the knee.

Only one placebo-controlled clinical trial has been performed to address the efficacy and safety of acetaminophen versus placebo in patients with OA. Amadio *et al*[3] conducted a 6-week, randomised, double-blind, crossover trial comparing 4000 mg/d of acetaminophen versus placebo in 25 knee OA patients. Significant improvement in pain at rest, pain on motion, and joint tenderness was observed in the active treatment group compared to placebo. There were no significant adverse effects reported.

(Table 7.1) (Visual Rx Faces 7.1)

Simple analgesics versus NSAIDS

A systematic review comparing tenoxicam with three other NSAIDs for OA found superiority of tenoxicam over piroxicam both for global efficacy (10 trials, 834 people; odds ratio 1·46, 1·08 to 2·03) and for global tolerability (seven trials, 974 people; 1·46, 1·01 to 2·15).[4] This result is at variance with a large RCT of 1328 people with OA or rheumatoid arthritis, which found no significant differences in global efficacy or tolerability between the two drugs; improvement was noted for 55% of patients receiving tenoxicam compared with 53% of patients on piroxicam (difference 2%, –5% to 9%).[5,6]

Several studies have been published since the Cochrane review publication. Eccles *et al* performed a meta-analysis of the previously discussed clinical trials comparing acetaminophen and NSAIDs.[7] They concluded that patients who received NSAIDs had greater improvement in pain at rest and at motion but no greater improvement in walk time and quality of life.

Pincus *et al* performed a 6 week, randomised, double blind, crossover trial comparing Arthrotec (diclofenac 153 mg/d plus misoprostol) and acetaminophen 4000 mg/d in 227 OA patients.[8] Improvement was statistically greater with Arthrotec than with acetaminophen, although patients with mild OA had similar improvements with both drugs. Even if acetaminophen was associated with fewer adverse events, Arthrotec was preferred by 60% of patients.

Altman *et al* (Abstract) performed a randomised double blind controlled trial comparing ibuprofen 1200 mg/d, acetaminophen 4000 mg/d, and placebo in 548 OA patients, and concluded to a similar efficacy of acetaminophen and ibuprofen in patients with mild to moderate pain, although ibuprofen was statistically superior to acetaminophen in patients with severe pain.[9]

Visual Rx Faces 7.1 NNT for acetaminophen compared to placebo

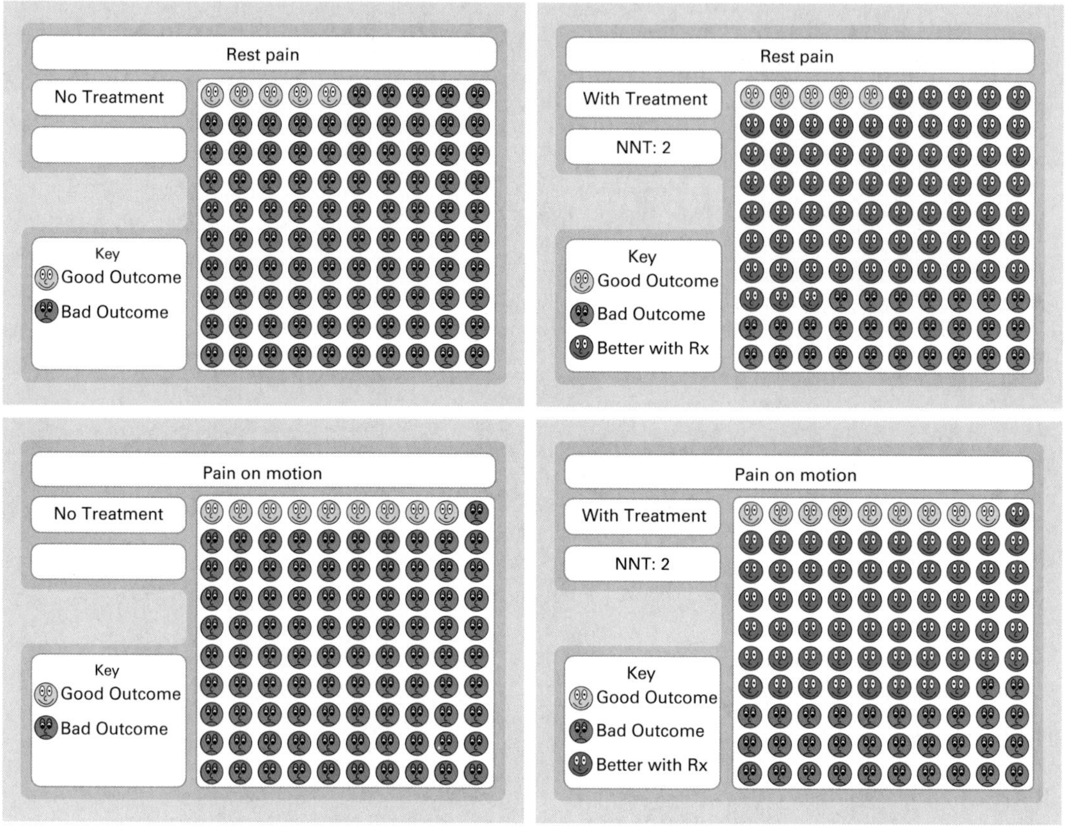

Rest pain
No Treatment
Key
Good Outcome
Bad Outcome

Rest pain
With Treatment
NNT: 2
Key
Good Outcome
Bad Outcome
Better with Rx

Pain on motion
No Treatment
Key
Good Outcome
Bad Outcome

Pain on motion
With Treatment
NNT: 2
Key
Good Outcome
Bad Outcome
Better with Rx

Temple *et al.* (Abstract) concluded that acetaminophen was effective in the treatment of knee OA pain and was well tolerated in doses of 4000 mg/d for up to 4 weeks and 2600 mg/d for up to 2 years.[10] They also concluded that an analgesic dose of acetaminophen (4000 mg/d) was similar in efficacy to an analgesic dose of ibuprofen (1200 mg/d) and to an anti-inflammatory dose of ibuprofen (2400 mg/d) for the treatment of the pain of knee OA with no significant adverse outcomes reported.

Simple analgesics versus coxibs

Geba *et al* performed a 6 week randomised, double blind, controlled trial comparing acetaminophen 4000 mg/d, celecoxib 200 mg/d and rofecoxib at doses of 12·5 mg/d or 25 mg/d in 379 patients with OA.[11] The rofecoxib 25 mg/d group showed greatest improvement with pain on walking, rest pain, night pain, morning stiffness, and global response than the other groups. At week 6, the percentage of patients who had a good or excellent patient global response to treatment on a 5-level Likert scale (cumulative incidence) were 39%, 46%, 56%, and 60% for the acetaminophen, celecoxib, 12·5 mg/d rofecoxib, and 25 mg/d rofecoxib groups, respectively. Changes between baseline and final, on a 0–100 WOMAC were for WOMAC were −24·9, −28·6, −28·0, −35·4 and for WOMAC pain subscale −19·5, −24·9, −24·3,

−29·7, for the acetaminophen, celecoxib, 12·5 mg/d rofecoxib and 25 mg/d rofecoxib groups, respectively. Changes were statistically significant between the acetaminophen group and the 25 mg/d rofecoxib group.

Peloso reviewed all the trials performed to address the efficacy and safety of opioids in patients with OA. All published trials demonstrated superiority of the opioids compared to placebo.[12] When acetaminophen is used as a comparator or rescue medication, opioids were superior analgesics. And these trials also suggest that opioids are superior to NSAIDs. However opioids are rarely considerd as first line symptomatic OA therapy.

Shamoon and Hochberg reviewed clinical trials of the efficacy and the safety of acetaminophen in the treatment of OA focusing on studies that compared acetaminophen to NSAIDs.[13]. They concluded that while NSAIDs play an important role in the management of patients with OA, their efficacy compared with analgesics such as acetaminophen is offset by a variety of adverse effects.

In the same year (2000) Gotzsche reviewed NSAIDs efficacy and safety.[14] He found no evidence that NSAIDs are more effective than simple analgesics, nor important differences in benefit between different NSAIDs or doses. Differences in toxicity related to increased doses and possibly to the nature of the NSAID itself was found. However, the coxibs have comparable efficacy to traditional dual inhibitor NSAIDs and have demonstrated a better gastrointestinal safety profile.[15]

However, when asked, many patients do have a considerable and statistically significant preference for NSAIDs compared with acetaminophen, even when both effectiveness and adverse effects are considered.[16]

Evidence summary: Silver

NSAIDs versus coxibs

Based on the observations of acetaminophen's efficacy, safety and cost, the authors recommend, as did the American College of Rheumatology and the European League Against Rheumatism, the use of analgesics such as acetaminophen in doses of up to 4 g per day for the initial pharmacological control of pain in patients with OA.[17] However, for patients who have severe pain and/or signs of inflammation, the use of NSAIDs including coxibs should be considered.[11,18]

Question 2

What is the level of symptomatic efficacy of specific anti-osteoarthritic drugs such as glucosamine sulphate, chondroitin sulphate, diacerein

Additional literature search

MEDLINE (Ovid): Database: MEDLINE <1966 to September Week 3 2002>:

(Please see primary search strategy 1 to 7, plus terms below)

8. slow acting drug. mp
9. antiosteoarthritic drug. mp
10. glucosamine. mp
11. exp. acetylglucosamine
12. n-acetylglucosamine. mp
13. n-acetyl-d-glucosamine. mp
14. avocado
15. soybeans
16. unsaponifiable
17. exp. chondroitin
18. chondroitin sulfate
19. diacerein

There are several RCTs assessing the symptomatic efficacy of different specific nutraceuticals but no meta-analysis has been conducted for any of these therapeutic agents. This literature review will therefore analyse the symptomatic efficacy of each agent separately.

Glucosamine sulphate

The Cochrane Library has published a systematic review combining the results of 16 RCTs assessing the efficacy of glucosamine for 2029 patients with OA.[19] The outcome variables included pain, range of motion, functional status, global assessment, radiographic assessment for changes in cartilage thickness, and health-related quality of life. Collectively, the 16 RCTs reviewed provide support for the symptomatic efficacy of glucosamine in the pharmacological management of OA. For pain, the pooled standardised mean difference (SMD) from seven RCTs ($n = 471$) for pain of glucosamine versus placebo 1.40 (95% CI 0·65, 2·14); for function (three RCTs $n = 563$) 0·63 (–0·044, 1·294).[20] The Cochrane Library review concluded that there is good evidence for both the symptomatic effectiveness and the safety of glucosamine for treating OA, however, the long term effectiveness and toxicity of glucosamine in OA remains unclear. As well, it is uncertain whether the different glucosamine preparations offered by different manufacturers are equally effective in the treatment of OA.[21]

Since the Cochrane meta-analysis, two RCTs and one meta-analysis assessing glucosamine have been published. The first RCT compared glucosamine versus placebo over a 60-day period in 98 patients and found no significant difference in resting pain or walking pain between the allocated groups.[22] The second RCT was a UK-based 6 month study which also failed to demonstrate the symptomatic efficacy of glucosamine compared to placebo ($n = 80$).[23] Finally, a recent meta-analysis of 15 placebo controlled RCTs assessing glucosamine and chondroitin preparations for OA symptoms concluded that although the trials evaluating pain and function demonstrated moderate to large effects, study methodological quality issues and likely publication bias suggest treatment effects may be exaggerated.[24] The aggregated effect size was 0·44 (95% CI 0·24–0·64). Similar results were observed when confining the models to trials with pain outcomes: 0·51 (0·05–0·96) and with function outcomes: 0·41 (0·14–0·69).

Evidence summary: Silver

One systematic review and two subsequent RCTs reveal mixed results. However, the results of the meta-analysis of the Cochrane Library lead to the conclusion that glucosamine has a symptomatic efficacy in osteoarthritis.

Chondroitin

The systematic quality assessment and meta-analysis of McAlindon *et al*, evaluating 15 RCTs assessing the efficacy of chondroitin in OA, concluded symptomatic efficacy of this drug versus placebo[24] (Table 7.2). The aggregated effect sizes was 0·96 (95% CI 0·63–1·30). Similar results were observed when confining the models to trials with pain outcomes: 0·86 (0·64–1·09) and to trials with function outcomes: 0·63 (0·32–0·94). However, the authors suggested that a possible publication bias might be amplifying the treatment effect found. Since the publication of this meta-analysis, a subsequent RCT (130 patients) found no significant difference between chondroitin sulphate (1 g daily) versus placebo over 6 months on the Lequesne scale.[25]

Evidence summary: Silver

The results of meta-analyses suggest symptomatic efficacy of chondroitin sulphate in OA with some concern about publication bias inflating results.

Glucosamine, chondroitin, and manganese combination

No RCTs of glucosamine plus chondroitin alone versus placebo were found, but two RCTs compare the combination of glucosamine–chondroitin plus manganese, a cofactor

Table 7.2 Number needed to treat for chondroitin versus placebo (McAlindon 2000)[24]

Outcome	Pooled standardised mean difference (95% CI)	% benefiting (95% CI) with chondroitin	NNT (95% CI)
Symptomatic relief	0·96 (0·63, 1·30) (note: significant for heterogeneity)	42% (30, 52)	3 (2, 4)
Symptomatic relief *	0·78 (0·60, 0·95)	35% (28, 45)	3 (3, 4)
Pain	0·86 (0·64, 1·09)	38% (30, 46)	3 (3, 4)
Function	0·63 (0·32, 0·95)	30% (15, 41)	4 (3, 7)

*Pain, Lequesne score, mobility, NSAID use (excluding the only intramuscular trial, after which heterogeneity was no longer statistically significant).

necessary for the efficient synthesis of proteoglycans.[26,27] The first RCT compared a combination of glucosamine plus chondroitin plus manganese ascorbate versus placebo in 34 patients with knee OA or degenerative low back pain over a 16-week treatment period.[26] The study found statistically significant improvements in disease score, self assessment, and pain score in patients allocated to active treatment compared with those allocated to placebo. In contrast, the second RCT, comparing a combination of glucosamine plus chondroitin plus manganese versus placebo over a period of 6 months in 93 knee OA patients, found no clear evidence of symptomatic effectiveness of the active treatment versus placebo.[27] The authors stratified the patients among their radiographic severity. In the mild to moderate cases (KL grade 2 or 3), 52% of patients in the treated group presented at least 25% of improvement in Lequesne index versus 28% of patients in the placebo group. But this positive result was not confirmed in the severe cases (KL grade 4) group (23% *v* 25%).

Evidence summary: Silver

Two RCTs gave inconsistent results.

Diacerein

Three RCTs have evaluated the efficacy and the safety of diacerein in patients with hip or knee OA.[28–30]

Diacerein versus placebo

There is evidence that diacerein has significant symptomatic (pain) effectiveness compared with placebo (two RCTs : $n = 772$).[28,29] At week 24, for the 100 mg/d group,[28] pain (VAS) standardised response mean (SRM) was 0·34, and function (WOMAC subscale) SRM 0·32. However, in a recent 3 year RCT, no statistically significant difference in the symptomatic variables between the diacerein group and the placebo group was observed ($n = 507$).[30]

Diacerein versus NSAIDs

When compared to NSAIDs, no statistically significant difference between the effectiveness of diacerein and tenoxicam in terms of pain and Lequesne index could be demonstrated.[29] In this 8 week RCT, patients who showed improvement of at least 30% in pain were 40·3%, 61·1%, 55·5%, 63·8%, and in function 29·2%, 52·8%, 40·3%, 56·9% in the placebo group, tenoxicam group, diacerein group, and diacerein plus tenoxicam group, respectively. The onset of action of diacerein was delayed (over 4 weeks) compared to that of the NSAID (under 2 weeks). These results may be due to the characteristics of the patients and the design of the trial. The patients in this 3 year structural trial had lower baseline levels of pain and functional impairment than did those of patients included in previous short-term (12–24 weeks) studies evaluating the symptomatic effects of diacerein. Moreover, during the study, symptomatic rescue treatments, such as analgesics and/or NSAIDs, were permitted, attenuating the potential beneficial effects of diacerein on symptoms. No differences were seen between these groups. The treatment was well tolerated and the most frequent adverse events were transient changes in bowel habits.

Evidence summary: Silver

Three RCTs against placebo gave mixed results.

Avocado/soybean unsaponifiables

Only two RCTs have evaluated the symptomatic effectiveness of avocado/soybean unsaponifiables (ASU) versus placebo in the treatment of knee or hip OA with contradictory results.[31,32] The first one (n = 163) failed to demonstrate any difference on clinical outcomes (pain, function, global assessment) between both groups at one year.[31] The second RCT (n = 164) provided evidence that ASU was symptomatically effective on pain outcomes compared to placebo at 6 months.[32]

Evidence summary: Silver

Two RCTs against placebo gave inconsistent results.

Glycosaminoglycan polysulphuric acid complex

The only RCT (n = 388) evaluating the effects of glycosaminoglycan polysulphuric acid complex (Rumalon) failed to demonstrate any structural efficacy at year 5.[33] In addition, no differences were found between Rumalon and placebo for Lequesne Algofunctional Index (LAI) pain on passive motion or consumption of NSAIDS.

Evidence summary: Silver

One RCT against placebo did not find evidence of benefit.

Evidence summary

Silver. Glucosamine, chondroitin.

Bronze. Diacerin, avocado/soybean unsaponifiables, glycosaminoglycan polysulphuric acid complex.

The literature reports that specific anti-osteoarthritic drugs such as glucosamine sulphate, chondroitin sulphate, and diacerein have a symptomatic effect compared to placebo. However, the level of evidence of their efficacy is limited due to methodological considerations in a number of these published reports, including lack of standardised case definitions and standardised outcome assessments, as well as insufficient information about study design. The ACR and the EULAR recommendations for the medical treatment of OA are not consistent; the ACR subcommittee (2000 update)[34] considers that it is premature to make specific recommendations about any of these treatments, while the EULAR task force considers that such drugs have a weak detectable symptomatic effect.

Question 3

What is the level of evidence of symptomatic efficacy of exercise?

Additional literature search

Cochrane Database of Systematic Reviews <2nd Quarter 2002>

MEDLINE (OVID): Database MEDLINE <1966 to June Week 2 2002>: osteoarthritis AND (exercise therapy):

1. osteoarthritis (all subheadings)
2. exercise therapy
3. 1 and 2

CINAHL (OVID): Database CINAHL <1982 to May week 5 2002>: osteoarthritis AND (exercise therapy):

1. osteoarthritis
2. exercise therapy
3. 1 and 2

Reference lists of retrieved articles and reviews were examined.

Many physicians have accepted graded exercise, as a potentially effective joint protective intervention for people with symptomatic osteoarthritis (OA) of the knee. In fact, both the ACR and the EULAR[35,36] strongly recommend exercise as the mainstay of non-pharmacological treatment. Three systematic reviews, combining the results of mostly small randomised trials comparing exercise with a non-exercise control group,[37–39] have recently been published.

The systematic review and meta-analysis conducted by Van Baar *et al*,[39] on randomised trials published up to September 1997, was able to combine the results of six trials conducted amongst people with OA of the hip or knee. After meta-analysis of the results for pain (six studies, mean small–moderate beneficial effect), self-reported disability (five studies, mean small beneficial effect), observed disability in walking (four studies, mean small beneficial effect), and patient's global assessment of effect (two studies, mean medium–large beneficial effect), the reviewers concluded that "the small number of good studies restricts drawing firm conclusions".

A subsequent systematic review conducted by Petrella[38] retrieved randomised trials conducted amongst people with OA published up until January 2000. The results for pain (14 studies), self-reported disability (six studies), walking (eight studies) and patient global assessment (two studies) were not quantitatively combined in a meta-analysis, but an extensive qualitative synthesis of the data provided by the studies for each outcome was reported. The review concluded there were "beneficial short term effects of exercise treatment in patients with OA knee".

The latest systematic review and meta-analysis[37] was able to retrieve 31 randomised trials conducted amongst people with OA knee published up until March 2001. Of the 31 retrieved studies, 14 met the inclusion criteria [40–53] (see Tables 7.2, 7.3). The 14 studies included provided data on 936 participants allocated to land-based therapeutic exercise and 697 participants allocated to a non-exercise control group. Only six of the 14 studies could demonstrate at least 80% power to detect a moderate treatment effect (0·5) at a significance level of 0·05.[42,43,47–50,53] Combining the results for the 14 included trials gave a standardised mean difference for exercise over control of 0·46 (95% CI 0·35–0·57) for self-reported pain and 0·33 (95% CI 0·23–0·43) for self-reported physical function (Tables 7.3, 7.4 and 7.5). These effects would be rated as moderate and small, respectively.[54]

The consistent finding of the three systematic studies including reviews was that land-based exercise results in small to moderate beneficial effect for people with OA knee. This should not be disappointing since people with chronic diseases can usually only attain small to medium effect sizes due to the inherent variability in the sample.[54]

Since the latest systematic review, the results of two small randomised trials have been published: one assessing a home-based programme of strength training[55] and one assessing the relative contribution of two forms

Table 7.3 Proportion of patients with OA knee benefiting from therapeutic land-based exercise (pooled data from Fransen, 2002)[37]

Outcome	Pooled standardised mean difference (95% CI)	% benefiting (95% CI) with exercise	NNT (95% CI)
Self-reported pain	−0·46 (−0·35, −0·57)	22% (16, 34)	5 (3, 6)
Self-reported function	−0·33 (−0·23, −0·43)*	16% (11, 21)	7 (5, 9)

*This estimate was significant for heterogeneity.

Table 7.4 Self-reported pain: standardised mean difference (SMD) and 95% confidence intervals (95% CI)

Study	Exercise (*n*)	Control (*n*)	Favours exercise	Favours control	SMD (95% CI)
Bautch[40]	15	15			1·20 (0·41, 1·98)
Deyle[41]	33	36			0·93 (0·43, 1·43)
Ettinger (A)[42]	144	75			0·53 (0·24, 0·81)
Ettinger (R)[42]	146	75			0·36 (0·08, 0·64)
Fransen[43]	83	43			0·62 (0·24, 0·99)
Hopman-Rock[44]	45	37			0·20 (−0·23, 0·64)
Kovar[45]	47	45			0·59 (0·17, 1·01)
Maurer[46]	49	49			0·19 (−0·21, 0·58)
Minor[47]	49	19			0·27 (−0·27, 0·80)
O'Reilly[48]	108	72			0·32 (0·02, 0·62)
Peloquin[49]	59	65			0·40 (0·04, 0·76)
Rogind[51]	11	12			0·50 (−0·33, 1·34)
Schilke[52]	10	10			1·06 (0·11, 2·01)
Van Baar[53]	54	59			0·55 (0·17, 0·92)
Overall	853	612			0·46 (0·35, 0·57)

−1 −5 0 5 1

of muscle strengthening.[56] The beneficial results of exercise are of a similar magnitude to those found in the systematic reviews.

Water-based exercise programmes were not included in the last two systematic reviews. However, a recent Cochrane systematic review evaluating randomised trials of hydrotherapy for patients with rheumatoid arthritis or OA did not include any studies conducted amongst people with OA knee.[57]

Several concerns in clinical trial methodology specific to the assessment of physical interventions such as exercise emerged from the above reviews. The primary concern is that the double blind "gold standard", specifically blinding of the therapist and the participant, is arguably unattainable for exercise. Given this limitation, it is of concern that many of the reviewed studies did not conduct – or report – blinded outcomes assessment is, on the other hand, the suspected lack of responsiveness of

Table 7.5 Self-reported physical function: standardised mean difference (SMD) and 95% confidence intervals (95% CI)

Study	Exercise (*n*)	Control (*n*)	Favours exercise / Favours control	SMD (95% CI)
Bautch[40]	15	15		–0·08 (–0·80, 0·63)
Deyle[41]	33	36		0·82 (0·32, 1·31)
Ettinger[42]	144	75		0·37 (0·09, 0·66)
Ettinger[42]	146	75		0·33 (0·05, 0·61)
Fransen[43]	83	43		0·39 (0·01, 0·76)
Hopman-Rock[44]	37	34		–0·18 (–0·65, 0·28)
Kovar[45]	47	45		1·10 (0·66, 1·54)
Maurer[46]	49	49		0·05 (–0·35, 0·44)
Minor[47]	49	19		0·48 (–0·05, 1·02)
O'Reilly[48]	108	72		0·29 (–0·01, 0·59)
Peloquin[49]	59	65		0·38 (0·02, 0·74)
Petrella[50]	91	88		0·22 (–0·07, 0·52)
Rogind[51]	11	12		0·22 (–0·60, 1·04)
Schilke[52]	10	10		0·91 (–0·02, 1·84)
Van Baar[53]	54	59		0·14 (–0·23, 0·51)
Overall	936	697		0·33 (0·23, 0·43)

–1 –5 0 5 1

self-reported physical function in early disease. People with early OA knee often have reduced lower limb muscle strength and aerobic capacity compared with their peers without the disease. However, these physiological impairments are frequently not yet sufficient to translate to reportable difficulties with activities of daily living, as important qualitative changes to functional movement patterns or adaptations to lifestyle or environment have been made. As clinical trials assessing exercise often target recruitment at early disease, important improvements in physiological function attributable to exercise will be undetected with self-report measures. Further specific aspects of study methodology that were highly recommended for future studies include: adequate sample sizes so that studies are sufficiently powered to demonstrate at least a moderate effect, analysis as "per intention to treat" and not just treatment completers, assessment of the sustainability of treatment effect, control of analgesia, and reporting of adverse effects. However, it was noted in the latest systematic review that the treatment effect of exercise may have been underestimated in the meta-analysis as many studies used an effective "complementary" non pharmacological strategy, such as education classes, as the control or "placebo" group.

Evidence summary: Gold

The three systematic reviews consistently provide evidence for small to moderate symptomatic efficacy (effect size versus placebo: 0·57, 0·59, 1·00) of (land-based) therapeutic exercise for people with OA of the knee. However, a continuing paucity of clinical trials in this area of research as well as substantial clinical heterogeneity in terms of participants recruited and interventions studied, precludes any specific recommendation regarding optimal treatment content (resistance, flexibility, aerobic) dosage (frequency, duration, intensity) or treatment delivery mode (individually provided treatments, group programmes or home-based exercise).

Question 4

Does an acute disease flare predict subsequent accelerated cartilage breakdown (which may be minimised by more aggressive therapy?)

Additional literature search

MEDLINE (Ovid): Database: MEDLINE <1966 to September Week 3 2002>:

1. osteoarthritis (all subheadings)
2. flare
3. 1 and 2
4. outcomes
5. and/1–4
6. progression
7. knee effusion.mp
8. 2 or 6
9. 1 and 8
10. 1 and 7
11. cartilage breakdown
12. acute
13. 12 or 8
14. 1 and 4 and 13
15. prognostic
16. 1 and 14
17. 7 and 16

In other words, are disease flares, defined as episodes of acute painful knee effusion, associated with an accelerated rate of joint space narrowing?

Several studies on cohorts of knee OA patients have assessed factors affecting radiographic disease progression,[58–60] but only a few have focused on the impact of acute flares.

There is evidence that knee effusion is associated with more severe symptomatic disease. In a cross-sectional study of 162 patients, variables reflecting an acute flare such as swelling, effusion, and increased joint temperature, were more reliable than variables reflecting disease chronicity for assessing clinical disease severity.[61] In the same way, a magnetic resonance imaging (MRI) study of 52 patients with OA knee has revealed that knee effusions increase in prevalence with increasing radiographic disease severity, ranging from 25% in those with mild radiographic disease to 100% in those with severe radiographic disease.[62] In contrast, Claessens *et al.* could not find any single clinical finding, including palpable effusion or swelling of the soft tissues, able to accurately predict the presence of radiographic knee OA.[63]

There is less evidence that knee effusion is associated with accelerated disease progression. In a 1 year follow up study of 736 patients with knee OA (353 completers), Dougados *et al*[64] found that the rate of joint space narrowing was better correlated with the treatments received, including synovial fluid aspiration, and that OA flares seemed to be correlated with the chondrolysis observed. A second prospective cohort study (350 OA knees) also found that joint space narrowing over a 2 year period occurred with increased frequency in patients with a history of effusions, and then particularly warm effusions (flares).[65] Lastly, in a 6 month follow up arthroscopic study of 46 patients with patellofemoral chondropathy, knee effusion presence at baseline and progression of chondropathy were positively correlated with the presence of synovitis at baseline.[66]

Acute flares seem to be associated with radiographic disease status and progression, assessed by joint space narrowing. Even if the level of evidence is moderate, this association suggests that loss of joint space width may not be a continuous phenomenon but occurring episodically during periods of disease flares.[67,68]

In our opinion, a flare may be a clinical marker of the OA disease process associated with a potential increased risk for accelerated cartilage breakdown. Therefore, it may be of benefit to focus, during these episodes, on the treatment of the flare with a combination of joint activity limitation, NSAIDs, and intra-articular injection of corticosteroids.[69]

Evidence summary: Bronze

Biological sense would suggest that flares should be treated aggressively. No RCTs to assess this were found.

Question 5

What is the level of evidence of symptomatic efficacy of intra-articular injections of corticosteroids?

Additional literature search

MEDLINE (Ovid): Database: MEDLINE <1966 to September Week 3 2002>:

(Please see primary search strategy 1 to 7, plus terms below)

8. injections, intra-articular
9. 7 and 8
10. hyaluronic acid
11. 7 and 10
12. steroids/tu
13. 7 and 12
14. 8 and 12

Intra-articular corticosteroids

Two systematic reviews assessing the efficacy of intra-articular corticosteroids for patients with knee OA were published in 1997. Kirwan and Rankin reviewed ten RCTs (search date not stated).[70] Common outcome measures, which allowed comparisons between the studies, were pain scores and the proportion of patients who improved compared with the pre-injection assessment (either in relation to pain or to the patient's overall assessment of their knee OA). This systematic review found that the intra-articular injection of glucocorticoids into the knee (one trial used four injections, the rest used single injections) provided some additional pain relief compared with placebo treatment. However, there were no significant differences between treatment groups occurring after more than 1 week of follow up. Interestingly, patient preference expressed at the end of the treatment period in one study did favour corticosteroids over placebo.[71]

Towheed and Hochberg summarised evidence from five RCTs of intra-articular steroids in knee OA patients published up to August 1994.[72] Using a quality rating system, critical analysis showed that none of the studies achieved a score of more than 3, out of a possible 8, for study design.[73] The review did conclude that intra-articular steroids were superior to placebo in short-term efficacy (< 1 month). This short-lived efficacy may be attenuated by a powerful response to placebo. In one study, for example, both placebo and treated groups showed a significant decrease in pain from week 1 to the final assessment at week 8.[74]

More recently, Ayral reviewed eight RCTs assessing intra-articular steroids versus placebo published up until October 2001[75] (see Table 7.6). Except for the two earliest studies, patients received a single corticosteroid injection. The steroids studied were hydrocortisone, prednisolone, triamcinolone hexatonide, methylprednisolone, and cortivazol. These different drugs have not been compared with one another. The clinical assessment of efficacy was pain relief. This review was able to conclude that there is evidence intra-articular steroid injections are effective, but that their benefit over placebo may be relatively short-lived, lasting only from 1 to 4 weeks.

There are no RCTs to assess whether the simple aspiration of the knee would not be as effective as injection.

Evidence summary: Silver

Systematic reviews of RCTs found that intra-articular steroids are effective in relieving pain in the short term.

Viscosupplementation

Viscosupplementation refers to the intra-articular injection of, in most cases, hyaluronic acid (HA), a high molecular weight polysaccharide which is a major component of synovial fluid and cartilage, in order to relieve pain and improve function. In OA, the molecular weight and concentration of HA is diminished. The concept of viscosupplementation suggests that intra-articular injection of HA could help restore the viscoelasticity of the synovial fluid.

The literature contains three systematic reviews and one additional RCT comparing hyaluronan preparations to placebo.[70,72,75,84] Most studies in humans have been carried out in patients with knee OA.

The first review identified 10 RCTs of hyaluronan in the knee joint (search date not stated) and found slightly greater benefit versus placebo at 1–6 months after treatment.[70] The second review (nine RCTs assessing biological agents, including HA) concluded that biological agents were superior to placebo and well tolerated over a mean follow-up of 48 weeks.[72] The third review evaluated separately the different hyaluronan preparations[75] Eight of nine RCTs found Hyalgan to be more effective than placebo for pain but also for function in three trials and for reduction in the number of intra-articular steroid injections in a one year trial. The three RCTs assessing Synvisc® also found this hyaluronan preparation superior to placebo. The results concerning the efficacy of Artz® compared to placebo are more contrasted. Of the three RCTs, only one found Artz more effective for pain and function compared with placebo.

Since publication of the previous reviews, one further RCT has been reported.[84] Brandt *et al* conducted a multicentre RCT evaluating the safety and the efficacy of Orthovisc® compared to physiologic saline in 226 patients. They found Orthovisc to be well tolerated and more effective than control in patients with a mild to moderate pain at baseline (Table 7.7).

Hyaluronan versus corticosteroids injections

In a systematic review comparing Hyalgan to various steroids, Ayral found five RCTs, three of which were unblinded, reporting a similar benefit to hyaluronic acid steroids at one month, but then followed by a superiority of Hyalgan after a few months.[75]

Hyaluronan versus NSAIDs

Three RCTs comparing hyaluronan with NSAIDs found that hyaluronan obtained a similar benefit as NSAIDs for pain, and in one trial for function, but with fewer gastrointestinal adverse effects.[85–87]

Evidence summary: Silver

RCTs show some evidence of long term pain reduction with intra-articular viscosupplementation versus placebo for up to 6 months after treatment.

The planned formal meta-analysis [88,89] of both intra-articular corticosteroids and viscosupplementation for knee OA by the Cochrane

Table 7.6 Intra-articular steroids versus placebo

Study	Corticosteroid	Control	Patient	Design	Injections	Duration (wk)	Results
Miller[76]	HC 50 mg	Placebo Novocaine Lactic acid Feigned injection	202	Parallel, single blind	5	24	Equal at wk 6 and wk 24 (pain)
Wright[77]	HC 25 mg	Placebo HC, TBA	25	Cross-over, double blind	4	4	wk 2: HC = P HC, TBA > P wk 4: HC (± TBA) = P (pain, tenderness, motion)
Cederlof[78]	Prednisolone 25 mg	Placebo	44	Parallel, double blind	1	8	Equal at wk 1, wk 3; wk 8 (pain, global assessment)
Friedman[79]	TH 20 mg	Placebo	34	Parallel, double blind	1	8	TH > P at 1 wk only (pain)
Dieppe[80]	TH 20 mg	Placebo	12 and 16	Parallel/cross-over, single blind	1	6 and 2	TH > P at 2 wk only (pain)
Gaffney[81]	TH 20 mg	Placebo	84	Parallel, double blind	1	6	TH > P at 1 wk only (pain)
Jones[82]	MP 40 mg	Placebo	59	Cross-over, double blind	1	8	MP > P at 3 wk only (pain)
Ravaud[83]	Cortivazol 3·75 mg	Placebo Cortivazol Lavage Lavage + cortivazol	98	Parallel, 2 x factorial, double blind	1	24	Cortivazol > P at wk 4 only (pain) Lavage (± Cortivazol) > P at wk 24 for pain

Abbreviations: HC = hydrocortisone ; HC,TBA = hydrocortisone tertiary butylacetate ; TH = triamcinolone hexacetonide ; MP = methylprednisolone; P = placebo.

Source: from Ayral X. In *Best Practice and Research Clinical Rheumatology* 2001;**15**(4):609–26, with permission

Collaboration will clarify the level of evidence supporting the symptomatic efficacy of these intra-articular treatments.

Question 6

Is the presence of joint effusion a predisposing factor for a better response to the intra-articular injection of steroids?

Additional literature search

MEDLINE (Ovid) : Database: MEDLINE <1966 to September Week 1 2002>:

(Please see primary search strategy 1 to 7, plus terms below)

8. injections, intra-articular
9. 7 and 8

Table 7.7 Number needed to treat for Orthovisc (efficacy data 27 weeks) (Brandt, 2001)[84]

Outcome	Improved with saline	Improved with Orthovisc	Relative risk of improvement with Orthovisc (95% CI)	Absolute Benefit Increase (95% CI)	NNT (95% CI)
Five or more units improvement in WOMAC pain score (approx. 50% improvement from baseline)	28/69 (41%)	38/66 (58%)	1·42 (1·00, 2·02)	0·17% (2, 34)	6 (4, 602)

10. steroids/tu
11. 8 and 10
12. knee effusion.mp
13. joint aspiration.mp
14. 8 and 13

An analysis by Jones and Doherty, examining a range of factors including function, psychosocial and disease-related features using logistic regression, failed to relate patient response to any of the baseline variables, including the presence of a joint effusion.[90] However, a significant predictor may have been missed due to the small sample size of the RCT. Only 59 knee OA patients were included in that placebo controlled crossover study.[91] For Friedman and Moore, the efficacy of steroids was also not related to the presence or to the absence of knee effusion.[92]

However, Kirwan and Rankin observed that practically all the RCTs in their review included aspiration of the joint to apparent dryness at the time of injection.[93] Therefore, the high placebo response observed may be the result of a true physiological reduction due to joint aspiration alone. In support of this, one single blinded trial ($n = 60$) reported a greater response to triamcinolone hexacetonide in patients with knee effusions who had synovial fluid successfully aspirated at the time of injection.[94] However, aspiration of the synovial fluid alone (compared with inability to aspirate synovial fluid) was not associated with a greater reduction in pain in the placebo group.

An explanation may be that the presence of knee effusion seems to be correlated with the presence of synovitis in osteoarthritis and that intra-articular steroids may be more effective for this inflammatory flare of the disease (see Question 4).[95,96] In support of this hypothesis, one RCT in 147 rheumatoid arthritis patients found a significant reduction in relapse in the group treated with complete synovial fluid aspiration before triamcinolone hexacetonide injection compared to the group without aspiration.[97] Another explanation may be that the greater pain and treatment efficacy demonstrated after successful aspiration of synovial fluid is related to the accuracy of the intra-articular injection.[91] Jones *et al* reported in a contrast radiography study that one-third of knee injections were extra-articular or uncertain and that aspiration of synovial fluid was associated with improved accuracy.[98]

Evidence summary: Silver

There is limited evidence from one RCT that the presence of hydarthrodial effusion is a predisposing factor for a better response to the intra-articular injection of steroids. However, *in our opinion* (see Question 4), knee effusion may reflect the presence of inflammatory synovitis, justifying the intra-articular injection of steroids.

Question 7

What is the level of evidence for the symptomatic efficacy of shoe insoles?

Additional literature search

Cochrane Library (CDSR, ACP Journal Club, DARE, CCTR):

1. osteoarthritis. mp [mp = ti, ot, ab, tx, kw, ct, sh, hw]
2. insoles
3. 1 and 2

MEDLINE (Ovid): Database: MEDLINE <1966 to July Week 3 2002>:

(Please see primary search strategy 1 to 7, plus terms below)

8. insole, orthoses (orthotic devices)
9. insole (shoe)
10. 7 and (8 or 9)

MEDLINE (PubMed): osteoarthritis, randomised, insoles (2).

Non-pharmacological treatments, such as insoles or orthoses, are recommended for the management of patients with knee OA.[99,100]. However, a literature search finds few published data on clinical outcomes and only two RCTs.

In the first RCT, Maillefert *et al* evaluated the symptomatic effect of insole wear for patients with medial compartment knee OA.[101] This 6 month study, comparing the clinical effects of laterally wedged insoles to neutrally wedged insoles, both with a capacity to absorb impact loading, failed to demonstrate the symptomatic efficacy of the laterally wedged insoles. However, the observed decrease in the use of NSAIDs and better treatment compliance in the laterally wedged insole group suggested a potential beneficial effect. These results were unchanged at a 2 year follow up assessment.[102]

In the second RCT, Toda *et al* evaluated the efficacy of laterally wedged insoles with or without elastic strapping in knee OA.[103] In this 8-week study, patients wearing the elastically strapped insoles significantly improved their pain score at the final assessment. This significant change was not found in the control group wearing inserted insoles without strapping.

Two other controlled trials of insoles, without randomisation, showed a short term improvement in the treatment group over the control group.[104,105]

Evidence summary: Silver

Two RCTs found mixed results on the symptomatic efficacy of insoles in knee OA.

Question 8

What is the symptomatic or structural efficacy of weight reduction?

Additional literature search

Cochrane Library Database of Systematic Reviews:

1. osteoarthritis
2. weight loss
3. 1 and 2

MEDLINE (Ovid): Database: MEDLINE <1966 to July Week 3 2002>:

(Please see primary search strategy 1 to 7, plus terms below)

8. weight loss. mp
9. weight reduction. mp
10. 7 and 8
11. 7 and 9

12. 1 and 8
13. 1 and 9
14. obesity
15. 7 and 14
16. 1 and 14

Several epidemiological studies have found that obesity is a major risk factor for the development and progression of knee OA.[106] Longitudinal data from the Framingham study have confirmed a causal relationship with obesity preceding the onset of OA.[107,108] In the Chinford study, obese women with unilateral knee OA had a greater risk of progression of structural disease in the affected knee and a greater risk of developing OA in the unaffected knee.[109] In general, this relationship is stronger in women than in men, especially in overweight post-menopausal women.[110,111]

In the Framingham Osteoarthritis Study, a decrease in body mass index (BMI) of at least 2 units in the preceding 10 years was associated with a 50% reduction in the risk of developing symptomatic knee OA.[112] Among women with a high risk for OA, due to elevated baseline BMI (greater than or equal to 25), weight loss markedly decreased the risk (for 2 units of BMI, 6% reduction in risk).

Avoidance of overweight is clearly important in terms of primary and, although there is good face validity to support weight reduction for secondary prevention, there are few clinical trials.[113]

One small RCT examined the use of weight loss mediation in subjects with knee OA and found a correlation between weight loss and improvements in symptoms.[114] Patients were randomised to an appetite suppressant, phentermine, or placebo and all patients participated in a weight loss programme. Weight loss (3–6 kg on average) correlated strongly with a reduction in an OA clinical score, the correlation being stronger for knee compared with hip OA.

A 6 month single blind RCT combined exercise with cognitive behavioural weight reduction and compared this intervention with exercise alone in subjects with knee OA (age ≥ 60 years).[115] Both groups lost weight (mean 8.5 kg in the exercise with weight reduction group versus 1·8 kg in the exercise alone group) and reported similar significant improvements in pain and disability. There was no clear benefit from the addition to exercise of the weight reduction programme, although this was a small study ($n = 24$).

A larger non-randomised study ($n = 126$) recently reported significant improvements in pain (VAS) and function (Lequesne algofunctional index) in subjects with knee OA who were able to lose more than 15% of initial body weight.[116]

One uncontrolled study examined the effect of weight loss on knee pain after gastric stapling.[117] There was a dramatic reduction in the prevalence of knee pain post-surgery (14 to 54%), however, these patients had lost an average of 45 kg in weight and did not necessarily have knee OA.

Lastly, a randomised unblinded study specifically evaluated the efficacy of change in body fat compared with a change in body weight in symptomatic knee OA.[118] Overweight patients (n = 22) were treated with a low calorie diet, with an appetite suppressant, NSAIDs, and received instruction in a walking programme. Controls got NSAIDs and the walking programme (n = 15) (Table 7.8). The patients in the diet group lost a mean of 3·9 kg over the course of 6 weeks, and also had significant improvement in remission score of Lequesne index of severity. Although this study had limitations, it provided the only data from a randomised trial demonstrating a relationship between loss of body fat (rather than loss of body weight) and improvement in symptoms of knee OA.[119]

Table 7.8 Number needed to treat for appetite suppressant, diet, NSAIDs, and walking versus NSAIDs and walking alone (Toda, 1998)[118]

Outcome	Improved with NSAIDs and walking alone	Improved with appetite suppressant, diet, NSAIDs, and walking	Relative risk of improvement with appetite suppressant and diet (95% CI)	Absolute Benefit Increase (95% CI)	NNT(95% CI)
% Improved. remission score (Lequesne index of severity)	4/15 (27%)	19/22 (86%)	3·24 (1·38, 7·62)	60% (27, 79)	2 (2, 4)

There are currently no published studies evaluating the structural effect of weight reduction on the rate of progression of knee OA.

The ACR recommends that overweight patients, especially if they are considered candidates for total knee arthroplasty, should be encouraged to participate in a comprehensive weight management programme.[120] Observational studies have found obesity to be associated with worse outcomes from joint replacement, in terms of self-assessed satisfaction and joint replacement failure rates. One systematic review identified 40 observational studies (number of people not stated) relating individual characteristics to outcome after hip replacement.[121] This review found that the following factors predicted better outcomes in terms of pain relief and function: age 45–75 years; weight less than 70 kg; good social support; higher educational level; and less preoperative morbidity. However, one prospective English cohort study (n = 176) found no difference in the quality of life after a primary hip replacement between the non-obese and moderately obese patients either at 1 or 3 years. However, the study reported no results in patients with a BMI greater than 40.[122] However, a Swedish cohort study found lower rates of long term implant survival in obese people.[123]

Evidence summary: Silver

There is limited evidence from RCTs of moderate symptomatic benefit from weight reduction for overweight and obese people with knee OA. Observational studies have demonstrated overweight is clearly associated with the risk of developing knee OA and is probably associated with poorer outcomes after joint replacement surgery.

No studies were found to assess the structural efficacy of weight reduction.

Question 9

Is there any evidence of a beneficial structural effect of any long term daily intake of oral drugs?

Additional literature search

MEDLINE (Ovid): Database: MEDLINE <1966 to December Week 3 2002>:

(Please see primary search strategy 1 to 7, plus terms below)

8. structural effect
9. progression
10. structure
11. structure progression
12. 7 and 8
13. 7 and 9
14. 7 and 10

NSAIDs

There is *in vitro* and *in vivo* evidence pointing to a possible beneficial structural effect of the use of NSAIDs, but there are presently no clinical data suggesting a beneficial structural effect for any available NSAID.[124,125] In fact, there are two RCTs suggesting a deleterious structural effect of daily, long term indomethacin intake. In the first RCT, 812 people with knee OA were treated with indomethacin 75 mg/d, tiaprofenic acid 600 mg/d or placebo. The indomethacin group showed a significantly higher rate of OA progression compared to the two other groups at 1 year.[126] The second RCT evaluated the time to arthroplasty of 105 patients with hip OA treated by indomethacin or azapropazone. The azapropazone group took longer than the indomethacin group to reach the arthroplasty end-point.[127] Another RCT, however, suggested a lack of such structural effect for long term daily use of other NSAIDs such as naproxen.[128]

Evidence summary: Silver

Three RCTs show conflicting results. However, deleterious structural effects have been evoked only with long term indomethacin intake. There is little evidence of a structural effect (beneficial or deleterious) with other NSAIDs.

Glucosamine sulphate

The Cochrane Library review collected only RCTs assessing the symptomatic efficacy of glucosamine in OA, but not the structural effects of glucosamine.[129]

A 3 year RCT evaluated the potential of glucosamine to protect the cartilage from further loss as defined by no change in radiographic joint space width.[130] This RCT ($n = 212$) showed a favourable response with no further loss of medial tibiofemoral joint space width (JSW) in subjects assigned to glucosamine over a 3 year period (Table 7.9). A debate emerged because of the potential bias in the radiological evaluation due to the fact that an improvement of symptoms might facilitate full knee extension through disappearance of the analgesic flexum. An increase of the radiological femorotibial inter-bone distance is then observed as the femur "rides up" on the cartilage rim.

More recently, a 3 year RCT demonstrated similar structural effects of glucosamine sulphate (1500 mg/d) versus placebo in 202 patients with knee OA (average JSW <4 mm at baseline).[131] Changes in radiographic minimum JSW were measured in the medial compartment of the tibiofemoral joint. Progressive joint space narrowing with placebo use was –0·19 mm (95% CI –0·29 to –0·09 mm) after 3 years. Conversely, there was no average change with glucosamine sulphate use (0·04 mm; 95% CI –0·06 to 0·14 mm) ($p = 0{\cdot}001$).

No statistically significant differences were found between groups in adverse events: any adverse event glucosamine 93%, placebo 94%;[130] glucosamine 66%, placebo 64%;[131] withdrawal due to adverse events: glucosamine 20%, placebo 17%.[130]

Despite the fact that the above two RCTs have shown a statistical significant difference in terms of changes over time in the radiological JSW between active and placebo drugs, the medical community is not convinced of the clinical relevance of such results.[132,133] Reasons include the validity of fully extended knee radiographs as an outcome measure, the threefold difference in the rate of narrowing between the two studies, the absence of results at an individual level (percentage of progressors) instead of at a group level (mean change in JSW), and a predefined data-driven definition of a clinically relevant definition of the size of the treatment effect (difference between groups in terms of percentage of progressors).

Evidence summary: Silver

Limited evidence from two RCTs suggest a beneficial structural effect of glucosamine sulphate, warranting further investigation.

Table 7.9 Number needed to treat for glucosamine versus placebo (Reginster, 2001)[130]

Outcome	Significant JSN with placebo	Significant JSN with glucosamine	Relative risk with glucosamine (95% CI)	ARR (65% CI)	NNT (95% CI)
Joint space narrowing >0·5 mm	32/106 (30%)	16/106 (15%)	0·50 (0·29, 0·85)	15% (4, 26)	7 (4,27)

Chondroitin

Uebelhart *et al* evaluated the minimum JSW of the medial femorotibial joint, as secondary outcome measure in a RCT in 60 patients with knee OA.[134] The radiographs were available in 26 people. At one year, JSW had significantly decreased in the placebo group and not in the chondroitin group. There was no intergroup comparison.

In a recent RCT, Mathieu compared the structural effect of chondroitin sulphates versus placebo in 300 patients with medial femorotibial OA.[135] The chondroitin group showed a stabilisation of minimum JSW compared to the placebo group at year two.

Evidence summary: Silver

Limited evidence from two RCTs suggests the need for a more definitive trial.

Diacerein

In a recent 3 year RCT study comparing the structural effects of diacerein versus placebo in 507 people with hip OA, the percentage of patients with a joint space narrowing of at least 0·5 mm and the rate of joint space narrowing at year 3 were lower in the diacerein group compared to the placebo group (Table 7.10).[136] These results suggest a structure-modifying effect of diacerein in hip OA.

Evidence summary: Silver

Limited evidence from one RCT suggests the need for a more definitive trial.

Avocado/soybean unsaponifiables

The only 2 year RCT (n = 163) evaluating the structural effects of avocado/soybean unsaponifiables (ASU) versus placebo in the treatment of hip OA failed to demonstrate a structural effect.[137]

Evidence summary: Silver

One RCT showed no effect.

Glycosaminoglycan polysulphuric acid complex

The only RCT ($n = 394$) evaluating the structural effects of glycosaminoglycan polysulphuric acid complex (Rumalon) in hip and knee OA failed to demonstrate any structural efficacy at year 5.[138]

Evidence summary: Silver

One RCT showed no effect.

Evidence summary: overall conclusion

The level of evidence of a beneficial structural effect of any long term daily intake of oral drugs in OA is low.

Question 10:

Are there any decision making tools to determine the optimal time for joint replacement surgery?

Additional literature search

MEDLINE (Ovid): Database: MEDLINE <1966 to December Week 3 2002>:

Table 7.10 Number needed to treat for diacerein versus placebo (3 year ITT data) (Dougados, 2001)[136]

Outcome	Significant JSN with placebo	Significant JSN with diacerein	Relative risk with diacerein (95% CI)	ARR (95% CI)	NNT (95% CI)
Joint space narrowing >0.5 mm	136/225 (60%)	112/221 (51%)	0.84 (0.71, 0.99)	10% (0·5, 19)	11 (6, 183)

(Please see primary search strategy 1 to 7, plus terms below)

8. arthroplasty, replacement
9. outcome assessment
10. indication. mp
11. 7 and 8
12. 1 and 8
13. or/9–10
14. 12 and
15. surgery
16. 1 and 15

Several indices or recommendations have been proposed to help determine the optimal time for total hip arthroplasty (THA) and total knee replacement (TKR) surgery.

Hip osteoarthritis

The National Institutes of Health (NIH) consensus development panel on total hip replacement has been both a data driven and experts' opinion approach.[139] The result of the consensus was that THA should be proposed to patients with radiographic evidence of joint damage and moderate to severe persistent pain or disability (or both) interfering with daily activities that is not substantially relieved by an extended course of non-surgical management. On the other hand, THA should not be recommended to patients with a high risk of infection or patients with poor health.

Hawker *et al* defined potential candidates for THA as patients with clinical and radiological evidence of hip OA and a Western Ontario and McMaster University Osteoarthritis Index (WOMAC) summary score ≥ 39 on a 0–100 scale.[140] However this arbitrary definition of severe OA, in their survey of 48 218 Canadian patients, may have been chosen to provide a conservative estimate of the potential need for arthroplasty.

Finally, Maillefert *et al* conducted a 3 year longitudinal study of patients with painful hip OA in order to propose a composite index for considering THA.[141] The variables included in the 0–100 index were: patient's global assessment, Lequesne index, analgesic and NSAIDs consumption, radiological joint space width, and joint space narrowing. However, the poor predictive value of the proposed composite index, using the selected cutoff, suggested there were other unmeasured factors determining access to surgery.

Knee osteoarthritis

While there are no published evidence-based indications for TKR, Dieppe *et al* have summarised indicators derived from the published results of three consensus groups of orthopedic surgeons.[142] Hardorn and Holmes, using a Delphi consensus technique, proposed the 0–100 New Zealand score, which included pain, functional impairment, movement, deformity, and other factors such as ability to work.[143] This scoring system has been proposed as an aid to surgical decision making, but a cut-off score to define the optimal time for surgery was not provided. Manusco *et al* reported no clear consensus from their postal survey of orthopaedic surgeons, but most agreement was achieved on severe daily pain, radiographic joint space narrowing, and high patient motivation as the key indications for TKR.[144] Co-morbidities and technical difficulties were considered as reasons for not doing the operation. Naylor and Williams developed algorithms, also using a Delphi technique, in which pain at rest, severity of functional impairment, problems with caregiving and the perceived likely improvement in function were the key determinants used to prioritise surgery.[145]

More recently, Woolhead *et al.* has published a work on the perspectives of the patients as to which factors should be prioritised.[146] Semi-structured interviews were conducted with 25 patients on a waiting list for TKR. In agreement with health professionals, the participants considered that pain and disability should be key criteria on which to prioritise people for a TKR. However, they also argued that a fair decision-making process should include factors specific to the patient's circumstances, such as the length and degree of suffering, whether there is a chance of return to work, dependants, and status of National Insurance contributions.

Whatever the OA localisation, there are no evidence-based indicators to decide the optimal time for surgery. *In our opinion*, the decision for total joint replacement in hip or knee OA has to take into account the following factors:

- symptomatic severity of the disease and health-related quality of life (pain, function);
- structural severity of the disease;
- age and comorbidity;
- patient's willingness to undergo joint replacement surgery;
- local healthcare system and patients health insurance coverage.

It is clear that more research is needed in this area.

Evidence summary: Bronze

There are no evidence-based criteria for deciding on the optimal time for joint replacement surgery.

References

1 Towheed T, Shea B, Wells G, Hochberg M. Analgesia and non-aspirin, non-steroidal anti-inflammatory drugs for osteoarthritis of the hip. *Cochrane Database Syst Rev* (2):CD000517, 2000. Available at: http://www.cochrane.org

2 Watson MC, Brookes ST, Kirwan JR, Faulkner A. Non-aspirin, non-steroidal anti-inflammatory drugs for osteoarthritis of the knee. *Cochrane Database Syst Rev* (2):CD000142, 2000. Available at: http://www.cochrane.org

3 Amadio P Jr, Cummings DM. Evaluation of acetaminophen in the management of osteoarthritis of the knee. *Curr Ther Res* 1983;**34**:59–66.

4 Riedemann PJ, Bersinic S, Cuddy J, Torrance GW, Tugwell PX. A study to determine the efficacy and safety of tenoxicam versus piroxicam, diclofenac and indomethacin in patients with osteoarthritis: a meta-analysis. *J Rheumatol* 1993;**20**:2095–103.

5 Simpson J, Golding DN, Freeman AM, *et al.* A large multicentre, parallel group, double-blind study comparing tenoxicam and piroxicam in the treatment of osteoarthritis and rheumatoid arthritis. *Br J Clin Pract* 1989;**43**:328–33

6 Dieppe P, Chard J, Faulkner A, Lohmander S. Osteoarthritis. *Clin Evidence* 1999;**2**:437–48.

7 Eccles M, Freemantle N, Mason J. North of England evidence based guideline development project: summary guideline for non-steroidal anti-inflammatory drugs versus basic analgesia in treating the pain of degenerative arthritis. The North of England Non-Steroidal Anti-Inflammatory Drug Guideline Development Group. *BMJ* 1998;**317**(7157):526–30.

8 Pincus T, Koch GG, Sokka T, *et al.* A randomised, double-blind, crossover clinical trial of diclofenac plus misoprostol versus acetaminophen in patients with osteoarthritis of the hip or knee. *Arthritis Rheum* 2001;**44**(7):1587–98.

9 Altman RD for the IAP Study Group. Ibuprofen, acetaminophen and placebo in osteoarthritis of the knee: a six-day double-blind study. *Arthritis Rheum* 1999;**42**:S403.

10 Temple AR, Reel LJ, Fox TM, Lynch JM. Long term use of acetaminophen in osteoarthritis pain. *Ann Rheum Dis* 2000;**59**:135.

11 Geba GP, Weaver AL, Polis AB, Dixon ME, Schnitzer TJ; Vioxx, Acetaminophen, Celecoxib Trial (VACT) Group.

Efficacy of rofecoxib, celecoxib, and acetaminophen in osteoarthritis of the knee: a randomised trial. *JAMA* 2002;**287**(1):64–71.

12 Peloso PM. Opioid therapy for osteoarthritis of the hip and knee: use it or lose it? *J Rheumatol* 2001;**28**(1):6–11.

13 Shamoon M, Hochberg MC. Treatment of osteoarthritis with acetaminophen: efficacy, safety, and comparison with nonsteroidal anti-inflammatory drugs. *Curr Rheumatol Rep* 2000;**2**(6):454–8.

14 Gotzsche PC. Non-steroidal anti-inflammatory drugs. *BMJ.* 2000;320(7241):1058–61.

15 Bombardier C. An evidence–based evaluation of the gastrointestinal safety of coxibs. *Am J Cardiol* 2002 21;**89**(6A):3D–9D

16 Wolfe F, Zhao S, Lane N. Preference for nonsteroidal antiinflammatory drugs over acetaminophen by rheumatic disease patients: a survey of 1,799 patients with osteoarthritis, rheumatoid arthritis, and fibromyalgia. *Arthritis Rheum* 2000;**43**(2):378–85.

17 Shamoon M, Hochberg MC. The role of acetaminophen in the management of patients with osteoarthritis. *Am J Med* 2001;**110**(3 suppl 1):46–9.

18 Hochberg MC, Dougados M. Pharmacological therapy of osteoarthritis. *Best Pract Res Clin Rheumatol* 2001;**15**(4): 583–93.

19 Towheed TE, Anastassiades TP, Shea B, Houpt J, Welch V, Hochberg MC. Glucosamine therapy for treating osteoarthritis. *Cochrane Database Syst Rev* (1):CD002946, 2001.

20 Reginster JY, Deroisy R, Rovati LC, *et al.* Long-term effects of glucosamine sulphate on osteoarthritis progression: a randomised, placebo-controlled clinical trial. *Lancet* 2001;**357**:251–6.

21 Houpt JB, McMillan R, Wein C, Paget-Dellio SD. Effect of glucosamine hydrochloride in the treatment of pain of osteoarthritis of the knee. *J Rheumatol* 1999;**26**:2423–30.

22 Rindone JP, Hiller D, Collacott E, Nordhaugen N, Arriola Randomised, controlled trial of glucosamine for treating osteoarthritis of the knee. *West J Med* 2000;**172**:91–4.

23 Hughes R, Carr A. A randomised, double-blind, placebo-controlled trial of glucosamine sulphate as an analgesic in osteoarthritis of the knee. *Rheumatology* 2002;**41**: 279–84.

24 McAlindon TE, LaValley MP, Gulin JP, Felson DT. Glucosamine and chondroitin for treatment of osteoarthritis: a systematic quality assessment and meta-analysis. *JAMA* 2000;**283**(11):1469–75.

25. Mazieres B, Combe B, Phan Van A, Tondut J, Grynfeltt M. Chondroitin sulfate in osteoarthritis of the knee: a prospective, double blind, placebo controlled multicenter clinical study. *J Rheumatol* 2001;**28**:173–81.

26. Leffler CT, Philippi AF, Leffler SG, Mosure JC, Kim PD. Glucosamine, chondroitin, and manganese ascorbate for degenerative joint disease of the knee or low back: a randomised, double-blind, placebo-controlled pilot study. *Mil Med* 1999;**164**:85–91

27. Das A Jr, Hammad TA. Efficacy of a combination of FCHG49 glucosamine hydrochloride, TRH122 low molecular weight sodium chondroitin sulfate and manganese ascorbate in the management of knee osteoarthritis. *Osteoarthritis Cartilage* 2000;**8**:343–50.

28. Pelletier JP, Yaron M, Haraoui B, Cohen P, Nahir MA, Choquette D, Wigler I, Rosner IA, Beaulieu AD. Efficacy and safety of diacerein in osteoarthritis of the knee: a double-blind, placebo-controlled trial. The Diacerein Study Group. *Arthritis Rheum* 2000;**43**(10):2339–48.

29. Nguyen M, Dougados M, Berdah L, Amor B. Diacerein in the treatment of osteoarthritis of the hip. *Arthritis Rheum* 1994;**37**(4):529–36.

30. Dougados M, Nguyen M, Berdah L, Mazieres B, Vignon E, Lequesne M. ECHODIAH Investigators Study Group. Evaluation of the structure-modifying effects of diacerein in hip osteoarthritis: ECHODIAH, a three-year, placebo-controlled trial. Evaluation of the Chondromodulating Effect of Diacerein in OA of the Hip. *Arthritis Rheum* 2001;**44**(11):2539–47.

31. Lequesne M, Maheu E, Cadet C, Dreiser RL. Structural effect of avocado/soybean unsaponifiables on joint space loss in osteoarthritis of the hip. *Arthritis Care Res* 2002;**47**(1):50–8.

32. Maheu E, Mazieres B, Valat JP, *et al.* Symptomatic efficacy of avocado/soybean unsaponifiables in the treatment of osteoarthritis of the knee and hip: a prospective, randomised, double-blind, placebo-controlled, multicenter clinical trial with a six-month treatment period and a two-month followup demonstrating a persistent effect. *Arthritis Rheum* 1998; **41**(1):81–91.

33. Pavelka K, Gatterova J, Gollerova V, Urbanova Z, Sedlackova M, Altman RD. A 5-year randomised controlled, double-blind study of glycosaminoglycan polysulphuric acid complex (Rumalon) as a structure

modifying therapy in osteoarthritis of the hip and knee. *Osteoarthritis Cartilage* 2000;**8**(5):335–42.

34. Recommendations for the medical management of osteoarthritis of the hip and knee: 2000 update. American College of Rheumatology Subcommittee on Osteoarthritis Guidelines. *Arthritis Rheum* 2000;**43**(9):1905–15.
35. American College of Rheumatology, Subcommittee on Osteoarthritis Guidelines. Recommendations for the medical management of osteoarthritis of the hip and knee. 2000 Update. *Arthritis Rheum* 2000;**43**:1905-15.
36. Pendleton A, Arden N, Dougados M, *et al.* EULAR recommendations for the management of knee osteoarthritis: report of a task force of the Standing Committee for International Clinical Studies Including Therapeutic Trials (ESCISIT). *Ann Rheum Dis* 2000;**59**: 936–44.
37. Fransen M, McConnell S, Bell M. Therapeutic exercise for people with osteoarthritis of the hip or knee. A systematic review. *J Rheumatol* 2002;**29**(8):1737–45.
38. Petrella RJ. Is exercise effective treatment for osteoarthritis of the knee? *Br J Sports Med* 2000;**34**:326–31.
39. van Baar ME, Assendelft WJ, Dekker J, Oostendorp RA, Bijlsma JW. Effectiveness of exercise therapy in patients with osteoarthritis of the hip or knee. *Arthritis Rheum* 1999;**42**:1361–9.
40. Bautch J, Malone D, Vailas A. Effects of exercise on knee joints with osteoarthritis: a pilot study of biologic markers. *Arthritis Care Res* 1997;**10**:48–55.
41. Deyle GD, Henderson NE, Matekel RL, Ryder MG, Garber MB, Allison SC. Effectiveness of manual physical therapy and exercise in osteoarthritis of the knee. A randomised, controlled trial. *Ann Intern Med* 2000;**132**:173–81.
42. Ettinger WH, Burns R, Messier SP, *et al.* A randomised trial comparing aerobic exercise and resistance exercise with a health education program in older adults with knee osteoarthritis. The Fitness Arthritis and Seniors Trial (FAST). *JAMA* 1997;**277**:25–31.
43. Fransen M, Crosbie J, Edmonds J. Physical Therapy is effective for patients with osteoarthritis of the knee: a randomised controlled clinical trial. *J Rheumatol* 2001;**28**: 156–64.
44. Hopman-Rock M, Westhoff M. The effects of a health educational and exercise program for older adults with osteoarthritis of the hip or knee. *J Rheumatol* 2000;**27**:1947–54.
45. Kovar PA, Allegrante JP, MacKenzie CR, Peterson MG, Gutin B, Charlson ME. Supervised fitness walking in patients with osteoarthritis of the knee. A randomised, controlled trial. *Ann Intern Med* 1992;**116**:529–34.
46. Maurer BT, Stern AG, Kinossian B, Cook KD, Schumacher HR. Osteoarthritis of the knee: isokinetic quadriceps exercise versus an educational intervention. *Arch Phys Med Rehab* 1999;**80**:1293–9.
47. Minor MA, Hewett JE, Webel RR, Anderson SK, Kay DR. Efficacy of physical conditioning exercise in patients with rheumatoid arthritis and osteoarthritis. *Arthritis Rheum* 1989;**32**:1396–405.
48. O'Reilly SC, Muir KR, Doherty M. Effectiveness of home exercise on pain and disability from osteoarthritis of the knee: a randomised controlled trial. *Ann Rheum Dis* 1999;**58**:15–19.
49. Peloquin L, Bravo G, Gauthier P, Lacombe G, Billiard J-S. Effects of a cross-training exercise program in persons with osteoarthritis of the knee. A randomised controlled trial. *J Clin Rheumatol* 1999;**5**:126–36.
50. Petrella RJ, Bartha C. Home based exercise therapy for older patients with knee osteoarthritis: a randomised clinical trial. *J Rheumatol* 2000;**27**(9):2215–21.
51. Rogind H, Bibow-Nielsen B, Jensen B, Moller HC, Frimodt-Moller H, Bliddal H. The effects of a physical training program on patients with osteoarthritis of the knees. *Arch Phys Med Rehab* 1998;**79**:1421–7.
52. Schilke JM, Johnson GO, Housh TJ, O'Dell JR. Effects of muscle-strength training on the functional status of patients with osteoarthritis of the knee joint. Nursing Research. 1996;**45**:68–72.
53. van Baar ME, Dekker J, Oostendorp RA, *et al.* The effectiveness of exercise therapy in patients with osteoarthritis of the hip or knee: a randomised clinical trial. *J Rheumatol* 1998;**25**:2432–9.
54. Cohen J. *Statistical power analysis for the behavioural sciences, rev. ed.* New York: Academic Press, 1977.
55. Baker KR, Nelson ME, Felson DT, Layne JE, Sarno R, Roubenoff R. The efficacy of home-based progressive strength training in older adults with knee osteoarthritis: a randomised controlled trial. *J Rheumatol* 2001;**28**: 1655–65.
56. Gur H, Cakin N, Akova B, Okay E, Kucukoglu S. Concentric versus combined concentric–eccentric isokinetic training: effects on functional capacity and

symptoms in patients with osteoarthrosis of the knee. *Arch Phys Med Rehab* 2002;**83**:308–16.

57. Verhagen AP, de Vet HCW, de Bie RA, Dessels AGH, Boers M, Knipschild PG. Balneotherapy for rheumatoid arthritis and osteoarthritis (Cochrane Review). In: Cochrane Collaboration. *Cochrane Library.* Issue 2, Oxford: Update Software; 2002.
58. Hart DJ, Doyle DV, Spector TD. Incidence and risk factors for radiographic knee osteoarthritis in middle-aged women: the Chingford Study. *Arthritis Rheum* 1999;**42**(1):17–24.
59. Spector TD, Dacre JE, Harris PA, Huskisson EC. Radiological progression of osteoarthritis: an 11 year follow up study of the knee. *Ann Rheum Dis* 1992;**51**(10):1107–10.
60. Hill CL, Gale DG, Chaisson CE, Skinner K, Kazis L, Gale ME, Felson DT. Knee effusions, popliteal cysts, and synovial thickening: association with knee pain in osteoarthritis. *J Rheumatol* 2001;**28**(6):1330–7.
61. Pavelka K, Gatterova J, Pavelka K Sr, *et al.* Correlation between knee roentgenogram changes and clinical symptoms in osteoarthritis. *Rev Rheum* 1992;**59**(9): 553–9.
62. Fernandez-Madrid F, Karvonen RL, Teitge RA, Miller PR, Negendank WG. MR features of osteoarthritis of the knee. *Magn Reson Imaging* 1994;**12**:703–9.
63. Claessens AA, Schouten JS, van den Ouweland FA, Valkenburg HA. Do clinical findings associate with radiographic osteoarthritis of the knee? *Ann Rheum Dis* 1990;**49**(10):771–4.
64. Dougados M, Gueguen A, Nguyen M, *et al.* Longitudinal radiologic evaluation of osteoarthritis of the knee. *J Rheumatol* 1992;**19**(3):378–84.
65. Ledingham J, Regan M, Jones A, Doherty M. Factors affecting radiographic progression of knee osteoarthritis. *Ann Rheum Dis* 1995;**54**(1):53–8.
66. Ayral X, Ravaud P, Bonvarlet JP, *et al.* Arthroscopic evaluation of post-traumatic patellofemoral chondropathy. *J Rheumatol* 1999;**26**:1140–7.
67. Creamer P. Intra-articular corticosteroid treatment in osteoarthritis. *Curr Opin Rheumatol* 1999;**11**(5):417–21.
68. Creamer P. Intra-articular corticosteroid injections in osteoarthritis: do they work and if so, how? *Ann Rheum Dis* 1997;**56**(11):634–6.
69. Ayral X. Injections in the treatment of osteoarthritis. *Best Pract Res Clin Rheumatol* 2001;**15**(4):609–26.
70. Kirwan JR, Rankin E. Intra-articular therapy in osteoarthritis. *Baillieres Clin Rheumatol* 1997;**11**(4): 769–94.
71. Jones A, Doherty M. Intra-articular corticosteroids are effective in osteoarthritis but there are no clinical predictors of response. *Ann Rheum Dis* 1996;**55**(11):829–32.
72. Towheed TE, Hochberg MC. A systematic review of randomised controlled trials of pharmacological therapy in osteoarthritis of the knee, with an emphasis on trial methodology. *Semin Arthritis Rheum* 1997;**26**(5):755–70.
73. Gotzche P. Methodology and overt hidden bias in reports of 196 double-blind trials of non-steroidal anti-inflammatory drugs in rheumatoid arthritis. *Control Clin Trials* 1989;**10**:31–56.
74 Friedman DM, Moore ME. The efficacy of intraarticular steroids in osteoarthritis: a double-blind study. *J Rheumatol* 1980;**7**(6):850–6.
75 Ayral X. Injections in the treatment of osteoarthritis. *Best Pract Res Clin Rheumatol* 2001;**15**(4):609–26.
76 Miller JH, White J, Norton TH. The value of intra-articular injections in osteoarthritis of the knee. *JBJS* 1958;**4013**:636–43.
77 Wright V, Chandler GN, Morison RA, Hartfall SJ. Intra-articular therapy in osteoarthritis. Comparison of hydrocortisone acetate and hydrocortisone tertiary-butyacetate. *Ann Rheum Dis* 1960;**19**:257–61.
78 Cederlof S, Jonson G. Intraarticular prednisolone injection for osteoarthritis of the knee. A double blind test with placebo. *Acta Chir Scand* 1966;**132**:532–6.
79 Friedman DM, Moore ME. The efficacy of intraarticular steroids in osteoarthritis: a double blind study. *J Rheum* 1980;**7**:850–6.
80 Dieppe PA, Sathapatayavongs B, Jones HE, *et al.* Intra-articular steroids in osteoarthritis. *Rheumatol Rehabil* 1980;**19**:212–17.
81 Gaffney K, Ledingham J, Perry JD. Intra-articular triamcinolone hexacetonide in knee osteoarthritis: factors influencing the clinical response. *Ann Rheum Dis* 1995;**54**:379–381.
82 Jones A, Doherty M. Intra-articular corticosteroids are effective in osteoarthritis but there are no predictors of response. *Ann Rheum Dis* 1996;**55**:829–32.
83 Ravaud P, Moulinier L, Giraudeau B, *et al.* Effects of joint lavage and steroids injection in patients with osteoarthritis of the knee. *Arthritis Rheum* 1999;**42**:475–82.

84 Brandt KD, Block JA, Michalski JP, Moreland LW, Caldwell JR, Lavin PT. Efficacy and safety of intraarticular sodium hyaluronate in knee osteoarthritis. ORTHOVISC Study Group. *Clin Orthop* 2001;**385**:130–43.

85 Altman RD, Moskowitz R. Intraarticular sodium hyaluronate (Hyalgan) in the treatment of patients with osteoarthritis of the knee: a randomised clinical trial. Hyalgan Study Group. *J Rheumatol* 1998;**25**(11): 2203–12.

86 Adams ME, Atkinson MH, Lussier AJ, *et al.* The role of viscosupplementation with hylan G-F 20 (Synvisc) in the treatment of osteoarthritis of the knee: a Canadian multicenter trial comparing hylan G-F 20 alone, hylan G-F 20 with non-steroidal anti-inflammatory drugs (NSAIDs) and NSAIDs alone. *Osteoarthritis Cartilage* 1995;**3**(4):213–25.

87 Petrella RJ, DiSilvestro MD, Hildebrand C. Effects of hyaluronate sodium on pain and physical functioning in osteoarthritis of the knee: a randomised, double-blind, placebo-controlled clinical trial. *Arch Intern Med* 2002;**162**(3):292–8.

88 Bellamy N, Campbell J, Wells G, Bourne R. Intra-articular corticosteroids for osteoarthritis of the knee [Protocol]. *Cochrane Database Syst Rev* (2), 2002; available at: http://www.cochrane.org

89 Bellamy N, Campbell J, Wells G, Bourne R. Viscosupplementation for osteoarthritis of the knee [Protocol]. *Cochrane Database Syst Rev* (2), 2002; available at: http://www.cochrane.org

90 Jones A, Doherty M. Intra-articular corticosteroids are effective in osteoarthritis but there are no clinical predictors of response. *Ann Rheum Dis* 1996;**55**(11): 829–32.

91 Ayral X. Injections in the treatment of osteoarthritis. *Best Pract Res Clin Rheumatol* 2001;**15**(4):609–26.

92 Friedman DM, Moore ME. The efficacy of intraarticular steroids in osteoarthritis: a double-blind study. *J Rheumatol* 1980;**7**(6):850–6.

93 Kirwan JR, Rankin E. Intra-articular therapy in osteoarthritis. *Baillieres Clin Rheumatol* 1997;**11**(4): 769–94.

94 Gaffney K, Ledingham J, Perry JD. Intra-articular triamcinolone hexacetonide in knee osteoarthritis: factors influencing the clinical response. *Ann Rheum Dis* 1995;**54**:379–81.

95 Ayral X, Ravaud P, Bonvarlet JP, *et al.* Arthroscopic evaluation of post-traumatic patellofemoral chondropathy. *J Rheumatol* 1999;**26**:1140–7.

96 Creamer P. Intra-articular corticosteroid treatment in osteoarthritis. *Curr Opin Rheumatol* 1999;**11**(5):417–21.

97 Weitoft T, Uddenfeldt P. Importance of synovial fluid aspiration when injecting intra-articular corticosteroids. *Ann Rheum Dis* 2000;**59**(3):233–5.

98 Jones A, Regan M, Ledingham J, Pattrick M, Manhire A, Doherty M. Importance of placement of intra-articular steroid injections. *BMJ* 1993;**307**:1329–30.

99 Pendleton A, Arden N, Dougados M, *et al.* EULAR recommendations for the management of knee osteoarthritis. Report of a task force of the Standing Committee for International Clinical Studies Including Therapeutic trials (ESCISIT). *Ann Rheum Dis* 2000;**59**: 936–44.

100 Hochberg MC, Altman RD, Brandt KD, Moscowitz RW. Design and conduct of clinical trials in osteoarthritis: preliminary recommendations from a task force of the Osteoarthritis Research Society. *J Rheumatol* 1997;**24**: 792–4.

101 Maillefert JF, Hudry C, Baron G, *et al.* Laterally elevated wedged insoles in the treatment of medial knee osteoarthritis: a prospective randomised controlled study. *Osteoarthritis Cart* 2001;**9**:738–45.

102 Pham T, Maillefert JF, Hudry C, *et al.* Laterally elevated wedged insoles in the treatment of medial knee osteoarthritis: a two-year prospective randomised controlled study. *Ann Rheum Dis* 2002;**61**(suppl 1):40 (abstract).

103 Toda Y, Segal N, Kato A, Yamamoto S, Irie M. Effect of a novel insole on the subtalar joint of patients with medial compartment osteoarthritis of the knee. *J Rheumatol* 2001;**28**:2705–10.

104 Sasaki T, Yasuda K. Clinical evaluation of the treatment of osteoarthritic knees using a newly designed wedged insole. *Clin Orthop* 1987;**221**:181–7.

105 Ogata K, Yasunaga M, Nomiyama H. The effects of wedged insoles on the thrust of osteoarthritic knees. *Int Orthop* 1997;**21**:308–12.

106 Hochberg MC, Altman RD, Brandt KD, *et al.* Guidelines for the medical management of osteoarthritis. Part II. Osteoarthritis of the knee. American College of Rheumatology. *Arthritis Rheum* 1995;**38**:1541–6.

107 Felson DT, Anderson JJ, Naimark A, Walker AM, Meenan RF. Obesity and knee osteoarthritis. The Framingham Study. *Ann Intern Med* 1988;**109**(1):18–24.

108 Felson DT, Zhang Y, Hannan MT, *et al.* Risk factors for incident radiographic knee osteoarthritis in the elderly: the Framingham Study. *Arthritis Rheum* 1997;**40**(4): 728–33.

109 Spector TD, Hart DJ, Doyle DV. Incidence and progression of osteoarthritis in women with unilateral knee disease in the general population: the effect of obesity. *Ann Rheum Dis* 1994;**53**(9):565–8.

110 Schouten JS, van den Ouweland FA, Valkenburg HA. A 12 year follow up study in the general population on prognostic factors of cartilage loss in osteoarthritis of the knee. *Ann Rheum Dis* 1992;**51**(8):932–7.

111 Balint G, Szebenyi B. Non-pharmacological therapies in osteoarthritis. *Baillieres Clin Rheumatol* 1997;**11**(4): 795–815.

112 Felson DT, Zhang Y, Anthony JM, Naimark A, Anderson JJ. Weight loss reduces the risk for symptomatic knee osteoarthritis in women. The Framingham Study. *Ann Intern Med* 1992;**116**:535–9.

113 O'Reilly S, Doherty M. Lifestyle changes in the management of osteoarthritis. *Best Pract Res Clin Rheumatol* 2001;**15**(4):559–68.

114 Williams RA, Foulsham BM. Weight reduction in osteoarthritis using phentermine. *Practitioner* 1981; **225**(1352):231–2.

115 Messier SP, Loeser RF, Mitchell MN, *et al.* Exercise and weight loss in obese older adults with knee osteoarthritis: a preliminary study. *J Am Geriatr Soc* 2000;**48**(9):1062–72.

116 Huang MH, Chen CH, Chen TW, Weng MC, Wang WT, Wang YL. The effects of weight reduction on the rehabilitation of patients with knee osteoarthritis and obesity. *Arthritis Care Research* 2000;**13**:398–405.

117 McGoey BV, Deitel M, Saplys RJ, Kliman ME. Effect of weight loss on musculoskeletal pain in the morbidly obese. *J Bone Joint Surg Br* 1990;**72**(2):322–3.

118 Toda Y, Toda T, Takemura S, Wada T, Morimoto T, Ogawa R. Change in body fat, but not body weight or metabolic correlates of obesity, is related to symptomatic relief of obese patients with knee osteoarthritis after a weight control program. *J Rheumatol* 1998;**25**(11): 2181–6.

119 Recommendations for the medical management of osteoarthritis of the hip and knee: 2000 update. American College of Rheumatology Subcommittee on Osteoarthritis Guidelines. *Arthritis Rheum* 2000;**43**(9):1905–15.

120 Hochberg MC, Altman RD, Brandt KD, *et al.* Guidelines for the medical management of osteoarthritis. Part II. Osteoarthritis of the knee. American College of Rheumatology. *Arthritis Rheum* 1995;**38**(11):1541–6.

121 Young NL, Cheah D, Waddell JP, *et al.* Patient characteristics that affect the outcome of total hip arthroplasty: a review. *Can J Surg* 1998;**41**:188–95.

122 Chan CL, Villar RN. Obesity and quality of life after primary hip arthroplasty. *J Bone Joint Surg Br* 1996;**78**:78–81.

123 Espehaug B, Havelin LI, Engesaeter LB, Langeland N, Vollset SE.. Patient-related risk-factors for early revision of total hip replacements. A population register-based case-control study of 674 revised hips. *Acta Orthop Scand* 1997;**68**:207–215.

124 Pelletier JP, Martel-Pelletier J. Effects of nimesulide and naproxen on the degradation and metalloprotease synthesis of human osteoarthritic cartilage. *Drugs* 1993;**46** Suppl 1:34–9.

125 Pelletier JP, Mineau F, Fernandes J, Kiansa K, Ranger P, Martel-Pelletier J. Two NSAIDs, nimesulide and naproxen, can reduce the synthesis of urokinase and IL-6 while increasing PAI-1, in human OA synovial fibroblasts. *Clin Exp Rheumatol* 1997;**15**(4):393–8.

126 Huskisson EC, Berry H, Gishen P, Jubb RW, Whitehead J. Effects on antiinflammatory drugs on the progression of osteoarthritis of the knee. LINK Study Group. Longitudinal Investigation of Nonsteroidal Antiinflammatory Drugs in Knee Osteoarthritis. *J.Rheumatol* 1995;**22**(10):1941–6.

127 Rashad S, Revell P, Hemingway A, Low F, Rainsford K, Walkes F. Effect of non-steroidal anti-inflammatory drugs on the course of osteoarthritis. *Lancet* 1989;**2**(8662): 519–22.

128 Williams HJ, Ward JR, Egger MJ, *et al.* Comparison of naproxen and acetaminophen in a two-year study of treatment of osteoarthritis of the knee. *Arthritis Rheum* 1993;**36**(9):1196–206.

129 Towheed TE, Anastassiades TP, Shea B, Houpt J, Welch V, Hochberg MC. Glucosamine therapy for treating osteoarthritis. *Cochrane Database Syst Rev* (1):CD002946, 2001.

130 Reginster JY, Deroisy R, Rovati LC, *et al.* Long-term effects of glucosamine sulphate on osteoarthritis progression: a randomised, placebo-controlled clinical trial. *Lancet* 2001;**357**:251–6.

131 Pavelka K, Gatterova J, Olejarova M, Machacek S, Giacovelli G, Rovati LC. Glucosamine sulfate use and delay of progression of knee osteoarthritis: a 3-year, randomised, placebo-controlled, double-blind study. *Arch Intern Med* 2002;**162**(18):2113–23.

132 Hochberg MC, Altman RD, Brandt KD, *et al.* Guidelines for the medical management of osteoarthritis. Part II. Osteoarthritis of the knee. American College of Rheumatology. *Arthritis Rheum* 1995;**38**(11):1541–6.

133 Recommendations for the medical management of osteoarthritis of the hip and knee: 2000 update. American College of Rheumatology Subcommittee on Osteoarthritis Guidelines. *Arthritis Rheum* 2000;**43**(9): 1905–15.

134 Uebelhart D, Thonar EJ, Delmas PD, Chantraine A, Vignon E. Effects of oral chondroitin sulfate on the progression of knee osteoarthritis: a pilot study. *Osteoarthritis Cartilage* 1998;**6** Suppl A:39–46.

135 Mathieu P. Radiological progression of internal femoro-tibial osteoarthritis in gonarthrosis. Chondro-protective effect of chondroitin sulfates ACS4-ACS6. *Presse Med* 2002;**31**(29):1386–90.

136 Dougados M, Nguyen M, Berdah L, Mazieres B, Vignon E, Lequesne M. ECHODIAH Investigators Study Group. Evaluation of the structure-modifying effects of diacerein in hip osteoarthritis: ECHODIAH, a three-year, placebo-controlled trial. Evaluation of the Chondromodulating Effect of Diacerein in OA of the Hip. *Arthritis Rheum* 2001;**44**(11):2539–47.

137 Lequesne M, Maheu E, Cadet C, Dreiser RL. Structural effect of avocado/soybean unsaponifiables on joint space loss in osteoarthritis of the hip. *Arthritis Care Research* 2002;**47**(1):50–8.

138 Pavelka K, Gatterova J, Gollerova V, Urbanova Z, Sedlackova M, Altman RD. A 5-year randomised controlled, double-blind study of glycosaminoglycan polysulphuric acid complex (Rumalon) as a structure modifying therapy in osteoarthritis of the hip and knee. *Osteoarthritis Cartilage* 2000;**8**(5):335–42.

139 NIH consensus conference: Total hip replacement. NIH Consensus Development Panel on Total Hip Replacement. *JAMA* 1995;**273**(24):1950–6.

140 Hawker GA, Wright JG, Coyte PC, *et al.* Differences between men and women in the rate of use of hip and knee arthroplasty. *N Engl J Med* 2000;**342**(14):1016–22.

141 Maillefert JF, Gueguen A, Nguyen M, *et al.* A composite index for total hip arthroplasty in patients with hip osteoarthritis. *J Rheumatol* 2002;**29**(2):347–52.

142 Dieppe P, Basler HD, Chard J, *et al.* Knee replacement surgery for osteoarthritis: effectiveness, practice variations, indications and possible determinants of utilization. *Rheumatology* 1999;**38**:73–83.

143 Hadorn D, Holmes A The New Zealand priority criteria project Part 1: Overview. *BMJ* 1997;**314**:131.

144 Manusco CA, Ranwat CS, Esdaile JM, Johanson NA, Charlson ME. Indications for total hip and total knee arthroplasties. Results of orthopaedic surveys. *J Arthroplasty* 1996;**1**:4–46.

145 Naylor CD, Williams JI. Primary hip and knee replacement surgery: Ontario criteria for case selection and surgical priority. *Qual Health Care* 1996;**5**:20–30.

146 Woolhead GM, Donovan JL, Chard JA, Dieppe PA. Who should have priority for a knee joint replacement? *Rheumatology* 2002;**41**(4):390–4.

Osteoarthritis
Summaries and decision aids

Osteoarthritis and pain killers
Summaries and decision aid

How well do painkillers work and how do they compare to anti-inflammatory drugs for treating osteoarthritis?

To answer this question, scientists found and analysed 6 high quality reviews (2 are Cochrane Systematic Reviews) and 6 more studies. People with osteoarthritis taking painkillers, non-steroidal anti-inflammatory drugs (NSAIDs) or sugar pills (placebo) were tested. These reviews and studies provide the best evidence we have today.

What is osteoarthritis and what drugs are used to decrease pain and swelling?

Osteoarthritis (OA) is the most common form of arthritis that can affect the hands, hips, shoulders, and knees. In OA, the cartilage that protects the ends of the bones breaks down and causes pain and swelling. Drug and non-drug treatments are used to relieve pain and/or swelling. There are two main types of drug treatments in OA: simple analgesics or painkillers, such as acetaminophen or paracetamol, are used to relieve pain but do not affect swelling and non-steroidal anti-inflammatory drugs (NSAIDs), such as ibuprofen, diclofenac and coxibs (rofecoxib and celecoxib), are used to relieve pain and decrease swelling.

How well do painkillers work and compare to anti-inflammatory drugs?

One study showed that acetaminophen improves pain and joint tenderness more than a sugar pill or placebo.

A Cochrane review and 3 other reviews plus 4 more studies found that NSAIDs work just as well as or better than acetaminophen. Two of the studies found that acetaminophen or NSAIDs help people who have mild to moderate pain but that NSAIDs work better than acetaminophen in people who have severe pain.

Were there any side effects with painkillers compared to anti-inflammatory drugs?

Two studies and 2 reviews showed that acetaminophen causes fewer side effects than NSAIDs, such as heartburn, nausea or vomiting, stomach pain and headaches. Serious side effects such as bleeding stomach ulcers or a hole in the lining of the gut also occur more often with NSAIDs.

What is the bottom line?

There is "Silver" level evidence that acetaminophen (in doses up to 4 grams per day) and NSAIDs improve pain and increase function in people with osteoarthritis of the knee and hip.

In people who have severe pain, NSAIDs will give more relief than acetaminophen. In people who have severe pain and who are more likely to have stomach problems, coxibs, also known as Cox-II inhibitors, which cause fewer serious stomach side effects, should be considered.

Based on Pham T, Fransen M, Ravaud P, Dougados M, Ottawa Methods Group. Osteoarthritis. In: *Evidence-based Rheumatology.* London: BMJ Books, 2003.

How well do painkillers work and how do they compare to anti-inflammatory drugs for treating osteoarthritis?

What is osteoarthritis and what medications are used to decrease pain and swelling?

Osteoarthritis (OA) is the most common form of arthritis. It can affect any joint of the body, such as the hands, hips, shoulders, and knees. In OA, the cartilage that protects the ends of the bones breaks down and causes pain, stiffness, and swelling. It is not known why pain occurs but it is thought that it may be because muscles and tendons work harder or in a different ways when the cartilage has broken down; because pieces of broken cartilage irritate soft tissue around the joint; or because bone rubs against bone. The pain and damage from OA limits people's ability to do daily activities at home and work and affects their wellbeing.

Drug and non-drug treatments are used to relieve pain and/or swelling. There are two main types of drug treatments for OA: simple analgesics or painkillers, such as acetaminophen or paracetamol (Tylenol) are used to relieve pain but do not affect swelling or inflammation; and non-steroidal anti-inflammatory drugs (NSAIDs) such as ibuprofen, diclofenac, and coxibs or Cox-II inhibitors (rofecoxib and celecoxib), are used to relieve pain and decrease swelling or inflammation.

How did the scientists find the information and analyse it?

To determine how well painkillers and anti-inflammatory drugs work, scientists searched for studies testing painkillers, and anti-inflammatory drugs in patients with OA. Unfortunately, not all studies or reviews found were of a high quality and so only those studies that met high standards were included in this summary.

Studies selected were randomised controlled trials where one group of patients received painkillers and was compared to another group of patients who received a placebo (a sugar pill) or another drug.

Which high quality reviews and studies were included?

There were 6 reviews (2 are Cochrane Systematic Reviews) and 6 studies included in this review that tested patients who had OA of the knee or hip. The studies tested the effects and safety of painkillers, such as acetaminophen; and of NSAIDs, such as ibuprofen, naproxen (Naprosyn), diclofenac and misoprostol (Arthrotec), etodalac, tenoxicam, piroxicam, celecoxib, and rofecoxib.

One of the best studies examined 227 patients with OA of knee or hip who received acetaminophen (1000 mg four times a day which is 4g a day) or an NSAID combined with another medicine to protect the stomach from ulcers (75 mg diclofenac plus 200 micrograms misoprostol, two times a day) for 6 weeks. This study examined the effects of the drugs by measuring pain, stiffness and physical function and by measuring the ability to do daily activities.

How well do painkillers (acetaminophen) work and compare to anti-inflammatory drugs (NSAIDs)?

Acetaminophen compared to placebo: One study showed that acetaminophen improves pain and joint tenderness more than a placebo.

Pain at rest: When taking acetaminophen, 73 out of 100 patients had less pain, but when taking a placebo 5 out of 100 patients had less pain.

Acetaminophen compared to NSAIDs

A Cochrane review and 3 other reviews plus 4 more studies compared patients taking NSAIDs with patients taking acetaminophen. It was found that NSAIDs work just as well as or better than acetaminophen. Two of the studies found that acetaminophen or NSAIDs help patients who have mild to moderate pain but that NSAIDs work better than acetaminophen in patients who have severe pain.

Specifically, the study that found the difference in the effect of NSAIDs for patients with mild/moderate pain and severe pain, showed :

- Patients with mild or moderate pain had less pain and functioned better with either acetaminophen or with an NSAID.
- On a pain, function, and stiffness scale from 0 to 100, patients with severe pain and taking NSAIDs, improved by about 14 more points than patients taking acetaminophen.
- In patients who tried each drug, 42 out of 100 patients said acetaminophen worked just as well as or better than an NSAID.

Were there any side effects with painkillers compared to anti-inflammatory drugs?

Common side effects: Two reviews plus one additional study showed that acetaminophen causes fewer side effects, such as heartburn, nausea or vomiting, stomach pain, and headache:

- 53 out of 100 patients had side effects with NSAIDs
- 46 out of 100 patients had side effects with acetaminophen.

Serious side effects: Bleeding stomach ulcers or a hole in the lining of the gut occur more often with NSAIDs. Normally, these side effects occur in 1 to 5 out of 100 patients. But some studies testing NSAIDs show that these serious side effects may occur more often than normal.

For those people who need to take NSAIDs because painkillers are not working and who are more likely to have stomach problems, coxibs, also known as Cox-II inhibitors (a type of NSAID), are safer for the stomach and intestines.

What is the bottom line?

There is "Silver" level evidence that acetaminophen (in doses up to 4 grams per day) and NSAIDs improve pain and increase function in people with osteoarthritis of the knee and hip.

In people who have severe pain, NSAIDs will give more relief than acetaminophen. In people who have severe pain and who are more likely to have stomach problems, coxibs, also known as Cox-II inhibitors, which cause fewer serious stomach side effects, should be considered.

Based on Pham T, Fransen M, Ravaud P, Dougados M, Ottawa Methods Group. Osteoarthritis. In: *Evidence-based Rheumatology.* London: BMJ Books, 2003.

Information about osteoarthritis treatment

What is osteoarthritis?

Osteoarthritis (OA) is the most common form of arthritis. It can affect any joint of the body such as the hands, hips, shoulders, and knees. In OA, the cartilage that protects the ends of the bones breaks down and causes pain, stiffness, and swelling. It is not known why pain occurs but it is thought that it may be because muscles and tendons work harder or in a different way when the cartilage has broken down; because pieces of broken cartilage irritate soft tissue around the joint; or because bone rubs against bone. The pain and damage from OA limits people's ability to do daily activities at home and work and affects their well-being.

The pain, stiffness and swelling usually come on slowly. However, the disease often progresses and if it is not treated, it may result in

- permanent damage to joints
- limited daily activities
- deformed joints
- need for surgery.

What can I do on my own to manage my disease?

✓ exercise ✓ hot/cold packs ✓ rest and relaxation ✓ maintain a healthy weight

What treatments are used for osteoarthritis?

Five kinds of treatment may be used alone or together. The common (generic) names of treatment are shown below.

1. *Pain medicines*
   - Acetaminophen
   - Codeine
   - Tramadol
2. *Aspirin and non-steroidal anti-inflammatory drugs (NSAIDs)*
   - Acetylsalicylic acid
   - Celecoxib
   - Diclofenac
   - Etodolac
   - Ibuprofen
   - Indomethacin
   - Ketoprofen
   - Naprosyn
   - Piroxicam
   - Rofecoxib
   - Sulindac
   - Tenoxicam
3. *Corticosteroid injections*
   - Cortisone
   - Hydrocortisone
4. *Viscosupplementation*
   - Hyaluronic acid
5. *Specific anti-osteoarthritic drugs*
   - Glucosamine sulphate
   - Diacerein
   - Condroitin

What about other treatments I have heard about?

There is not enough evidence about the effects of some treatments. For example:

- Acupuncture
- Avocado/soybean unsaponifiables
- Glycosaminoglycan polysulphuric acid complex
- Electropuncture
- Electrical stimulation
- Thermotherapy
- Ultrasound
- Shoe insoles
- Manganese

What are my choices? How can I decide?

Treatment for your disease will depend on your condition. You need to know the good points (pros) and bad points (cons) about each treatment before you can decide.

Osteoarthritis decision aid

Should I take non-steroidal anti-inflammatory drugs (NSAIDs)?

This guide can help you make decisions about the treatment your doctor is asking you to consider.

It will help you to:

1. Clarify what you need to decide.
2. Consider the pros and cons of different choices.
3. Decide what role you want to have in choosing your treatment.
4. Identify what you need to help you make the decision.
5. Plan the next steps.
6. Share your thinking with your doctor.

Step 1: Clarify what you need to decide

What is the decision?

Should I start taking non-steroidal anti-inflammatory drugs (NSAIDs) when painkillers are not working?

NSAIDs may be taken as a pill daily.

When does this decision have to be made? Check ✓ one

☐ within days ☐ within weeks ☐ within months

How far along are you with this decision? Check ✓ one

☐ I have not thought about it yet

☐ I am considering the choices

☐ I am close to making a choice

☐ I have already made a choice

Step 2: Consider the pros and cons of different choices

What does the research show?

NSAIDs are classified as: **Trade-off between benefits and harms**

There is "Silver" level evidence from 6 reviews (2 are Cochrane Systematic Reviews) and 4 more studies of people with osteoarthritis of the knee and hip who took pain medicines, NSAIDs or placebo (sugar pills). These studies found pros and cons that are listed in the chart below.

What do I think of the pros and cons of non-steroidal anti-inflammatory drugs (NSAIDs)?

1. Review the common pros and cons.
2. Add any other pros and cons that are important to you.
3. Show how important each pro and con is to you by circling from one (*) star if it is a little important to you, to up to five (*****) stars if it is very important to you.

PROS AND CONS OF NON-STEROIDAL ANTI-INFLAMMATORY DRUGS (NSAIDS)

PROS (number of people affected)	How important is it to you?	CONS (number of people affected)	How important is it to you?
Improves pain, function and stiffness by 14 more points on a scale of 0 to 100 with an NSAID than with a painkiller	* * * * *	Common side effects: heartburn, nausea or vomiting, stomach cramps, constipation 53 out of 100 people had side effects with NSAIDs 46 out of 100 people had side effects with painkillers	* * * * *
Other pros:	* * * * *	Serious long term side effects and rare serious harms: 1 to 5 more people out of 100 people will get a bleeding stomach ulcer or a hole in the lining of their gut	* * * * *
		Personal cost of medicine	* * * * *
		More clinic visits and blood tests needed	* * * * *
		Other cons:	* * * * *

What do you think about taking NSAIDs? Check ✓ one.

☐ Willing to consider this treatment
Pros are more important to me than the cons

☐ Unsure

☐ Not willing to consider this treatment
Cons are more important to me than the pros

Step 3: Choose the role you want to have in choosing your treatment. Check ✓ one

☐ I prefer to decide on my own after listening to the opinions of others

☐ I prefer to share the decision with: ______________________

☐ I prefer someone else to decide for me, namely: ______________

Step 4. Identify what you need to help you make the decision

What I know	Do you know enough about your condition to make a choice?	☐ Yes	☐ No	☐ Unsure
	Do you know which options are available to you?	☐ Yes	☐ No	☐ Unsure
	Do you know the good points (pros) of each option?	☐ Yes	☐ No	☐ Unsure
	Do you know the bad points (cons) of each option?	☐ Yes	☐ No	☐ Unsure
What's important	Are you clear about which **pros** are most *important to you?*	☐ Yes	☐ No	☐ Unsure
	Are you clear about which **cons** are most *important to you?*	☐ Yes	☐ No	☐ Unsure
How others help	Do you have enough support from others to make a choice?	☐ Yes	☐ No	☐ Unsure
	Are you choosing without pressure from others?	☐ Yes	☐ No	☐ Unsure
	Do you have enough advice to make a choice?	☐ Yes	☐ No	☐ Unsure
How sure I feel	Are you clear about the best choice for you?	☐ Yes	☐ No	☐ Unsure
	Do you feel sure about what to choose?	☐ Yes	☐ No	☐ Unsure

If you answered No or Unsure to many of these questions, you should talk to your doctor.

Step 5: Plan the next steps

What do you need to do before you make this decision?

For example: talk to your doctor, read more about this treatment or other treatments for osteoarthritis.

Step 6: Share the information on this form with your doctor

It will help your doctor understand what you think about this treatment.

8
Postmenopausal osteoporosis

Ann Cranney, Lee S Simon, Peter Tugwell, Rick Adachi, Gordon Guyatt, Ottawa Methods Group

Introduction

Osteoporosis is a major public health problem, with 70% of postmenopausal women meeting criteria for osteoporosis by age 80. The burden of osteoporotic fractures is anticipated to increase over the next few decades as the population ages.[1] Low bone density, prior history of fragility fractures, and age are an independent predictors of future fractures and therapy should be directed at women (>65 years) with osteoporosis as defined by the WHO criteria (T score of less than −2·5 SD) or a previous history of fragility fracture.[2] The choice of therapies for women with postmenopausal osteoporosis should be as evidence-based as possible.

One of the strongest levels of evidence comes from meta-analyses, which can result in a more precise unbiased estimate of the treatment effect.[3] A well-conducted large RCT that is adequately powered for fractures can also constitute strong evidence. In this chapter we present the evidence for anti-fracture efficacy of osteoporosis therapies. For each therapy we review results from systematic reviews/ meta-analyses or RCTs that have been conducted. Outcomes include bone mineral density (BMD), fractures, both vertebral, non-vertebral, and pain. Therapies presented include calcium, vitamin D, calcitonin, alendronate, risedronate, etidronate, raloxifene, hormone replacement therapy, and parathyroid hormone. Hip protector pads represent a non-pharmaceutical option to reduce the incidence of hip fractures in older women and we summarise the results of the efficacy of hip protector pads.

Methodology

The systematic reviews followed the Cochrane Collaboration methodology for conducting a systematic review.[4] Eligibility criteria, subgroup, and sensitivity analysis were specified a priori. Eligibility criteria included RCTs of postmenopausal women with osteoporosis or osteopenia of at least one year in duration. Outcomes included fracture (vertebral and non-vertebral), bone mineral density, and adverse effects. We used the Cochrane Collaboration search strategy to identify relevant studies for each therapy.[5,6] Regression analyses allowed us to determine for which doses and years we could pool data and we chose the most parsimonious model.[1] Subgroup analysis according to population was performed by: prevention (normal or near normal bone mineral density) versus treatment (BMD T score <−2·0 SD); dosage (varied depending on the particular intervention), and duration of treatment.[3]

Outcomes

Reduction of incident fractures (vertebral and non-vertebral) was the primary outcome in each systematic review. Clinical trials in osteoporosis have been adequately powered to detect changes in fracture rates over the past few years.

Question 1

What is the number needed to treat to prevent one non-vertebral fracture with the various anti-osteoporosis therapies?

Number needed to treat

We have estimated the 5 year baseline risk of fracture in an untreated high risk population from a fracture risk model developed by Black *et al.*[7] High risk is defined as age 65–69 with a previous history of fracture and a bone mineral density T score of <2·5 (score of 6 on a fracture index).[7] Lifetime fracture risk estimates are those of an average 50-year-old woman.[8] Number needed to treat has been calculated as (1/event rate*(1–RR)). Bone mineral density is a surrogate outcome measure for osteoporosis interventions and an independent risk factor for fracture. Studies on the efficacy of SERMs (selective (o)estrogen receptor modulators), other anti-resorptive agents and sodium fluoride, have shown that there is not a clear relationship between bone mineral density and fracture.[9,10] Adverse effects were evaluated through total withdrawals and specific events related the adverse effect profiles of each intervention.

Summary

This chapter will present a summary of recent systematic reviews and meta-analyses of osteoporosis interventions, including calcium and vitamin D, bisphosphonates, hormone replacement therapy (HRT), selective oestrogen receptor modulators (SERMs), calcitonin, parathyroid hormone, and hip protector pads.

Since these reviews do not include head-to-head fracture trials of different therapies, we are not able to draw conclusions about the relative efficacy of different therapies. Baseline populations may differ in responsiveness (bone density, prevalent fracture).

We use the case presentations to illustrate how different medications may be selected depending on the desired outcome, risk profile, and preferences of the individual woman.

Case presentation

A 68-year-old woman presents to your office with a recent history of lower thoracic pain, which occurred after she slipped on ice. Spine X-rays done by her family doctor revealed compression fractures of T10 and T12 with a 40% loss of height. Her BMD of the total hip area was –2·7 SD. Risk factors for osteoporosis included low body mass index, a maternal history of hip fracture, and a previous wrist fracture at age 55 after slipping on her driveway. She did not take hormone replacement therapy after menopause. This woman has an increased risk of further vertebral fractures in addition to an increased lifetime risk of hip fracture.

Question 2

(a) What therapies would reduce her risk of subsequent vertebral and non-vertebral fractures?

(b) What therapies would be beneficial to reduce the pain related to acute vertebral fracture?

Case presentation

A 57-year-old woman has osteopenia on her bone mineral density. She has a family history of breast cancer. Her weight is 145 lb. She has no previous history of fractures.

Question 3

What options to prevent further bone loss and osteoporosis should this patient consider?

Calcium

Introduction

Calcium is the simplest and least expensive preventive strategy for osteoporotic fractures. The NIH Consensus Development Conference approved a statement that calcium intake for older adults be maintained at 1000–1500 mg per day.[11] However, the impact of calcium supplementation alone on the reduction of fractures is less clear. We present the results of a recent systematic review by Shea *et al.*[12]

Literature search

1. osteoporosis, postmenopausal/
2. osteoporosis/
3. osteoporosis.tw.
4. exp bone density/
5. bone loss$.tw.
6. (bone adj2 densit$).tw.
7. or/2–6
8. exp menopause/
9. post-menopaus$.tw.
10. postmenopaus$.tw.
11. or/8–10
12. 7 and 11
13. 1 or 12
14. calcium/
15. calcium carbonate/
16. calcium, dietary/
17. (calcite or calcium).tw.
18. or/14–17
19. 13 and 18
20. meta-analysis.pt,sh.
21. (meta-anal: or metaanal:).tw.
22. (quantitativ: review: or quantitativ: overview:).tw.
23. (methodologic: review: or methodologic: overview:).tw.
24. (systematic: review: or systematic: overview).tw.
25. review.pt. and medline.tw.
26. or/20–25
27. 19 and 26
28. clinical trial.pt.
29. randomised controlled trial.pt.
30. tu.fs.
31. dt.fs.
32. random$.tw.
33. (double adj blind$).tw.
34. placebo$.tw.
35. or/28–34
36. 19 and 35

Outcomes

Fracture

Vertebral fracture: The pooled relative risk (RR) for vertebral fractures from five trials (n = 576)[12,13] with calcium was consistent with a non-significant trend toward reduction in vertebral fractures with a RR of 0·77 (95% CI 0·54–1·09), p = 0·14.

Non-vertebral fracture: Only two trials (n = 222) reported non-vertebral fractures with very few events and the confidence interval was very wide: RR of 0·86 (95% CI 0·43–1·72), p = 0·66.[13,14]

Bone mineral density

The pooled results of 9 trials (n = 845) comparing calcium to placebo resulted in an increase in bone density of 1·66% (95% CI 0·92–2·39), p<0·01, heterogeneity p value 0·02 for the lumbar spine. Increases at the other sites included 1·64% (95% CI 0·70–2·57), p < 0·01 for the femoral neck and 1·91 (95% CI 0·33–3·50), p = 0·02 for the distal radius.

Evidence summary: Silver

The systematic review, which pooled data from five RCTs, found evidence which suggests that calcium alone reduces the risk of vertebral fractures, however the 95% CI overlapped 1·0.

This systematic review did not find a significant reduction of non-vertebral fractures with calcium. The systematic review found that calcium increases bone density at the lumbar spine by 1·5 to 2%.

Case presentations
As a lifestyle change, the women in both Questions 2 and 3 would benefit by increasing their total calcium intake to 1000 to1500 mg per day, unless either has a history of hypercalcaemia, or hypercalciuria.[11]

Vitamin D
Introduction

Guidelines have recommended that vitamin D be given to postmenopausal women for prevention and treatment of osteoporosis.[11]. Bone loss in elderly women may be associated with secondary hyperparathyroidism, which can be related to vitamin D deficiency. There are a number of different formulations of vitamin D but they can be grouped into standard (cholecalciferol) and hydroxylated (both 1,25 OH and 1 alpha hydroxy-vitamin D_3). The risks associated with low dose vitamin D are small and the recommended dose would be 800 to 1000 IU per day.

Gillespie *et al* performed a systematic review of the effect of vitamin D on fractures and adverse effects, but did not evaluate the impact on bone mineral density.[15]

Literature search

1. osteoporosis, postmenopausal/
2. osteoporosis/
3. osteoporosis.tw.
4. exp bone density/
5. bone loss$.tw.
6. (bone adj2 densit$).tw.
7. or/2–6
8. exp menopause/
9. post-menopaus$.tw.
10. postmenopaus$.tw.
11. or/8–10
12. 7 and 11
13. exp Vitamin D/
14. vitamin d.tw.
15. Cholecalciferol.tw.
16. Dihydrotachysterol.tw.
17. Ergosterol.tw.
18. vitamin d.rn.
19. or/13–18
20. 12 and 19
21. meta-analysis.pt,sh.
22. (meta-anal: or metaanal:).tw.
23. (quantitativ: review: or quantitativ: overview:).tw.
24. (methodologic: review: or methodologic: overview:).tw.
25. (systematic: review: or systematic: overview). tw.
26. review.pt. and medline.tw.
27. or/21–26
28. clinical trial.pt.
29. randomised controlled trial.pt.
30. tu.fs.
31. dt.fs.
32. random$.tw.
33. (double adj blind$).tw.
34. placebo$.tw.
35. or/28–34
36. 20 and 27
37. 20 and 35

Outcomes
Fractures

In a meta-analysis of vitamin D, eight trials (n = 1130) measured the effect of vitamin D on **vertebral fractures**, with the majority of the trials using hydroxylated D, (1- alpha, or 1,25).[16] The pooled estimate indicated a 37% relative risk reduction in vertebral fractures: RR of 0·63 (95% CI 0·45–0·88), $p < 0{\cdot}01$ (Table 8.1).

Table 8.1 Five year (high risk woman) and lifetime risk of fracture, relative risk, and NNT with vitamin D (Papadimitropoulos *et al*, 2002)[16]

Outcome	5 year and lifetime risk of fracture in untreated population	5 year and lifetime risk in a treated population	Relative risk with treatment (95% CI)	NNT
Vertebral fracture	5 year: 7·1%	5 year: 4·5	0·63	5 year: 38
	Lifetime: 9·6%	Lifetime: 6·0	(0·45–0·88)	LIfetime: 28

Six trials (*n* = 6187) evaluated the effect on **non-vertebral fractures** and the pooled estimate of 0·77 (95% CI 0·57–1·04), p = 0·09 suggested a 23% reduction. However, the upper bound of the confidence interval included a relative risk increase of 4%, which is consistent with a non-significant reduction. The between trial heterogeneity was significant.

There is evidence, however, from individual large RCTs (Gold level) that vitamin D reduces the incidence of non-vertebral fractures in elderly women.[17]

Bone density

The effect of standard vitamin D is small, with the greatest impact on the lumbar spine: four trials WMD (weighted mean difference) of 0·86 (95% CI 0·17–1·54), p = 0·01 and femoral neck, five trials (0·98, 95% CI of 0·10–1·85), p = 0·03. Larger effects on BMD are seen with hydroxylated vitamin D at doses greater than 0·50 micrograms.

Adverse effects

The pooled relative risk for withdrawals due to adverse effects from 12 trials was 1·37 (95% CI 1·01– 1·88) and this was similar in standard and hydroxylated vitamin D trials.

Other benefits

Vitamin D deficiency has been associated with lower muscle strength and increased body sway and could predispose to an increased frequency of falls. Vitamin D treatment may assist in fall prevention through improvement in muscle strength and postural control.[18]

Evidence summary: Silver

The pooled results of the systematic review found a non-statistically significant reduction in non-vertebral fractures. However, there is evidence from individual large RCTs that vitamin D reduces non-vertebral fractures in both community-dwelling and institutionalised elderly women.[17,19] The systematic review of vitamin D (standard and hydroxylated) found a statistically significant reduction in vertebral fractures, however there were a number of trials with methodological limitations. Vitamin D has a positive if small impact on bone density of the lumbar spine, and femoral neck.

Case presentations

The women in both Questions 2 and 3 would benefit from taking 800 IU of vitamin D daily.

Etidronate

Introduction

Etidronate is a first-generation bisphosphonate that may improve bone mineral density and reduce incident fractures by inhibiting osteoclast-mediated resorption. Etidronate has potential to cause dose-related inhibition of mineralisation and cause osteomalacia. Therefore it is given on a cyclical schedule every 3 months.

A meta-analysis by Cardona in 1997 used the number of fractures instead of the number of women with fractures.[20] The authors did not come to any conclusion about the relative efficacy of either medication. We present the results of a more recent meta-analysis.[21]

Literature search

1. osteoporosis, postmenopausal/
2. osteoporosis/
3. osteoporosis.tw.
4. exp bone density/
5. bone loss$.tw.
6. (bone adj2 densit$).tw.
7. or/2–6
8. exp menopause/
9. post-menopaus$.tw.
10. postmenopaus$.tw.
11. or/8–10
12. 7 and 11
13. 1 or 12
14. etidronic acid/
15. etidronate.tw,rn.
16. (xidifon or xidiphon$).tw.
17. (ehdp or ethanehydroxydiphosphonate).tw.
18. or/14–17
19. 13 and 18
20. meta-analysis.pt,sh.
21. (meta-anal: or metaanal:).tw.
22. (quantitativ: review: or quantitativ: overview:).tw.
23. (methodologic: review: or methodologic: overview:) tw.
24. (systematic: review: or systematic: overview).tw.
25. review.pt. and medline.tw.
26. or/20–25
27. 19 and 26
28. clinical trial.pt.
29. randomised controlled trial.pt.
30. tu.fs.
31. dt.fs.
32. random$.tw.
33. (double adj blind$).tw.
34. placebo$.tw.
35. or/28–34
36. 19 and 35

Outcomes

Fracture

Nine RCTs ($n = 1076$) assessed the efficacy of etidronate at a dose of 400 mg on morphometric (radiographic) **vertebral fractures** after 2 years.[22–28] The weighted relative risk (RR) was 0·63 (95% CI 0·44–0·92), $p = 0{\cdot}02$, or a relative risk reduction of 37%[21] (Table 8.2) (Visual Rx Faces 8.1).

Seven randomised placebo controlled trials ($n = 867$) assessed the efficacy of etidronate on **non-vertebral fractures** after 2 years. The weighted RR was 0·99 (95% CI 0·69–1·42), $p = 0{\cdot}97$, suggesting no effect on non-vertebral fractures. Pooled data from four trials that had hip fracture data resulted in a pooled relative risk of 1·18 (95% CI 0·38–3·64).

Bone mineral density

Ten trials ($n = 875$) evaluated the impact of etidronate 400 mg on the **lumbar spine** and the pooled percent difference compared to placebo was 4·06 (95% CI 3·12–5·00), $p < 0{\cdot}01$, heterogeneity $p = 0{\cdot}10$.

Eight randomised placebo controlled trials ($n = 800$) assessed the efficacy of etidronate on **femoral neck** BMD. The duration of the included trials was 1 to 3 years. The weighted mean difference was 2·35% (95% CI 1·66–3·04), $p < 0{\cdot}01$, heterogeneity $p = 0{\cdot}40$.

Adverse effects

Withdrawals due to adverse effects from eight trials showed a relative risk of 0·93 (95% CI 0·70–1·23).

Evidence summary: Silver

The systematic review of seven RCTs with non-vertebral fractures did not find benefit for non-vertebral fracture reduction with etidronate despite an increase in femoral neck BMD. The systemic review of nine RCTs found that etidronate was efficacious in reducing vertebral

Table 8.2 NNT for five year (high risk woman) and lifetime risk of fracture in women treated with etidronate compared to no treatment (Cranney *et al*, 2001)[21]

Outcome	5 year and lifetime risk of fracture in untreated population	5 year and lifetime risk in a treated population	Relative risk with treatment (95% CI)	NNT for 5 years
Vertebral fracture	5 year: 7·1%	5 year: 4·5%	0·63	5 year: 38
	Lifetime: 9·6%	Lifetime: 6·0%	(0·44–0·92)	Lifetime: 28

Visual Rx Faces 8.1 NNT for five year and lifetime risk of fracture for women treated with etidronate compared to no treatment

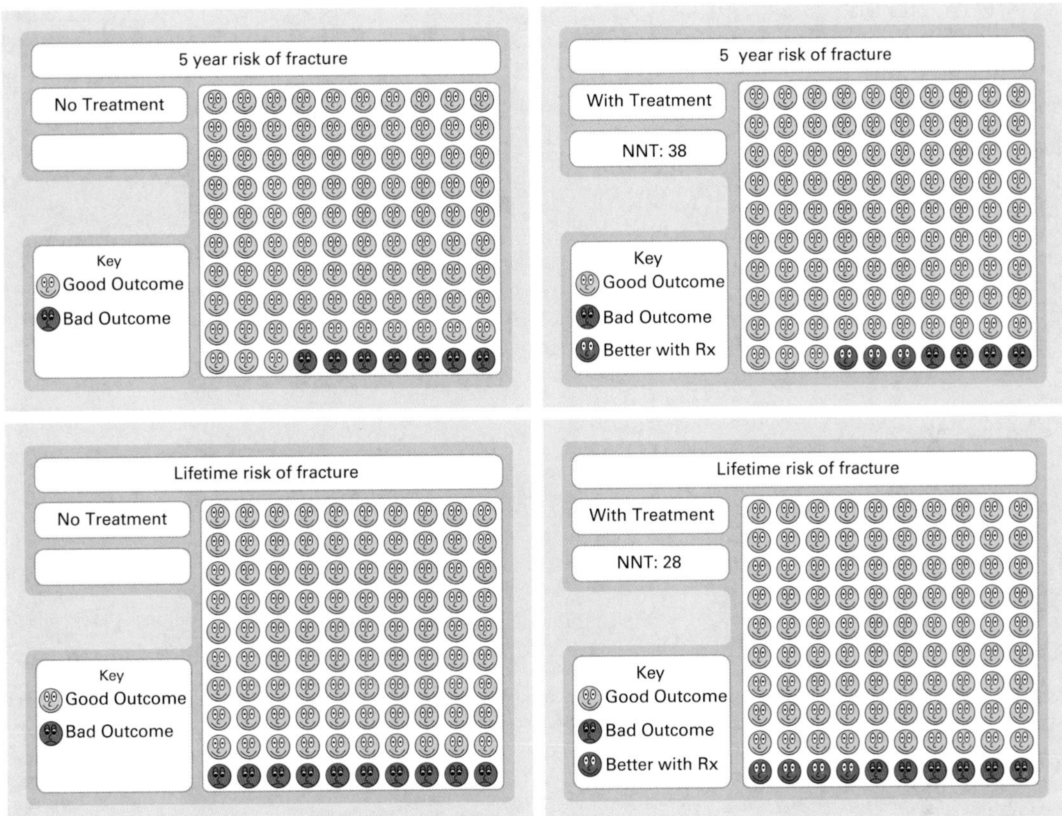

fractures. This is supported by the improvement in lumbar spine BMD.

Case presentation

Etidronate would be an option to reduce the risk of vertebral fracture of the woman in either Question 2 or Question 3, but the evidence does not suggest that etidronate will reduce her risk of non-vertebral fractures.

Alendronate

Introduction

Alendronate sodium is a second-generation nitrogen-containing bisphosphonate that does not impair bone mineralisation at doses that inhibit bone resorption.[29] Alendronate can induce apoptosis in osteoclasts through an effect on the mevalonic acid pathway and interference with protein prenylation.

Table 8.3 NNT for five year (high risk woman) and lifetime risk of fracture, with alendronate compared with no treatment (Cranney *et al*, 2002)[31]

Outcome	5 year and lifetime risk of fracture in untreated population	5 year and lifetime risk in a treated population	Relative risk with treatment (95% CI)	NNT
Vertebral fracture	5 year: 7·1%	5 year: 3·6%	0·52	5 year: 29
	Lifetime: 9·6%	Lifetime: 5·9%	(0·43–0·65)	Lifetime: 22
Non-vertebral	5 year: 19·8%	5 year: 10·1%	0·51	5 year: 10
fracture	Lifetime: 42·1%	Lifetime: 21·5%	(0·38–0·69)	Lifetime: 5

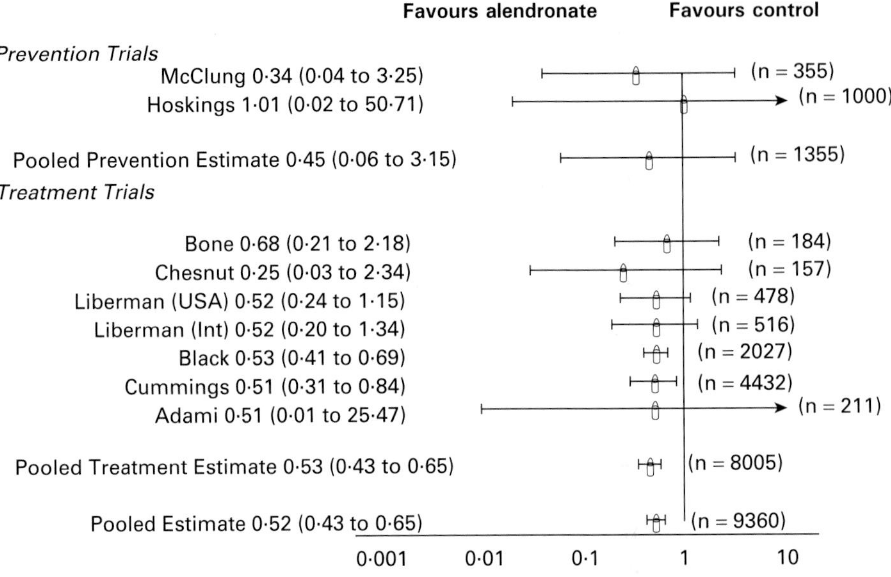

Figure 8.1 Pooled estimate of relative risk for vertebral fractures.

A systematic review by Karpf *et al* demonstrated a reduction in non-vertebral fractures with alendronate; however, the upper bound of the 95% CI bordered on no effect.[30] The results of a more recent meta-analysis are presented[31] (Table 8.3, Figure 8.1).

Literature search (Visual Rx Faces 8.2)

1. osteoporosis, postmenopausal/
2. osteoporosis/
3. osteoporosis.tw.
4. exp bone density/
5. bone loss$.tw.
6. (bone adj2 densit$).tw.
7. or/2–6
8. exp menopause/
9. post-menopaus$.tw.
10. postmenopaus$.tw.
11. or/8–10
12. 7 and 11
13. 1 or 12

Visual Rx Faces 8.2 NNT for 5 year (high risk woman) and lifetime risk of fracture with alendranate compared to no treatment

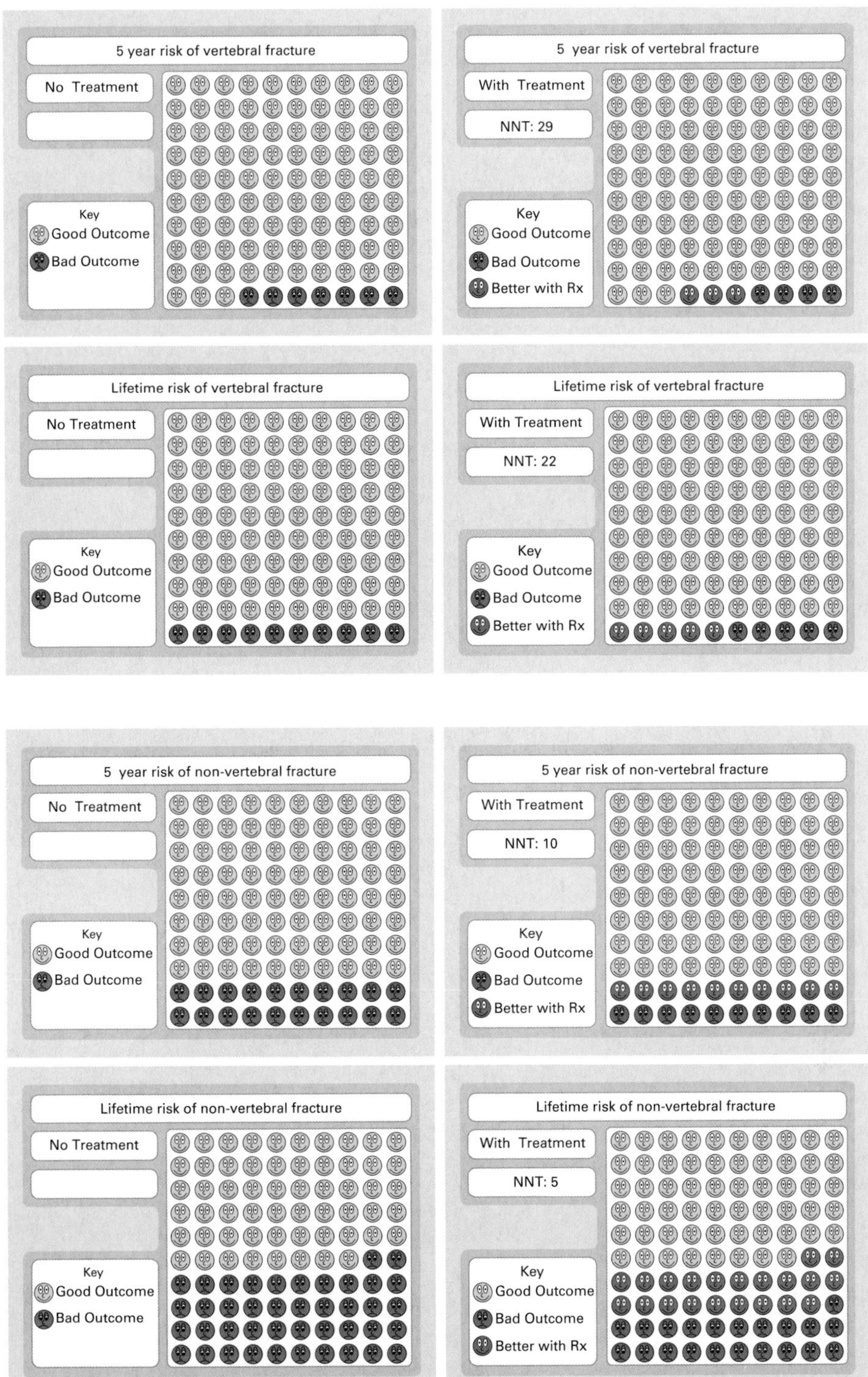

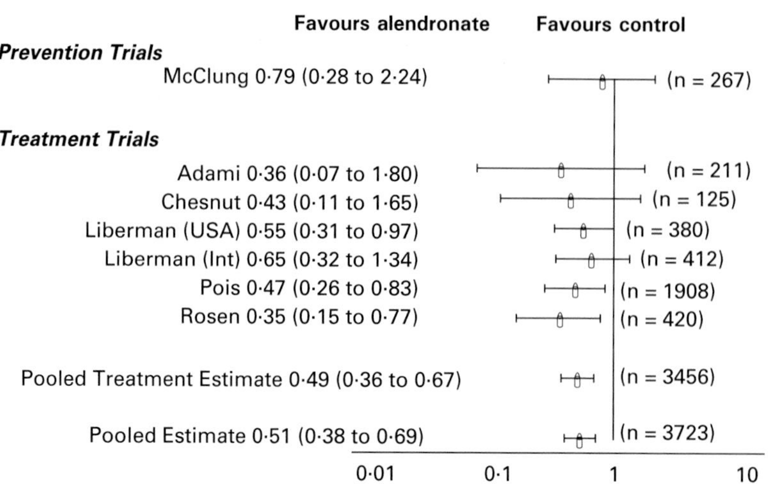

Figure 8.2 Pooled estimate of relative risk for non-vertebral fractures.

14. alendronate/
15. alendronate.tw,rn.
16. fosamax.tw.
17. aminohydroxybutane bisphosphonate.tw.
18. or/14–17
19. 13 and 18
20. meta-analysis.pt,sh.
21. (meta-anal: or metaanal:).tw.
22. (quantitativ: review: or quantitativ: overview:). tw.
23. (methodologic: review: or methodologic: overview:).tw.
24. (systematic: review: or systematic: overview). tw.
25. review.pt. and medline.tw.
26. or/20–25
27. 19 and 26
28. clinical trial.pt.
29. randomised controlled trial.pt.
30. tu.fs.
31. dt.fs.
32. random$.tw.
33. (double adj blind$).tw.
34. placebo$.tw
35. or/28–34
36. 19 and 35

Outcomes

Fracture

The pooled estimate of the relative risk of morphometric **vertebral fractures** with alendronate doses of 5– 40 mg from eight trials ($n = 8603$) was 0·52 (95%CI 0·43–0·65, $p < 0·01$), which was very consistent across the trials[32–39] (Figure 8·1).

About 7 out of 100 high risk women will have vertebral fractures in 5 years if left untreated (red faces). If these 100 women were treated with alendronate, about 4 women out of 100 will develop vertebral fractures. Therefore, 3 out of 100 women benefit from treatment. The NNT for a high risk population to prevent one vertebral fracture over 5 years and lifetime is 29 and 22 women, respectively.

For **non-vertebral fractures** the pooled estimate from six trials[34,36,38–40]) ($n = 3723$) of doses 10–40 mg was 0·51 (95% CI 0·38–0·69, $p < 0·01$) (Figure 8·2). With doses of 5 mg of alendronate ($n = 3723$, eight trials), the pooled RR for non-vertebral fractures was 0·87 (95% CI 0·73, 1·02, $p = 0·09$).

Table 8.4 NNT for five year and lifetime risk of fracture with Residronate compared to no treatment (Cranney 2002)[44]

Outcome	5 year and lifetime risk of fracture in untreated population	5 year and lifetime risk in a treated population	Absolute risk reduction	Relative risk with treatment (95% CI)	NNT
Vertebral fracture	5 year: 7·1%	5 year: 4·6%	5 year: 2·5%	0·65	5 year: 40
	Lifetime: 9·6%	Lifetime: 6·2%	Lifetime: 3·4%	(0·54–0·77)	Lifetime: 30
Non-vertebral	5 year: 19·8%	5 year: 14·5%	5 year: 5·3%	0·73	5 year: 19
fracture	Lifetime: 42·1%	Lifetime: 30·6%	Lifetime: 11·5	(0·61–0·87)	Lifetime: 9
(including hip)					

The 5 year and lifetime benefit on non-vertebral fractures of treating 100 high risk women with alendronate are also shown. About 20 women out of 100 high risk women will have non-vertebral fractures in 5 years if left untreated (red faces). If these 100 women were treated with alendronate, about 10 women out of 100 will develop non-vertebral fractures. Therefore, 10 women out of 100 benefit from treatment. The NNT for high risk women to prevent one non-vertebral fracture over 5 years and lifetime is 10 and 5 women, respectively.

For **hip fractures**, the pooled relative risk from six trials ($n = 3723$) for alendronate 10–40 mg was 0·45 (0·18–1·13, p = 0·09). This p-value indicates that there is a 9 in 100 chance that this pooled estimate of RR was found by chance. When we pooled across studies with 5 mg or greater the pooled relative risk was 0·63 (0·43–0·92).

Adverse effects

The most common adverse effects of alendronate are heartburn and ulcers of the oesophagus. The pooled estimate of the RR of discontinuing medication as a result of adverse effects from eight trials was 1·15 (95% CI 0·93–1·42).

Bone mineral density

Alendronate produced consistent increases in bone density at the **lumbar spine** and **femoral neck**. After 3 years the increase in bone density relative to placebo was 7·48 (95% CI 6·12–8·85, p < 0·01) and 5·60 (95% CI 4·80–6·39, p < 0·01). In addition, there is 10 year data that alendronate continues to increase bone mineral density.

The impact of alendronate on **forearm** bone density was less but was increased relative to placebo, with a pooled difference of 2·08 (95% CI 1·53–2·63, p < 0·01) after 2–4 years.

Evidence summary: Platinum

A systematic review of alendronate RCTs found that alendronate reduces the rate of both vertebral and non-vertebral fractures in postmenopausal women with osteoporosis. Alendronate has a consistent effect on bone density of the lumbar spine, femoral neck, and forearm compared to placebo.

Case presentation

Alendronate would be an appropriate choice for the woman in Question 2 to decrease her risk of both subsequent vertebral fractures and non-vertebral fractures. It could also be used as an option to prevent bone loss for the woman in Question 3.

Risedronate

Introduction

Risedronate, a third-generation pyridinyl bisphosphonate, acts to inhibit osteoclast mediated bone resorption and also acts on the mevalonic acic pathway.[41] There are multiple studies that demonstrate a positive impact on fracture and bone mineral density at 2·5 and 5 mg doses and for 1 to 3 years of treatment duration.[42,43] We present a summary of the results of a recent meta-analysis of residronate (Table 8.4).[44]

Literature search

1. osteoporosis, postmenopausal/
2. osteoporosis/
3. osteoporosis.tw.
4. exp bone density/
5. bone loss$.tw.
6. (bone adj2 densit$).tw.
7. or/2–6
8. exp menopause/
9. post-menopaus$.tw.
10. postmenopaus$.tw.
11. or/8–10
12. 7 and 11
13. 1 or 12
14. risedronate.tw.
15. 13 and 14
16. meta-analysis.pt,sh.
17. (meta-anal: or metaanal:).tw.
18. (quantitativ: review: or quantitativ: overview:).tw.
19. (methodologic: review: or methodologic: overview:).tw.
20. (systematic: review: or systematic: overview).tw.
21. review.pt. and medline.tw.
22. or/16–21
23. 15 and 22
24. clinical trial.pt.
25. randomised controlled trial.pt.
26. tu.fs.
27. dt.fs.
28. random$.tw.
29. (double adj blind$).tw.
30. placebo$.tw.
31. or/24–30
32. 15 and 31

Outcomes

Fracture

Five randomised placebo controlled trials assessed the efficacy of risedronate on radiographic **vertebral fractures** ($n = 2604$).[42,43,45–47] The weighted relative risk (RR) was 0·65 (95% CI 0·54–0·77, $p < 0{\cdot}01$). Using the 5 mg dose alone, resulted in a similar RR of 0·62 (95% CI 0·51, 0·76).

Seven randomised placebo controlled trials ($n = 12\,958$) estimated the weighted RR on **non-vertebral fracture**.[42,43,45–49] The pooled RR from these trials was 0·73 (95% CI 0·61, 0·87, $p < 0{\cdot}01$). If the results were restricted to the 5 mg dose, the pooled relative risk was 0·68 (95% CI 0·53, 0·87) consistent with a 32% reduction. A methodological limitation of these studies was the high loss to follow up.

Bone mineral density

Six randomised placebo controlled trials ($n = 2138$) were available that assessed the efficacy of risedronate with a dose of 5 mg. The weighted mean difference after 1·5 to 3 years of therapy was 4·54% (95% CI 4·12–4·97, $p < 0{\cdot}01$). The results were not heterogeneous.

Femoral neck

There were six randomised placebo controlled trials ($n = 2337$) available that assessed the efficacy of risedronate after 18 months to 3 years of treatment with 5 mg daily. The weighted mean difference on femoral neck was 2·75% (95% CI 2·32–3·17, $p < 0{\cdot}01$).

Adverse effects

The pooled relative risk of discontinuing medication due to adverse effects, from eight trials, was 0·94 (95% 0·80–1·10, $p = 0{\cdot}2$). The relative risk for discontinuing medication due to gastrointestinal adverse effect was 0·97 (95%

CI 0·90–1·04). The pooled relative risks for dyspepsia and oesophagitis were similar.

Evidence summary: Silver

The systematic review of risedronate found a reduction of 27–32% (seven trials) in non-vertebral fractures and 35–38% (five trials) in vertebral fractures in women with postmenopausal osteoporosis. This is supported by an increase in bone density at the lumbar spine and femoral neck.

Case presentation

Risedronate would be another option for the woman in Question 2, if she would like to reduce her risk of both subsequent vertebral and non-vertebral fractures.

Hormone replacement therapy

Introduction

Until recently, hormone replacement therapy (HRT) was recommended as first line therapy for osteoporosis. There is evidence that HRT improves bone density because the majority of the trials have used BMD as the primary outcome measure. Until recently there was Silver level evidence suggesting a reduction in hip fractures of 25–50% from observational studies.[50]

The recent HERS trial, which was designed to evaluate the impact of HRT on coronary heart disease, showed no impact of HRT on fractures, although only 20% of these women were osteoporotic.[51] The results presented below are from the recent meta-analysis by Wells *et al*.[52]

Outcomes

Fractures

Wells *et al* pooled the results from five trials (n = 3018) that evaluated **vertebral fractures**.[53–57] The resulting pooled estimate was 0·66 (95% CI 0·41–1·07), which is consistent with a 34% reduction in radiographic vertebral fractures, although the results were not significant.

In the meta-analysis by Wells *et al.* six trials (n = 3986) measured the effect of HRT on non-vertebral fractures.[37,54–58] The pooled results of comparing HRT and placebo groups resulted in a relative risk of 0·87 (95% CI 0·71–1·08), indicating a non-significant relative risk reduction of 13%.

A meta-analysis of **non-vertebral fractures** by Torgerson found that the pooled relative risk from 22 trials was consistent with a 27% reduction in non-vertebral fractures with HRT in comparison to control.[59]

Bone mineral density

A recent meta-analysis pooled the results of 56 randomised trials of HRT.[52] After two years of treatment, the pooled percentage change in bone mineral density was 6·8% (95%CI 5·63–7·9), 4·5% (95% CI 3·68–5·36), and 4·1 % (95% CI 3·45–4·80) at the lumbar spine, forearm, and femoral neck respectively ($p < 0·01$).

There also was a significant dose–response relationship seen when we grouped the doses of oestrogen into low (Premarin = 0·3 mg, medium (equivalent to Premarin 0·625 mg) and high (Premarin = 0·9 mg).[52]

Women's Health Initiative

The Women's Health Initiative (WHI) is a 15 year randomised controlled prevention trial of HRT. The HRT arm of the WHI (n = 16 608) was stopped prematurely in July 2002 due to a statistically significant increased risk of breast cancer. There was a reduced relative risk of hip fracture (HR 0·66, 95% CI 0·45–0·98) and a reduction in vertebral fracture (HR 0·66, 95% CI 0·44–0·98) (Table 8.5, Faces 8.4). There was also a significant reduction in colorectal cancer and an increased risk of coronary heart disease (HR 1·29, 95% CI 1·02–1·63), stroke, and

Visual Rx Faces 8.3 NNT for five year (high risk woman) and lifetime risk of fracture with HRT compared to no

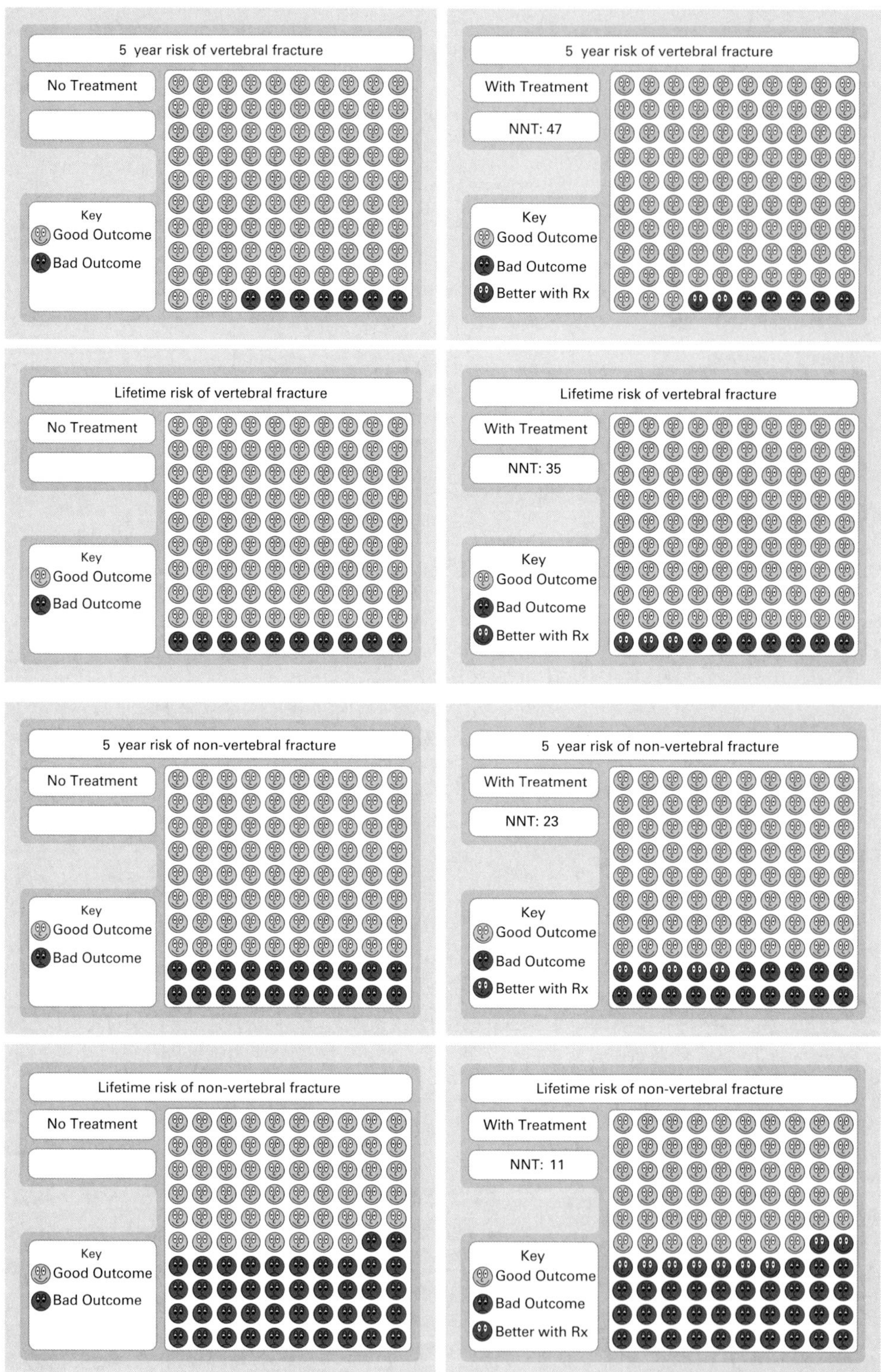

Table 8.5 NNT for five year (high risk woman) and lifetime risk of fracture with HRT compared to no treatment

Outcome	5 year and lifetime risk of fracture in untreated population	5 year and lifetime risk in a treated population	Relative risk with treatment (95% CI)	NNT
Vertebral fracture	5 year: 7·1% Lifetime: 9·6%	5 year: 5·0% Lifetime: 6·7%	0·70 (0·52–0·94)	5 year: 47 Lifetime: 35
Non-vertebral fracture (including hip)	5 year: 19·8% Lifetime: 42·1%	5 year: 15·4% Lifetime: 32·8%	0·78 (0·64–0·96)	5 year: 23 Lifetime: 11
Hip (1 trial, Women's Health Initiative 2002 CEE 0·625 mg + MPA 2·5 mg daily)[60]	5 year: 3·9% Lifetime 17·0%	5 year: 2·6% Lifetime: 11·2%	0·66 (0·45, 0·98)	5 year: 75 Lifetime: 17

Visual Rx Faces 8.4 NNT for hip fracture with HRT compared to no treatment

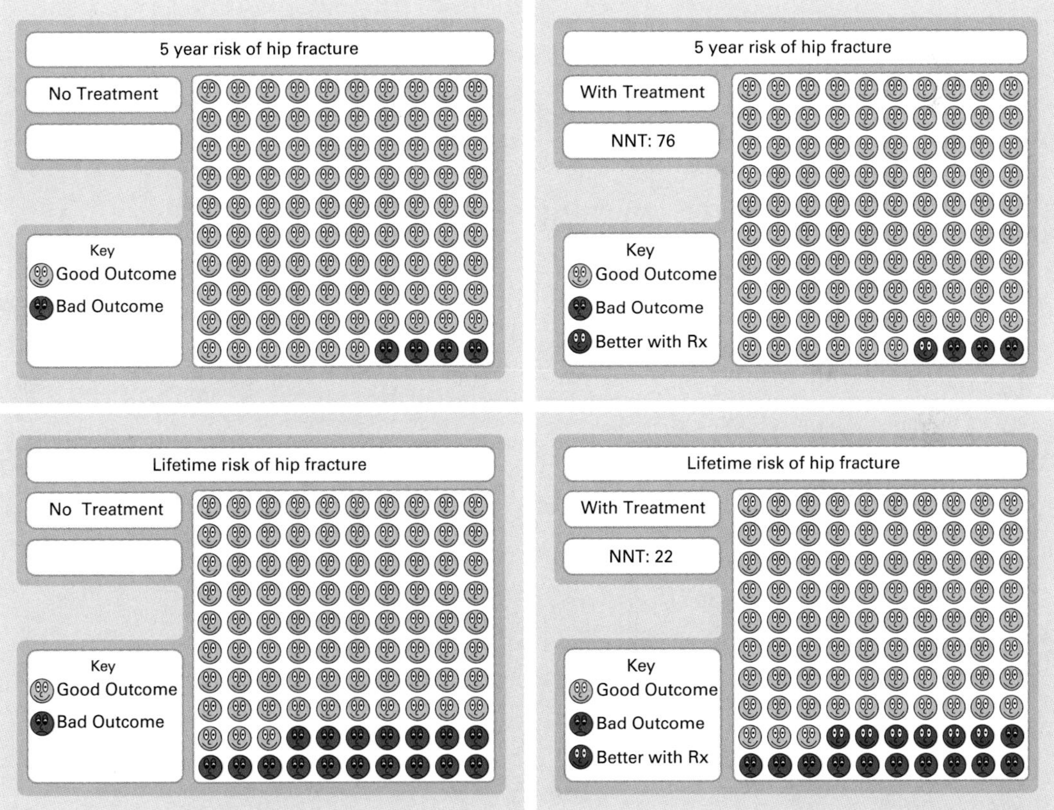

Table 8.6 Number needed to harm for HRT (for one preparation – oral CEE 0·625 mg + MPA 2·5 mg) (Women's Health Initiative, 2002)[60]

Outcome	% in placebo group	% for CEE + continuous MPA (95% CI)	Relative risk for CEE + continuous MPA	Absolute risk increase (95% CI)	NNH (95% CI)
Coronary heart disease (CHD death or non-fatal MI)	122/8102 (1·5%)	164/8506 (1·9%)	1·28 (1·02, 1·63)	0·4% (0·0, 0·8)	236 (121, 3874)
Stroke (fatal + non-fatal)	85/8102 (1·0%)	127/8506 (1·5%)	1·42 (1·07, 1·85)	0·4% (0·1, 0·8)	225 (126, 976)
Venous thromboembolic disease (DVT, PE)	67/8102 (0·8%)	151/8506 (1·8%)	2·15 (1·58, 2·82)	0·9% (0·6, 1·3)	105 (77, 164)
Invasive breast cancer	124/8102 (1·5%)	166/8506 (2·0%)	1·28 (1·00, 1·59)	0·4% (0·0, 0·8)	237 (121, 4565)

Table 8.7 NNT for five year (high risk woman) and lifetime risk of fracture with raloxifene compared to no treatment (Cranney *et al*, 2002)[62]

Outcome	5 year and lifetime risk of fracture in untreated population	5 year and lifetime risk in a treated population	Relative risk with treatment (95% CI)	NNT (95% CI)
Vertebral fracture: one trial; (Ettinger[10])	5 year: 7·1% Lifetime: 9·6%	5 year: 4·3% Lifetime: 5·8%	0·60 (0·50–0·70)	5 year: 35 Lifetime: 26

pulmonary embolism[60] (Table 8.6). There was no increase in overall mortality in the HRT arm compared to the placebo arm. When we pooled the results of the WHI with other trials that evaluated fractures the pooled relative risks became significant. The pooled relative risk for vertebral fractures was 0·70 (0·52–0·94) and for non-vertebral fractures the pooled relative risk was 0·78 (0·64–0·96).

Evidence summary: Gold

A systematic review of seven RCTs found that HRT lowers the risk of non-vertebral fractures by 22% and vertebral fractures by 30%. The WHI RCT alone found a 34% reduction in non-vertebral fractures. This is supported by the evidence that HRT increases bone density relative to placebo at the lumbar spine, femoral neck and forearm.

Case presentation

HRT may be an option for the woman in Question 2 if she wants to decrease her risk of further fractures, however the risk/benefit ratio for combined oestrogen/progestin therapy is not favourable for long term treatment. Further data on the risk/benefit ratio of oestrogen alone will be available when the oestrogen arm of the WHI study is complete. If she has severe postmenopausal symptoms she may consider taking HRT for a period of time. The woman in question 3 may choose to avoid HRT because of concerns regarding breast cancer.

Raloxifene

Introduction

Raloxifene hydrochloride is a non-steroidal benzothiophene, which is classified as a

Table 8.8 Number needed to harm for raloxifene (Cranney *et al.*, 2002)[62]

Outcome	Risk in untreated population	Risk in a treated population	Relative risk with treatment (95% CI)	NNH (95% CI)
Thromboembolic events	0·3%	0·9%	3·29 (1·60, 6·73)	157
Hot flashes	8·5%	13·5%	1·53 (1·34, 1·74)	20

selective oestrogen receptor modulator.[61] It exerts selective agonist or antagonist effects with oestrogen-like effects on bone and lipid metabolism, and oestrogen antagonist effects on the breast and uterus. The literature suggests that raloxifene is a less potent agent than newer bisphosphonates, with respect to effects on bone mineral density.[61] Here we report the results of a recent meta-analysis examining the efficacy of raloxifene with respect to fracture reduction and bone mineral density.[62]

Literature search

1. osteoporosis, postmenopausal/
2. osteoporosis/
3. osteoporosis.tw.
4. exp bone density/
5. bone loss$.tw.
6. (bone adj2 densit$).tw.
7. or/2–6
8. exp menopause/
9. post-menopaus$.tw.
10. postmenopaus$.tw.
11. or/8–10
12. 7 and 11
13. 1 or 12
14. raloxifene/
15. raloxifene.tw,rn.
16. (evista or keoxifene).tw.
17. or/14–16
18. 13 and 17
19. meta-analysis.pt,sh.
20. (meta-anal: or metaanal:).tw.
21. (quantitativ: review: or quantitativ: overview:).tw.
22. (methodologic: review: or methodologic: overview:).tw.
23. (systematic: review: or systematic: overview).tw.
24. review.pt. and medline.tw.
25. or/19–24
26. 18 and 25
27. clinical trial.pt.
28. randomised controlled trial.pt.
29. tu.fs.
30. dt.fs.
31. random$.tw.
32. (double adj blind$).tw.
33. placebo$.tw.
34. or/27–33
35. 18 and 34

Outcomes

Fracture

Two randomised controlled trials ($n = 7848$) assessed the efficacy of raloxifene on **vertebral fractures**.[10] The trials included one large multicentre trial ($n = 7705$)[10] and one small trial ($n = 143$) with contrasting estimates of relative risk (RR). The RR for vertebral fractures for the larger trial was 0·60 (0·50–0·70, $p < 0{\cdot}01$) (Table 8.7). The smaller trial, by Lufkin *et al*, was not powered to evaluate fractures and had a relative risk of 1·16 (95% CI 0·77 to 1·76, $p = 0{\cdot}48$). For this reason we did not pool the results of the two trials but used the results from the MORE trial.

The one large randomised controlled trial ($n = 7705$) assessed **non-vertebral fractures**, and the RR was 0·92 (95% CI 0·79–1·06, $p = 0{\cdot}24$). For the smaller trial the RR of non-vertebral fractures was 0·52 (95% CI 0·12–2·18, $p = 0{\cdot}37$).

Bone mineral density

There were seven randomised placebo controlled trials ($n = 6428$) available that assessed the efficacy of raloxifene after one year of treatment at 60 mg daily.[10,63–68] The weighted mean difference was 1.82% (95% CI 1·50–2·14, $p < 0{\cdot}001$). After two years of treatment (five trials, $n = 6238$) the estimate increased to 2·38 (95% CI 2·32–2·53, $p < 0{\cdot}001$).[31] Heterogeneity of treatment effect was not significant.

Femoral neck: There were three randomised placebo controlled trials ($n = 5320$) available that assessed the efficacy of raloxifene after one year of treatment at 60 mg daily.[64,67,68] The weighted mean difference was 1·33% (95% CI 1·09–1·58, $p < 0{\cdot}001$). After two years of treatment (three trials, $n = 5518$), the estimate increased to 1·98 (95% CI 1·79–2·18, $p < 0{\cdot}001$). There was no heterogeneity of treatment effect.

Forearm: Two randomised placebo controlled trials ($n = 204$) were pooled to assess the efficacy of raloxifene after one year of treatment at 60 mg. The weighted mean difference was 0·61 (95% CI –0·17 to 1·40, $p = 0{\cdot}12$, heterogeneity $p = 0{\cdot}76$). After two years of treatment (one trial (n=108) the estimate increased to 1·93 (95% CI 0·23–3·63, $p = 0{\cdot}03$).[66]

Adverse effects

The withdrawal due to adverse effects was 1·15 (95% CI 1·00–1·33). The pooled relative risk for hot flashes from four trials ($n = 9360$) was 1·53 (95% CI 1·34–1·74, $p < 0{\cdot}0001$). For breast pain the pooled relative risk was 0.97 (95% CI 0·75–1·24, $p = 0{\cdot}79$). The pooled relative risk of thromboembolic events from two trials ($n = 8680$) was 3·29 (95% CI 1·60–6·73) for raloxifene compared to placebo.[10,62]

Evidence summary: Silver

Raloxifene at a dose of 60 mg appears to have a small but consistent effect on bone mineral density. Despite the small impact on bone mineral density, there is Gold level evidence from one large RCT that raloxifene reduces vertebral fractures. At this time there is no support for reduction of non-vertebral fractures, suggesting that larger effects on bone mineral density are necessary to reduce the risk of hip fractures, although there are ongoing large trials that are designed to evaluate hip fracture as a secondary outcome.

Case presentation

Raloxifene would be a valid treatment option for the woman in Question 2, to lower her risk of vertebral fractures, especially if she was unable to tolerate bisphosphonates or wanted to take a therapy that could lower her risk of breast cancer. Raloxifene would be an option for the prevention of further bone loss or treatment of mild osteoporosis, such as for the woman in Question 3.

Calcitonin

Introduction

Calcitonin is a polypeptide hormone classified as an anti-resorptive agent. It acts by inhibiting and reducing the lifespan of osteoclasts. A number of trials have demonstrated the efficacy of calcitonin for the prevention of trabecular bone loss in postmenopausal osteoporosis. In addition, calcitonin has also been shown to have an analgesic effect in women with established osteoporosis and vertebral fracture in multiple studies. Here we present the results of a recent meta-analysis.[69]

Literature search

1. osteoporosis, postmenopausal/
2. osteoporosis/
3. osteoporosis.tw.
4. exp bone density/
5. bone loss$.tw.
6. (bone adj2 densit$).tw.
7. or/2–6
8. exp menopause/
9. post-menopaus$.tw.
10. postmenopaus$.tw.
11. or/8–10
12. 7 and 11
13. 1 or 12
14. calcitonin/
15. calcitonin.tw,rn
16. (calcitrin or thyrocalcitonin).tw.
17. miacalcin.tw.
18. or/14–17
19. 13 and 18
20. meta-analysis.pt,sh.
21. (meta-anal: or metaanal:).tw.
22. (quantitativ: review: or quantitativ: overview:).tw.
23. (methodologic: review: or methodologic: overview:).tw.
24. (systematic: review: or systematic: overview).tw.
25. review.pt. and medline.tw.
26. or/20–25
27. 19 and 26
28. clinical trial.pt.
29. randomised controlled trial.pt.
30. tu.fs.
31. dt.fs.
32. random$.tw.
33. (double adj blind$).tw.
34. placebo$.tw.
35. or/28–34
36. 19 and 35

Outcomes

Fractures

In three small trials (total $n = 269$) that studied **vertebral fracture** outcomes at 1 and 2 years we found data suggesting large treatment effects, suggesting the possibility of publication bias.[70–72] Data were also available for fracture outcomes at five years from a larger trial, Prevent Recurrence of Osteoporotic Fractures (PROOF). Because of the variability in the results between the smaller studies and the PROOF trial we chose not to pool the data. We elected to use the PROOF trial estimate as we felt this treatment effect was the most representative. The relative risk ($n = 1108$) for vertebral fracture at 5 years was 0·79 (95% CI 0·62 –1·00). Unfortunately, the PROOF trial had a large number of subjects lost to follow up (60%) and failed to maintain blinding.[73]

In our meta-analysis three studies assessed **non-vertebral fracture** as an outcome measure. However, this included two trials of small sample size with larger treatment effects, suggesting the possibility of publication bias. Again, we agreed that the point estimate of the treatment effect from the PROOF trial was the most representative. Data from the PROOF trial were available for fracture outcomes at 5 years.[73] The relative risk for **non-vertebral fracture** at 5 years was 0·80 (95% CI 0·59–1·15) ($n = 1245$).

Bone mineral density

In our meta-analysis 12 trials were pooled to estimate the weighted mean difference of the percentage change from baseline between calcitonin (700 IU weekly) and placebo on **lumbar spine** bone mineral density after one year of treatment.[51] The pooled estimate ($n = 1124$) was 3·75% (95% CI 1·98–5·53, $p < 0·001$, heterogeneity $p < 0·001$). Data from eight publications were pooled to assess the efficacy of calcitonin (1400 IU weekly) versus placebo.

Table 8.9 NNT for five year (high risk woman) and lifetime risk of fracture with PTH compared to no treatment (Neer *et al*, 2001)[82]

Outcome	5 year and lifetime risk of fracture in untreated population	5 year and lifetime risk in a treated population	Relative risk with treatment (95% CI)	NNT
Vertebral fracture	5 year: 7·1%	5 year: 2·5%	0·35	5 year: 22 (18, 28)
(20 microgram PTH)	Lifetime: 9·6%	Lifetime: 3·4%	(0·22–0·50)	LIfetime: 16 (13, 21)
Vertebral fracture	5 year: 7·1%	5 year: 2·2%	0·31	5 year: 20 (18, 26)
(40 microgram PTH)	Lifetime: 9·6%	Lifetime: 3·0%	(0·23–0·46)	LIfetime: 15 (14, 19)
Non-vertebral	5 year: 19·8%	5 year: 12·9%	0·65	5 year: 14 (9, 253)
fracture	Lifetime: 42·1%	Lifetime: 27·4%	(0·43–0·98)	Lifetime: 7 (4, 119)
(including hip)				
(20 microgram PTH)				
Non-vertebral	5 year: 19·8%	5 year: 12·1%	0·62	5 year: 13 (9, 101)
fracture	Lifetime: 42·1%	Lifetime: 26·1%	(0·41–0·95)	Lifetime: 6 (4, 48)
(including hip)				
(40 microgram PTH)				

The weighted mean (n = 866) was 3·14% (95% CI 1·33–4·94, p < 0·001, heterogeneity p < 0·001).

Our systematic review of the literature revealed that very few publications have fully assessed the effect of calcitonin versus placebo on **femoral neck** bone mineral density after one year of treatment. Three publications (n = 111) were pooled to assess calcitonin (700 IU weekly).

The weighted mean difference was 6·78% (95% CI 1·55–12·01, p < 0·01, heterogeneity p < 0.001). Two publications (n = 92) were pooled to estimate the weighted mean difference for calcitonin (1400 IU weekly).[71,74] The weighted mean difference was 2·11% (95% CI –4·20 to 8·43, p = 0·5, heterogeneity p < 0·01).

Our meta-analysis combined data from five publications to estimate the efficacy of calcitonin (700 IU weekly) versus placebo on **forearm** bone mineral density.[75,76] The weighted mean difference (n = 230) was 2·61% (95% CI –0·84 to 6·05, p = 0·14, with significant heterogeneity p < 0·001). Four trials were used to estimate the weighted mean difference of calcitonin (1400 IU weekly).[76] The weighted mean difference (n = 161) was 0·33% (95% CI –0·57 to 1·23, p = 0·5).

Pain

Back pain, as a result of vertebral fracture, is a common manifestation of osteoporosis. Calcitonin may affect pain immediately after acute vertebral fracture through increasing plasma beta-endorphin levels.[77] In our meta-analysis we found four trials (n = 212) that used a visual analogue scale to assess pain in subjects with acute vertebral fracture.[78] A percentage change from baseline in pain score was calculated and a pooled measurement derived. The overall effect size was –44·84% (95% CI –55·71 to –34·33, p < 0·01, heterogeneity non-significant), suggesting that calcitonin results in short term pain relief after acute vertebral fracture.

Adverse effects

The pooled relative risk from four trials for rhinitis was 1·72 (95% CI 0·92 to 3·23, p = 0·09).[69]

Evidence summary: Silver

There is silver level evidence that calcitonin reduces vertebral fractures with a risk reduction of approximately 20%. There were methodological weaknesses of the PROOF calcitonin trial, including failure to conceal allocation, blinding, and large losses to follow up. There was no evidence that calcitonin reduced non-vertebral fractures. Calcitonin improves BMD at the lumbar spine and femoral neck. There was no significant treatment effect of calcitonin on forearm BMD. There is evidence for the use of calcitonin for the reduction of acute pain following vertebral fracture.

Case presentation

Calcitonin could be used as a second line treatment if the goal was to prevent vertebral fractures, particularly if the woman in Question 2 was unable to tolerate other antiresorptive agents. Calcitonin may be useful to treat acute pain related to the vertebral fracture for the woman in Question 2.

Parathyroid hormone

Introduction

Human parathyroid hormone (hPTH) represents a new class of drugs for the management of postmenopausal osteoporosis.[79] hPTH (Recombinant) has an anabolic effect if given intermittently and appears to build architecturally normal bone.[80] Currently, hPTH is given via daily subcutaneous self-injection but alternative forms of delivery are currently being explored. A number of trials have used hPTH in combination with antiresorptive drugs.[79,81] One large RCT has evaluated the effect of hPTH in different doses in comparison to placebo.[82]

Literature search

1. osteoporosis, postmenopausal/
2. osteoporosis/
3. osteoporosis.tw.
4. exp bone density/
5. bone loss$.tw.
6. (bone adj2 densit$).tw.
7. or/2–6
8. exp menopause/
9. post-menopaus$.tw.
10. postmenopaus$.tw.
11. or/8–10
12. 7 and 11
13. 1 or 12
14. exp parathyroid hormone/ or parathyroid hormones/
15. parathyroid hormone.tw.
16. (parathormone or parathyrin or hpth).tw.
17. or/14–16
18. 13 and 17
19. meta-analysis.pt,sh.
20. (meta-anal: or meta-anal:).tw.
21. (quantitativ: review: or quantitativ: overview:).tw.
22. (methodologic: review: or methodologic: overview:).tw.
23. (systematic: review: or systematic: overview).tw.
24. review.pt. and medline.tw.
25. or/19–24
26. 18 and 25
27. clinical trial.pt.
28. randomised controlled trial.pt.
29. tu.fs.
30. dt.fs.
31. random$.tw.
32. (double adj blind$).tw.
33. placebo$.tw.
34. or/27–33
35. 18 and 34

Outcomes

Fractures

One large randomised placebo controlled trial evaluated the efficacy of the N-terminal rhPTH (1–34) in postmenopausal women with prevalent **vertebral fractures** ($n = 1637$).[82] The relative risk

Table 8.10 Number needed to harm for PTH (Neer *et al*, 2001)[82]

Outcome	Risk in placebo group	Relative risk with treatment (95% CI)	Risk in a treated population	Absolute risk increase (95% CI)	NNH (95% CI)
Hypercalcaemia (20 microgram PTH)	11/544 (2%)	5·48 (2·92, 10·32)	60/541 (11%)	9·1% (6·2, 12·1)	11 (8, 16)
Hypercalcaemia (40 microgram PTH)	11/544 (2%)	13·89 (7·62, 25·30)	155/552 (28%)	26·1% (22·1, 30)	3 (3, 4)

(RR) of incident vertebral fractures was 0·35 (95% CI 0·22–0·50, p < 0·001 and 0·31 95% CI 0·23–0·46, p < 0·001) for 20 micrograms ($n = 892$) and 40 micrograms ($n = 882$) daily, respectively (Table 8.9).

The estimated RR of incident **non-vertebral fractures** was 0·65 (0·43–0·98, p = 0·04) and 0·62 (95% CI 0·41–0·95, p = 0·03 for 20 micrograms ($n = 1096$) and 40 micrograms ($n = 1096$) of hPTH 1–34 daily, respectively (Table 8.9).

Bone mineral density

Two randomised placebo controlled trials ($n = 913$) evaluated the efficacy of hPTH (1–34) on bone mineral density of the lumbar spine. One 2 year study was very large ($n = 892$)[82] and the second was very small ($n = 31$).[81] The PTH analogue varied between studies; (1–34)[82] versus (1–84).[81] In addition, dosing was very different between the two studies; 20 and 40 micrograms versus 50, 75, and 100 micrograms daily.

Lumbar spine: The results from Neer *et al* ($n = 892$) suggested a mean difference of 8·60% (95% CI 7·74–9·46, p < 0·001) and 12·60% (95% CI 11·55–13·65, p < 0·001 for 20 and 40 micrograms, respectively.[82]

Femoral neck: The results from the Neer trial ($n = 892$) suggested a mean difference of 3·50% (95% CI 2·77– 4·23, p < 0·01) and 5·80% (95% CI 5·00–6·60, p < 0·01) for 20 and 40 microgram doses, respectively.

Forearm: Neer *et al* evaluated the efficacy of hPTH (1–34) on bone mineral density of the distal forearm.[82] The weighted mean difference of hPTH compared to control was 1·50% (95% CI 0·48–2·52, p = 0·004) and 0·10% (95% CI–1·00 to 1·20, p = 0·9) for 20 and 40 micrograms daily, respectively. There was greater bone loss in the hPTH arms than in controls at the radial shaft.

Adverse effects

Withdrawals due to adverse effects were 1·46 (95% CI 0·92, 2·15) from the Neer trial. In the Neer trial, hypercalcaemia in a dose dependent fashion was noted with hPTH (2% in controls and 11% and 28% in 20 micrograms and 40 microgram dose, respectively).

Rats that were given almost lifetime daily injections of hPTH (1–34) manifested increased osteosarcoma in a dose-dependent fashion as a result of PTH administration.[82] However, this effect is not apparent in primate models. There is no evidence that the decrease in a radius BMD translates into an increase in radial fractures. The long term effects of daily hPTH are uncertain and require further research.

Evidence summary: Silver

There is Silver level evidence that hPTH increases BMD in the lumbar spine, and femoral neck. There is Silver level evidence that PTH results in a risk reduction for vertebral fractures of 67% and non-vertebral fractures of 38%.

Case presentation

hPTH would be an option for the woman in Question 2, with a prevalent vertebral fracture and low bone density, to increase her bone density and decrease her risk of future fractures.

Hip protector pads

Introduction

Nursing home residents are at increased risk of hip fracture for multiple reasons. Hip protector pads are a non-pharmacological intervention that can reduce the incidence of hip fractures in institutionalised and potentially community dwelling elderly people. Hip protectors attenuate the impact on the proximal femur during falls by absorbing and shunting the force.[83]

A Cochrane review by Parker *et al* suggested that the use of hip protectors might reduce the relative risk of hip fracture by 76% (RR 0·24, 95% 0·09 to 0·65).[84] We pooled the results from all five trials that evaluated hip protectors in an institutionalised setting,[85–90] and found that hip protectors reduced the relative risk of hip fractures.

There are methodological limitations in a number of the trials. More recent trials have shown conflicting results on hip fracture reduction.[91,92] Unfortunately, compliance with hip protector pads is limited, with estimates as low as 24·4% at 1 year, which is even lower than compliance estimates with pharmaceutical interventions.[86]

Further research to evaluate efficacy and compliance of hip protectors.[91]

Evidence summary: Silver

There is Silver level evidence from systematic reviews that hip protectors may reduce the risk of hip fractures in institutionalised elderly people, although their efficacy in those elderly people dwelling in the community is uncertain. Compliance with hip protectors is sub-optimal and further research on methods to increase compliance is necessary.

References

1 Papadimitropoulos E, Coyte PC, Josse RG, Greenwood CE. Current and projected rates of hip fracture in Canada. *CMAJ* 1997;**157**:1257–363.

2 Marshall D, Johnell O. Meta-analysis of how well measures of bone mineral density predict occurrence of osteoporotic fractures by postural instability and bone density. *BMJ* 1996;**3**:1254–9.

3 Cranney A, Tugwell P, Wells G, Guyatt G. Meta-analyses of therapies for postmenopausal osteoporosis. I. Systematic reviews of randomised trials in osteoporosis: introduction and methodology. *Endocrin Rev* 2002;**23**(4):496–507.

4 Clarke M, Oxman AD. *The Cochrane Reviewer's Handbook 1999 Review Manager.* Cochrane Collaboration version 4·0. Oxford: Update, 2003.

5 Dickersin K, Scherer R, Lefebvre C. Identifying relevant studies for systematic reviews. *BMJ* 1994;**309**:1286–91.

6 Haynes R, Wilczynski N, McKibbon KA, Walker CJ, Sinclair JC. Developing optimal search strategies for detecting clinically sound strategies in MEDLINE. *J Am Med Info Assoc* 1994;**1**(1):447–58.

7 Black DM, Steinbuch M, Palmero L, Dargent-Molina P, Lindsay R, Hoseyni MS. An assessment tool for predicting fracture risk in postmenopausal women. *Osteoporos Int* 2001;**12**(7):519–28.

8 Doherty DA, Sanders KM, Kotowicz MA, Prince RL. Lifetime and five-year age-specific risks of first and subsequent osteoporotic fractures in postmenopausal women. *Osteoporos Int* 2001;**12**(1):16–23.

9 Guyatt GH, Cranney A, Griffith L, *et al.* Summary of meta-analyses of therapies for postmenopausal osteoporosis and the relationship between bone density and fractures. *Endocrinol Metab Clin North Am* 2002;**31**(3):659–79, xii.

10 Ettinger B, Black DM, Mitlak BH, *et al.* Reduction of vertebral fracture risk in postmenopausal women with osteoporosis treated with raloxifene. *JAMA* 1999;**282**(7):637–45.

11 NIH Consensus Statement – Osteoporosis prevention, diagnosis, and therapy. *JAMA* 2000;**285**:785–95.

12 Shea B, Wells G, Cranney A, *et al.* Meta-analyses of therapies for postmenopausal osteoporosis. VII. Meta-analysis of calcium supplementation for the prevention of postmenopausal osteoporosis. *Endocrin Rev* 2002;**23**(4): 552–9.

13 Riggs BL, O'Fallon WM, Muhs J, O'Connor MK, Kumar R, Melton III LJ. Long-term effects of calcium supplementation on serum parathyroid hormone level, bone turnover, and bone loss in elderly women. *J Bone Miner Res* 1998;**13**(2):168–74.

14 Chevalley T, Nydegger V, Slosman D, *et al.* Effects on calcium supplements on femoral bone mineral density and vertebral fracture rate in vitamin-D-replete elderly patients. *Osteoporos Int* 1994;**4**:245–52.

15 Gillespie WJ, Henry DA, O'Connell DL, Roberston J. Vitamin D and vitamin D analogues for preventing fractures associated with involutional and post-menopausal osteoporosis. In: Cochrane Collaboration. *Cochrane Library.* Issue 1. Oxford: Update Software, 1999:1–17.

16 Papadimitropoulos E, Wells G, Shea B, *et al.* Meta-analyses of therapies for postmenopausal osteoporosis. VIII: Meta-analysis of the efficacy of vitamin D treatment in preventing osteoporosis in postmenopausal women. *Endocrin Rev* 2002;**23**(4):560–9.

17 Chapuy MC, Arlot ME, Duboeuf F, *et al.* Vitamin D3 and calcium to prevent hip fractures in elderly women. *N Engl J Med* 1992;**327**:1637–42.

18 Pfeifer MB, Begerow B, Minne HW. Vitamin D and muscle function. *Osteoporos Int* 2002;**13**:187–94.

19 Dawson-Hughes B, Harris S, Krall E, Dallal GE. Effect of calcium and vitamin D supplementation on bone density in men and women 65 years of age or older. *N Engl J Med* 1997;**337**:670–6.

20 Cardona JM, Pastor E. Calcitonin versus etidronate for the treatment of postmenopausal osteoporosis: a meta-analysis of published clinical trials. *Osteoporos Int* 1997;**7**:165–74.

21 Cranney A, Guyatt G, Krolicki N, *et al.* A meta-analysis of etidronate for the treatment of postmenopausal osteoporosis. *Osteoporos Int* 2001;**12**(2):140–51.

22 Montessori ML, Scheele WH, Netelenbos JC, Kerkhoff JF, Bakker K. The use of etidronate and calcium versus calcium alone in the treatment of postmenopausal osteopenia: results of three years of treatment. *Osteoporos Int* 1997;**7**:52–8.

23 Pacifici R, McMurtry C, Vered I, Rupich R, Avioli LV. Coherence therapy does not prevent axial bone loss in osteoporotic women: a preliminary comparative study. *J Clin Endocrinol Metab* 1988;**66**:747–53.

24 Storm T, Thamsborg G, Steiniche T, Genant HK, Sorensen OH. Effect of intermittent cyclical etidronate therapy on bone mass and fracture rate in women with postmenopausal osteoporosis. *N Engl J Med* 1990;**322**:1265–71.

25 Lyritis GP, Tsakalakos N, Paspati I, Skarantavos GR, Galanos A, Androulakis C. The effect of a modified etidronate cyclical regimen on postmenopausal osteoporosis: a four-year study. *Clin Rheumatol* 1997;**16**:354–60.

26 Watts NB, Harris ST, Genant HK, *et al.* Intermittent cyclical etidronate treatment of postmenopausal osteoporosis. *N Engl J Med* 1990;**323**:73–9.

27 Herd RJ, Balena R, Blake GM, Ryan PJ, Fogelman I. The prevention of early postmenopausal bone loss by cyclical etidronate therapy: a 2-year, double-blind, placebo-controlled study. *Am J Med* 1997;**103**:92–9.

28 Pouilles JM, Tremollieres F, Roux C, *et al.* Effects of cyclical etidronate therapy on bone loss in early postmenopausal women who are not undergoing hormonal replacement therapy. *Osteoporos Int* 1997;**7**:213–18.

29 Jeal W, Barradell LB, McTavish D. Alendronate. A review of its pharmacological properties and therapeutic efficacy in postmenopausal osteoporosis. *Drugs* 1997;**53**:415–34.

30 Karpf DB, Shapiro DR, Seeman E, *et al.* Prevention of nonvertebral fractures by alendronate. A meta-analysis. Alendronate Osteoporosis Treatment Study Groups. *JAMA* 1997;**277**:1159–64.

31 Cranney A, Wells G, Willan A, *et al.* Meta-analyses of therapies for postmenopausal osteoporosis. II. Meta-analysis of alendronate for the treatment of postmenopausal women. *Endocrin Rev* 2002;**23**(4):508–16.

32 Black DM, Cummings SR, Karpf DB, *et al.* Randomised trial of effect of alendronate on risk of fracture in women with existing vertebral fractures. Fracture Intervention Trial Research Group. *Lancet* 1996;**348**:1535–41.

33 Cummings SR, Black DM, Thompson DE for the FIT group. Alendronate reduces the risk of vertebral fractures in women without pre-existing vertebral fractures: results of the fracture intervention trial. *J Bone Miner Res* 1998;**12**:S149.

34 Liberman UA, Weiss SR, Broll J, *et al.* Effect of oral alendronate on bone mineral density and the incidence of fractures in postmenopausal osteoporosis. The Alendronate Phase III Osteoporosis Treatment Study Group. *N Engl J Med* 1995;**333**:1437–43.

35 Bone HG, Downs RW, Jr., Tucci JR, *et al.* Dose–response relationships for alendronate treatment in osteoporotic elderly women. Alendronate Elderly Osteoporosis Study Centers. *J Clin Endocrinol Metabol* 1997;**82**:265–74.

36 McClung M, Clemmesen B, Daifotis A, *et al.* Alendronate prevents postmenopausal bone loss in women without osteoporosis. A double-blind, randomised, controlled trial. Alendronate Osteoporosis Prevention Study Group. *Ann Intern Med* 1998;**128**:253–61.

37 Hosking D, Chilvers CE, Christiansen C, *et al.* Prevention of bone loss with alendronate in postmenopausal women under 60 years of age. Early Postmenopausal Intervention Cohort Study Group. *N Engl J Med* 1998;**338**:485–92.

38 Adami S, Passeri M, Ortolani S, *et al.* Effects of oral alendronate and intranasal salmon calcitonin on bone mass and biochemical markers of bone turnover in postmenopausal women with osteoporosis. *Bone* 1995;**17**:383–90.

39 Chesnut CH, McClung MR, Ensrud KE, *et al.* Alendronate treatment of the postmenopausal osteoporotic woman: effect of multiple dosages on bone mass and bone remodeling. *Am J Med* 1995;**99**:144–52.

40 Pols HAP for the FOSIT group. A multinational placebo-controlled study of alendronate in postmenopausal women with osteoporosis – results from the FOSIT group. *J Bone Miner Res* 1997;**12**:S172.

41 Goa KL, Balfour JA. Residronate. *Drugs Aging* 1998;**13**:83–91.

42 Harris ST, Watts NB, Genant HK, *et al.* Effects of risedronate treatment on vertebral and nonvertebral fractures in women with postmenopausal osteoporosis – a randomised controlled trial. *JAMA* 1999;**282**(14):1344–52.

43 Reginster JY, Minne H, Sorensen O, *et al.* Randomised trial of the effects of risedronate on vertebral fractures in women with established postmenopausal osteoporosis. *Osteoporos Int* 2000;**1**:83–91.

44 Cranney A, Tugwell P, Adachi J, *et al.* Meta-analyses of therapies for postmenopausal osteoporosis. III. Meta-analysis of risedronate for the treatment of postmenopausal osteoporosis. *Endocr Rev* 2002;**23**(4):517–23.

45 Mortensen L, Charles P, Bekker PJ, Digennaro J, Johnston CC. Risedronate increases bone mass in an early postmenopausal population: two years of treatment plus one year of follow-up. *J Clin Endocrinol Metabol* 1998;**83**:396–402.

46 Clemmesen B, Ravn P, Zegels B, Taquet AN, Christiansen C, Reginster JY. A 2-year phase II study with 1-year of follow-up of risedronate (NE–58095) in postmenopausal osteoporosis. *Osteoporos Int* 1997;**7**:488–95.

47 Fogelman I, Ribot C, Smith R, Ethgen D, Sod E, Reginster JY. Risedronate reverses bone loss in postmenopausal women with low bone mass: results from a multinational, double-blind, placebo-controlled trial. *J Clin Endocrinol Metabol* 2000;**85**:1895–900.

48 McClung MR, Geusens P, Miller PD, *et al.* Effect of risedronate on the risk of hip fracture in elderly women. *N Engl J Med* 2001;**344**(5):333–40.

49 McClung M, Bensen W, Bolognese M, *et al.* Residronate increases bone mineral density at the hip, spine, and radius in postmenopausal women with low bone mass. *Osteoporos Int* 1998;**8**(3):111.

50 Grady D, Rubin SM, Petitti DB, *et al.* Hormone therapy to prevent disease and prolong life in postmenopausal women. *Ann Intern Med* 1992;**117**:1016–37.

51 Cauley JA, Black DM, Barrett-Connor E, *et al.* Effects of hormone replacement therapy on clinical fractures and height loss: The Heart and Estrogen/Progestin Replacement Study (HERS). *Am J Med* 2001;**110**:442–50.

52 Wells G, Tugwell P, Shea B, *et al.* V. Meta-analysis of the efficacy of hormone replacement therapy in treating and preventing osteoporosis in postmenopausal women. *Endocrin Rev* 2002;**23**(4):529–39.

53 Lufkin EG, Wahner HW, O'Fallon WM, *et al.* Treatment of postmenopausal osteoporosis with transdermal estrogen. *Ann Intern Med* 1992;**117**(1):1–9.

54 Greenspan S, Bankhurst A, Bell N, *et al.* Effects of alendronate and estrogen alone and in combination on bone mass and turnover in postmenopausal osteoporosis. *J Bone Miner Res* 1998;**S174**:Abstract.

55 Alexandersen P, Riis BJ, Christiansen C. Monofluro-phosphate combined with hormone replacement therapy induces a synergistic effect on bone mass by dissociating bone formation and resorption in post-menopausal women: a randomised study. *J Clin Endocrinol Metabol* 1999;**84**:3013–20.

56 Hulley S, Grady D, Bush T, *et al.* Randomised trial of estrogen plus progestin for secondary prevention of coronary heart disease in postmenopausal women. *JAMA* 1998;**280**:605–13.

57 Wimalawansa SJ. A four-year randomised controlled trial of hormone replacement and bisphosphonate, alone or in combination in women with postmenopausal osteoporosis. *Am J Med* 1998;**104**:219–26.

58 Komulainen M, Tuppurainen MT, Kroger H, *et al.* HRT and vitamin D in prevention of nonvertebral fractures in postmenopausal women: a 5-year randomised trial. *Maturitas* 1998;**31**(1):45–54.

59 Torgerson DJ, Bell-Syer SEM. Hormone replacement therapy and prevention of nonvertebral fractures. *JAMA* 2001;**285**(22):2891–7.

60 Writing Group for the Women's Health Initiative Investigators. Risks and benefits of estrogen plus progestin in healthy postmenopausal women. Principal results from the Women's Health Initiative randomised controlled trial. *JAMA* 2002;**288**:321–33.

61 Riggs BL, Hartmann LC. Selective estrogen-receptor modulators – mechanisms of action and application to clinical practice. *N Engl J Med* 2003;**348**:618–29.

62 Cranney A, Tugwell P, Zytaruk N, *et al.* Meta-analyses of therapies for postmenopausal osteoporosis. IV. Meta-analysis of raloxifene for the prevention and treatment of postmenopausal osteoporosis. *Endocr Rev* 2002;**23**(4):524–8.

63 Adachi JD. GGGH – A long-term comparison of raloxifene HCl, placebo, and premarin in the prevention of osteoporosis in postmenopausal, hysterectomised women. FDA, 2001.

64 Pavo I, Masanauskaite D, Rojinskaya L, *et al.* Effects of raloxifene versus placebo on bone mineral density in postmenopausal women in the absence of calcium supplementation. *J Bone Miner Res* 1999;**14**:S410.

65 Johnston CC. Long-term effects of raloxifene on bone mineral density, bone turnover, and serum lipid levels in early postmenopausal women: three-year data from 2 double-blind, randomised, placebo-controlled trials. *Arch Intern Med* 2000;**160**(22):3444–50.

66 Lufkin EG, Whitaker MD, Nickelesen T, *et al.* Treatment of established postmenopausal osteoporosis with raloxifene: a randomised trial. *J Bone Miner Res* 1998;**13**:1747–54.

67 Meunier PJ, Vignot E, Gernero P, *et al.* Treatment of postmenopausal women with osteoporosis or low bone density with raloxifene. *Osteoporos Int* 1999;**10**(4):330–6.

68 Johnell O, Scheele W, Lu Y, *et al.* Effects of raloxifene (RLX), alendronate (ALN and RLX + ALN on bone mineral density (BMD and biochemical markers bone turnover in postmenopausal women with osteoporosis. *J Bone Miner Res* 1999;**14**(S157).

69 Cranney A, Tugwell P, Zytaruk N, *et al.* Meta-analyses of therapies for postmenopausal osteoporosis. VI. Meta-analysis of calcitonin for the treatment of postmenopausal osteoporosis. *Endocrin Rev* 2002;**23**(4):540–51.

70 Hizmetli S, Elden H, Kaptanoglu E, Nacitarhan V, Kocagil S. The effect of different doses of calcitonin on bone mineral density and fracture risk in postmenopausal osteoporosis. *Int J Clin Pract* 1998;**52**(7):453–5.

71 Gennari C, Chierichetti SM, Bigassi. Comparative effects on bone mineral content of calcium plus salmon calcitonin given in two different regimens in postmenopausal osteoporosis. *Curr Ther Res* 1985;**38**:455–62.

72 Overgaard K, Hansen MA, Jenson SB, Christiansen J. Effect of salcatonin given intranasally on bone mass and fracture rates in established osteoporosis: a dose–response study. *Br Med J* 1992;**305**:556–61.

73 Chestnut CH, Silverman S, Andriano K, *et al.* A randomised trial of nasal spray salmon calcitonin in postmenopausal women with established osteoporosis: The prevent recurrence of osteoporotic fractures study. *Am J Med* 2000;**109**:267–76.

74 Thamsburg G, Jenson SB, Kollerup G, Hauge EM, Melsen F, Sorensen OH. Effect of nasal salmon calcitonin on bone remodeling and bone mass in postmenopausal osteoporosis. *Bone* 1996;**18**(2):207–12.

75 Perrone G, Galoppi, Valente M. Intranasal salmon calcitonin in postmenopausal osteoporosis: effect of different therapeutic regimens on vertebral and peripheral bone density. *Gynecol Obstet Invest* 1992;**33**:168–71.

76 Thamsburg G, Storm TL, Sykulski R, Brinch E, Nielson HK, Sorensen OH. Effect of different doses of nasal calcitonin on bone mass. *Calcified Tissue Int* 1991;**48**:302–7.

77 Ploskder GL, McTavish D. Intranasal salcatonin: a review of its pharmacological properties and role in the management of postmenopausal osteoporosis. *Drugs Aging* 2001;**8**:378–400.

78 Lyritis GP, Tsakalakos N, Magiasis B, Karachalios T, Tsekoura M. Analgesic effect of salmon calcitonin in osteoporotic vertebral fractures: A double blind placebo-controlled clinical study. *Calcified Tissue Int* 1991;**49**:369–72.

79 Crandall C. Parathyroid hormone for treatment of osteoporosis. *Arch Intern Med* 2002;**162**:2297–309.

80 Rosen CJ, Bilezikian JP. Anabolic therapy for osteoporosis. *J Clin Endocrinol Metabol* 2001;**86**:957–64.

81 Rittmaster RS, Bolognese M, Ettinger MP, *et al.* Enhancement of bone mass in osteoporotic women with parathyroid hormone followed by alendronate. *J Clin Endocrinol Metabol* 2000;**85**(6):2129–34.

82 Neer RM, Arnaud CD, Aznchetta JR, *et al.* Effect of parathyroid hormone (1–34) on fractures and bone mineral density in postmenopausal women with osteoporosis. *N Engl J Med* 2001;**344**:1434–41.

83 Parkkari J, Kannus P, Heikkila J, Poutala J, Sievanen H, Vuori I. Energy-shunting external hip protector attenuates the peak femoral impact force below the theoretical fracture threshold: an in vitro biomechanical study under falling conditions of the elderly. *J Bone Miner Res* 1995;**10**(10):1437–42.

84 Parker MJ, Gillespie LD, Gillespie WJ. Hip protectors for preventing hip fractures in the elderly (Cochrane Review).In: Cochrane Collaboration. Cochrane Database of Systematic Reviews (computer file)(4):CD001255 2000.

85 Waldegger L, Cranney A, Man-Son-Hing M, Coyle D. Cost-effectiveness of hip protectors in institutional dwelling elderly. *Osteoporos Int* 2003;**14**(3):243–50.

86 Lauritzen JB, Petersen MM, Lund B. Effect of external hip protectors on hip fractures. *Lancet* 1993;**341**(8836): 11–13.

87 Chan DK, Hillier G, Coore M, *et al.* Effectiveness and acceptability of a newly designed hip protector: a pilot study. *Arch Gerontol Geriatr* 2000;**30**(12):25–34.

88 Harada A, Okuizumi H. Hip fracture prevention trial using hip protector in Japanese elderly. *Osteoporos Int* 1998;**8**(Suppl 3):121 Abstract.

89 Kannus P, Parkkari J, Niemi S, *et al.* Prevention of hip fracture in elderly people with use of a hip protector. *N Engl J Med* 2000;**343**(21):1506–13.

90 Ekman A, Mallmin H, Michaelsson K, Ljunghall S. External hip protectors to prevent osteoporotic hip fractures. *Lancet* 1997;**350**(9077):563–4.

91 Meyer G, Warnke A, Bender R, Mulhauser I. Effect on hip fractures of increased use of hip protectors in nursing homes: cluster randomised controlled trial. *BMJ* 2003;**326**:76–80.

92 Van Schoor NM, Smit JH, Twisk JWR, Bouter LM, Lips P. Prevention of hip fractures by external hip portectors, a randomised controlled trial. *JAMA* 2003;**289**(15):1957–62.

Osteoporosis
Summaries and decision aids

Osteoporosis and etidronate
Summaries and decision aid

How well does etidronate work to treat and prevent osteoporosis in women after menopause?

To answer this question, scientists found and analysed 13 high quality studies (from a Cochrane Systematic Review). These studies tested over 1000 women after menopause who received a placebo (sugar pill) or received 400 mg of etidronate for 14 to 20 days followed by calcium supplements with or without vitamin D, in a cycle about every 3 months. These studies provide the best evidence we have today.

What is osteoporosis and how can etidronate help?

Osteoporosis is a condition of weak, brittle bones that break easily. In osteoporosis, breaks or fractures of the spine and hip or wrist (non-spinal fractures) may occur and often without a fall. Etidronate is a bisphosphonate – a drug that is often prescribed to women after menopause to decrease fractures (or breaks) by slowing the loss of bone. There is some debate about whether etidronate decreases all types of fractures, such as hip and non-spinal fractures.

How well did etidronate decrease fractures and increase bone density?

After 2 years, fewer women after menopause have spine fractures when receiving etidronate than a placebo but there was no difference in the number of women with hip and non-spinal (wrist, forearm, etc.) fractures. This was true for women who have osteoporosis.

Over 3 to 4 years, bone mineral density in the spine, hip, and total body increased more in all women after menopause who received etidronate than in women who received placebo. The greatest increases were seen at 4 years but there were not many people tested at 4 years.

Were there any side effects?

Side effects such as heartburn, diarrhoea and leg cramps may occur. However, the number of people who stopped taking etidronate due to side effects was about equal to the number of people who stopped taking a placebo (sugar pill).

What is the bottom line?

There is "Silver" level evidence that in women after menopause with osteoporosis, etidronate at 400 mg daily for 14 days followed by calcium with or without vitamin D taken in a cycle every 3 months over 2 years prevents or decreases spine fractures but not hip or non-spinal fractures.

After 3 years, etidronate increases bone density in the lower spine and hip.

Most women do not appear to have side effects that would cause them to stop taking etidronate.

From Cranney A, Simon LS, Tugwell P, Adachi R, Ottawa Methods Group. Osteoporosis. In: *Evidence-based Rheumatology.* London: BMJ Books, 2003.

How well does etidronate work to treat and prevent osteoporosis in women after menopause?

What is osteoporosis and how can etidronate help?

Osteoporosis is a condition of weak, brittle bones that break easily. In osteoporosis, breaks or fractures of the spine and hip, wrist or forearm (non-spinal fractures) may occur and often without a fall. Osteoporosis is detected using a bone density test that measures the amount of bone loss. A result that is at least 2·5 "standard deviations" below normal confirms the diagnosis. This means people have lost at least 25 per cent of their bone mass or density. Drugs have been developed to slow the bone loss.

Etidronate is a bisphosphonate drug and an "antiresorptive agent" that was developed for women after menopause (postmenopausal women) to decrease fractures. Etidronate works to slow bone loss or "resorption" and is provided every 3 months followed by calcium because it may stop bones from building and it may cause osteomalacia (soft bones). There is some debate about whether etidronate decreases all types of fractures, such as hip and non-spinal fractures.

How did the scientists find the information and analyse it?

To find out just how well etidronate works, the scientists searched for studies testing etidronate. Unfortunately, not all studies found were of a high quality and so only those studies that met high standards were examined.

- Studies had to be randomised controlled trials – where postmenopausal women receiving etidronate were compared to postmenopausal women receiving a placebo (a sugar pill) for at least one year.
- Studies had to show how well etidronate works by measuring bone mineral density (BMD) and the number of fractures (or breaks), as well as indicate side effects.

Which high quality studies were included in the summary?

Thirteen high quality studies were examined (available in a Cochrane Systematic Review). The studies included 1267 postmenopausal women who received 400 mg of etidronate for 14 to 20 days followed by calcium supplements with or without vitamin D, in a cycle about every 3 months. Eight studies provided etidronate to women with normal to near normal bone density to prevent bone loss and fractures and 5 studies provided etidronate to women who already had bone losses (low bone mineral density – BMD).

How well did etidronate decrease fractures and increase bone density?

Spine fractures: Fewer postmenopausal women have spine fractures over a lifetime when receiving etidronate than no treatment or a placebo:

- 6 out of 100 women receiving etidronate have a spine fracture
- 10 out of 100 women receiving no treatment or a placebo (sugar pill) have a spine fracture.

This means that 4 more women out of 100 benefited from taking etidronate than a placebo

Hip and non-spinal fractures: The number of postmenopausal women who had hip and non-spinal fractures (wrist, etc.) when receiving etidronate was about equal to the number receiving a placebo:

- 11 out of 100 women receiving etidronate had non-spinal fractures
- 12 out 100 women receiving a placebo (or sugar pill) had non-spinal fractures.

Specifically, the number of women taking etidronate who had a hip fracture was about equal to the number of women taking a placebo (2 compared to 1 woman).

Bone mineral density (BMD): Bone mineral density was measured in the lower spine, hip, total body, and forearm.

Over 3 to 4 years, all measurements of bone mineral density increased more in postmenopausal women who received etidronate than in women who received placebo. The increase was substantial in the lower spine, hip and total body but smaller in the forearm.

The increases in bone mineral density were greatest at 4 years but the number of patients tested at 4 years was small.

Were there any side effects?

Side effects such as heartburn, diarrheoa and leg cramps may occur.

After 2 to 4years, the number of women who stopped taking etidronate due to side effects was about equal to the number of women who stopped taking a placebo (3 compared to 2).

What did the scientists conclude about etidronate?

There is "Silver" level evidence that in women after menopause with osteoporosis, etidronate at 400 mg daily for 14 days followed by calcium with or without vitamin D taken in a cycle every 3 months over 2 years, prevents or decreases spine fractures but not non-spinal fractures.

After 3 years, etidronate increases bone density in the lower spine and hip.

Most women do not appear to have side effects that would cause them to stop taking etidronate.

From Cranney A, Simon LS, Tugwell P, Adachi R, Ottawa Methods Group. Osteoporosis. In *Evidence-based Rheumatology.* London: BMJ Books, 2003.

Information about osteoporosis and treatment

What is osteoporosis?

Osteoporosis is a condition of weak, brittle bones that break easily. The most common breaks or fractures are in the spine, hip, or wrist and these may occur without a fall. Osteoporosis is detected using a bone density test that measures the amount of bone loss. A result that is at least 2·5 "standard deviations" below normal confirms the diagnosis. This means people have lost at least 25 per cent of their bone mass or density.

Hip fractures can cause severe disability or death.

- Among 100 women with normal bone density, about **15** may break a hip in their lifetime.
- Among 100 women with low bone density, about **35 to 75** may break a hip in their lifetime.

This number depends on *amount of bone loss*, *age*, and other risk factors, such as:

- *major bone-related risks:* previous broken bones since age 50 (not from trauma); family history of fracture (e.g. mother who broke a hip, wrist, spine)
- *major fall-related risks:* poor health; unable to rise from a chair without help; use of sleeping pills.

Spine fractures are more common, disabling, and painful. They can cause stooped posture and loss of height of up to 6 inches.

To find out your personal risk of broken bones, ask your doctor.

What can I do on my own to manage my disease?

✓ Calcium and vitamin D ✓ Regular impact exercises (e.g. walking)

What treatments are used for osteoporosis?

Three kinds of treatment may be used alone or together. The common (generic) names of treatment are shown below.

1. *Bone-specific drugs*
   - Alendronate
   - Calcitonin
   - Etidronate
   - Risedronate
2. *Hormones that affect bones and other organs*
   - Parathyroid hormone
   - Raloxifene
   - Hormone replacement therapy (oestrogen and progestin)
3. *Other*
   - Hip protector pads

What about other treatments I have heard about?

There is not enough evidence about the effects of some treatments. Other treatments do not work. For example:

- Calcitonin for non-spinal fractures
- Etidronate for non-spinal fractures
- Raloxifene for non-spinal fractures

What are my choices? How can I decide?

Treatment for your disease will depend on your condition. You need to know the good points (pros) and bad points (cons) about each treatment before you can decide.

Osteoporosis decision aid

Should I take etidronate?

This guide can help you make decisions about the treatment your doctor is asking you to consider.

It will help you to:

1. Clarify what you need to decide.
2. Consider the pros and cons of different choices.
3. Decide what role you want to have in choosing your treatment.
4. Identify what you need to help you make the decision.
5. Plan the next steps.
6. Share your thinking with your doctor.

Step 1: Clarify what you need to decide

What is the decision?

Should I take etidronate to slow bone loss or prevent breaks?

Etidronate may be taken as a pill daily for 2 weeks and followed by 3 months of calcium pills taken daily.

When does this decision have to be made? Check ✓ one

☐ within days ☐ within weeks ☐ within months

How far along are you with this decision? Check ✓ one

☐ I have not thought about it yet

☐ I am considering the choices

☐ I am close to making a choice

☐ I have already made a choice

Step 2: Consider the pros and cons of different choices

What does the research show?

Etidronate is classified as: **Likely beneficial**

There is "Silver" level evidence from 13 studies (available in a Cochrane Systematic Review) of 1267 women after menopause testing etidronate. The studies lasted up to 4 years. The women had osteoporosis (low bone density) or normal to near normal bone density. These studies found pros and cons that are listed in the chart below.

What do I think of the pros and cons of etidronate?

1. Review the common pros and cons that are shown below.
2. Add any other pros and cons that are important to you.
3. Show how important each pro and con is to you by circling from one (*) star if it is a little important to you, to up to five (*****) stars if it is very important to you.

PROS AND CONS OF ETIDRONATE TREATMENT

PROS (number of people affected)	How important is it to you?	CONS (number of people affected)	How important is it to you?
Fewer broken bones in the spine 4 less women out of 100 have a spine fracture over their lifetime with etidronate	* * * * *	May not decrease broken bones in the hip or wrist	* * * * *
Increases bone density	* * * * *	Side effects: heartburn, stomach irritation, diarrhoea, leg cramps	* * * * *
Cyclical 3 month schedule 2 weeks of etidronate then 3 months of a calcium supplement	* * * * *	Must take 2 hours before or after a meal	* * * * *
Flexible dosing and no need to stand or sit for 1 hour afterwards May be taken mid-morning, afternoon or evening	* * * * *	Personal cost of medicine	* * * * *
Other pros:	* * * * *	Other cons:	* * * * *

What do you think of taking etidronate? Check ✓ one

☐	☐	☐
Willing to consider this treatment Pros are more important to me than the Cons	Unsure	Not willing to consider this treatment Cons are more important to me than the Pros

Step 3: Choose the role you want to have in choosing your treatment Check ✓ one

☐ I prefer to decide on my own after listening to the opinions of others

☐ I prefer to share the decision with: ____________________

☐ I prefer someone else to decide for me, namely: ____________

Step 4: Identify what you need to help you make the decision

What I know	Do you know enough about your condition to make a choice?	☐ Yes	☐ No	☐ Unsure
	Do you know which options are available to you?	☐ Yes	☐ No	☐ Unsure
	Do you know the good points (pros) of each option?	☐ Yes	☐ No	☐ Unsure
	Do you know the bad points (cons) of each option?	☐ Yes	☐ No	☐ Unsure
What's important	Are you clear about which **pros** are most *important to you?*	☐ Yes	☐ No	☐ Unsure
	Are you clear about which **cons** are most *important to you?*	☐ Yes	☐ No	☐ Unsure
How others help	Do you have enough support from others to make a choice?	☐ Yes	☐ No	☐ Unsure
	Are you choosing without pressure from others?	☐ Yes	☐ No	☐ Unsure
	Do you have enough advice to make a choice?	☐ Yes	☐ No	☐ Unsure
How sure I feel	Are you clear about the best choice for you?	☐ Yes	☐ No	☐ Unsure
	Do you feel sure about what to choose?	☐ Yes	☐ No	☐ Unsure

If you answered No or Unsure to many of these questions, you should talk to your doctor.

Step 5: Plan the next steps

What do you need to do before you make this decision?

For example: talk to your doctor, read more about this treatment or other treatments for osteoporosis.

Step 6: Share the information on this form with your doctor

It will help your doctor understand what you think about this treatment.

Osteoporosis and alendronate
Summaries and decision aid

How well does alendronate (Fosamax) work to treat and prevent osteoporosis in women after menopause?

To answer this question, scientists found and analysed 11 studies testing alendronate in over 12 500 women after menopause. Women received 5 to 40 mg of alendronate as a pill daily for 1 to 4 years. These studies provide the best evidence we have today.

What is osteoporosis and how can alendronate help?

Osteoporosis is a condition of weak brittle bones that break easily. Breaks or fractures of the spine and hip or wrist (non-spinal fractures) may occur and often without a fall. Alendronate is a bisphosphonate and "antiresorptive agent" used to decrease fractures by slowing bone loss. There is some debate about whether alendronate decreases fractures, in women with normal or near normal bone density.

How well did alendronate decrease fractures and increase bone density?

In women after menopause who have osteoporosis, alendronate decreased the number of **spine** fractures more than a placebo or sugar pill. 10 to 40 mg of alendronate daily decreased the number of **non-spinal fractures** (such as wrist and hip) more than a placebo or sugar pill in women with osteoporosis, but not in women who have normal to near normal bone density.

Bone mineral density increased in the spine, hip and somewhat in the forearm.

Were there any side effects?

Heartburn or ulcers in the oesophagus or gullet may occur. But the number of women who stopped taking alendronate due to side effects was no different than the number of women who stopped taking a placebo.

What is the bottom line?

There is "Platinum" level evidence that women after menopause with osteoporosis, have fewer spine fractures when taking alendronate at 5 to 40 mg daily for 2 to 3 years. Women after menopause with osteoporosis have fewer hip and non-spinal fractures with 10 to 40 mg of alendronate for 2 to 3 years.

Alendronate for 2 to 3 years, increases bone mineral density.

Side effects such as heartburn or ulcers in the oesophagus or gullet may occur.

From Cranney A, Simon LS, Tugwell P, Adachi R, Ottawa Methods Group. Osteoporosis. In: *Evidence-based Rheumatology*. London: BMJ Books, 2003.

How well does alendronate (Fosamax) work to treat and prevent osteoporosis in women after menopause?

What is osteoporosis and how can alendronate help?

Osteoporosis is a condition of weak brittle bones that break easily. In osteoporosis, breaks or fractures of the spine and hip, wrist or forearm (non-spinal fractures) may occur and often without a fall. Osteoporosis is detected using a bone density test that measures the amount of bone loss. A result that is at least 2·5 "standard deviations" below normal confirms the diagnosis. This means people have lost at least 25 per cent of their bone mass or density. Drugs have been developed to slow the bone loss.

Alendronate is a bisphosphonate drug and an "antiresorptive agent" that was developed for women after menopause to decrease fractures. Alendronate works by slowing bone loss or "resorption" and does not interfere with bone building or mineralisation. There is some debate about whether alendronate increases bone density in women after menopause who have normal to near normal bone density or who already have bone loss (as in osteoporosis) and whether it decrease all types of fractures, such as spine and non-spinal fractures.

How did the scientists find the information and analyse it?

To find out just how well alendronate works, the scientists searched for studies testing alendronate. Unfortunately, not all studies found were of a high quality and so only those studies that met high standards were examined in this summary.

- Studies had to be randomised controlled trials – where a group of women after menopause (post menopausal) received alendronate and was compared to postmenopausal women who received a placebo (or sugar pill) for at least one year.
- Studies had to show how well alendronate works by measuring bone mineral density (BMD) and the number of fractures (or breaks).

Which high quality studies were examined in the summary?

Eleven high quality studies were examined. The studies included 12 855 women after menopause (postmenopausal women) receiving 5 to 40 mg of alendronate daily for 1 to 4 years. Two studies provided alendronate to women with normal to near normal bone density to prevent bone loss and fractures and 9 studies provided alendronate to women who already had bone losses (or low bone mineral density – BMD). Some studies included women who already had a spine fracture.

How well did alendronate decrease fractures and increase bone density?

Spine fractures: Over a lifetime, in women who have normal to near normal bone density or osteoporosis:

- 5 out of 100 women receiving 5 to 40 mg of alendronate daily will have a spine fracture
- 10 out of 100 women receiving no treatment or a placebo (sugar pill) will have a spine fracture.

This means that 5 out of 100 more women benefit from taking alendronate than a placebo.

Hip and non-spinal fractures (wrist, etc.): Over a lifetime, in women who have **osteoporosis**:

- 21 out of 100 women receiving 10 to 40 mg of alendronate daily will have a hip fracture or other non-spinal fracture
- 42 out of 100 women receiving no treatment or a placebo (sugar pill) will have a hip fracture or other non-spinal fracture.

This means that 21 out of 100 more women benefited from taking alendronate than a placebo.

In women who have **normal to near normal** bone density:

- the benefit of taking alendronate to prevent hip fracture or other non-spinal fractures is still in question since most of these women are at a lower risk of having a fracture.

The number of women taking 10 to 40 mg of alendronate daily over 2 to 3 years who will have a hip fracture is no different than the number of women taking a placebo (2 out of 100 compared to 4 out of 100 women). These numbers may also be due to chance and not to treatment with alendronate.

Bone mineral density (BMD): Bone mineral density increased in the lower spine and in the hip in **postmenopausal women** who had normal to near normal bone density and in women with osteoporosis who received 5 to 40 mg of alendronate. The increase in the bone density of the forearm was also increased but not as much as in the lower spine and hip.

Despite the fact that bone density increased after each year, the amount of the increase was less after each year.

Were there any side effects?

Side effects such as heartburn or ulcers in the oesophagus (or gullet) may occur. But the number of women who stopped taking alendronate due to side effects was no different than the number of women who stopped taking a placebo.

In the biggest study, 7 out of 100 women taking 5 to 40 mg of alendronate and 6 out of 100 women taking a placebo stopped their medication.

It will be long before we can assess the rare and late side effects of alendronate.

What is the bottom line?

There is "Platinum" level of evidence that women after menopause with normal to near normal bone density or osteoporosis, have fewer spine fractures when taking alendronate at 5 to 40 mg daily for 2 to 3 years.

Women after menopause with osteoporosis have fewer hip fractures and other non-spinal fractures with 10 to 40 mg of alendronate for 2 to 3 years. It is unclear whether women with normal or near normal bone density have fewer non-spinal fractures with alendronate.

Alendronate, at 10 to 40 mg daily for 2 to 3 years, increases bone mineral density in women after menopause with normal to near normal bone density or osteoporosis. This effect appeared to increase with larger doses of alendronate over longer periods of treatment.

Side effects such as heartburn or ulcers in the oesophagus (or gullet) may occur . However after 2 to 3 years of taking the pills, women after menopause do not appear to experience side effects that would cause them to stop taking alendronate. It is not certain yet what are the rare side effects of alendronate.

From Cranney A, Simon LS, Tugwell P, Adachi R, Ottawa Methods Group. Osteoporosis. In: *Evidence-based Rheumatology.* London: BMJ Books, 2003.

Information about osteoporosis and treatment

What is osteoporosis?

Osteoporosis is a condition of weak brittle bones that break easily. The most common breaks or fractures are in the spine, hip, or wrist and these may occur without a fall. Osteoporosis is detected using a bone density test that measures the amount of bone loss. A result that is at least 2·5 "standard deviations" below normal confirms the diagnosis. This means people have lost at least 25 per cent of their bone mass or density.

Hip fractures can cause severe disability or death.

- Among 100 women with normal bone density, about **15** may break a hip in their lifetime.
- Among 100 women with low bone density, about **35 to 75** may break a hip in their lifetime.

This number depends on amount of bone loss, age, and other risk factors, such as:

- *major bone-related risks:* previous broken bones since age 50 (not from trauma); family history of fracture (e.g. mother who broke a hip, wrist, spine)
- *major fall-related risks:* poor health; unable to rise from a chair without help; use of sleeping pills.

Spine fractures are more common, disabling, and painful. They can cause stooped posture and loss of height of up to 6 inches.

To find out your personal risk of broken bones, ask your doctor.

What can I do on my own to manage my disease?

✓ Calcium and vitamin D

✓ Regular impact exercises (e.g. walking)

What treatments are used for osteoporosis?

Three kinds of treatment may be used alone or together. The common (generic) names of treatment are shown below.

1. *Bone-specific drugs*
   - Alendronate
   - Calcitonin
   - Etidronate
   - Risedronate
2. *Hormones that affect bones and other organs*
   - Parathyroid hormone
   - Raloxifene
   - Hormone replacement therapy (oestrogen and progestin)
3. *Other*
   - Hip protector pads

What about other treatments I have heard about?

There is not enough evidence about the effects of some treatments. Other treatments do not work. For example:

- Calcitonin non-spinal fractures
- Etidronate for non-spinal fractures
- Raloxifene for non-spinal fractures

What are my choices? How can I decide?

Treatment for your disease will depend on your condition. You need to know the good points (pros) and bad points (cons) about each treatment before you can decide.

Osteoporosis decision aid

Should I take alendronate?

This guide can help you make decisions about the treatment your doctor is asking you to consider.

It will help you to:

1. Clarify what you need to decide.
2. Consider the pros and cons of different choices.
3. Decide what role you want to have in choosing your treatment.
4. Identify what you need to help you make the decision.
5. Plan the next steps.
6. Share your thinking with your doctor.

Step 1: Clarify what you need to decide

What is the decision?

Should I take alendronate to slow bone loss or prevent breaks?

Alendronate may be taken as a pill daily or once a week.

When does this decision have to be made? Check ✓ one

☐ within days ☐ within weeks ☐ within months

How far along are you with this decision? Check ✓ one

☐ I have not thought about it yet

☐ I am considering the choices

☐ I am close to making a choice

☐ I have already made a choice

Step 2: Consider the pros and cons of different choices

What does the research show?

Alendronate is classified as: **Beneficial**

There is "Platinum" level evidence from 11 studies of 12 855 women after menopause that tested alendronate and lasted up to 4 years. The women had osteoporosis (low bone density) or normal to near normal bone density. These studies found pros and cons that are listed in the chart below.

What do I think of the pros and cons of alendronate?

1. Review the common pros and cons that are shown below.
2. Add any other pros and cons that are important to you.
3. Show how important each pro and con is to you by circling from one (*) star if it is a little important to you, to up to five (*****) stars if it is very important to you.

PROS AND CONS OF ALENDRONATE TREATMENT

PROS (number of people affected)	How important is it to you?	CONS (number of people affected)	How important is it to you?
Fewer broken bones in the spine 5 less women out of 100 have breaks in their spine over a lifetime with alendronate	* * * * *	Side effects: heartburn, **stomach irritation**	* * * * *
Fewer broken bones in the hip or wrist 21 less women out of 100 with **osteoporosis** have breaks in their hip or wrist over a lifetime	* * * * *	Increases chance of developing ulcers in the oesophagus or gullet	* * * * *
Increases bone density	* * * * *	Must be taken in morning 1 hour before eating and sit or stand after taking the pill	* * * * *
Flexible dosing may be taken once a week	* * * * *	**Personal cost of medicine**	* * * * *
Other pros	* * * * *	Other cons	* * * * *

What do you think about taking alendronate? Check ✓ one

☐ Willing to consider this treatment
Pros are more important to me than the Cons

☐ Unsure

☐ Not willing to consider this treatment
Cons are more important to me than the Pros

Step 3: Choose the role you want to have in choosing your treatment Check ✓ one

☐ I prefer to decide on my own after listening to the opinions of others

☐ I prefer to share the decision with: ______________________

☐ I prefer someone else to decide for me, namely: ______________

Step 4: Identify what you need to help you make the decision

What I know	Do you know enough about your condition to make a choice?	☐ Yes	☐ No	☐ Unsure
	Do you know which options are available to you?	☐ Yes	☐ No	☐ Unsure
	Do you know the good points (pros) of each option?	☐ Yes	☐ No	☐ Unsure
	Do you know the bad points (cons) of each option?	☐ Yes	☐ No	☐ Unsure
What's important	Are you clear about which **pros** are most *important to you?*	☐ Yes	☐ No	☐ Unsure
	Are you clear about which **cons** are most *important to you?*	☐ Yes	☐ No	☐ Unsure
How others help	Do you have enough support from others to make a choice?	☐ Yes	☐ No	☐ Unsure
	Are you choosing without pressure from others?	☐ Yes	☐ No	☐ Unsure
	Do you have enough advice to make a choice?	☐ Yes	☐ No	☐ Unsure
How sure I feel	Are you clear about the best choice for you?	☐ Yes	☐ No	☐ Unsure
	Do you feel sure about what to choose?	☐ Yes	☐ No	☐ Unsure

If you answered No or Unsure to many of these questions, you should talk to your doctor.

Step 5: Plan the next steps

What do you need to do before you make this decision?

For example: talk to your doctor, read more about this treatment or other treatments for osteoporosis.

Step 6: Share the information on this form with your doctor

It will help your doctor understand what you think about this treatment.

Osteoporosis and hormone replacement therapy (HRT) Summaries and decision aid

How well does hormone replacement therapy (HRT) work to treat and prevent osteoporosis in women after menopause?

To answer this question, scientists found and analysed 2 reviews of the literature and 1 large study (Women's Health Initiative study) testing HRT in over 25 000 women after menopause. Women received HRT, placebo or vitamin D and calcium. These studies provide the best evidence today.

What is osteoporosis and how can HRT help?

Osteoporosis is a condition of weak brittle bones that break easily. In osteoporosis, breaks or fractures of the spine and hip, wrist or forearm (non-spinal fractures) may occur and often without a fall. After menopause, women make less sex hormones, such as oestrogen and progestin, that help keep bones strong. HRT provides extra oestrogen and/or progestin to the body to slow down bone loss.

How well did HRT decrease fractures and increase bone density?

One review and the Women's Health Initiative study showed that the chances of having **spine fractures** are less when taking HRT than when taking a placebo or calcium and vitamin D. Two reviews and the Women's Health Initiative study showed that the chances of having **non-spinal fractures (wrist, hip, etc.)** are less when taking HRT than when taking a placebo.

Bone mineral density increased about the same in the spine, forearm and hip when taking HRT for 2 years.

Were there any side effects?

Side effects such as depression, headaches, breast tenderness, premenstrual syndrome, skin irritation, and weight gain can occur with HRT. The Women's Health Initiative study showed that HRT may increase the chances of developing breast cancer, heart disease, stroke, and blood clots, but decrease the chances of developing colorectal cancer (bowel cancer).

What is the bottom line?

There is "Gold" level evidence that hormone replacement therapy increases bone density more than a placebo or no treatment in the lower spine, forearm, and hip. Hormone replacement therapy also decreases the chances of spine fractures and non-spinal fractures.

Hormone replacement therapy may increase the chances of developing breast cancer, heart disease, stroke, and blood clots but decreases the chances of bowel cancer. But taking hormone replacement therapy for a short period of time may be helpful to decrease symptoms of menopause and decrease the risk of fractures.

From Cranney A, Simon LS, Tugwell P, Adachi R, Ottawa Methods Group. Osteoporosis. In: *Evidence-based Rheumatology.* London: BMJ Books, 2003.

How well does hormone replacement therapy (HRT) work to treat and prevent osteoporosis in women after menopause?

What is osteoporosis and how can hormone replacement therapy help?

Osteoporosis is a condition of weak, brittle bones that break easily. In osteoporosis, breaks or fractures of the spine and hip, wrist or forearm (non-spinal fractures) may occur and often withour a fall. Osteoporosis is detected using a bone density test that measures the amount of bone loss. A result that is a least 2·5 "standard deviations" below normal confirms the diagnosis. This means people have lost at least 25 per cent of their bone mass or density. Treatments have been developed to slow the bone loss and try to promote bone building.

After menopause, women make less sex hormones, such as oestrogen and progestin, that help keep bones strong. Hormone replacement therapy provides extra oestrogen and/or progestin to the body to slow down bone loss.

How did the scientists find the information and analyse it?

To find out just how well hormone replacement therapy works, the scientists searched for studies testing hormone replacement therapy. Unfortunately, not all studies found were of a high quality and so only those studies that met high standards were examined in this summary.

- Studies had to be randomised controlled trials – where a group of women after menopause (postmenopausal) received hormone replacement therapy and was compared to postmenopausal women who received a placebo (or sugar pill) or calcium and vitamin D, for at least one year.
- Studies had to show how well hormone replacement therapy works by measuring bone mineral density (BMD) and the number of fractures (or breaks).

Which high quality studies were examined in the summary?

Two reviews and 1 additional study were included in this summary.

- One review of the medical literature examined 57 high quality studies. The studies included over 9900 women after menopause (postmenopausal women) receiving different types of hormone replacement therapy including oestrogen and/or progestin for, on average, 1 to 2 years. Forty-seven studies provided hormone replacement therapy to women with normal to near normal bone density to prevent bone loss and fractures and 10 studies provided hormone replacement therapy to treat women who already had bone losses (or low bone mineral density – BMD).
- Another review examined 22 studies.
- The additional study called the Women's Health Initative was just recently completed and tested one type of hormone replacement therapy in over 16 600 postmenopausal women.

How well did hormone replacement therapy decrease fractures and increase bone density?

Spline fractures: Results from five studies in the first review that tested over 3000 women and the additional recent Women's Health Initiative study showed that the chances of having spine fractures over a lifetime are less when taking hormone replacement therapy than when taking a placebo or calcium and vitamin D:

- 7 out of 100 women receiving hormone replacement therapy will have a spine fracture over their lifetime
- 10 out of 100 women receiving no treatment or a placebo (sugar pill) will have a spine fracture over their lifetime.

This means that 3 out of 100 more women benefited from taking hormone replacement than a placebo

Hip and non-spinal fractures (wrist, etc.): Results from six studies in the first review that tested 3986 women combined with the Women's Health Initiative study, and results from another review showed that the chances of having non-spinal fractures over a lifetime are less when taking hormone replacement therapy than when taking no treatment or a placebo:

- 33 out of 100 women receiving hormone replacement therapy will have a non-spinal fracture over their lifetime
- 42 out of 100 women receiving no treatment or a placebo (sugar pill) will have a non-spinal fracture over their lifetime.

This means that 9 out of 100 more women benefited from taking hormone replacement therapy than a placebo

For hip fractures specifically, the Women's Health Initiative study showed that the chances of having a hip fracture over a lifetime are less when taking hormone replacement therapy than when taking a placebo:

- 11 out of 100 women receiving hormone replacement therapy will have a hip fracture over their lifetime
- 17 out of 100 women reveiving no treatment orn placebo (sugar pill) will have a spine fracture over their lifetime.

This means that 8 out of 100 women benefited from taking hormone replacement therapy than a placebo

Bone mineral density (BMD): Bone mineral density increased by about the same amount in the lower spine, forearm, and hip when taking hormone replacement therapy after 2 years. This increase in bone density was larger with higher doses of hormone replacement therapy.

Were there any side effects?

Side effects such as depression, headaches, breast tenderness, premenstrual syndrome, sking irritation, and weigh gain can occur with hormone replacement therapy.

The Women's Health Initiative study showed that hormone replacement therapy may increase the chances of developing breast cancer, heart disease, stroke, and blood clots.

Breast cancer:

- 20 out of 1000 women with hormone replacement therapy developed breast cancer:
- 15 out of 1000 women with a placebo or sugar pill developed breaset cancer.

Heart disease:

- 19 out of 1000 women developed heart disease with hormone replacement therapy
- 15 out of 1000 women developed heart disease with a placebo or sugar pill.

Stroke:

- 15 out of 1000 women had a stroke with hormone replacement therapy
- 10 out of 1000 women had a stoke with a placebo or sugar pill.

Blood clots:

- 18 out of 1000 women had blood clots with hormone replacement therapy
- 8 out of 1000 women had blood clots with a placebo or sugar pill.

But the Women's health Initiative study showed that hormone replacement therapy may decrease the chances of developing colorectal cancer (cancer of the bowels).

Bowel cancer:

- 5 out of 1000 women had cancer of the bowels with a hormone replacement therapy
- 8 out of 1000 women had cancer of the bowels with a placebo or sugar pill.

What is the bottom line?

There is "Gold" level evidence that hormone replacement therapy increases bone density more than a placebo or no treatment in the lower spine, forearm and hip.

There is "Gold" level evidence that hormone replacement therapy also decreases the chances of spine fractures and hip fracture and other non-spinal fractures.

Hormone replacement therapy increases the chances of developing breast cancer, heart disease, stroke, and blood clots but decreases the chances of bowel cancer.

The cons outweigh the pros of hormone replacement therapy in the long term. But taking hormone replacement therapy for a short period of time may be helpful to decrease symptoms of menopause and decrease the risk of fractures.

From Cranney A, Simon LS, Tugwell P, Adachi R, Ottawa Methods Group. Osteoporosis. In: *Evidence-based Rheumatology.* London: BMJ Books, 2003.

Information about osteoporosis and treatment

What is osteoporosis?

Osteoporosis is a condition of weak, brittle bones that break easily. The most common breaks or fractures are in the spine, hip, wrist or forearm, and these may occur without a fall. Osteoporosis is detected using a bone density test that measures the amount of bone loss. A result that is at least 2·5 "standard deviations" below normal confirms the diagnosis. This means people have lost at least 25 per cent of their bone mass or density.

Hip fractures can cause severe disability or death.

- Among 100 women with normal bone density, about **15** may break a hip in their lifetime.
- Among 100 women with low bone density, about **35 to 75** may break a hip in their lifetime.

This number depends on *amount of bone loss*, *age*, and other risk factors, such as:

- *major bone-related risks:* previous broken bones since age 50 (not from trauma); family history of fracture (e.g. mother who broke a hip, wrist, spine)
- *major fall-related risks:* poor health; unable to rise from a chair without help; use of sleeping pills.

Spine fractures are more common, disabling, and painful. They can cause stooped posture and loss of height of up to 6 inches.

To find out your personal risk of broken bones, ask your doctor.

What can I do on my own to manage my disease?

✓ Calcium and vitamin D ✓ Regular impact exercises (e.g. walking)

What treatments are used for osteoporosis?

Three kinds of treatment may be used alone or together. The common (generic) names of treatment are shown below.

1. *Bone-specific drugs*
   - Alendronate
   - Calcitonin
   - Etidronate
   - Risedronate
2. *Hormones that affect bones and other organs*
   - Parathyroid hormone
   - Raloxifene
   - Hormone replacement therapy (oestrogen and progestin)
3. *Other*
   - Hip protector pads

What about other treatments I have heard about?

There is not enough evidence about the effects of some treatments. Other treatments do not work. For example:

- Calcitonin for non-spinal fractures
- Etidronate for non-spinal fractures
- Raloxifene for non-spinal fractures

What are my choices? How can I decide?

Treatment for your disease will depend on your condition. You need to know the good points (pros) and bad points (cons) about each treatment before you can decide.

Osteoporosis decision aid

Should I take hormone replacement therapy (HRT)?

This guide can help you make decisions about the treatment your doctor is asking you to consider.

It will help you to:

1. Clarify what you need to decide.
2. Consider the pros and cons of different choices.
3. Decide what role you want to have in choosing your treatment.
4. Identify what you need to help you make the decision.
5. Plan the next steps.
6. Share your thinking with your doctor.

Step 1: Clarify what you need to decide

What is the decision?

Should I take hormone replacement therapy (HRT) to slow bone loss or prevent breaks?

Hormone replacement therapy (HRT) may be a combination of oestrogen and/or progestin and may be taken as pills, creams, injections or patches.

When does this decision have to be made? Check ✓ one

☐ within days ☐ within weeks ☐ within months

How far along are you with this decision? Check ✓ one

☐ I have not thought about it yet

☐ I am considering the choices

☐ I am close to making a choice

☐ I have already made a choice

Step 2: Consider the pros and cons of different choices

What does the research show?

Hormone replacement therapy (HRT) is classified as: **Trade-off between benefits and harms**

There is "Gold" level evidence from 1 large study and 2 reviews with over 25 000 women after menopause that tested hormone replacement therapy (HRT) and lasted up to 4 years. The women had osteoporosis (low bone density) or normal to near normal bone density. These studies found pros and cons that are listed in the chart below.

What do I think of the pros and cons of hormone replacement therapy (HRT)?

1. Review the common pros and cons that are shown below.
2. Add any other pros and cons that are important to you.
3. Show how important each pro and con is to you by circling from one (*) star if it is a little important to you, to up to five (*****) stars if it is very important to you.

PROS AND CONS OF HORMONE REPLACEMENT THERAPY (HRT)

PROS (number of people affected)	How important is it to you?	CONS (number of people affected)	How important is it to you?
Fewer broken bones in the spine 3 less women out of 100 have a break in the spine over their lifetime by taking HRT compared to no treatment	* * * * *	**Side effects: depression, headaches, breast tenderness, premenstrual** syndrome, skin irritation, and weight gain	* * * * *
Fewer broken bones in the hip or wrist 9 less women out of 100 have a break in the hip or wrist over their lifetime when taking HRT compared to no treatment	* * * * *	Long term harms with hormone replacement therapy: Breast cancer (in 5 out of 1000 more women) Heart disease (in 4 out of 1000 more women Stroke (in 5 out of 1000 more women) Blood clots (in 10 out of 1000 more women)	* * * * *
Increases bone density	* * * * *	**Personal cost of medicine**	* * * * *
May decrease the changes of bowel **cancer (colorectal cancer)** 3 out of 1000 less women with HRT compared to placedo	* * * * *	Regular menstrual periods	* * * * *
Other pros:	* * * * *	Other cons:	* * * * *

What do you think of hormone replacement therapy (HRT)? Check ✓ one

☐	☐	☐
Willing to consider this treatment Pros are more important to me than the Cons	Unsure	Not willing to consider this treatment Cons are more important to me than the Pros

Step 3: Choose the role you want to have in choosing your treatment. Check ✓ one

☐ I prefer to decide on my own after listening to the opinions of others

☐ I prefer to share the decision with: ____________________

☐ I prefer someone else to decide for me, namely: ______________

Step 4: Identify what you need to help you make the decision

What I know	Do you know enough about your condition to make a choice?	☐ Yes ☐ No ☐ Unsure
	Do you know which options are available to you?	☐ Yes ☐ No ☐ Unsure
	Do you know the good points (pros) of each option?	☐ Yes ☐ No ☐ Unsure
	Do you know the bad points (cons) of each option?	☐ Yes ☐ No ☐ Unsure
What's important	Are you clear about which **pros** are most *important to you?*	☐ Yes ☐ No ☐ Unsure
	Are you clear about which **cons** are most *important to you?*	☐ Yes ☐ No ☐ Unsure
How others help	Do you have enough support from others to make a choice?	☐ Yes ☐ No ☐ Unsure
	Are you choosing without pressure from others?	☐ Yes ☐ No ☐ Unsure
	Do you have enough advice to make a choice?	☐ Yes ☐ No ☐ Unsure
How sure I feel	Are you clear about the best choice for you?	☐ Yes ☐ No ☐ Unsure
	Do you feel sure about what to choose?	☐ Yes ☐ No ☐ Unsure

If you answered No or Unsure to many of these questions, you should talk to your doctor.

Step 5: Plan the next steps

What do you need to do before you make this decision?

For example: talk to your doctor, read more about this treatment or other treatments for osteoporosis.

Step 6: Share the information on this form with your doctor

It will help your doctor understand what you think about this treatment.

9
Rheumatoid arthritis

Maria E. Suarez-Almazor, Manathip Osiri, Paul Emery, Ottawa Methods Group

Introduction

Rheumatoid arthritis (RA) is a chronic inflammatory joint disease that affects around 0·5–1% of the population worldwide.[1] It is characterised by chronic symmetric polyarthritis that can result in progressive joint destruction and disability. Rheumatoid arthritis has a harmful effect on patients' functional ability, work productivity, quality of life, and life expectancy, with additional detrimental consequences on patient families and society at large. The course of RA is variable and difficult to predict; some patients have a progressive unremitting course, while others may experience flares and remissions. About 10% of patients will experience a single episode of polyarthritis, which resolves after a few months, or a few years. The past decade has seen a shift in the treatment recommendations for RA, with an emphasis on early and aggressive treatment with disease modifying antirheumatic drugs (DMARDs), as single drugs or in combination.[2,3] Early treatment of RA with DMARDs has been shown to retard joint inflammation and destruction, as well as to improve the functional status and quality of life of the patient. Published guidelines for the treatment of RA recommend early DMARD therapy.[4]

In addition to a more aggressive and early therapeutic approach, the treatment of RA has also been modified in the past few years by the development of selectively targeted drugs such as COX-2 selective inhibitors and biologic agents. Although these therapies have been proven to be effective, questions remain about their risk–benefit ratios and overall cost-effectiveness when compared to the standard treatments.

In this chapter, we report a summary of the existing evidence for ten clinical questions that relate to the treatment of patients with RA (see Box below). We present three different patient scenarios to illustrate the major therapeutic decisions faced by patients and their physicians throughout the course of the disease.

Ten clinical questions related to treatment of patients with RA

Case presentation 1

- **Question 1:** Should patients with early RA initiate DMARD therapy once their diagnosis is established?
- **Question 2:** What are the relative benefits and harms of the various DMARDs?
- **Question 3:** Is there a benefit in treating patients with early RA with a combination of DMARDs, instead of a single drug?
- **Question 4:** Should patients with early RA be treated with a biologic agent?
- **Question 5:** Are low dose oral corticosteroids beneficial in the treatment of patients with RA?

- **Question 6:** Are COX-2 inhibitors a better therapeutic choice than non-selective COX-inhibitors in patients with RA?
- **Question 7:** Should patients with RA be referred to education programmes?
- **Question 8:** Are non-pharmacological modalities effective in patients with RA?

Case presentation 2

- **Question 9:** What is the treatment of choice in a patient who has partially failed methotrexate therapy?

Case presentation 3

- **Question 10:** For how long should patients with RA continue to receive DMARD?

Methodology

The best evidence for therapeutic efficacy is derived from systematic reviews of randomised clinical trials (RCTs), with or without meta-analysis, because they critically synthesise and combine evidence from all available sources, using a systematic, unbiased approach. These sources include individual RCTs, observational studies, such as cohort studies and small case series and case reports. We are reporting here, for the most part, evidence, based on the results of systematic reviews and randomised trials. Most of the interventions discussed in this chapter have been tested experimentally in trials, so, for the most part, we are not reporting data from studies of lower methodological quality. We have only used evidence from cohorts for issues related to longer term outcomes that cannot be easily studied in clinical trials. Our initial searches for each question have included the Cochrane Database of Systematic Reviews, and Clinical Evidence. Beyond those searches, we have conducted searches in MEDLINE to retrieve additional data, subsequent to the publication of the systematic reviews, and also for interventions for which no systematic review was found. For these searches, we have used broad search terms: RA and the name of the intervention under study (for example, RA and infliximab).

Outcomes

The progression and outcome of RA cannot be assessed with a single measure. There are two major components that have to be measured, disease activity and disease damage. Some of the currently used measures assess disease activity (for example, ESR), others assess damage (for example, radiographic changes), and some assess outcomes that can be a result of both disease activity and damage (for example, functional impairment). Two expert groups, the American College of Rheumatology and OMERACT (Outcome Measures for Rheumatology Clinical Trials), have standardised which outcome measures should be used to evaluate disease activity and progression in the RA patients included in clinical trials. These outcomes were later endorsed by the World Health Organisation (WHO) and the International League of Association on Rheumatology (ILAR).[5] They include the following: number of tender joints, number of swollen joints, pain, physician global assessment, patient global assessment, functional status, acute phase reactants (ESR, CRP), and radiographic damage. The American College of Rheumatology has developed composite measures of improvement, which were published in 1995.[6] For an ACR20 response, improvement occurs with at least a 20% reduction in the number of tender and swollen joints and a 20% improvement in three or more of the following: pain, functional status, acute phase reactants, physician global assessment, and patient global assessment; ACR50 and ACR70 responses respectively require a minimum of 50% or 70% improvement in these same parameters. Similar criteria for improvement have been developed by the European League against

Rheumatism (EULAR), which have validity comparable to the ACR criteria.[7]

In this chapter we include two measures that help make trial results more understandable for practising clinicians: the number needed to treat (NNT) and the number needed to harm (NNH). Both can be helpful in decision making in daily clinical practice. The NNT is the estimated number of patients that have to be treated with an intervention in order to prevent one additional bad outcome, or to gain one additional good outcome. It is calculated as the inverse of the absolute risk reduction (ARR) (NNT = 1/ARR).[8–10] The ARR is the difference in the rate of outcomes between the experimental treatment group and the control group. The NNT is usually calculated from a dichotomous outcome (for example, event rate) and should be accompanied by a finite 95% confidence interval (95% CI) to provide the level of certainty on the benefit from the experimental treatment.[8,9] Similarly, the NNH is the estimated number of patients who have to be treated before an adverse event occurs; that is, how many patients will not develop the event for each patient who does. Most recent trials in patients with RA use the ACR composite improvement indices as primary endpoints; NNT can be easily calculated from these indices. For trials reporting only continuous measures of disease activity or damage, such as number of tender joints or ESR, NNT (and its 95% confidence intervals) can be calculated from the mean changes in these outcomes, using the method proposed by Norman *et al.*[11]

Evaluating the evidence

Case presentation 1

Mrs S., aged 48 years, developed symmetric polyarthritis of her wrists, finger joints, knees, and ankles 6 months ago. She has early morning stiffness in these joints, which lasts two hours. She works as a secretary, and her arthritis affects her work substantially. Her joint pain and swelling have not improved with over-the-counter analgesics. Mrs S. is otherwise healthy, does not smoke, and only drinks alcoholic beverages socially. Physical examination reveals tender and swollen wrists, metacarpophalangeal and proximal interphalangeal joints, elbows, knees, and ankles. The range of motion of her shoulder joints and wrists is limited. No joint deformity is observed. Laboratory tests show mild anaemia with thrombocytosis, an erythrocyte sedimentation rate (ESR) of 60 mm/hr, and a positive serum rheumatoid factor (163 IU/ml). Other blood chemistry is normal. Hand radiographs show periarticular soft tissue swelling and erosions at the base of the left 3rd proximal phalanx and the right 4th metacarpal bone. A diagnosis of early RA is made and the patient receives a prescription for naproxen 250 mg bid. Mrs S. comes back after 4 weeks, reporting slight improvement in her joint pain and morning stiffness; her physical examination reveals continuing swelling of the affected joints.

Introduction

When a patient initially presents with a diagnosis of early RA, the treating physician and the patient face several treatment questions: when should DMARD therapy be initiated, what are the benefits and harms of the various DMARDs, what is the efficacy of the newer biologic agents, are COX-2 inhibitors more appropriate than non-selective NSAIDs, and should non-pharmacological approaches be recommended. Questions 1–8 apply to this patient, and cover these issues.

Traditionally, most clinical trials for a new DMARD have been conducted in patients with longstanding RA and not in those in the early stage of the disease. Thus, there are some limitations in extrapolating the existing data to patients with early RA, but because of the paucity of trials conducted exclusively in patients with newly developed disease, we have presented the evidence for individual interventions, as tested in patients with RA in general. For each drug, we have reported the benefits and harms associated with the intervention and have included the outcome measures proposed by OMERACT and the American College of Rheumatology. In addition, for more recent trials, we have presented the evidence related to improvement using the composite response indices ACR20, ACR50, and ACR70. Where possible, we have reported evidence specific for patients with early RA.

Question 1

Should patients with early RA initiate DMARD therapy once their diagnosis is established?

About 10% of patients with polyarthritis experience a short illness that resolves and remains largely quiescent.[12] Early treatment may expose them to adverse effects unnecessarily. The early introduction of DMARDs requires an accurate diagnosis of RA. Most RCTs comparing commonly used DMARDs to placebo show efficacy of the drug. However, for the most part, these trials have short duration (≤ 12 months), do not provide evidence for the potential long term effects of a delay in initiating DMARD therapy, and do not provide evidence for whether patients receiving placebo for a short period of time will eventually "catch-up" to patients treated earlier. To answer this question, we report the evidence from studies that have specifically examined the longer term effects (≥12 months) of delaying DMARD therapy.

Literature search

There were no systematic reviews in the Cochrane Database of Systematic Reviews. We found two systematic reviews and three additional trials specifically evaluating the effects of delaying DMARD therapy in patients with early RA. In addition, we report the results of a cohort study, which compares the results of two cohorts of RA patients with patients originally included in a RCT and followed for a longer period of time.

Outcome

There are two systematic reviews that evaluate the therapeutic value of treating patients with early RA.[13,14] The reviews did not pool the data. In addition, we found another three studies not included in the reviews.[15–17] The first systematic review included three delayed treatment trials.[13] The second review reported four delayed treatment trials (including the three in the previous one) with a total of 776 patients.[14] The first small RCT[18] included 23 patients and found that early intramuscular gold treatment reduced radiological progression, compared to a delay in treatment onset of 6 to 12 months. The second trial reported on 75 patients (137 enrolled in the original trial) and found that early oral gold administration for two years, compared to placebo, significantly reduced the number of swollen joints, the radiological progression, and the functional decline.[19] The third trial included 440 patients, but their disease duration was variable, and not all had early disease; nevertheless, a delay in the onset of gold therapy was associated with a decrease in physical function after 5 years.[20] The last trial in the review examined 238 patients with recently diagnosed RA and found that early administration of methotrexate, parenteral gold, or antimalarials significantly improved tender and swollen joints, pain and function.[21] Tsakonas *et al* reported a prospective 3 year follow up of 119 patients with early RA, originally included in a RCT of hydroxychloroquine versus placebo, and found that a 9 month delay in instituting DMARD treatment had a significant detrimental effect on pain intensity and patient global wellbeing.[15] A

RCT, including 38 patients with disease duration of less than a year, compared minocycline to a placebo.[16] All participants were given DMARDs at the end of the 3 month study. After a 4 year follow up, eight patients who originally received minocycline were in remission compared to one in the placebo group (p = 0·02); the need for DMARDs at 4 years was also reduced in the minocycline group.

For the COBRA study by Boers *et al*,[17] 155 patients with early RA were randomised to receive combined step-down prednisolone plus methotrexate and sulphasalazine, or sulphasalazine alone in a 56 week, double blind RCT. The combined treatment group improved significantly in number of swollen joints, ESR, and functional ability at 28 weeks, but at 56 weeks, after prednisolone and MTX were discontinued, disease activity in both groups was comparable. Radiographic progression was significantly slower, and new erosions were fewer in the combined treatment group than in those treated with sulphasalazine alone at 28, 56, and 80 weeks. A follow up study of the COBRA trial by Landewé *et al*[22] showed that the patients initially randomised to the combined treatment group still had a lower rate of radiographic progression at 5 years, although the COBRA therapy was stopped. During the trial period, the mean Sharp score increased by 12·4 points/year in the sulphasalazine alone group and 6.6 points/year in the combined treatment group, compared with 8·6 and 5·6 points per year thereafter, respectively. The rate of joint damage did not catch up to that of the sulphasalazine monotherapy group. These findings suggest that the rate of radiographic progression is set at the very early stages of RA, and that effective interventions must be administered within a narrow time frame, that is, a "window of opportunity".

Lard *et al* investigated the effect of early versus delayed DMARD therapy in cohorts of patients with early RA, including patients originally involved in the COBRA trial.[23] They showed that a more aggressive treatment using combination therapy decreased the deleterious effect of a delay in institution of therapy, suggesting that recently diagnosed patients who have had untreated disease for longer periods of time may benefit from a more aggressive approach. They also assessed the relationship between outcomes and the presence of a shared epitope (SE).[24] In the cohort study, one cohort of patients was promptly treated with chloroquine or sulphasalazine (median lag time to DMARD treatment 15 days), and the other, only after showing a lack of response to analgesics (median lag time 123 days). At two years, the radiographic progression was significantly less in the early treatment group. Subgroup analysis was performed to evaluate the relationship between having a SE allele, and the effect of delaying DMARD therapy. In the cohort study, the presence of SE alleles did not affect the radiological progression of patients treated early with DMARDs, but in those with delayed treatment, it was associated with a higher damage score. In the COBRA follow-up, the combination treatment group had a lower rate of radiographic progression regardless of the SE status, but for those treated with sulphasalazine alone, a higher joint damage score was observed in those carrying SE alleles.[24] Thus, there is some evidence (Silver) that patients with SE alleles may be at higher risk of an adverse outcome if DMARD therapy is delayed.

An additional trial in 195 patients[25] comparing treatment with a single DMARD to a combination regime, found that a delay in therapy was the only significant predictor for remission in patients receiving a single drug; this was not observed in those receiving combination therapy.

The ACR guidelines for the management of RA state that the majority of patients with newly diagnosed RA should be started on DMARD therapy within 3 months of diagnosis.

Evidence summary: Gold

Evidence from systematic reviews and subsequent RCTs suggests that patients with active RA should start treatment with DMARDs early in the course of their disease.

Case presentation 1

The patient in Case 1 showed some improvement with NSAIDs, but she continues to have persistent disease activity and has developed radiological erosions. NSAIDs can partially control joint inflammation and pain, but they do not modify the natural course of RA. This woman should be encouraged to start a DMARD. The next questions will evaluate the evidence for different DMARDs.

Question 2

What are the relative benefits and harms of the various DMARDs?

Very few RCTs of DMARDs have been conducted in DMARD-naive patients with early disease, such as the woman in Case 1. Most of the evidence has been obtained in trials including patients with variable disease duration, and in the majority, the patients included had already received one or more previous DMARDs. Therefore, the efficacy and toxicity of the various DMARDs are reviewed here in relation to the evidence for RA in general. An additional issue in the evaluation of DMARDs is that for the older agents, most placebo controlled trials were small and of mediocre quality, whereas for the newer ones, the trials often compare different drugs head to head, and are larger and better designed. We have included the evidence for each DMARD separately, followed by a section on the comparative efficacy of these drugs, and a review of RCTs conducted in patients with early disease.

Literature search

We found several systematic reviews in the Cochrane Database of Systematic Reviews, and some additional ones published in journals, addressing the efficacy of different DMARDs. In addition, by searching the literature using broad search terms as described previously, we found several additional RCTs published subsequently to the systematic reviews.

Outcome

Methotrexate

We found one systematic review (five RCTs, 219 patients) of low dose methotrexate for 12–18 weeks (usually < 20 mg/wk) versus placebo.[26] It found a significant improvement with methotrexate in the number of swollen and tender joints, pain score, physician and patient global assessment, and functional status. There was no significant difference in ESR. We found two subsequent RCTs of methotrexate versus leflunomide versus placebo, which found similar results as the review when comparing methotrexate to the placebo arm.[27,28] Methotrexate improved quality of life compared to placebo.

We found one systematic review comparing RCTs of various DMARDs, including nine methotrexate arms with 274 patients.[29] This systematic review, however, did not compare trials with the same interventions head to head, and pooled all of the arms for each intervention comparing them to the pooled placebo arms. This methodology does not respect the randomisation process, and the results are not as robust; the treatment arms pooled in this fashion have to be considered cohorts, and the evidence can only be rated as

Silver. The review found no consistent differences between methotrexate and other DMARDs. One subsequent RCT (483 patients) found that methotrexate was not significantly different from leflunomide over one year.[28] Another large subsequent RCT (999 patients) found that leflunomide improved some outcomes more than did methotrexate.[27] In the leflunomide trials, no substantial differences in radiological progression were observed between methotrexate and leflunomide.

Two 52 week trials in patients with early disease compared methotrexate with sulphasalazine and with the combination of these two drugs and found no significant differences between the two drugs.[30,31] Two other subsequent RCTs compared methotrexate with parenteral gold, each including 141 and 174 patients respectively.[32,33] No significant differences were observed between the two drugs.

Three additional systematic reviews comparing various DMARDs were found, but are not included here because they were eclipsed by a more recent update,[34] they did not directly answer our question,[35] or they were available only in abstract form.[36]

One systematic review (search date 1991) of observational studies comparing methotrexate to other DMARDs on radiological progression found a significant benefit from methotrexate only when compared with azathioprine (p = 0·049).[37] It found no significant differences between methotrexate and parenteral gold.

The systematic review of methotrexate versus placebo found that more patients on methotrexate withdrew because of adverse events (22% *v* 7%).[26] The adverse effects were mainly liver enzyme abnormalities (11% with methotrexate versus 2·6% with placebo; RR 4·5, 95% CI 1·6–11·0). Other common adverse effects were mucocutaneous, gastrointestinal, or haematologic complaints. One systematic review of observational studies and RCTs compared the withdrawal rates over 60 months.[38] It found that methotrexate had the lowest discontinuation rate compared to other DMARDs: 36% of patients remained on methotrexate compared to 23% on gold and 22% on sulphasalazine. Methotrexate also had the lowest rate of withdrawals because of adverse events.

Some serious adverse events have been reported in case series; their incidence rate is too low to be adequately studied in RCTs, but they should be considered because of their clinical importance. A systematic review of pancytopenia identified 99 cases, with risk factors being renal failure and co-administration of trimethoprim-sulphamethoxazole and salazosulphapyridine. Pulmonary toxicity, hepatic fibrosis, and serious infections occasionally occur, even at the low dosages usually administered in RA. A systematic review found that concurrent administration of folic acid decreased the risk of gastrointestinal and mucocutaneous adverse effects (51% with folic acid versus 83% without folic acid) with no adverse impact on the efficacy of methotrexate.[39] Although some studies reported an increased risk of tumours with methotrexate, results have not been consistent.[40] In a large cohort study, methotrexate was shown to reduce mortality in patients with RA.[41]

Evidence summary: Gold

Systematic reviews including nine RCTs and additional RCTs not in the review found consistent clinical benefits with methotrexate (Visual Rx Faces 9.1).

The 2002 ACR guidelines for the medical management of RA recommend methotrexate as the DMARD to be used first in patients with very active disease.[4] The ACR guidelines for monitoring therapy should be followed.[42]

Visual Rx Faces 9.1 NNT for MTX versus placebo

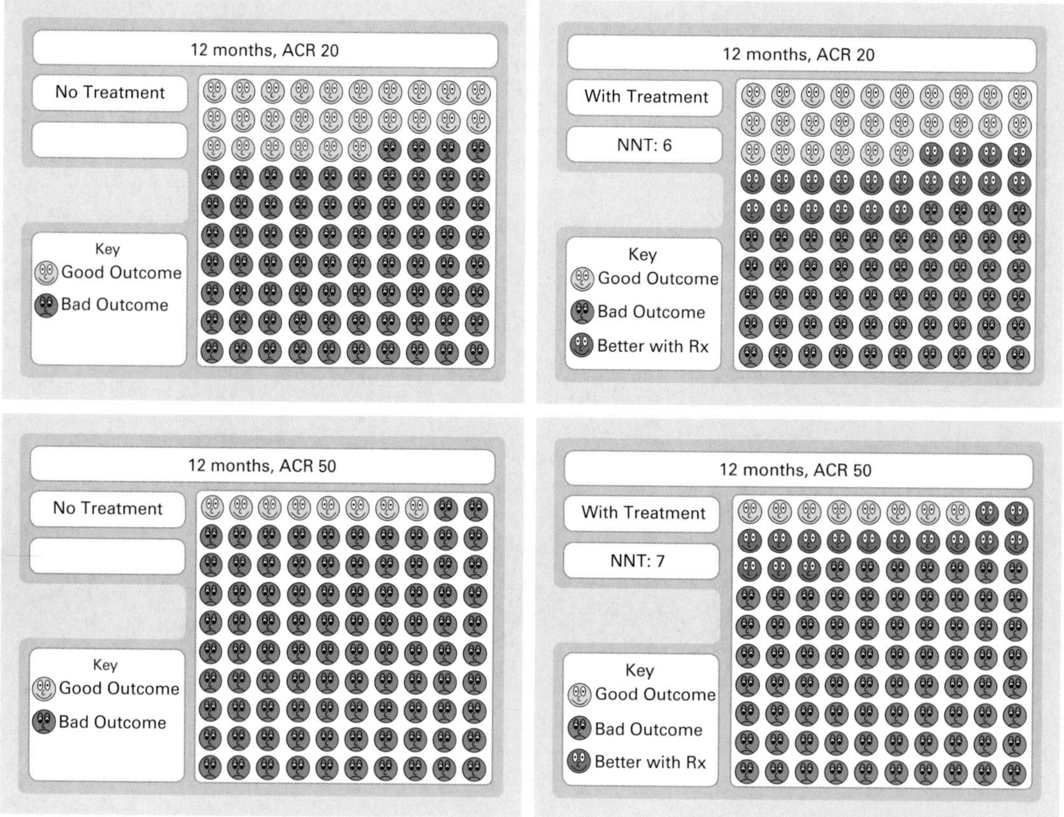

> ***Case presentation 1***
> Methotrexate is the DMARD that we would first recommend to the patient in Case 1. Although there are no placebo controlled trials restricted to early patients, systematic reviews and subsequent RCTs found consistent clinical benefit from methotrexate across early and late patient presentations.

Sulphasalazine

We found two systematic reviews [43,44] and one subsequent RCT comparing sulphasalazine to leflunomide and placebo.[45] The first review (six RCTs, 252 patients) of sulphasalazine given for 6 months found improvement in the number of tender and swollen joints, pain score, and ESR.[43] Only two RCTs (155 patients) included global assessments, and they found no significant effect. None evaluated functional status. The second review of placebo controlled trials (eight RCTs, 903 patients) found better results with sulphasalazine on all outcome measures (decrease in number of swollen joints: 51% in the sulphasalazine group versus 26% in the placebo group; $p < 0{\cdot}0001$).[44] The subsequent RCT found that sulphasalazine (133 patients) versus placebo (92 patients) significantly improved patient and physician global assessment.[45]

One of the systematic reviews[44] and three additional RCTs compared sulphasalazine versus other DMARDs.[45–47] The systematic review found no significant difference between sulphasalazine and hydroxychloroquine in improvement on the number of swollen joints (37% *v* 28%, $p = 0{\cdot}38$) or ESR (43% *v* 26%; $p = 0{\cdot}10$). One additional RCT (60 patients), comparing sulphasalazine versus hydroxychloroquine, found that sulphasalazine was significantly better in controlling radiological damage, although progression occurred with both drugs (median erosion scores at week 48: 16 with hydroxychloroquine versus 5 with sulphasalazine; $p < 0{\cdot}02$);[46] however, hydroxychloroquine was given at a lower dose than is usually recommended. One subsequent RCT (358 patients over 24 weeks) of sulphasalazine versus leflunomide versus placebo found no significant difference between sulphasalazine and leflunomide in tender joint count, swollen joint count, or pain (on a visual analogue scale).[45] No differences were observed in radiological progression. One longer-term follow-up of a RCT comparing sulphasalazine versus penicillamine (200 patients) found significantly better functional status with sulphasalazine after 12 years;[47] however, differences were small, and many patients had changed treatment or died during the 12 years. In the 52-week combination trials in early disease, which also compared methotrexate to sulphasalazine, head to head, no differences were observed between the two drugs.[30,31]

Common adverse effects in the systematic reviews and RCTs included gastrointestinal discomfort, rash, and liver enzyme abnormalities.[43] More serious haematological or hepatic toxicity was uncommon. Reversible leucopenia or agranulocytosis was occasionally observed. Treatment was discontinued for adverse effects less often than with other DMARDs, with the exception of antimalarials. The comparative systematic review of observational studies and RCTs found that the proportion of patients who remained on the same treatment over 5 years was lower with sulphasalazine than with methotrexate, but was the same as with parenteral gold.[38] More patients withdrew because of adverse effects on parenteral gold than with sulphasalazine, but fewer withdrew with methotrexate.

Evidence summary: Gold

Systematic reviews that included eight RCTs found that sulphasalazine is more effective than placebo in reducing disease activity and joint inflammation. In the short term, sulphasalazine has similar effects on radiological progression and improvement of function as methotrexate and leflunomide. Longer-term observational studies demonstrate that patients are more likely to remain on methotrexate than sulphasalazine, suggesting that sulphasalazine may lose some effectiveness over time, compared to methotrexate.

Case presentation 1

Sulphasalazine could be an option for the patient in Case 1, although there is some evidence from observational studies that methotrexate may be more effective in the longer term. Sulphasalazine should be considered as an option for DMARD naive patients who may have a contraindication to receive methotrexate (for example, elevated liver enzymes).

Antimalarials

We found one systematic review of four RCTs of hydroxychloroquine given for 6–12 months compared to placebo (592 patients).[48] It reported a significant improvement in the number of swollen and tender joints, pain score, physician and patient global assessment, and ESR. One RCT (119 patients) assessed functional status and found no significant difference. The comparative systematic review of various DMARDS[29] found no significant difference between antimalarials and other drugs. Individual RCTs comparing antimalarials with other DMARDs found no consistent advantage for any one drug, although some found better results with penicillamine and sulphasalazine. We found no RCTs that adequately compared chloroquine versus hydroxychloroquine. One older RCT included both drugs but did not report a direct comparison.[49]

The systematic review of placebo controlled RCTs found no significant difference in the number of withdrawals because of adverse effects.[48] No participants discontinued treatment because of ocular adverse effects, and mild toxicity was reported in only one person. One long-term retrospective observational study of 97 patients found that more patients receiving chloroquine developed retinopathy compared to hydroxychloroquine (19·4% *v* 0%).[50] We found no good evidence on the optimal frequency for eye examinations; expert opinion ranges from every six months to two years. One RCT found that the most common non-ocular adverse effects were gastrointestinal disturbances, occurring in about 25% of patients.[51] Skin reactions and renal abnormalities occasionally occur. Mild neurological abnormalities include non-specific symptoms such as vertigo and blurred vision. Cardiomyopathy and severe neurological disease are extremely rare.

One five-year RCT (541 patients) compared hydroxychloroquine versus penicillamine versus parenteral gold versus auranofin.[52] It found that at 5 years, significantly more patients continued to take pencillamine (53%) than hydroxychloroquine (30%), but similar numbers of patients continued to take parenteral gold (34%) and auranofin (31%). A systematic review of RCTs and observational studies found that over two years, patients with RA were more likely to continue on methotrexate than on antimalarials, but they were more likely to continue on antimalarials than on parenteral gold or sulphasalazine.[38] Most patients discontinued antimalarial treatment because of lack of efficacy.

Evidence summary: Gold

One systematic review that includes four RCTS found that hydroxychloroquine reduces disease activity and joint inflammation, compared to placebo, in patients with RA. Two RCTs found no evidence of benefit on functional status and radiological progression. Two systematic reviews found mixed results regarding differences in short-term efficacy between antimalarials and other DMARDs.

Case presentation 1

The woman in Case 1 has persistent disease severity and radiological erosions, so we would recommend methotrexate over antimalarials.

Parenteral gold

We found one systematic review (four RCTs, 415 patients) of parenteral gold for 6 months versus placebo.[53] It found significant improvement in the number of swollen joints, patient and physician global assessments, and ESR. Functional status was not evaluated. Another review (nine RCTs and one observational study) that included radiological assessment found that parenteral gold decreased the radiological progression compared to placebo.[54]

We found one systematic review of various DMARDs, described in the sections above,[29] and two subsequent RCTs.[32,55] The review found no consistent differences between parenteral gold and other DMARDs. Some RCTs found that parenteral gold was more effective, but also more toxic, than its oral counterpart, auranofin. A few RCTs comparing parenteral gold versus methotrexate found no major differences in short-term disease activity between parenteral gold and methotrexate.[32,33] Another RCT found no significant differences in radiological damage or self-assessment of disease activity between gold and ciclosporin.[55]

The systematic review of parenteral gold versus placebo found that more patients receiving gold discontinued treatment because of adverse events, including dermatitis, stomatitis, proteinuria, and haematological changes. At six months, 30% of patients receiving parenteral gold had withdrawn, compared to 15% receiving placebo: (RR 1·9; 95% CI 1·3–2·8).[53] The subsequent RCT found that more patients withdrew due to toxicity with parenteral gold than with methotrexate (43% *v* 19%).[32] The systematic review of observational studies and RCTs found that the proportion of patients who remained on the same treatment over five years was lower with gold than with methotrexate, and it was similar with sulphasalazine.[38] More patients withdrew because of adverse effects on parenteral gold than with sulphasalazine or methotrexate. Life threatening reactions, such as aplastic anaemia, are rare, but have been reported in observational studies and necessitate close monitoring. Use of parenteral gold is limited by toxicity, and also by the need for parental administration and frequent toxicity monitoring.

Evidence summary: Silver

One systematic review that included four RCTS found that parenteral gold versus placebo reduces disease activity and joint inflammation, and slows radiological progression in patients with RA. We found no evidence on long term functional status. The evidence indicates that increased rates of withdrawal due to toxicity occurred with parenteral gold compared with methotrexate or sulphasalazine.

Case presentation 1

We would not recommend parenteral gold to the patient in Case 1 as the first DMARD option because of its more serious toxicity profile and because of the inconvenience of intramuscular injections and frequent monitoring.

Penicillamine

We found one systematic review of penicillamine versus placebo (six RCTs, 683 patients).[56] It found significant improvement in the number of swollen joints and ESR. Only some of the RCTs evaluated global assessment and functional status, and results were inconclusive. The systematic review of RCTs comparing various DMARDs included penicillamine arms with 583 patients.[29] It found no consistent differences in efficacy between penicillamine and other drugs, although some trials found penicillamine to be superior to antimalarials.

The review reported increased withdrawals because of adverse reactions with penicillamine (20·1% for penicillamine 500–1000 mg/day *v* 8·7% with placebo; RR 2·4, 95% CI 1·4–4·1).[56] Adverse events were common and sometimes serious, and they included mucocutaneous reactions, altered taste, gastrointestinal events, proteinuria, haematologic effects, myositis, and autoimmune induced disease. The adverse events most frequently responsible for penicillamine discontinuation were haematologic 6·6%, mucosal/cutaneous 4·9%, impaired/loss of taste 4·7%, renal 4·1%, and gastrointestinal 2·3%.

Evidence summary: Gold

One systematic review that included six RCTs found that penicillamine reduces disease activity and joint inflammation compared to placebo. We found no evidence of its effect on radiological progression or long term functional status. One systematic review has found no consistent difference between penicillamine and other DMARDs. The use of penicillamine is limited by the frequency of serious adverse effects. Observational studies found that most patients discontinued the drug within the first two years of treatment. Use of this drug is declining.

Case presentation 1

We would not recommend penicillamine to the patient in Case 1.

Leflunomide

We found two systematic reviews on the efficacy of leflunomide versus placebo, methotrexate or sulphasalazine.[57,58] They found that leflunomide improved disease activity, function, quality of life, and radiological progression. The first systematic review[57] included the data from four RCTs[27,28,45,59] while the other systematic review[58] included four RCTs,[27,28,45,59] two of them with two year follow ups.[60,61] These trials involved 1144 patients randomised to leflunomide, 312 to placebo, 680 to methotrexate, and 132 to sulphasalazine in the first year of trials. Leflunomide significantly improved the number of tender and swollen joints; pain; global assessments; function; ESR; ACR20, 50, and 70 response rates; and delayed radiographic changes compared to placebo. When compared to methotrexate and sulphasalazine at 12 months of treatment, leflunomide was not better than these two DMARDs in improving disease activity, ACR response rate, or radiographic progression. One exception was observed; leflunomide significantly improved disease activity measures compared to sulphasalazine at 24 months, but there was no difference in the rate of radiographic progression.

Withdrawals due to adverse events in the leflunomide group were significantly higher than in the placebo group (RR 2·73, 95% CI 1·67–4·47), but not in the methotrexate group at 12 months (RR 1·56, 95% CI 0·95–2·55), or at two years (RR 1·19; 95% CI 0·89–1·6), or in the sulphasalazine group (RR 0·77, 95% CI 0·45–1·33). Major reported adverse events from leflunomide included gastrointestinal symptoms (diarrhoea, dyspepsia, nausea/vomiting, abdominal pain, oral ulcers), elevated liver function tests, allergic reactions, alopecia, infections, weight loss, and hypertension. GI symptoms, elevated liver enzymes, allergic reactions, and alopecia were significantly higher for leflunomide than placebo. Most adverse events from leflunomide were not significantly different from those from methotrexate and sulphasalazine.

We found no evidence on long term adverse effects.

Evidence summary: Platinum

A systematic review that included six RCTs found that leflunomide was as effective as methotrexate and sulphasalazine in reducing disease activity, improving function, and retarding radiological progression over 12 months, and had a different toxicity profile. Relative toxicity in comparison to other DMARDs needs to be established in longer term comparative studies.

Case presentation 1

Because leflunomide is a new drug and has limited data on long term toxicity, we would not recommend it as the first choice for the woman in Case 1.

Ciclosporin

We found one systematic review comparing ciclosporin to placebo for a minimum of 4 months (three RCTs, 318 patients).[62] It found significant improvement in the number of tender and swollen joints, and in pain and functional status. It found limited evidence that radiological progression was also reduced.

The review reported that ciclosporin was associated with more adverse events than placebo including gum hyperplasia (9·1% *v* 0%), paraesthesia (13·8% *v* 6·3%; RR 2·2, 95% CI 1·1–4·5), nausea (25·8% *v* 13·8%; RR 1·9, 95% CI 1·2–3·0), headache (16·4% *v* 4·9%; RR 3·3, 95% CI 0·96–11·5), and tremor (30·8% *v* 6·0%; RR 5·1, 95% CI 2·5–10·5). Patients have also developed nephropathy (potentially irreversible) hypertension, hypertrichosis, and hepatotoxicity. It has been suggested that ciclosporin may be associated with an increased risk of infections and tumours.

Evidence summary: Gold

A systematic review including three RCTs found that ciclosporin is effective in the treatment of RA. Because of its serious toxicity profile ciclosporin is usually reserved for patients who do not respond to other less toxic DMARDs.

Case presentation 1

We would not recommend ciclosporin in Case 1.

Azathioprine

We found one systematic review (three RCTs of azathioprine versus placebo, 81 patients).[63] It found a significant short term benefit in tender joint score, favouring azathioprine. No other outcome was reported by all trials. The systematic review of RCTs for various DMARDs[29] found limited evidence that azathioprine had about the same effect as that of antimalarials, but less than other DMARDs.

The review found that patients on azathioprine were significantly more likely to withdraw than were those on placebo (RR 4·6, 95% CI 1·2–17·9). The most common adverse events were gastrointestinal, mucocutaneous, and haematologic. An increased risk of liver abnormalities, infection, and cancer has been reported in observational studies and case series.

Evidence summary: Silver

One systematic review that included three RCTs found that azathioprine reduces disease activity compared to placebo. We found no evidence on radiological progression or long term functional status. We found no evidence that it is superior to other DMARDs. A high level of toxicity limits its usefulness. Because of its toxicity profile, azathioprine tends to be reserved for patients who have not responded to other DMARDs.

Case presentation 1

We would not recommend azathioprine for the patient in Case 1.

Cyclophosphamide

We found one systematic review comparing cyclophosphamide to placebo for 6 months (two RCTs, 70 patients).[64] It reported a significant reduction in the number of tender and swollen joints compared to placebo. One RCT reported radiological progression, which appeared to be delayed in the cyclophosphamide group. We found no evidence of its effect on functional status.

The review reported adverse effects including nausea or vomiting (58%), alopecia (26%), and dysuria (26%).[64] Other severe reactions reported in observational studies include leucopenia, thrombocytopenia, anaemia, amenorrhoea, haemorrhagic cystitis, and increased risk of infections such as herpes zoster. One long term (20 years) observational study reported that prolonged use was associated with increased risk of cancer, in particular bladder cancer.[65]

Evidence summary: Silver

One systematic review including two RCTs found that cyclophosphamide is more effective than placebo in reducing disease activity and joint inflammation in patients with RA. It may also reduce the rate of radiological progression, but evidence was limited. We found no evidence of its effect on long term functional status. Because of its cytotoxic effects, cyclophosphamide is usually reserved for patients who have not responded to other DMARDs.

Case presentation 1

We would not recommend cyclophosphamide for the patient in Case 1.

Minocycline

We found no systematic review. We found three RCTs of minocycline versus placebo.[16,66,67] They found that minocycline improved control of disease activity. The largest RCT (219 patients) compared minocycline versus placebo over 48 weeks.[67] It found that more patients had improvement in swollen joints (54% with minocycline versus 39% with placebo; $p < 0{\cdot}03$) and joint tenderness (56% with minocycline versus 41% with placebo; $p < 0{\cdot}03$). The second RCT (80 patients) compared minocycline versus placebo over 24 weeks.[67] It found a significant improvement on a composite measure of clinical and laboratory outcomes. The third RCT (43 patients) found that minocycline was superior to placebo: 13% of patients on minocycline did not improve compared to 55% with placebo.[16]

One RCT ($n = 60$) found minocycline to be more effective than hydroxychloroquine, with ACR50 responses after 2 years of 60% and 33% respectively.[68]

The largest RCT reported adverse reactions including nausea (50% with minocycline versus 13% with placebo), dyspepsia, dizziness (40% with minocycline versus 15% with placebo), and skin pigmentation.[66] Other reported important but rare events are hepatitis and drug-induced systemic lupus erythematosus.

Evidence summary: Silver

Three RCTs have found that when compared to placebo, minocycline improves control of disease activity in patients with RA. The magnitude of the beneficial effects of minocycline seems moderate, perhaps somewhat higher than that observed with antimalarials.

Case presentation 1

We would not recommend minocycline as the first choice for the patient in Case 1. There is no evidence to suggest better efficacy than methotrexate or sulphasalazine.

Auranofin

We found one systematic review (nine RCTs, 1049 patients).[69] It found significantly better results with auranofin for tender joints, swollen joint scores, pain, and ESR.

Comparisons with other DMARDs were reported in a systematic review (26 auranofin treatment arms with 1500 patients)[29] and a subsequent RCT.[70] The review found that auranofin was significantly less effective than other DMARDs (antimalarials, methotrexate, penicillamine, sulphasalazine, azathioprine) using efficacy/toxicity trade-off plots, but the review did not compare efficacy within RCTs directly.[29] The subsequent RCT (200 patients) of auranofin versus sulphasalazine found that patients were more than twice as likely to continue with sulphasalazine than with auranofin over 5 years (31% with sulphasalazine versus 15% with auranofin; $p < 0{\cdot}05$).[70]

The review found that the most common adverse events of auranofin were gastrointestinal (OR 3.0, 95% CI 1·4–6·5), particularly diarrhoea (OR 3·0, 95% CI 1·3–7·1).[69] It found that withdrawals because of haematologic or renal effects were rare (1% each). A review of adverse events found that serious events, such as those associated with parenteral gold, were rare with auranofin (participants developing serious organ specific toxicity < 0·5%; blood 0·2%, renal 0·1%, lung 0·1%, and hepatic 0·4%).[71]

Evidence summary: Gold

One systematic review that included nine RCTs found that auranofin reduces disease activity and joint inflammation compared to placebo, but found no evidence on radiological progression or long term functional status. Limited evidence from RCTs suggests that auranofin is less effective than other DMARDs (Silver). The lack of good comparative efficacy results means that auranofin is now used rarely.

Case presentation 1

We would not recommend auranofin for the patient in Case 1 because it appears to be less effective than other DMARDs.

Comparisons among DMARDs

We found a 1992 systematic review of comparative RCTs,[29] including 66 clinical trials that contained 117 treatment groups. This review did not compare trials with the same interventions head to head, and pooled the arms for each intervention, comparing them to the pooled placebo arms. This methodology does not respect the randomisation process, and the level of evidence of these results can only be considered to be silver. Auranofin was less efficacious than methotrexate, parenteral gold, penicillamine, and sulphasalazine, and slightly, but not significantly, weaker than antimalarial agents ($p = 0{\cdot}11$). No major differences were observed between methotrexate, parenteral gold, pencillamine, and sulphasalazine. Parenteral gold had higher toxicity rates and higher total dropout rates than any other drug. Antimalarials and auranofin had relatively low rates of toxicity.

A more recent study examined the effects of DMARDs according to NNT and NNH.[72] Only more recent trials reporting ACR improvement criteria were included to allow calculations of NNT. Table 9.1 shows the results of this review, with some additional data from other RCTs and systematic reviews. No statistically significant differences were observed among DMARDs in the NNTs.

Observational cohort studies have shown that once patients are treated in clinical practice, methotrexate has the longest continuation rates. A systematic review of observational studies and RCTs compared withdrawal rates over 60 months.[38] Methotrexate had the lowest discontinuation rate compared to other DMARDs, and had also the lowest rate of withdrawals because of adverse events.

DMARDs in early RA

There has been no consensus on the definition of early RA. Several clinical trials have used a cut-off point for disease duration of less than 1–3 years, mostly 2 years.[3] Data from radiological outcome studies have shown that radiographic damage of hands and feet occurs early in the course of RA. Approximately 75% of RA patients develop joint damage after 2 years.[73] For the purpose of this review, we are using a duration of disease of 2 years or less to define early disease.

Table 9.1 Number needed to treat (NNT) and number needed to harm (NNH) for single DMARD in RA clinical trials

Study	Active treatment	Comparator	Criteria for NNT	NNT (95% CI)	NNH (95% CI) (criterion: toxicity withdrawals)
Early RA					
Esdaile[51]	HCQ	Placebo	Paulus criteria at 36 wk	5 (3, 26)	111 (NS)
Marchesoni[89]	MTX	CsA	ACR20 at 24 mth	3 (2, 5)	10 (NS)
			ACR50 at 24 mth	3 (2, 13)	
			ACR70 at 24 mth	8 (NS)	
O'Dell[16]	MIN	Placebo	ACR50 at 6 mth	2 (2, 4)	25 (NS)
O'Dell[68]	MIN	HCQ	ACR20 at 2 yr	5 (3, 10)	33 (NS)
			ACR50 at 2 yr	4 (3, 8)	
			ACR70 at 2 yr	7 (4, 34)	
Rau[78]	MTX	IM gold	Remission at 12 mth	8 (5, 100)	3 (2, 5)
Van Everdingen[113]	PDN 10 mg/day	Placebo	ACR20 at 24 mth	13 (NS)	10 (NS)*
Established RA					
Smolen[45]	SSZ	Placebo	ACR20 at 24 wk	4 (3, 7)	8 (4, 25)
			ACR 50 at 24 wk		
Strand[28]	MTX	Placebo	ACR20 at 12 mth	5 (4, 12)	50 (NS)
			ACR50 at 12 mth	7 (5, 13)	
			ACR70 at 12 mth	20 (NS)	
Williams[132]	MTX	Placebo	Paulus criteria at 18 wk	3 (3, 5)	6 (4, 14)
Osiri[58]	LEF	Placebo	ACR20 at 12 mth	4 (3, 6)	10 (6, 16)
			ACR50 at 12 mth	4 (3, 6)	
			ACR70 at 12 mth	7 (5, 12)	167
	LEF	MTX	ACR20 at 24 mth	100 (NS)	16 (10, 50)
			ACR50 at 24 mth	8 (NS)	
	LEF	SSZ	ACR20 at 24 mth	5 (3, 17)	25 (NS)
			ACR50 at 24 mth	4 (3, 10)	
			ACR70 at 24 mth	15 (NS)	
Suarez-Almazor[63]	AZA	Placebo	Mean change of TJC at 16–24 wk	3 (2, 9)	5 (2, 38)
Ward[133]	AUR	Placebo	Paulus criteria at 20 wk	7 (NS)	35 (NS)
	IM gold	Placebo	Paulus criteria at 20 wk	1 (3, 15)	7 (4, 142)
Townes[134]	CYC	Placebo	Predefined clinical response criteria at 36 wk	2 (2, 5)	10 (NS)

(*Continued*)

Table 9.1 (*Continued*)

Study	Active treatment	Comparator	Criteria for NNT	NNT (95% CI)	NNH (95% CI) (criterion: toxicity withdrawals)
Williams[135]	D-P 500–1000 mg/day	Placebo	Predefined clinical response criteria at 36 wk	3 (2, 5)	9 (5, 38)
Suarez-Almazor[56]	D-P (>1000 mg/day)	Placebo	Mean change of TJC at 36 wk	6 (3, 35)	5 (3, 16)
Wells[62]	CsA A	Placebo	Mean change of TJC at 6 mth	5 (3, 10)	2 (2, 3)**

Abbreviations: MTX, methotrexate; HCQ, hydroxychloroquine; MIN, minocycline; PDN, prednisone; SSZ, sulphasalazine; LEF, leflunomide; AZA, azathioprine; AUR, auranofin; CYC, cyclophoshamide; D-P, D-penicillinamine; CsA, ciclosporin A; NS = not significant.

* Rate of osteoporotic fracture, ** Rate of hypertrichosis.

There are several RCTs comparing the efficacy of different single DMARDs in early RA[16,51,68,74–79] (Table 9.2). Five RCTs compared the efficacy of a DMARD compared to placebo in early RA. Two studies assessed sulphasalazine compared to placebo,[76,79] two others hydroxychloroquine[51,75] and the remaining two, minocycline and auranofin.[16,74] The other RCTs compared the efficacy among various DMARDs.[68,77,78]

In the first RCT comparing sulphasalazine and placebo at 6 months, sulphasalazine was significantly better than placebo in improving swollen and tender joints, and ESR. The mean changes from baseline in the number of swollen and tender joints were 10·4 joints for patients receiving sulphasalazine and 7·6 joints for patients receiving placebo.[79] In the other study that compared sulphasalazine with placebo at 48 weeks,[76] sulphasalazine also significantly reduced the number of swollen joints, Ritchie index, patient global assessment, and pain index. Radiographic progression was lower in the sulphasalazine group, but the statistical difference did not reach significance.

The HERA Study Group investigated the efficacy of hydroxychloroquine compared with placebo at 36 weeks.[51] Hydroxychloroquine significantly improved the number of tender and swollen joints, grip strength, pain index, and physical function, compared to placebo. Withdrawals due to adverse events in the hydroxychloroquine and placebo groups were one and two, respectively. The other RCT comparing hydroxychloroquine to placebo at 12 months showed that hydroxychloropine was superior in improving Ritchie index, synovitis score, grip strength, duration of morning stiffness, and ESR. At 12 months, median change in the synovitis score from baseline in the hydroxychloroquine-treated group was 6·5 and in the placebo group 3. Withdrawal rates from adverse events were similar in both groups.[75]

Borg *et al* studied the efficacy of auranofin compared to placebo in the treatment of early RA after 2 years of treatment. Patients in the auranofin group improved significantly in the number of swollen joints, physical function, and mental depression.[74] Radiographic progression was slower in the auranofin-treated group than the placebo group. Median changes from baseline in the number of swollen joints were –64 and –37 in the auranofin group and placebo groups, respectively.

Table 9.2 Randomised clinical trials of DMARD therapy in early RA

Study	Design and duration	Sample	Treatment	Outcomes
Australian Multicentre Clinical Trial Group[79]	Double blind, RCT; 6 mth	105 patients with early, non-erosive RA, disease duration of < 12 mth	SSZ *v* placebo	Significant improvement in the number of swollen and tender joints, Ritchie articular index, ESR, CRP and RF titre
Hannonen[76]	Double blind, RCT; 48 wk	80 patients with RA; disease duration of < 12 mth	SSZ *v* placebo	Significant improvement in disease activity; trend to delay radiographic progression compared to placebo
HERA Study Group[51]	Double blind, RCT; 36 wk	120 patients with RA; disease duration of < 2 yr; DMARD-naïve	HCQ *v* placebo	Significant improvement in joint indices, pain and function
Davis[75]	Double blind, RCT; 12 mth	104 patients with RA, median disease duration of 12–17 mth	HCQ *v* placebo	Significant improvement Ritchie index, morning stiffness, grip strength, synovitis score and ESR
O'Dell[16]	Double blind, RCT; 6 mth	46 patients with RA; disease duration of < 1 yr	MIN *v* placebo	Significant improvement in disease activity
Borg[74]	Double blind, RCT, placebo controlled trial; 24 mth	138 patients with RA; disease duration of < 2 yr	Early treatment with AUR *v* 8-mth delayed DMARD treatment	Significant improvement in joint swelling, function (HAQ) and delayed radiographic progression
O'Dell[68]	Double-blind, RCT; 2 yr	60 patients with RA; DMARD- naïve, disease duration of < 1 yr	MIN *v* HCQ	MIN superior HCQ in improving ACR50 response rate
van Jaarsveld[77]	Open RCT; 2 yr	313 patients with RA; disease duration of < 1 yr	Strategy 1: HCQ or AUR Strategy 2: IM gold or D-P Strategy 3: MTX or SSZ	All strategies improved joint score, pain, ESR, function and remission rates. Radiographic damage in all strategies progressed significantly, especially in patients treated with strategy 1

(*Continued*)

Table 9.2 (*Continued*)

Study	Design and duration	Sample	Treatment	Outcomes
Rau[78]	Double blind, RCT; 12 mth	174 patients with RA; disease duration of <2 yr	MTX IM gold	Similar improvement in joint counts. More patients achieved remission with RA gold, but MTX was better tolerated

Abbreviations: as Table 9.1.

Minocycline was shown to be more effective than placebo in patients with disease duration less than one year.[16] Minocycline was also compared to hydroxychlorquine for the treatment of patients with early RA with positive RF in a 2 year double blind RCT.[68] Minocycline was more efficacious than hydroxychloroquine in the number of patients achieving the ACR50 response rate (60% *v* 33%; p = 0·04). Patients in the minocycline group received less prednisone. Ten to 20% of patients treated with minocycline developed hyperpigmentation of the skin.

Rau *et al* studied the one-year radiographic progression in a RCT, comparing methotrexate and gold in patients with early RA. Both treatment groups demonstrated radiographic progression, but there was no significant difference in the rate of progression.[33,78]

Evidence summary: Silver

Based on the combined data from RCTs and observational studies, methotrexate is the most commonly used DMARD. The evidence shows that its efficacy is similar or better than other DMARDs, and its safety profile is acceptable. Long term observational studies that measure effectiveness in clinical practice show that methrotrexate has the lowest discontinuation rate among DMARDs, suggesting it has the best long term effectiveness.

Methotrexate is the first choice for patients with very active disease. For patients with milder disease activity, sulphasalazine or antimalarials could also be used initially.

Case presentation 1

The woman in Case 1 has persistent disease activity and evidence of joint damage, with radiological erosions, so we would recommend methotrexate as the initial DMARD.

Question 3

Is there a benefit in treating patients with RA with a combination of DMARDs, instead of a single drug?

A number of RCTs have examined the efficacy and toxicity of combining two or more DMARDs compared to the administration of a single drug. Many of these studies have been performed in patients with longer duration of disease; therefore, we are reviewing the efficacy of combination therapy in general here, but we have also added a section about trials conducted on patients with shorter duration of disease.

Literature search

We found one systematic review (20 RCTs, 1956 patients)[80] and several subsequent RCTs. An additional meta-analysis pooled data from RCTs comparing single versus combination drug treatments.[81] However, the analysis did not provide adequate data on specific combinations.

Outcome

The review concluded that many combinations of DMARDs may be useful.[80] Some RCTs included in the review found no significant differences between combinations of different agents and monotherapy. Nine of the RCTs (1240 patients) compared methotrexate plus another DMARD, versus methotrexate alone or the other DMARD alone. A wide range of other DMARDs was included. The review found that some methotrexate combinations (methotrexate + ciclosporin, methotrexate + sulphasalazine + hydroxychloroquine) were more beneficial than treatment with a single drug.[80] However, many possible combinations were tested in small studies, with inadequate power to reach robust conclusions. Some other subsequent RCTs have also found that combinations of different DMARDs (antimalarials, sulphasalazine, methotrexate, ciclosporin, and steroids) had greater beneficial effects than monotherapy.[17,82–87]

A 1996 RCT found that the combination of methotrexate, sulphasalazine, and hydroxychloroquine was more effective than monotherapy.[84] A more recent RCT (171 patients with disease duration >6 months) found that methotrexate plus hydroxychloroquine plus sulphasalazine increased ACR20 response rates at 2 years, compared with either methotrexate plus hydroxychloroquine, or methotrexate plus sulphasalazine (ACR20 response 78% with triple combination versus 60% with methotrexate + hydroxychloroquine versus 49% with methotrexate + sulphasalazine; $p = 0{\cdot}002$ for first comparison, $p = 0{\cdot}05$ for second comparison).[87]

Several RCTs have compared the efficacy of combination therapy to single DMARDs in early RA (Table 9.3). The combination strategies have included a fixed combination of DMARDs throughout the trial, combined "step-up" DMARDs and combined "step-down" DMARDs. In the step-up strategy, a single DMARD is prescribed for a period of time, and if the response is suboptimal, another DMARD is added. The combined step-down regimen starts with multiple DMARDs (with or without steroids) and is continued until the disease activity is controlled; the more toxic DMARDs and steroids are then tapered off.

Four RCTs have evaluated fixed combinations in early RA.[25,30,31,83,85] Haagsma *et al* and Dougados *et al* assessed the efficacy sulphasalazine and methotrexate in combination compared to sulphasalazine and methotrexate as single drugs in RCTs lasting 52 weeks.[30,31] No substantial differences were observed between the single drugs and the combination therapy in the ACR response rates, the EULAR response rates, the Disease Activity Score (DAS), or other outcome measues, including radiological progression. Möttönen *et al* reported the efficacy of combined sulphasalazine, methotrexate, hydroxychloroquine, and prednisolone compared to a single DMARD (sulphasalazine or methotrexate) in an open RCT.[25,83] At 2 years, the remission rate in the combination group was significantly higher (37%) than in the single DMARD groups (18%), and ACR50 response rates were not significantly different between groups. Radiographic progression was slower in the combination group; the median increment in the Larsen score (a radiographic index) was 2 versus 10 in the single DMARD group.

Visual Rx Faces 9.2 NNT for combination DMARDs compared to methotrexate

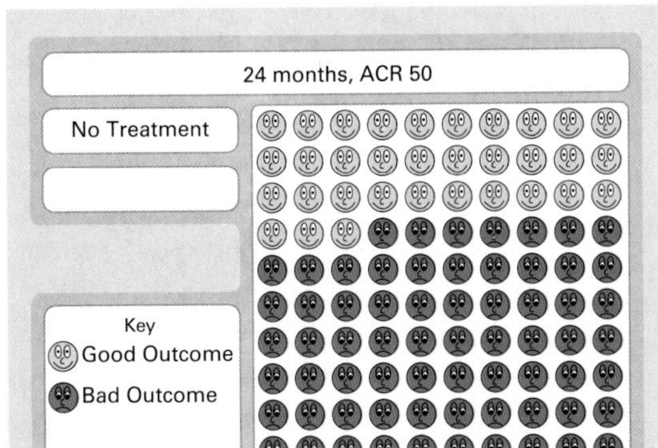

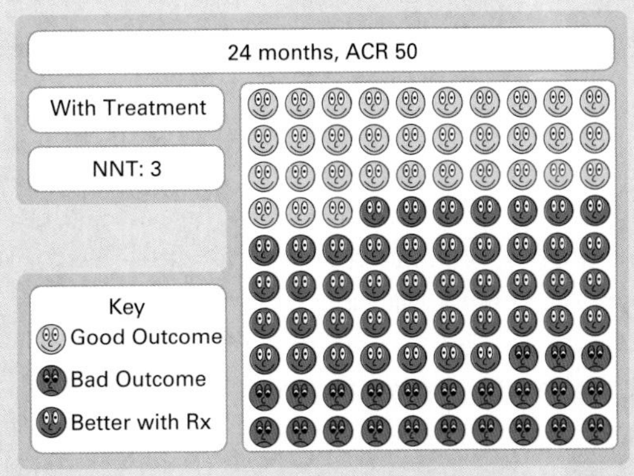

Another trial compared the efficacy of combination therapy with methotrexate, ciclosporin, and intra-articular methylprednisolone with sulphasalazine alone at 48 weeks of treatment.[85] Although the patients in the combined treatment group achieved a more rapid control of disease activity than the sulphasalazine-treated group during the first 12 weeks, the ACR20 response rates (58% with combination therapy versus 45% with sulphasalazine) and the remission rates (43% versus 36% respectively) were not significantly different at the end of study. The number of swollen joints was significantly lower in the combination group at the end of 48 weeks, but no other outcomes were significantly different between groups.

One trial evaluated a combination step-up regimen of methotrexate, ciclosporin, and sulphasalazine compared to sulphasalazine alone for 18 months.[88] Patients were randomly assigned to receive methotrexate, ciclosporin or sulphasalazine for 6 months, and if the response did not reach the ACR50 response criteria, patients who received methotrexate or ciclosporin were given the combination therapy (methotrexate and ciclosporin). Sulphasalazine was added to the combination regimen after 12 months if the response was not satisfactory. At 6 months, the ACR50 response rate in the methotrexate group was 57%, 31% in the ciclosporin group, and 33% in the sulphasalazine group. At 12 months, after starting combination regimen, 67% of patients receiving methotrexate + ciclosporin, 76% on ciclosporin + methotrexate, and 24% on sulphasalazine alone had achieved an ACR50 response. At 18 months, 90% of the patients receiving methotrexate (1) + ciclosporin (2) + sulphasalazine (3), 88% of those receiving ciclosporin (1) + methotrexate (2) + sulphasalazine (3), and only 24% of the sulphasalazine-alone group had achieved an ACR50 response. Withdrawals due to adverse events were similar in all three groups.

The first RCT reporting the efficacy of a step-down strategy found better outcomes of combined prednisolone, methotrexate, and sulphasalazine compared to sulphasalazine alone (COBRA trial).[17] Patients were randomly assigned, in a double blind fashion, to receive either combination therapy with prednisolone (60 mg/d in week 1 then tapered off at

Table 9.3 Randomised clinical trials of combination DMARD therapy is early RA

Study	Design and duration	Population studied	Treatment	Outcomes
Boers[17]	Double blind, RCT; 56 wk	155 patients with active RA; disease duration of ≤ 2 yr	Combined step-down PDN + MTX + SSZ *v* SSZ	Combined step-down treatment significantly improved disease activity and delayed joint erosion compared to SSZ alone
Dougados[30]	Double blind, RCT; 52 wk	205 patients with RA; disease duration ≤12 mth	Combined SSZ + MTX *v* SSZ *v* MTX	No significant differences in DAS, ACR20 response rates and radiological progression
Ferraccioli[88]	Open, RCT; 3 yr	126 patients with RA; mean disease duration of 1–2 yr	Combined step-up MTX + CsA + SSZ *v* combined step-up CsA + MTX + SSZ *v* SSZ	Combined step-up MTX + CsA + SSZ significantly increased ACR50 response rate compared to SSZ alone
Haagsma[31]	Double blind, RCT; 52 wk	105 patients with RA; disease duration of ≤ 12 mth	Combined SSZ + MTX *v* SSZ *v* MTX	No significant difference in DAS, ACR20 response rate, Ritchie articular index, number of swollen joints and ESR among the three groups
Marchesoni[89]	Single blind (assessor), RCT; 18 mth	57 patients with non-erosive RA; disease duration of 6–24 mth	CsA *v* MTX after combined CsA and MTX treatment for 6 mth	MTX significantly improved ACR20, 50, and 70 response rates at 24 mth with a lower rate of dropouts
Möttönen[25,83]	Open, RCT; 2 yr	195 patients with RA; disease duration of < 2 yr	Combination DMARD (SSZ + MTX + HCQ + PDN) *v* single DMARD	Remission rate and ACR50 response rate were higher in combination DMARD group; 4-mth delay to single DMARD significantly decreased remission rate
Proudman[85]	Open, RCT; 48 wk	82 patients with RA; DMARD-naïve, disease duration of < 12 mth	Combined CsA + MTX + IA methylPDN *v* SSZ	Combined DMARDs and IA steroid led to a more rapid disease suppression but had no effect on ACR response or remission rate

Abbreviations: as Table 9.1.

week 28), methotrexate (7·5 mg/week and discontinued at week 40), and sulphasalazine (2 g/d), or monotherapy with sulphasalazine alone. At 28 weeks, patients in the combination regimen showed significantly better outcomes, including disease activity measures, function, and ESR, than patients receiving monotherapy with sulphasalazine alone. The ACR20 (72% *v* 49%) and ACR50 (49% *v* 27%) response rates were significantly higher in the combination group than in the sulphasalazine group. At 56 and 80 weeks, after prednisolone and methotrexate were discontinued, there were no longer any differences in the disease activity and function measures between both groups. However, the rate of radiographic damage was significantly lower in the combination group. This finding was confirmed in the follow up study at 5 years.[22]

A second RCT reporting the results of a step-down regimen assessed the efficacy of an initial combination regime of methotrexate and ciclosporin, followed by either methotrexate or ciclosporin alone after 6 months.[89] At 18 months, 64% of patients receiving ciclosporin and 15% of those receiving methotrexate had withdrawn from the study. The main reason for withdrawals from the ciclosporin group was lack of efficacy. Three patients taking ciclosporin and one in the methotrexate group withdrew from the study because of adverse effects. The ACR20 response rate in the ciclosporin group was 41% compared to 89% in the methotrexate group; ACR50 response rates were 36% and 70%, respectively. The rate of radiographic progression was not significantly different between the two groups.

The toxicity of combination treatments depends on the drugs used, with monitoring for the most toxic part of the combination. The adverse effects of combination treatments may be greater than the sum of individual treatments because of potential interactions.

Table 9.4 shows the NNT and NNH for various DMARD combinations in trials of patients with early RA that have measured ACR response rates; when reported, we have included the NNT for ACR50 and ACR70 responses as well.

Evidence summary: Gold

One systematic review and several subsequent RCTs have found that combining certain DMARDs is more effective than using individual drugs alone (Visual Rx Faces 9.2). However, the balance between benefits and harm varies between combinations, and this balance should be considered in patients with early disease. We found no consistent evidence that any DMARD combination treatment is more effective than any one of the other combination treatments. There is a controversy about whether to initiate combination therapy early in the course of the disease, using a "step-down" approach, or whether to start treatment with a single drug, and then use a sequential "step-up" strategy. The ACR guidelines for the management of RA recommend starting methotrexate as monotherapy, or as a component of combination therapy, for patients whose treatment has not included this drug.

Case presentation 1

For this patient, there is no conclusive evidence that initiating combination therapy would be better in the long term than initiating methotrexate alone. Careful consideration of patient preferences in relation to potential risks and benefits with these strategies should guide the recommendation.

Question 4

Should patients with early RA be treated with a biologic agent?

In the past few years, a number of biologic therapies that target specific cytokines involved in the pathogenesis of RA have been developed. The efficacy and safety of some of these agents have been tested in placebo-controlled RCTs, and these agents have now been approved around the world for the treatment of RA. These biologic therapies include agents directed against tumour necrosis factor-α (TNF-α) (etanercept, infliximab, and adalimumab) and interleukin-1 (IL-1) (anakinra).

Table 9.4 Number needed to treat (NNT) and number needed to harm (NNH) for DMARD combinations

Study	Active treatment	Comparator	Criteria for NNT	NNT (95% CI)	NNH (95% CI) (criterion: toxicity withdrawals)
Early RA					
Boers[17]	Combined step-down PDN + MTX + SSZ	SSZ	ACR20 at 28 wk	5 (3, 13)	20 (NS)
Ferraccioli[88]	Combined step-up MTX + CsA + SSZ	SSZ	ACR50 at 18 mth	2 (2, 2)	8 (NS)
Dougados[30]	Combined SSZ + MTX	SSZ MTX	ACR20 at 52 wk ACR20 at 52 wk	20 (NS) 20 (NS)	100 (NS)* 33 (NS)
Haagsma[31]	Combined SSZ + MTX	SSZ MTX	ACR20 at 52 wk ACR20 at 52 wk	25 (NS) 17 (NS)	7 (NS) 12 (NS)
Möttönen[25]	Combined SSZ + MTX + HCQ + PDN	Single DMARD	ACR20 at 2 yr ACR50 at 2 yr Remission rate at 2 yr	17 (NS) 8 (NS) 6 (4, 17)	100 (NS)
Proudman[85]	Combined CsA + MTX + IA methylPDN	SSZ	ACR20 at 48 wk ACR50 at 48 wk	8 (NS) 12 (NS)	50 (NS)

Abbreviations: as Table 9.1.

*NNH reversed (comparator more withdrawals than combination).

Literature search

We found one systematic review of infliximab in the Cochrane Database,[90] one systematic review of adalimumab,[91] and one systematic review of anakinra.[92] We found an additional non-English language review of TNF-α inhibitors, which has not been translated.[93]

Outcome

There have been no head-to-head comparisons of biologic agents, so each has been reviewed separately. Table 9.5 shows the NNT and NNH for the various agents reviewed below. Only etanercept has been tested in patients with early RA, with results similar to those observed in patients with disease of longer duration.

Etanercept

We found two 6 month placebo controlled RCTs.[94,95] One RCT (234 patients who had failed to respond to other DMARDs) compared two doses of etanercept (25 mg and 10 mg, both given twice weekly) versus placebo.[94] More patients improved by at least 20% (ACR20 criteria) with etanercept 25 mg than with the lower dose or with placebo (59% with high dose etanercept versus 51% with low dose etanercept versus 11% with placebo; 10 mg versus placebo, $p < 0{\cdot}001$; 25 mg versus placebo, $p < 0{\cdot}001$; 25 mg versus 10 mg, $p = 0{\cdot}2$). Improvement by at least 50% (ACR50 criteria) was found in 40% of patients with high dose etanercept, in 24% with low dose etanercept, and in 5% with placebo (10 mg versus placebo; $p < 0{\cdot}001$; 25 mg versus placebo; $p < 0{\cdot}001$; 25 mg versus 10 mg; $p = 0{\cdot}03$). The RCT also found that etanercept improved functional status (disability index: 25 mg versus placebo; $p < 0{\cdot}05$) and quality of life (general health status: 25 mg versus placebo; $p < 0{\cdot}05$). The second RCT (89 patients with inadequate response to methotrexate) compared etanercept (25 mg/wk) versus

Table 9.5 Number needed to treat (NNT) and number needed to harm (NNH) for RCTs of biologic agents

Study	Active treatment	Comparator	Criteria for NNT	NNT (95% CI)	NNH (95% CI) (criterion: toxicity withdrawals)
Early RA					
Bathon[96]	ETA 25 mg	MTX	ACR20 at 12 mth	5 (4–9)	16 (9–100)
			ACR50 at 12 mth	20 (NS)	
			ACR70 at 12 mth	34 (NS)	
Genovese[97]	ETA 25 mg	MTX	ACR20 at 2 yr	8 (NS)	N/A
Established RA					
Maini[99]	IFX 3 mg/kg q 8 wk + MTX	MTX	ACR20 at 30 wk	4 (3–7)	100 (NS)
			ACR50 at 30 wk	5 (4–10)	
			ACR70 at 30 wk	13 (7–50)	
Lipsky[101]	IFX 3 mg/kg q 8 wk + MTX	MTX	ACR20 at 54 wk	4 (3–9)	50 (NS)
			ACR50 at 54 wk	8 (5–34)	
			ACR70 at 54 wk	13 (7–100)	
Weinblatt[103]	ADA 40 mg + MTX	MTX	ACR20 at 24 wk	2 (2–3)	33 (NS)
			ACR50 at 24 wk	3 (2–3)	
			ACR70 at 24 wk	5 (3–10)	
Moreland[94]	ETA 25 mg	Placebo	ACR20 at 6 mth	2 (2–2)	2 (2–4)*
			ACR50 at 6 mth	3 (2–3)	
			ACR70 at 6 mth	6 (4–12)	
Weinblatt[95]	ETA 25 mg + MTX	MTX	ACR20 at 24 wk	3 (2–4)	2 (2–5)*
			ACR50 at 24 wk	3 (2–5)	
			ACR70 at 24 wk	7 (4–20)	
Cohen[107]	ANK 1 mg/kg/d + MTX	MTX	ACR20 at 24 wk	6 (3–50)	10 (NS)
			ACR50 at 24 wk	5 (4–15)	
			ACR70 at 24 wk	10 (6–50)	

ADA, adalimumab; ANK, anakinra; ETA, etanercept; IFX, infliximab; MTX, methotrexate.

N/A, not available.

*NNH was calculated from the rate of injection site reaction.

placebo.[95] Patients were allowed to continue methotrexate. More patients achieved ACR20 criteria with etanercept than with placebo (71% *v* 27%; $p < 0.001$). A 12 month RCT (632 patients with early RA) compared methotrexate versus two doses of etanercept (10 mg and 25 mg, both given twice weekly).[96] It found significantly more patients achieved ACR20, ACR50, and ACR70 responses with etanercept 25 mg versus methotrexate at 6 months. By 12 months, there was no significant difference (72% *v* 65%; $p = 0.16$). The higher dose etancercept was significantly better than the lower dose in terms of ACR20, ACR50, and ACR70 response at 12 months ($p < 0.03$ for all comparisons). Continued improvement and delay of radiological progression were reported in the 2 year continuation study.[97] The most common adverse effect was mild injection site reaction (42–49% in the treated group versus 7–13% in the placebo group). Other adverse effects included upper respiratory symptoms or infections, headache, and diarrhoea. Autoantibodies to double stranded DNA developed in 5–9% of the treated group. Less than 1% of patients developed malignancies or infections in the 6 month trials. Reactivation of demyelinating disease has been described.

Infliximab

We found one systematic review in the Cochrane Database.[90] The review included two trials (*n* = 529) comparing infliximab with placebo, for a minimum duration of 6 months.[98,99] We found an additional RCT of 4 weeks' duration.[100] The first RCT in the review (101 patients) compared 1, 3, or 10 mg/kg infliximab with or without methotrexate versus placebo.[98] It found a greater improvement with 3 or 10 mg/kg infliximab versus placebo (ACR20 improvement: 60% in patients taking 3 or 10 mg/kg infliximab versus 15% in patients taking placebo).[98] The second RCT was a large multicentre study (428 patients with active disease not responsive to methotrexate) that compared five groups over 7 months: placebo versus infliximab at 3 mg/kg or 10 mg/kg, administered every 4 or 8 weeks.[99] All continued to receive methotrexate. ACR20 criteria were reached by 50–58% who received infliximab/methotrexate and by 20% of the methotrexate/placebo group. ACR50 was attained by 26–31% of the patients receiving infliximab and by 5% in the placebo group ($p < 0{\cdot}001$). Longer term results at 54 weeks found that all infliximab groups significantly improved versus placebo in terms of ACR20, ACR50, and ACR70 criteria (all results $p < 0{\cdot}05$)[101] (Visual Rx Faces 9.3). The additional RCT of 4 weeks' duration (73 patients) compared infliximab 1 mg/kg versus infliximab 10 mg/kg versus placebo over 4 weeks, and showed similar results favouring infliximab.[100] In the RCTs, common adverse reactions were upper respiratory infections, headache, diarrhoea, and abdominal pain. Reactions during or immediately after the injection (headache, nausea, and urticaria) were also observed in the placebo groups, but were more frequent with infliximab. Antibodies to double stranded DNA were found in about 16% of patients taking infliximab. The rates of serious adverse effects in treated and placebo groups were not significantly different, but there was insufficient power to detect clinically important differences. Worldwide, over 150 cases of reactivation of tuberculosis have been documented, and patients should be screened for previous tuberculosis before treatment.

Adalimumab

We found one review of adalimumab, including the results of five studies, but not all were published as full papers.[91] Two of the trials compared adalimumab with placebo and were reported as full publications. The first study compared a single dose of adalimumab, at 0·5, 1, 3, 5 and 10 mg/kg, with placebo (*n* = 120; 89 on adalimumab and 31 on placebo).[102] Patients did not receive any concomitant DMARDs. Efficacy was measured on day 29 after the injection. ACR20 response rate for increasing dosages of adalimumab were 47%, 67%, 78%, 67%, and 83% respectively, compared to 16% for placebo. The second RCT (ARMADA trial) was a 24 week study including 271 patients, randomly assigned to receive adalimumab at 20, 40, or 80 mg, or placebo.[103] All patients were receiving methotrexate and continued this therapy at a stable dose. ACR20 response rates with increasing dosages of adalimumab were 48%, 67%, and 66%, compared to 14% in the placebo group. In both trials, adalimumab was well tolerated; adverse event rates did not differ between the adalimumab and placebo groups.

Anakinra

We found one systematic review of anakinra (without meta-analysis), which included 4 RCTs.[92] Two of the trials were of short duration[104,105] and the other two ran for 24 weeks.[106,107] One 24 week

Visual Rx Faces 9.3 NNT for infliximab + MTX compared to MTX

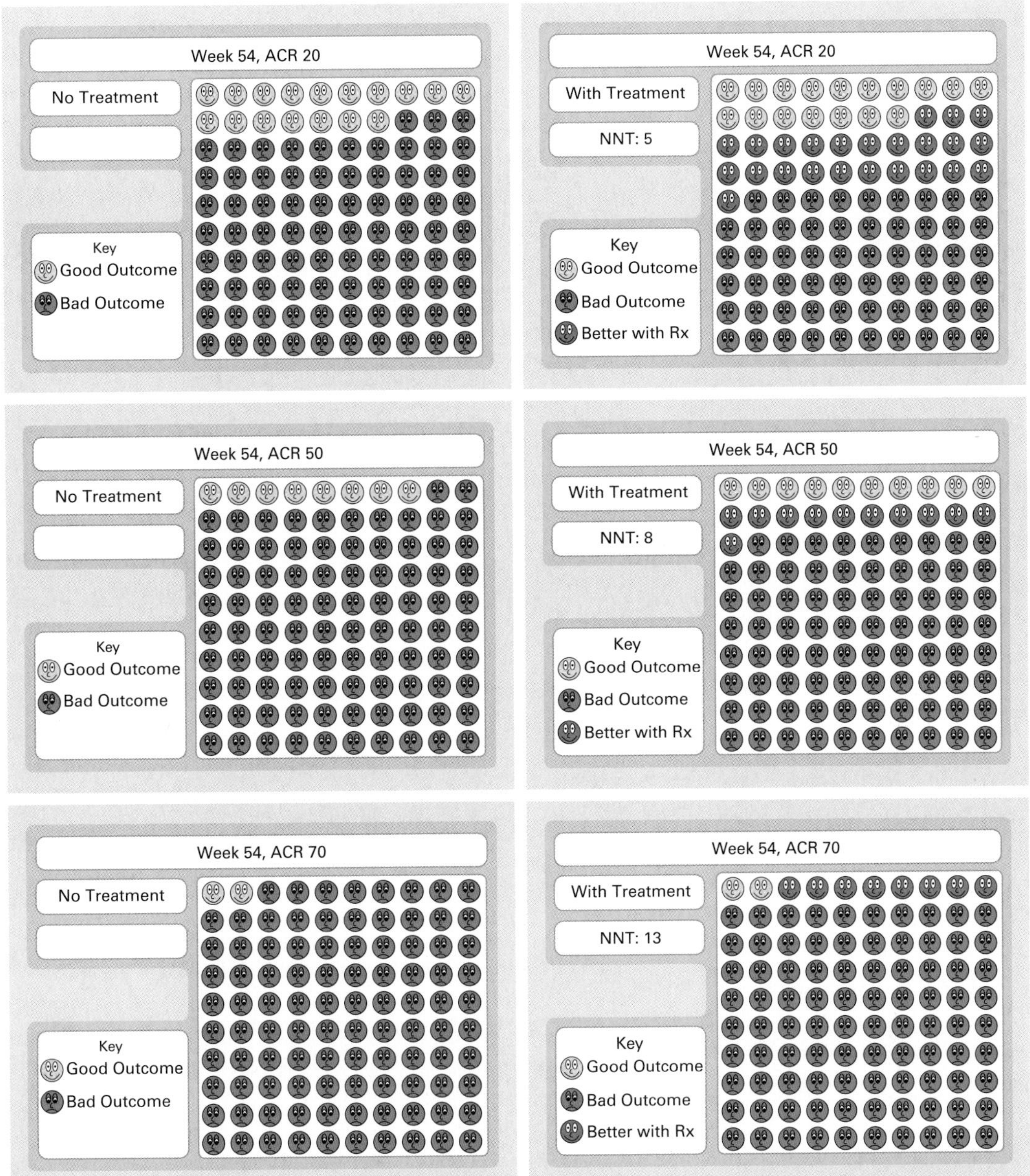

trial (*n* = 472) compared anakinra at dosages of 30 mg, 75 mg, and 150 mg to placebo.[106] More patients in the anakinra group achieved ACR20 responses than those on placebo (43% *v* 27%, p = 0·01). In addition, all anakinra groups had a significant reduction in radiological progression. A longer term evaluation of the patients included in this trial showed that anakinra was well tolerated over a period of 76 weeks.[108] The other trial (*n* = 419) compared anakinra at dosages of 0·04, 0·1, 0·4, 1·0, or 2·0 mg/kg against placebo;[107] all patients were receiving methotrexate as well. The ACR20 response rate in the placebo group was 19%, compared to 46% in the 1·0 mg/kg anakinra group (p = 0·001) and 38% in the 2·0 mg/kg group (p = 0·007). In the RCTs, there were no differences observed in the number of withdrawals due to adverse reactions between anakinra and placebo. The most common adverse event was injection-site reaction. The long term safety follow up of one of the trials showed that anakinra was well tolerated over a period of one year.[108]

Evidence summary: Gold

Systematic reviews and RCTs have found that TNF-α and IL-1 inhibitors (etanercept, infliximab, adalumimab, anakinra) improve symptoms and reduce disease activity and joint inflammation. TNF-α inhibitors may be more efficacious than anakinra, but additional, longer term data is needed to compare these drugs. Short term toxicity is relatively low, but long term safety less clear. Problems have been identified with reactivation of demyelinating disease and tuberculosis.

These drugs are generally restricted to patients who have failed conventional disease modifying antirheumatic drugs and are used in secondary care. Their effects on disease activity occurred within weeks, unlike other DMARDs that may take several months to have an effect.

The ACR guidelines recommend biologic agents as an option for those patients who have shown suboptimal methotrexate response.

Case presentation 1

The patient presented in Case 1 is DMARD naive; we would not recommend a biologic agent for this patient as her initial therapy because of the high cost of these drugs, and the uncertainty in relation to their long term effects.

Question 5

Are low dose oral corticosteroids beneficial in the treatment of patients with RA?

Literature search

We found two systematic reviews.[109,110]

Outcome

The first review (search date 1997, 10 RCTs, 402 patients) compared short term treatment with a low dose of prednisolone (15 mg/day for several weeks) against placebo or non-steroidal anti-inflammatory drugs.[109] It found that, in the short term, prednisolone had a greater effect than did placebo or non-steroidal anti-inflammatory drugs in controlling disease activity. Prednisolone versus placebo improved pain, grip strength, and joint tenderness (WMD for the number of tender joints –12, 95% CI –18 to –6). The second review (search date 1998, 7 RCTs, 508 patients) evaluated longer term treatment with corticosteroids (for at least 3 months).[110] It found that longer term treatment with prednisolone was superior to placebo (WMD for tender joints –0.37, 95% CI –0·59 to –0·14; swollen joints –0·41, 95% CI –0·67 to –0·16; pain –0·43, 95% CI –0·74 to –0·12; and functional status –0·57, 95% CI –0·92 to –0·22). The review also found that prednisolone was comparable to aspirin or chloroquine. One RCT (128 patients) included in the review evaluated radiological damage.[111] It found a significant decrease in the rate of progression in patients treated with prednisolone 7.5 mg daily versus placebo over 2 years. The follow up study of patients in this RCT found that joint destruction resumed after discontinuing prednisolone.[112] One systematic review (search date 1998, 1 RCT, 56 patients with RA diagnosed at age ≥ 60 years) found no significant difference between oral prednisolone and chloroquine in improving disease activity.[110] An additional RCT compared prednisone 10 mg/day with placebo in 81 patients with early RA.[113] Patients in the prednisone group showed significantly less radiological progression after 6 months than those receiving placebo.

Serious long term adverse effects of corticosteroids include hypertension, diabetes, osteoporosis, infections, gastrointestinal ulcers, obesity, and hirsutism. Observational studies of patients with RA have suggested that mortality may be increased by long term treatment with steroids.[114] However, many of those studies included patients receiving dosages greater than 7·5 mg daily, which are higher than those currently recommended. One systematic review found that bone loss was limited when lower dosages were prescribed.[115]

Evidence summary: Gold

Two systematic reviews, including 10 RCTs, have found benefit from both short and longer term treatment (> 3 months) with low dose oral corticosteroids. Short term treatment reduces disease activity and joint inflammation. Longer term treatment may reduce radiological progression while treatment continues. However, long term use is associated with considerable adverse effects.

ACR guidelines suggest the decision to give oral corticosteroids should balance the potential for increased co-morbidity, which is affected by individual risk factors, and the potential improvement in disease activity.

Case presentation 1

For this patient, low dose corticosteroids could be an option, in addition to the DMARD treatment, but the benefit/risk ratio, and the uncertainty about overall effectiveness in the long-term, should be carefully discussed.

Question 6

Are COX-2 inhibitors a better therapeutic choice than non-selective COX-inhibitors in patients with RA?

Non-steroidal anti-inflammatory drugs (NSAIDs) have long been used to control the symptoms of RA. Traditional non-selective NSAIDs inhibit both cyclo-oxygenase isoenzymes COX-1 and COX-2. COX-1 regulates platelet activation, renal function, and gastrointestinal protection, and a major drawback of non-selective NSAIDs is the high incidence of serious upper gastrointestinal events (ulcers and bleeds). COX-2 is primarily involved in inflammatory processes. A new class of drugs, selective COX-2 inhibitors, was recently introduced in the market, under the expectation that selective COX-2 inhibition will decrease inflammation, without the associated gastrointestinal events observed with non-selective NSAIDs

Literature search

We found two systematic reviews in the Cochrane Database, one for celecoxib and one for rofecoxib. In addition, we found RCTs that included patients with osteoarthritis as well, but reported results related to the safety profile of these drugs, which can be relevant to patients with RA.

Outcome

The celecoxib review[116] included five RCTs with 4465 participants; three of the studies included patients with osteoarthitis as well (only trials that reported separate results for patients with RA and osteoarthritis were included). In the various trials, celecoxib was compared to placebo, naproxen, diclofenac, and ibuprofen. In terms of efficacy, when compared to placebo, celecoxib was significantly superior. No statistically significant differences were observed when it was compared to other NSAIDs (naproxen, diclofenac or ibuprofen). The 6 month analysis showed a reduced rate of upper gastrointestinal events, but this reduction was not evident beyond 6 months. The largest celecoxib RCT, the 6 month CLASS study, which assessed 7968 patients, was not included in the review because it did not provide separate results for RA and osteoarthritis patients.[117] The CLASS study compared celecoxib to ibuprofen or diclofenac, and showed that the overall rates of upper gastrointestinal ulcer events in the celecoxib group was not significantly different from the rates observed in the ibuprofen group (0·76% *v* 1·45%, p = 0.09); subgroup analyses showed that the difference was significant for patients who were not receiving aspirin. In patients receiving aspirin, no differences were observed. The rofecoxib review[118] included two RCTs with 8734 participants. One trial compared rofecoxib to placebo (8 weeks, 658 patients), and the other to naproxen.[119,120] The efficacy of rofecoxib was significantly better than that of placebo, and similar to that of naproxen. The safety profile of rofecoxib was similar to that observed in patients receiving placebo. Rofecoxib was statistically superior to naproxen and reduced by half the number of upper gastrointestinal events (RR = 0·46; 95% CI = 0·34–0·63). However, rofecoxib increased the risk of a cardiovascular event, when compared to naproxen: 1·1% *v* 0·47% respectively (RR = 2·4; 95% CI = 1·4–4·0). This included an increase in the risk of a non-fatal myocardial infarction (0·44% *v* 0·10%; RR = 4·5; 95% CI = 1·5–13·2).

Evidence summary: Gold

Seven RCTs included in two systematic reviews showed that celecoxib and rofecoxib are superior to placebo in controlling RA symptoms, and their efficacy is similar to the efficacy observed with other non-selective NSAIDs. COX-2 inhibitors appear to reduce the risk of upper gastrointestinal events compared to other NSAIDs, but the evidence is somewhat conflicting. For celecoxib, this decrease may be short-lived and appears to be significant only for patients not receiving aspirin. Rofecoxib decreases the risk of upper gastrointestinal lesions compared to naproxen, but increases the risk of cardiovascular events.

The evidence related to the risk–benefit ratios of COX-2 inhibitors is uncertain. The potential advantage of selective COX-2 inhibitors, through reduction of gastrointestinal adverse events, has to be balanced against their increased costs compared to non-selective NSAIDs, the evidence suggesting that the reduced risk for gastrointestinal complications may only be short-lived, and the increase in cardiovascular events.

The ACR guidelines recommend the use of a selective COX-2 inhibitor, or a combination of an NSAID with a gastroprotective agent for RA patients at risk of serious gastrointestinal effects.

Case presentation 1

The patient does not appear to be at increased risk for gastrointestinal events. Because of the high cost and potential cardiovascular morbidity associated with these agents, we would not recommend their use at this time.

Question 7

Should patients with RA be referred to education programmes?

Literature search

We found one systematic review of patient education programmes for RA in the Cochrane Database. We found an additional systematic review examining the efficacy of disease management programmes in RA, which included patient education as one of the interventions.

Outcome

The Cochrane Review included 24 RCTs with relevant data.[121] Moderately sized effects were observed for patient global assessment in the short term. Small short term effects were observed for physical function, joint counts, and psychological status. No significant long term effects were observed. The systematic review of disease management programmes, which included 11 studies,[122] found a small benefit that did not reach statistical significance. Only more intensive ongoing interventions, lasting more than 5 weeks, showed statistically significant improvement in patients' functional status.

Evidence summary: Gold

The systematic review of 24 RCTs of patient education programmes appears to have shown significant but small beneficial effects in patients with RA. No longer term benefits were observed.

The ACR guidelines recommend that patients with RA learn and accept the consequences of living with RA, and participate fully in disease management decision making. There are no known deleterious effects from education programmes, but there appear to be some small benefits; in addition, the impact on psychosocial well-being has not been well studied to date.

Case presentation 1

We would recommend that the patient be offered information about patient education programmes so that she may elect to join one of them.

Question 8

Are non-pharmacological modalities effective in patients with RA?

Literature search

We found several systematic reviews in the Cochrane Database examining the effects of various physical and non-pharmacological modalities on RA.

Outcome

Two studies (n = 84) were included in a systematic review of acupuncture and electroacupuncture for RA.[123] No significant benefits were observed in the study reporting the effect of acupuncture. In the second study, using electroacupuncture, a significant decrease in knee pain 24 hours post-treatment was observed in the group receiving electroacupuncture.

A systematic review of ultrasound in RA included two controlled clinical trials (80 patients).[124] Ultrasound of the hand significantly increased grip strength. No significant differences were observed in other measures. The methodological quality of the trials was low.

A systematic review of thermotherapy in patients with RA included seven studies (328 patients).[125] The interventions examined were ice pack applications, cryotherapy, and faradic baths. No significant beneficial effects were observed, compared to controls, in joint counts, pain, range of motion, grip strength, or hand function. No harmful effects were observed.

One systematic review assessed the efficacy of electrical stimulation for improving muscle strength and function in patients with RA.[126] Only one RCT met the inclusion criteria. The results showed that electrical stimulation increased grip strength and fatigue resistance in patients with RA, but the methodological quality of the trial was low.

One systematic review examined the role of dynamic exercise in RA (6 RCTs; n = 251).[127] The exercise programme had to include exercise with an intensity level exceeding 60% of maximal heart rate during at least 20 minutes, twice a week, and for 6 weeks or more. The review included six trials, and no meta-analysis was performed. The review concluded that dynamic exercise increased aerobic capacity and muscle strength, with no detrimental effects on pain and disease activity. No clear effects were observed on functional ability.

Evidence summary: Silver

Dynamic exercise increases aerobic capacity and muscle strength in patients with RA with no detrimental effects on their disease status. There is no evidence to show that other non-pharmacological physical modalities have substantial beneficial effects in the treatment of RA. Ultrasound may increase hand strength in patients with RA, and electroacupuncture may produce short-term relief. The methodological quality of these studies is poor. Additional larger, better designed studies are needed.

Case presentation 1

Dynamic exercise could be an option for this patient. Although beneficial effects on RA outcomes have not been observed, dynamic exercise increases muscle strength and aerobic capacity, with no detrimental effects on disease activity. At present, we would not recommend any of the other non-pharmacological therapies.

Case presentation 2

Mr T. is a 55-year-old male and developed RA 5 years ago. He was started on NSAIDS, oral prednisone 5 mg/day, and oral methotrexate, which was progressively increased to a weekly dose of 15 mg. He had a very good response, with significant reduction of his joint pain and swelling. Mr T. is an electrician, who had stopped working because of his RA, but was able to return to full-time work with this regime. About a year ago, his condition started to progressively worsen, his joint pain and swelling increased, his functional status declined, and he started having difficulties once again with his daily activities and work. His physical examination shows symmetrical polyarthritis and some limitation in the range of motion of shoulders, wrists, and proximal interphalangeal joints. His hand radiographs show multiple erosions in the proximal interphalangeal and metacarpophalangeal joints. Overall, his clinical status is slightly better than when he started methotrexate therapy, but there has been a clear decline in the past months.

Introduction

Most patients with RA are initially treated with methotrexate. However, long term cohort studies have shown that methotrexate failure rates, although lower than the rates observed with other DMARDs, remain high. Approximately 50% of the patients will have discontinued methotrexate therapy after 5 years, because of lack of efficacy or adverse events. Many patients, who initially respond to methotrexate, show progressive resistance and partial response in subsequent years. In the past, patients who failed one DMARD therapy were switched to a different drug. When the response has been partial, but not optimal, an alternative is to "step up" the treatment by adding one or more DMARDs.

Question 9

What is the treatment of choice in a patient who has partially failed methotrexate therapy?

Literature search

Studies evaluating the comparative performance of DMARDs and biologic agents have been reviewed in previous sections. In addition, we found one systematic review of "step-up" trials following methotrexate failure.

Outcome

The step-up systematic review[128] included four placebo controlled trials of at least 6 months' duration. The drugs evaluated in the trials included ciclosporin, leflunomide, etanercept, and infliximab. All drugs were significantly better than placebo (remaining in methotrexate therapy alone). No significant differences in efficacy (ACR20 response) were observed among drugs. The NNT for the various strategies were as follows: ciclosporin 3, 95% CI 2–6; leflunomide 4, 95% CI 3–6; etanercept 2, 95% CI 1–4; and infliximab 3, 95% CI 2–4.

No trial has compared a step-up approach with switching DMARDs. It is still uncertain whether the improvements in response by adding a DMARD could also be achieved by switching to this other DMARD and discontinuing methotrexate.

Evidence summary: Gold

A systematic review, including four RCTs, found that several different DMARDs can be added to methotrexate in patients with partial response to improve efficacy. The evidence does not show any significant differences between DMARDs. The decision to add a particular DMARD to methotrexate should also take into consideration potential toxicity and costs.

The ACR guidelines recommend that patients with a suboptimal methotrexate response receive combination therapy, be switched to another DMARD monotherapy, or receive a biologic agent (as monotherapy or in combination).

Case presentation 2

There is no evidence to choose one of these alternatives over another. We would recommend that the treating physician discuss the various alternatives and potential benefits and risks with the patient in Case 2. Other co-morbidities that may impact on the development of adverse events with any of these approaches should be considered.

Case presentation 3

Fifty-eight-year-old Mrs M. has had seropositive RA for the past 8 years. She was initially treated with antimalarials and had a partial response to this treatment, with a decrease in joint pain and swelling. After 3 years, her arthritis started to get progressively worse, and she developed radiographic erosions in both hands. The antimalarials were discontinued, and she was started on sulphasalazine. Mrs M. was unable to tolerate sulphasalazine because of gastrointestinal adverse events, so this treatment was discontinued after a few months, and since her arthritis was still active and she was experiencing some functional decline, she was started on oral methotrexate, 10 mg per week. She had an excellent response, with substantial pain decrease and major improvement in her joint swelling. She was able to get back to her daily activities and work with no discomfort. After 2 years of treatment with methotrexate, she experienced a flare, with an increase in joint swelling, pain, and significant morning stiffness. The methotrexate dose was progressively increased to 20 mg per week. In a few months, her disease activity was controlled, and the methotrexate dose was decreased to 15 mg per week. For the past 2 years, Mrs M. has been mostly asymptomatic and only complains of occasional joint pain and morning stiffness. Her physical examination reveals no joint swelling and just a minor decrease in the range of motion of the small joints of her hands, which results in some difficulty in closing her fists. Her hand radiographs show slight radiological progression, with a few more erosions in the proximal interphalageal joints, when compared to her radiographs from 5 years before. Her laboratory tests, including CBC and ESR are normal. Mrs M. wonders if it would be reasonable for her to discontinue treatment with methotrexate, since she has been asymptomatic for the past 2 years.

Question 10

For how long should patients with RA continue to receive DMARD?

Literature search

Evidence from the effects of discontinuing DMARDs has been, for the most part, observational. We found one RCT of discontinuation versus continuation of DMARD treatment.

Outcome

Clinical practice now means that most people with RA are taking a DMARD for the long term, and this will limit our ability to answer this question. We found one non-systematic review of 122 studies of disease modifying antirheumatic drugs (DMARDs) (including 57 single or double blinded RCTs, 35 open label RCTs, and 19 observational studies; 16 071 people).[129] It found that 90% of participants had been followed for one year or less. Short term clinical trials in people with rheumatoid arthritis found beneficial effects for most DMARDs, but in the longer-term, effectiveness of these drugs seemed to decline. Observational studies have found that after a few years, most people discontinued the prescribed DMARD, either because of toxicity or lack of effectiveness. We found limited evidence suggesting that discontinuing DMARDs, even for people in remission, may result in disease exacerbation or flare. Few RCTs have followed people for more than one year, and most people discontinue treatment with an individual drug within a few years because of toxicity or lack of effectiveness. These effects may vary according to the DMARD being discontinued. One RCT (285 people who had been on second line treatment for a median of 5 years and in remission) compared continuation of second line treatment versus placebo.[130] It found that at 52 weeks, significantly more people on placebo had a flare (22% with active treatment versus 38% with placebo; RR 0·57, 95% CI 0·39–0·84).

Effects may vary according to DMARDs being discontinued, with some evidence that methotrexate has a shorter time to relapse. In a RCT of 84 patients allocated to methotrexate or gold, patients with early RA stopping gold because of adverse effects showed longer sustained remission than patients stopping methotrexate.[131]

Evidence summary: Silver

One RCT found a significant increase in flares among people in remission who discontinued disease modifying antirheumatic drugs.

Recommendation for case presentation 3

For Case 3 we would recommend that the risks of discontinuing therapy be clearly explained to the patient. If the patient is intent in discontinuing treatment, tapering off should be slow, and under close monitoring to promptly identify a relapse.

References

1 Gabriel SE. The epidemiology of rheumatoid arthritis. *Rheum Dis Clin North Am* 2001;**27**(2):269–281.

2 Wilske KR, Healey LA. Remodeling the pyramid – a concept whose time has come. *J Rheumatol* 1989;**16**(5):565–7.

3 Boers M. Rheumatoid arthritis. Treatment of early disease. *Rheum Dis Clin North Am* 2001;**27**(2):405–14.

4 Guidelines for the management of rheumatoid arthritis: 2002 Update. *Arthritis Rheum* 2002;**46**(2):328–46.

5 Boers M, Tugwell P, Felson DT, *et al.* World Health Organization and International League of Associations for Rheumatology core endpoints for symptom modifying antirheumatic drugs in rheumatoid arthritis clinical trials. *J Rheumatol* Suppl 1994;**41**:86–9.

6 Felson DT, Anderson JJ, Boers M, *et al.* American College of Rheumatology. Preliminary definition of improvement in rheumatoid arthritis. *Arthritis Rheum* 1995;**38**(6):727–35.

7 van Gestel AM, Anderson JJ, van Riel PL, *et al.* ACR and EULAR improvement criteria have comparable validity in rheumatoid arthritis trials. American College of Rheumatology European League of Associations for Rheumatology. *J Rheumatol* 1999;**26**(3):705–11.

8 Cook RJ, Sackett DL. The number needed to treat: a clinically useful measure of treatment effect. *BMJ* 1995;**310**(6977):452–4.

9 Laupacis A, Sackett DL, Roberts RS. An assessment of clinically useful measures of the consequences of treatment. *N Engl J Med* 1988;**318**(26):1728–33.

10 Sackett DL, Straus S, Richardson SW, Rosenberg W, Haynes BR. Therapy. *Evidence-based medicine. How to practice and teach EBM, 2nd ed.* Edinburgh: Churchill Livingstone, 2000:105–53.

11 Norman GR, Sridhar FG, Guyatt GH, Walter SD. Relation of distribution- and anchor-based approaches in interpretation of changes in health-related quality of life. *Med Care* 2001;**39**(10):1039–47.

12 Green M, Marzo-Ortega H, McGonagle D, *et al.* Persistence of mild, early inflammatory arthritis: the importance of disease duration, rheumatoid factor, and the shared epitope. *Arthritis Rheum* 1999;**42**(10):2184–8.

13 Emery P, Breedveld FC, Dougados M, Kalden JR, Schiff MH, Smolen JS. Early referral recommendation for newly diagnosed rheumatoid arthritis: evidence based development of a clinical guide. *Ann Rheum Dis* 2002;**61**(4):290–7.

14 Quinn MA, Conaghan PG, Emery P. The therapeutic approach of early intervention for rheumatoid arthritis: what is the evidence? *Rheumatology (Oxford)* 2001;**40**(11):1211–20.

15 Tsakonas E, Fitzgerald AA, Fitzcharles MA, *et al.* Consequences of delayed therapy with second-line agents in rheumatoid arthritis: a 3 year followup on the hydroxychloroquine in early rheumatoid arthritis (HERA study). *J Rheumatol* 2000;**27**(3):623–9.

16 O'Dell JR, Haire CE, Palmer W, *et al.* Treatment of early rheumatoid arthritis with minocycline or placebo: results of a randomised, double-blind, placebo-controlled trial. *Arthritis Rheum* 1997;**40**(5):842–8.

17 Boers M, Verhoeven AC, Markusse HM, *et al.* Randomised comparison of combined step-down prednisolone, methotrexate and sulphasalazine with sulphasalazine alone in early rheumatoid arthritis. *Lancet* 1997;**350**(9074):309–18.

18 Buckland-Wright JC, Clarke GS, Chikanza IC, Grahame R. Quantitative microfocal radiography detects changes in erosion area in patients with early rheumatoid arthritis treated with myocrisine. *J Rheumatol* 1993;**20**(2):243–7.

19 Egsmose C, Lund B, Borg G, *et al.* Patients with rheumatoid arthritis benefit from early 2nd line therapy: 5 year followup of a prospective double blind placebo controlled study. *J Rheumatol* 1995;**22**(12):2208–13.

20 Munro R, Hampson R, McEntegart A, *et al.* Improved functional outcome in patients with early rheumatoid arthritis treated with intramuscular gold: results of a five year prospective study. *Ann Rheum Dis* 1998;**57**(2):88–93.

21 van der Heide A, Jacobs JW, Bijlsma JW, *et al.* The effectiveness of early treatment with "second-line" antirheumatic drugs. A randomised, controlled trial. *Ann Intern Med* 1996;**124**(8):699–707.

22 Landewe RB, Boers M, Verhoeven AC, *et al.* COBRA combination therapy in patients with early rheumatoid arthritis: long-term structural benefits of a brief intervention. *Arthritis Rheum* 2002;**46**(2):347–56.

23 Lard LR, Visser H, Speyer I, *et al.* Early versus delayed treatment in patients with recent-onset rheumatoid arthritis: comparison of two cohorts who received different treatment strategies. *Am J Med* 2001;**111**(6):446–51.

24 Lard LR, Boers M, Verhoeven A, *et al.* Early and aggressive treatment of rheumatoid arthritis patients affects the association of HLA class II antigens with progression of joint damage. *Arthritis Rheum* 2002;**46**(4):899–905.

25 Möttönen T, Hannonen P, Korpela M, *et al.* Delay to institution of therapy and induction of remission using single-drug or combination-disease-modifying antirheumatic drug therapy in early rheumatoid arthritis. *Arthritis Rheum* 2002;**46**(4):894–8.

26 Suarez-Almazor ME, Belseck E, Shea B, Wells G, Tugwell P. Methotrexate for rheumatoid arthritis. *Cochrane Database Syst Rev* 2000;(2):CD000957.

27 Emery P, Breedveld FC, Lemmel EM, *et al.* A comparison of the efficacy and safety of leflunomide and methotrexate for the treatment of rheumatoid arthritis. *Rheumatology (Oxford)* 2000;**39**(6):655–65.

28 Strand V, Cohen S, Schiff M, *et al.* Treatment of active rheumatoid arthritis with leflunomide compared with placebo and methotrexate. Leflunomide Rheumatoid Arthritis Investigators Group. *Arch Intern Med* 1999;**159**(21):2542–50.

29 Felson DT, Anderson JJ, Meenan RF. Use of short-term efficacy/toxicity tradeoffs to select second-line drugs in rheumatoid arthritis. A metaanalysis of published clinical trials. *Arthritis Rheum* 1992;**35**(10):1117–25.

30 Dougados M, Combe B, Cantagrel A, *et al.* Combination therapy in early rheumatoid arthritis: a randomised, controlled, double blind 52 week clinical trial of

sulphasalazine and methotrexate compared with the single components. *Ann Rheum Dis* 1999;**58**(4):220–5.

31 Haagsma CJ, van Riel PL, de Jong AJ, van de Putte LB. Combination of sulphasalazine and methotrexate versus the single components in early rheumatoid arthritis: a randomised, controlled, double-blind, 52 week clinical trial. *Br J Rheumatol* 1997;**36**(10):1082–8.

32 Hamilton J, McInnes IB, Thomson EA, *et al.* Comparative study of intramuscular gold and methotrexate in a rheumatoid arthritis population from a socially deprived area. *Ann Rheum Dis* 2001;**60**(6):566–72.

33 Rau R, Herborn G, Menninger H, Sangha O. Radiographic outcome after three years of patients with early erosive rheumatoid arthritis treated with intramuscular methotrexate or parenteral gold. Extension of a one-year double-blind study in 174 patients. *Rheumatology (Oxford)* 2002;**41**(2):196–204.

34 Felson DT, Anderson JJ, Meenan RF. The comparative efficacy and toxicity of second-line drugs in rheumatoid arthritis. Results of two metaanalyses. *Arthritis Rheum* 1990;**33**(10):1449–61.

35 Gotzsche PC, Podenphant J, Olesen M, Halberg P. Meta-analysis of second-line antirheumatic drugs: sample size bias and uncertain benefit. *J Clin Epidemiol* 1992;**45**(6): 587–94.

36 Suarez-Almazor ME, Belseck E, Wells G, Shea B, Tugwell P. Meta-analyses of placebo controlled trials of disease-modifying antirheumatic drugs (DMARD for the treatment of rheumatoid arthritis (RA). *Arthritis Rheum* 1998;**41**: S153.

37 Alarcon GS, Lopez-Mendez A, Walter J, *et al.* Radiographic evidence of disease progression in methotrexate treated and nonmethotrexate disease modifying antirheumatic drug treated rheumatoid arthritis patients: a meta-analysis. *J Rheumatol* 1992;**19**(12):1868–73.

38 Maetzel A, Wong A, Strand V, Tugwell P, Wells G, Bombardier C. Meta-analysis of treatment termination rates among rheumatoid arthritis patients receiving disease-modifying anti-rheumatic drugs. *Rheumatology (Oxford)* 2000;**39**(9):975–81.

39 Ortiz Z, Shea B, Suarez-Almazor ME, Moher D, Wells GA, Tugwell P. The efficacy of folic acid and folinic acid in reducing methotrexate gastrointestinal toxicity in rheumatoid arthritis. A metaanalysis of randomised controlled trials. *J Rheumatol* 1998;**25**(1):36–43.

40 Beauparlant P, Papp K, Haraoui B. The incidence of cancer associated with the treatment of rheumatoid arthritis. *Semin Arthritis Rheum* 1999;**29**(3):148–58.

41 Choi HK, Hernan MA, Seeger JD, Robins JM, Wolfe F. Methotrexate and mortality in patients with rheumatoid arthritis: a prospective study. *Lancet* 2002;**359**(9313): 1173–7.

42 Guidelines for monitoring drug therapy in rheumatoid arthritis. American College of Rheumatology Ad Hoc Committee on Clinical Guidelines. *Arthritis Rheum* 1996;**39**(5):723–31.

43 Suarez-Almazor ME, Belseck E, Shea B, Wells G, Tugwell P. Sulfasalazine for rheumatoid arthritis. *Cochrane Database Syst Rev* 2000;(2):CD000958.

44 Weinblatt ME, Reda D, Henderson W, *et al.* Sulfasalazine treatment for rheumatoid arthritis: a metaanalysis of 15 randomised trials. *J Rheumatol* 1999;**26**(10):2123–30.

45 Smolen JS, Kalden JR, Scott DL, *et al.* Efficacy and safety of leflunomide compared with placebo and sulphasalazine in active rheumatoid arthritis: a double-blind, randomised, multicentre trial. European Leflunomide Study Group. *Lancet* 1999;**353**(9149): 259–66.

46 van der Heijde DM, van Riel PL, Nuver-Zwart IH, Gribnau FW, vad de Putte LB. Effects of hydroxychloroquine and sulphasalazine on progression of joint damage in rheumatoid arthritis. *Lancet* 1989;**1**(8646):1036–8.

47 Capell HA, Maiden N, Madhok R, Hampson R, Thomson EA. Intention-to-treat analysis of 200 patients with rheumatoid arthritis 12 years after random allocation to either sulfasalazine or penicillamine. *J Rheumatol* 1998;**25**(10):1880–6.

48 Suarez-Almazor ME, Belseck E, Shea B, Homik J, Wells G, Tugwell P. Antimalarials for treating rheumatoid arthritis. *Cochrane Database Syst Rev* 2000;(4): CD000959.

49 Scull E. Chloroquine and hydroxychloroquine therapy in rheumatoid arthritis. *Arthritis Rheum* 1962;**5**:30–6.

50 Finbloom DS, Silver K, Newsome DA, Gunkel R. Comparison of hydroxychloroquine and chloroquine use and the development of retinal toxicity. *J Rheumatol* 1985;**12**(4):692–4.

51 Esdaile JM, Suissa S, Shiroky JB, *et al.* A randomised trial of hydroxychloroquine in early rheumatoid arthritis: the HERA study. *Am J Med* 1995;**98**:156–68.

52 Jessop JD, O'Sullivan MM, Lewis PA, *et al.* A long-term five-year randomised controlled trial of hydroxychloroquine, sodium aurothiomalate, auranofin and penicillamine in the treatment of patients with rheumatoid arthritis. *Br J Rheumatol* 1998;**37**(9): 992–1002.

53 Clark P, Tugwell P, Bennet K, *et al.* Injectable gold for rheumatoid arthritis. *Cochrane Database Syst Rev* 2000;(2):CD000520.

54 Rau R. Does parenteral gold retard radiological progression in rheumatoid arthritis? *Z Rheumatol* 1996;**55**:307–18.

55 Kvien TK, Zeidler HK, Hannonen P, *et al.* Long term efficacy and safety of cyclosporin versus parenteral gold in early rheumatoid arthritis: a three year study of radiographic progression, renal function, and arterial hypertension. *Ann Rheum Dis* 2002;**61**:511–16.

56 Suarez-Almazor ME, Spooner C, Belseck E. Penicillamine for rheumatoid arthritis. *Cochrane Database Syst Rev* 2000;(2):CD001460.

57 Hewitson PJ, Debroe S, McBride A, Milne R. Leflunomide and rheumatoid arthritis: a systematic review of effectiveness, safety and cost implications. *J Clin Pharm Ther* 2000;**25**(4):295–302.

58 Osiri M, Shea B, Robinson V, *et al.* Leflunomide for treating rheumatoid arthritis. *Cochrane Database Syst Rev* 2003;(1):CD002047.

59 Mladenovic V, Domljan Z, Rozman B, *et al.* Safety and effectiveness of leflunomide in the treatment of patients with active rheumatoid arthritis. Results of a randomised, placebo-controlled, phase II study. *Arthritis Rheum* 1995;**38**(11):1595–603.

60 Scott DL, Smolen JS, Kalden JR, *et al.* Treatment of active rheumatoid arthritis with leflunomide: two year follow up of a double blind, placebo controlled trial versus sulfasalazine. *Ann Rheum Dis* 2001;**60**(10):913–23.

61 Cohen S, Cannon GW, Schiff M, *et al.* Two-year, blinded, randomised, controlled trial of treatment of active rheumatoid arthritis with leflunomide compared with methotrexate. Utilization of Leflunomide in the Treatment of Rheumatoid Arthritis Trial Investigator Group. *Arthritis Rheum* 2001;**44**(9):1984–92.

62 Wells G, Haguenauer D, Shea B, *et al.* Cyclosporin for rheumatoid arthritis. The Cochrane Library [3]. 2000. *Cochrane Database Syst Rev* 2000;(3):CD00846.

63 Suarez-Almazor ME, Spooner C, Belseck E. Azathioprine for rheumatoid arthritis. *Cochrane Database Syst Rev* 2000;(2):CD001461.

64 Suarez-Almazor ME, Belseck E, Shea B, Wells G, Tugwell P. Cyclophosphamide for rheumatoid arthritis. *Cochrane Database Syst Rev* 2000;(2):CD001157.

65 Radis CD, Kahl LE, Baker GL, *et al.* Effects of cyclophosphamide on the development of malignancy and on long-term survival of patients with rheumatoid arthritis. A 20-year followup study. *Arthritis Rheum* 1995;**38**(8):1120–7.

66 Kloppenburg M, Breedveld FC, Terwiel JP, Mallee C, Dijkmans BA. Minocycline in active rheumatoid arthritis. A double-blind, placebo-controlled trial. *Arthritis Rheum* 1994;**37**(5):629–36.

67 Tilley BC, Alarcon GS, Heyse SP, *et al.* Minocycline in rheumatoid arthritis. A 48-week, double-blind, placebo-controlled trial. MIRA Trial Group. *Ann Intern Med* 1995;**122**(2):81–9.

68 O'Dell JR, Blakely KW, Mallek JA, *et al.* Treatment of early seropositive rheumatoid arthritis: a two-year, double-blind comparison of minocycline and hydroxychloroquine. *Arthritis Rheum* 2001;**44**(10):2235–41.

69 Suarez-Almazor ME, Spooner CH, Belseck E, Shea B. Auranofin versus placebo in rheumatoid arthritis. *Cochrane Database Syst Rev* 2000;(2):CD002048.

70 McEntegart A, Porter D, Capell HA, Thomson EA. Sulfasalazine has a better efficacy/toxicity profile than auranofin – evidence from a 5 year prospective, randomised trial. *J Rheumatol* 1996;**23**(11):1887–90.

71 Singh G, Fries JF, Williams CA, Zatarain E, Spitz P, Bloch DA. Toxicity profiles of disease modifying antirheumatic drugs in rheumatoid arthritis. *J Rheumatol* 1991;**18**(2): 188–94.

72 Osiri M, Suarez-Almazor M, Wells G, Robinson V, Tugwell P. Number needed to treat (NNT): Implication in Rheumatology Clinical Practice. *Ann Rheum Dis* 2003;**62**(4):316–21

73 van der Heijde DM. Joint erosions and patients with early rheumatoid arthritis. *Br J Rheumatol* 1995;**34** Suppl 2:74–8.

74 Borg G, Allander E, Berg E, Brodin U, From A, Trang L. Auranofin treatment in early rheumatoid arthritis may postpone early retirement. Results from a 2-year double blind trial. *J Rheumatol* 1991;**18**(7):1015–20.

75 Davis MJ, Dawes PT, Fowler PD, Clarke S, Fisher J, Shadforth MF. Should disease-modifying agents be used in mild rheumatoid arthritis? *Br J Rheumatol* 1991;**30**(6):451–4.

76 Hannonen P, Mottonen T, Hakola M, Oka M. Sulfasalazine in early rheumatoid arthritis. A 48-week double-blind, prospective, placebo-controlled study. *Arthritis Rheum* 1993;**36**(11):1501–9.

77 van Jaarsveld CH, Jacobs JW, van der Veen MJ, *et al.* Aggressive treatment in early rheumatoid arthritis: a randomised controlled trial. On behalf of the Rheumatic Research Foundation Utrecht, The Netherlands. *Ann Rheum Dis* 2000;**59**(6):468–77.

78 Rau R, Herborn G, Menninger H, Blechschmidt J. Comparison of intramuscular methotrexate and gold sodium thiomalate in the treatment of early erosive rheumatoid arthritis: 12 month data of a double-blind parallel study of 174 patients. *Br J Rheumatol* 1997;**36**(3):345–52.

79 Sulfasalazine in early rheumatoid arthritis. The Australian Multicentre Clinical Trial Group. *J Rheumatol* 1992;**19**(11):1672–7.

80 Verhoeven AC, Boers M, Tugwell P. Combination therapy in rheumatoid arthritis: updated systematic review. *Br J Rheumatol* 1998;**37**(6):612–19.

81 Felson DT, Anderson JJ, Meenan RF. The efficacy and toxicity of combination therapy in rheumatoid arthritis. A meta-analysis. *Arthritis Rheum* 1994;**37**(10):1487–91.

82 Calguneri M, Pay S, Caliskaner Z, *et al.* Combination therapy versus monotherapy for the treatment of patients with rheumatoid arthritis. *Clin Exp Rheumatol* 1999;**17**(6): 699–704.

83 Möttönen T, Hannonen P, Leirisalo-Repo M, Nissila M, Kautiainen H, Korpela M *et al.* Comparison of combination therapy with single-drug therapy in early rheumatoid arthritis: a randomised trial. FIN–RACo trial group. *Lancet* 1999;**353**(9164):1568–73.

84 O'Dell JR, Haire CE, Erikson N, *et al.* Treatment of rheumatoid arthritis with methotrexate alone, sulfasalazine and hydroxychloroquine, or a combination of all three medications. *N Engl J Med* 1996;**334**(20): 1287–91.

85 Proudman SM, Conaghan PG, Richardson C, Griffiths B, Green MJ, McGonagle D *et al.* Treatment of poor-prognosis early rheumatoid arthritis. A randomised study of treatment with methotrexate, cyclosporin A, and intraarticular corticosteroids compared with sulfasalazine alone. *Arthritis Rheum* 2000;**43**(8):1809–19.

86 van den Borne BE, Landewe RB, Goei The HS, *et al.* Combination therapy in recent onset rheumatoid arthritis: a randomised double blind trial of the addition of low dose cyclosporine to patients treated with low dose chloroquine. *J Rheumatol* 1998;**25**(8):1493–8.

87 O'Dell JR, Leff R, Paulsen G, *et al.* Treatment of rheumatoid arthritis with methotrexate and hydroxychloroquine, methotrexate and sulfasalazine, or a combination of the three medications: results of a two-year, randomised, double-blind, placebo-controlled trial. *Arthritis Rheum* 2002;**46**(5):1164–70.

88 Ferraccioli GF, Gremese E, Tomietto P, *et al.* Analysis of improvements, full responses, remission and toxicity in rheumatoid patients treated with step-up combination therapy (methotrexate, cyclosporin A, sulphasalazine) or monotherapy for three years. *Rheumatology (Oxford)* S2002;**41**(8):892–8.

89 Marchesoni A, Battafarano N, Arreghini M, *et al.* Step-down approach using either cyclosporin A or methotrexate as maintenance therapy in early rheumatoid arthritis. *Arthritis Rheum* 2002;**47**(1):59–66.

90 Blumenauer B, Judd M, Wells G, *et al.* Infliximab for the treatment of rheumatoid arthritis. *Cochrane Database Syst Rev* 2002;(3):CD003785.

91 Rau R. Adalimumab (a fully human anti-tumour necrosis factor alpha monoclonal antibody) in the treatment of active rheumatoid arthritis: the initial results of five trials. *Ann Rheum Dis* 2002;**61** Suppl 2:ii70–ii73.

92 Calabrese LH. Anakinra treatment of patients with rheumatoid arthritis. *Ann Pharmacother* 2002;**36**(7–8): 1204–9.

93 Reneses S, Pestana L. (Systematic review of clinical trials on the treatment of rheumatoid arthritis with tumour necrosis factor alpha inhibitors.) *Med Clin (Barc)* 2001;**116**(16):620–8.

94 Moreland LW, Schiff MH, Baumgartner SW, *et al.* Etanercept therapy in rheumatoid arthritis. A randomised, controlled trial. *Ann Intern Med* 1999;**130**(6):478–86.

95 Weinblatt ME, Kremer JM, Bankhurst AD, *et al.* A trial of etanercept, a recombinant tumor necrosis factor receptor:Fc fusion protein, in patients with rheumatoid arthritis receiving methotrexate. *N Engl J Med* 1999;**340**(4):253–9.

96 Bathon JM, Martin RW, Fleischmann RM, *et al.* A comparison of etanercept and methotrexate in patients with early rheumatoid arthritis. *N Engl J Med* 2000;**343**(22):1586–93.

97 Genovese MC, Bathon JM, Martin RW, *et al.* Etanercept versus methotrexate in patients with early rheumatoid arthritis: two-year radiographic and clinical outcomes. *Arthritis Rheum* 2002;**46**(6):1443–50.

98 Maini RN, Breedveld FC, Kalden JR, *et al.* Therapeutic efficacy of multiple intravenous infusions of anti-tumor necrosis factor alpha monoclonal antibody combined with low-dose weekly methotrexate in rheumatoid arthritis. *Arthritis Rheum* 1998;**41**(9):1552–63.

99 Maini R, St Clair EW, Breedveld F, *et al.* Infliximab (chimeric anti-tumour necrosis factor alpha) monoclonal antibody versus placebo in rheumatoid arthritis patients receiving concomitant methotrexate: a randomised phase III trial. ATTRACT Study Group. *Lancet* 1999;**354**(9194):1932–9.

100 Elliott MJ, Maini RN, Feldmann M, *et al.* Randomised double-blind comparison of chimeric monoclonal antibody to tumour necrosis factor alpha (cA2 versus placebo in rheumatoid arthritis). *Lancet* 1994;**344**(8930): 1105–10.

101 Lipsky PE, van der Heijde DM, St Clair EW, *et al.* Infliximab and methotrexate in the treatment of rheumatoid arthritis. Anti-Tumor Necrosis Factor Trial in Rheumatoid Arthritis with Concomitant Therapy Study Group. *N Engl J Med* 2000;**343**(22):1594–602.

102 den Broeder A, van de PL, Rau R, *et al.* A single dose, placebo controlled study of the fully human anti-tumor necrosis factor-alpha antibody adalimumab (D2E7)in patients with rheumatoid arthritis. *J Rheumatol* 2002;**29**(11):2288–98.

103 Weinblatt ME, Keystone EC, Furst DE, *et al.* Adalimumab, a fully human anti-tumor necrosis factor alpha monoclonal antibody, for the treatment of rheumatoid arthritis in patients taking concomitant methotrexate: the ARMADA trial. *Arthritis Rheum* 2003;**48**(1):35–45.

104 Campion GV, Lebsack ME, Lookabaugh J, *et al.* Dose–range and dose–frequency study of recombinant human interleukin-1 receptor antagonist in patients with rheumatoid arthritis. The IL-1Ra Arthritis Study Group. *Arthritis Rheum* 1996;**39**(7):1092–101.

105 Drevlow BE, Lovis R, Haag MA, *et al.* Recombinant human interleukin-1 receptor type I in the treatment of patients with active rheumatoid arthritis. *Arthritis Rheum* 1996;**39**(2):257–65.

106 Jiang Y, Genant HK, Watt I, *et al.* A multicenter, double-blind, dose-ranging, randomised, placebo- controlled study of recombinant human interleukin-1 receptor antagonist in patients with rheumatoid arthritis: radiologic progression and correlation of Genant and Larsen scores. *Arthritis Rheum* 2000;**43**(5):1001–9.

107 Cohen S, Hurd E, Cush J, *et al.* Treatment of rheumatoid arthritis with anakinra, a recombinant human interleukin-1 receptor antagonist, in combination with methotrexate: results of a twenty-four-week, multicenter, randomised, double-blind, placebo-controlled trial. *Arthritis Rheum* 2002;**46**(3):614–24.

108 Nuki G, Bresnihan B, Bear MB, McCabe D. Long-term safety and maintenance of clinical improvement following treatment with anakinra (recombinant human interleukin-1 receptor antagonist) in patients with rheumatoid arthritis: extension phase of a randomised, double-blind, placebo-controlled trial. *Arthritis Rheum* 2002;**46**(11):2838–46.

109 Gotzsche PC, Johansen HK. Meta-analysis of short-term low dose prednisolone versus placebo and non-steroidal anti-inflammatory drugs in rheumatoid arthritis. *BMJ* 1998;**316**(7134):811–18.

110 Criswell LA, Saag KG, Sems KM, *et al.* Moderate-term, low-dose corticosteroids for rheumatoid arthritis. *Cochrane Database Syst Rev* 2000;(2):CD001158.

111 Kirwan JR. The effect of glucocorticoids on joint destruction in rheumatoid arthritis. The Arthritis and Rheumatism Council Low-Dose Glucocorticoid Study Group. *N Engl J Med* 1995;**333**(3):142–6.

112 Hickling P, Jacoby RK, Kirwan JR. Joint destruction after glucocorticoids are withdrawn in early rheumatoid arthritis. Arthritis and Rheumatism Council Low Dose Glucocorticoid Study Group. *Br J Rheumatol* 1998;**37**(9): 930–6.

113 Van Everdingen AA, Jacobs JW, Van Reesema DRS, *et al.* Low-dose prednisolone therapy for patients with early active rheumatoid arthritis. *Ann Intern Med* 2002; **136**:1–12.

114 Wolfe F, Mitchell DM, Sibley JT, *et al.* The mortality of rheumatoid arthritis. *Arthritis Rheum* 1994;**37**(4):481–94.

115 Verhoeven AC, Boers M. Limited bone loss due to corticosteroids; a systematic review of prospective studies in rheumatoid arthritis and other diseases. *J Rheumatol* 1997;**24**(8):1495–503.

116 Garner S, Fidan D, Frankish R, *et al.* Celecoxib for rheumatoid arthritis. *Cochrane Database Syst Rev* 2003;(4):CD003831.

117 Silverstein FE, Faich G, Goldstein JL, *et al.* Gastrointestinal toxicity with celecoxib vs nonsteroidal anti-inflammatory drugs for osteoarthritis and rheumatoid arthritis: the CLASS study: A randomised controlled trial. Celecoxib Long-term Arthritis Safety Study. *JAMA* 2000;**284**(10):1247–55.

118 Garner S, Fidan D, Frankish R, *et al.* Rofecoxib for the treatment of rheumatoid arthritis. *Cochrane Database Syst Rev* 2002;(3):CD003685.

119 Bombardier C, Laine L, Reicin A, *et al.* Comparison of upper gastrointestinal toxicity of rofecoxib and naproxen in patients with rheumatoid arthritis. VIGOR Study Group. *N Engl J Med* 2000;**343**(21):1520–8.

120 Schnitzer TJ, Truitt K, Fleischmann R, *et al.* The safety profile, tolerability, and effective dose range of rofecoxib in the treatment of rheumatoid arthritis. Phase II Rofecoxib Rheumatoid Arthritis Study Group. *Clin Ther* 1999;**21**(10):1688–702.

121 Riemsma RP, Kirwan JR, Taal E, Rasker JJ. Patient education for adults with rheumatoid arthritis. *Cochrane Database Syst Rev* 2002;(3):CD003688.

122 Badamgarav E, Croft JD, Hohlbauch A, *et al.* Effectiveness of disease management programs in rheumatoid arthritis. *Arthritis Rheum* 2003;**49**(3):377–87.

123 Casimiro L, Brosseau L, Milne S, Robinson V, Wells G, Tugwell P. Acupuncture and electroacupuncture for the treatment of RA. *Cochrane Database Syst Rev* 2002;(3):CD003788.

124 Casimiro L, Brosseau L, Robinson V, *et al.* Therapeutic ultrasound for the treatment of rheumatoid arthritis. Cochrane Database Systematic Review 2002;(3): CD003787.

125 Robinson V, Brosseau L, Casimiro L, *et al.* Thermotherapy for treating rheumatoid arthritis. *Cochrane Database Syst Rev* 2002;(2):CD002826.

126 Brosseau LU, Pelland LU, Casimiro LY, Robinson VI, Tugwell PE, Wells GE. Electrical stimulation for the treatment of rheumatoid arthritis. *Cochrane Database Syst Rev* 2002;(2):CD003687.

127 Van Den Ende CH, Vliet Vlieland TP, Munneke M, Hazes JM. Dynamic exercise therapy for rheumatoid arthritis. *Cochrane Database Syst Rev* 2000;(2):CD000322.

128 Hochberg MC, Tracy JK, Flores RH. "Stepping-up" from methotrexate: a systematic review of randomised placebo controlled trials in patients with rheumatoid arthritis with an incomplete response to methotrexate. *Ann Rheum Dis* 2001;**60** Suppl 3:iii51–iii54.

129 Hawley DJ, Wolfe F. Are the results of controlled clinical trials and observational studies of second line therapy in rheumatoid arthritis valid and generalizable as measures of rheumatoid arthritis outcome: analysis of 122 studies. *J Rheumatol* 1991;**18**(7):1008–14.

130 ten Wolde S, Breedveld FC, Hermans J, *et al.* Randomised placebo-controlled study of stopping second-line drugs in rheumatoid arthritis. *Lancet* 1996;**347**(8998):347–52.

131 Sander O, Herborn G, Bock E, Rau R. Prospective six year follow up of patients withdrawn from a randomised study comparing parenteral gold salt and methotrexate. *Ann Rheum Dis* 1999;**58**(5):281–7.

132 Williams HJ, Willkens RF, Samuelson CO, Jr., Alarcon GS, Guttadauria M, Yarboro C *et al.* Comparison of low-dose oral pulse methotrexate and placebo in the treatment of rheumatoid arthritis. A controlled clinical trial. *Arthritis Rheum* 1985;**28**(7):721–30.

133 Ward JR, Williams HJ, Egger MJ, *et al.* Comparison of auranofin, gold sodium thiomalate, and placebo in the treatment of rheumatoid arthritis. A controlled clinical trial. *Arthritis Rheum* 1983;**26**(11):1303–15.

134 Townes AS, Sowa JM, Shulman LE. Controlled trial of cyclophosphamide in rheumatoid arthritis. *Arthritis Rheum* 1976;**19**(3):563–73.

135 Williams HJ, Ward JR, Reading JC, *et al.* Low-dose D-penicillamine therapy in rheumatoid arthritis. A controlled, double-blind clinical trial. *Arthritis Rheum* 1983;**26**(5):581–92.

Rheumatoid arthritis
Summaries and decision aids

Rheumatoid arthritis and methotrexate
Summaries and decision aid

How well does methotrexate (MTX) work for treating rheumatoid arthritis and how safe is it?

To answer this question, scientists found and analysed 7 reviews (2 were Cochrane reviews) and 8 more studies. People with rheumatoid arthritis taking methotrexate at 15 to 20 mg/week were tested up to 1 year. These studies provide the best evidence we have today.

What is methotrexate and why is it prescribed?

Rheumatoid arthritis is a disease in which the body's immune system attacks its own healthy tissues. The attack happens mostly in the joints of the feet and hands and causes redness, pain, swelling, and heat around the joint. Methotrexate is a disease modifying anti-rheumatic drug (DMARD) that is often prescribed when painkillers are not working well.

How well did methotrexate work?

Studies and reviews showed that patients receiving methotrexate for up to 1 year had less pain, functioned better, had fewer swollen and tender joints, and had less disease activity overall as reported by themselves and their doctors. Methotrexate also worked as well as parenteral gold, sulphasalazine and leflunomide. But some studies showed that leflunomide worked better.

X-rays showed that the progress of the disease slowed or stopped in many patients receiving methotrexate. Some studies show that methotrexate works just as well to slow progress as parenteral gold, sulphasalazine and leflunomide, and better than azathioprine.

What side effects occurred with methotrexate?

Side effects, such as diarrhoea, lung infections, headache, nausea, heartburn, rash, and changes in liver enzymes, may occur. It is not clear whether it increases the chance of developing tumours. People stopped taking other DMARDs, such as gold and sulphasalazine, due to side effects more often than they stopped taking methotrexate.

What is the bottom line?

There is "Gold" level evidence that methotrexate decreases pain, improves function, decreases the number of swollen and tender joints and disease activity and slows the progress of rheumatoid arthritis. It works just as well as other DMARDs and sometimes better. Methotrexate is recommended to be used first in people with very active disease.

Stomach and intestinal side effects, as well as headache, rash and high liver enzyme levels may occur when taking methotrexate but people continue to take methotrexate despite the side effects.

Based on Suarez-Almazor M, Osiri M, Emery P, Ottawa Methods Group. Rheumatoid arthritis. In *Evidence-based Rheumatology*. London: BMJ Books, 2003.

How well does methotrexate (MTX) work for treating rheumatoid arthritis and how safe is it?

What is methotrexate and why is it prescribed?

Rheumatoid arthritis is a disease in which the body's immune system attacks its own healthy tissues. The attack happens mostly in the joints of the feet and hands and causes redness, pain, swelling, and heat around the joint. There also can be damage to cartilage, bone, tendons, and ligaments. The pain and damage from rheumatoid arthritis limits people's ability to carry out daily activities at home and work and affects their wellbeing.

Painkillers or analgesics are often prescribed to decrease joint pain and swelling. But sometimes these drugs do not work well and disease modifying antirheumatic drugs or DMARDs are often prescribed. DMARDs work to decrease pain and swelling and slow the progress of rheumatoid arthritis. Methotrexate is a DMARD that is often prescribed early in the treatment of rheumatoid arthritis. Methotrexate can also cause side effects and therefore it is important to know how well methotrexate works and how safe it is.

How did the scientists find the information and analyse it?

The scientists searched for studies and reviews of the medical literature that tested methotrexate in people with rheumatoid arthritis. Not all studies and reviews found were of a high quality and so only those studies that met high standards were selected.

Studies were randomised controlled trials – where a group of patients receiving methotrexate were compared to a group of patients receiving a sugar pill (placebo) or another drug. The reviews were done systematically and examined the results from randomised controlled trials.

Which high quality studies and reviews were examined in this summary?

Seven high quality reviews of the literature (including 2 Cochrane Reviews) and 8 more high quality studies were examined. These studies and reviews tested patients with rheumatoid arthritis who did not improve with painkillers such as acetaminophen (Tylenol). The studies compared methotrexate to a sugar pill (placebo) or to another DMARD to find out how well methotrexate works.

One of the reviews and 3 of the studies specifically measured the effect of methotrexate on the progress of rheumatoid arthritis as seen on *x*-rays.

Five of the reviews and 2 of the studies tested the side effects of methotrexate.

How well did methotrexate work?

The studies and reviews showed that patients receiving methotrexate at less than 20 mg/week for 12 to 18 weeks had less pain and better function, had fewer swollen and tender joints, reported less disease activity overall and their physicians reported that they had less disease activity overall as well. The benefits of methotrexate were better than the benefits with a sugar pill (placebo).

One study showed that after 1 year of receiving methotrexate at (7·5–15 mg/week) patients had a 20%, 50%, and 70% improvement in symptoms of rheumatoid arthritis.

ACR 20 response:

- 46 out of 100 patients showed a 20% improvement with methotrexate
- 26 out of 100 patients showed a 20% improvement with a placebo.

This means 20 more patients benefited with methotrexate than with placebo.

ACR 50 response:

- 23 out of 100 patients showed a 50% improvement with methotrexate
- 8 out of 100 patients showed a 50% improvement with a placebo.

This means 15 more patients benefited with methotrexate than with placebo.

ACR 70 response:

- 9 out of 100 patients showed a 70% improvement with methotrexate
- 4 out of 100 patients showed a 70% improvement with a placebo.

Only a few patients show a 70% improvement with methotrexate, not very different than with placebo.

The reviews and studies that compared methotrexate to other DMARDs showed that methotrexate worked just a well as other DMARDs such as parenteral gold and sulphasalazine. However, some studies showed that methotrexate worked just as well as leflunomide, while other studies showed that leflunomide worked better.

X-rays showed that the progress of the disease slowed or stopped in many patients receiving methotrexate. In one study, about 70 out of 100 patients had little to no progress in the disease with methotrexate over 2 years. Some studies show that methotrexate works just as well as other DMARDs such as parenteral gold, sulphasalazine, and leflunomide to slow progress, while other studies show that methotrexate is better than other DMARDs, such as azathioprine.

What side effects occurred with methotrexate?

Side effects such as diarrhoea, lung infections, headache, nausea, heartburn, and rash occurred.

One recent study showed that the number of patients who stopped taking methotrexate or a placebo because of side effects was about equal:

- 10 out of 100 patients stopped taking methotrexate due to side effects
- 9 out of 100 patients stopped taking a placebo due to side effects.

Changes in liver enzymes may also occur when receiving methotrexate (4 out of 100 patients had abnormal liver enzyme levels with methotrexate compared to 2 out of 100 patients with a placebo). It is not clear whether there is a higher chance of developing tumours when receiving methotrexate. A Cochrane review showed that taking folic acid while receiving methotrexate may decrease the side effects.

Another review showed that patients stopped taking other medications, such as gold and sulphasalazine, due to side effects more often than they stopped taking methotrexate due to side effects.

What is the bottom line?

There is "Gold" level evidence that methotrexate decreases pain, improves function, decreases the number of swollen and tender joints and disease activity and slows the progress of rheumatoid arthritis. It works just as well as other DMARDs and sometimes better. Methotrexate recommended to be used first in people with very active disease.

Stomach and intestinal side effects, as well as headache, rash, and high liver enzyme levels may occur when taking methotrexate but people continue to take methotrexate despite the side effects.

Based on Suarez-Almazor M, Osiri M, Emery P, Ottawa Methods Group. Rheumatoid arthritis. In: *Evidence-based Rheumatology*. London: BMJ Books, 2003.

Information about rheumatoid arthritis and treatment

What is rheumatoid arthritis?

Rheumatoid arthritis is a disease in which the body's immune system attacks its own healthy tissues. The attack happens mostly in the joints of the feet and hands, causing redness, pain, swelling, and heat around the joint. There also can be damage to cartilage, bone, tendons, and ligaments. The pain and damage from rheumatoid arthritis limits people's ability to do daily activities at home and work and affects their well-being.

The pain and swelling sometimes gets worse and then gets better on its own. However, if the disease progresses or if it is moderate or severe rheumatoid arthritis and is not treated, it may result in:

- limited daily activities
- deformed joints
- permanent damage to joints
- need for surgery.

What can I do on my own to manage my disease?

✓ exercise ✓ hot/cold packs ✓ relaxation ✓ activity with less stress on joints

What treatments are used for rheumatoid arthritis?

Four kinds of treatment may be used alone or together. The common (generic) names of treatment are shown below.

1. *Pain medicine, aspirin, and non-steroidal anti-inflammatory drugs (NSAIDs)*
   - Acetylsalicylic acid
   - Acetaminophen
   - Celecoxib
   - Diclofenac
   - Etodolac
   - Ibuprofen
   - Indomethacin
   - Ketoprofen
   - Naproxen
   - Piroxicam
   - Rofecoxib
   - Sulindac
   - Tenoxicam
2. *Disease modifying antirheumatic drugs (DMARDs)*
   - Antimalarials
   - Auranofin
   - Azathioprine
   - Cloroquine
   - Cyclophosphamide
   - Ciclosporin
   - Leflunomide
   - Methotrexate
   - Minocycline
   - Parenteral Gold
   - Penicillamine
   - Sulphasalazine
3. *Biologic agents*
   - Etanercept
   - Infliximab
   - Adalimimab
   - Anakinra
4. *Oral corticosteroids*
   - Prednisolone
   - Prednisone

What about other treatments I have heard about?

There is not enough evidence about the effects of some treatments. Other treatments do not work. For example:

- Acupuncture
- Electropuncture
- Ultrasound
- Thermotherapy
- Electrical stimulation

What are my choices? How can I decide?

Treatment for your disease will depend on your condition. You need to know the good points (pros) and the bad points (cons) about each treatment before you can decide.

Rheumatoid Arthritis (RA) decision aid

Should I take methotrexate?

This guide can help you make decisions about the treatment your doctor is asking you to consider.

It will help you to:

1. Clarify what you need to decide
2. Consider the pros and cons of different choices
3. Decide what role you want to have in choosing your treatment
4. Identify what you need to help you make the decision
5. Plan the next steps
6. Share your thinking with your doctor.

Step 1: Clarify what you need to decide

What is the decision?

Should I start taking methotrexate when pain killers such as acetaminophen are not working to control rheumatoid arthritis?

Methotrexate is an injection given at set times within a month or taken as a pill.

When does this decision have to be made? Check ✓one

☐ within days ☐ within weeks ☐ within months

How far along are you with this decision? Check ✓one

☐ I have not thought about it yet

☐ I am considering the choices

☐ I am close to making a choice

☐ I have already made a choice

Step 2. Consider the pros and cons of different choices

What does the research show?

Methotrexate is classified as: Beneficial

There is "Gold" level evidence from 7 reviews (2 are Cochrane Reviews) and 8 more studies of people with rheumatoid arthritis. Studies lasted up to 2 years. These studies found pros and cons that are listed in the chart below.

What do I think of the pros and cons of methotrexate?

1. Review the common pros and cons.
2. Add any other pros and cons that are important to you.
3. Show how important each pro and con is to you by circling from one (*) star if it is a little important to you, to up to five (*****) stars if it is very important to you.

PROS AND CONS OF METHOTREXATE TREATMENT

PROS (number of people affected)	How important is it to you?	CONS (number of people affected)	How important is it to you?
Improves pain and function 46 out of 100 are helped at least a little 23 out of 100 people are helped a lot	* * * * *	Side effects: diarrhoea, lung infections, headache, nausea, heartburn, and rash 10 out of 100 people had side effects with methotrexate	* * * * *
Slows progress of disease 70 out of 100 people show improvement on *x*-rays	* * * * *	Unsure of long term side effects and rare serious harms (such as cancer)	* * * * *
Same effect as other DMARDs	* * * * *	Extra clinic visits and blood tests needed	* * * * *
More people stay on methotrexate longer compared to other DMARDs	* * * * *	Cost of medicine	* * * * *
Other pros:	* * * * *	Other cons:	* * * * *

***What do you think about taking methotrexate?* Check ✓one**

☐ Willing to consider this treatment
Pros are more important to me than the Cons

☐ Unsure

☐ Not willing to consider this treatment
Cons are more important to me than the Pros

Step 3: Choose the role you want to have in choosing your treatment. Check ✓ one

☐ I prefer to decide on my own after listening to the opinions of others

☐ I prefer to share the decision with: ______________________

☐ I prefer someone else to decide for me, namely: ______________

Step 4: Identify what you need to help you make the decision

What I know	Do you know enough about your condition to make a choice?	☐ Yes ☐ No ☐ Unsure
	Do you know which options are available to you?	☐ Yes ☐ No ☐ Unsure
	Do you know the good points (pros) of each option?	☐ Yes ☐ No ☐ Unsure
	Do you know the bad points (cons) of each option?	☐ Yes ☐ No ☐ Unsure
What's important	Are you clear about which **pros** are most *important to you?*	☐ Yes ☐ No ☐ Unsure
	Are you clear about which **cons** are most *important to you?*	☐ Yes ☐ No ☐ Unsure
How others help	Do you have enough support from others to make a choice?	☐ Yes ☐ No ☐ Unsure
	Are you choosing without pressure from others?	☐ Yes ☐ No ☐ Unsure
	Do you have enough advice to make a choice?	☐ Yes ☐ No ☐ Unsure
How sure I feel	Are you clear about the best choice for you?	☐ Yes ☐ No ☐ Unsure
	Do you feel sure about what to choose?	☐ Yes ☐ No ☐ Unsure

If you answered No or Unsure to many of these questions, you should talk to your doctor.

Step 5: Plan the next steps

What do you need to do before you make this decision?

For example – talk to your doctor, read more about this treatment or other treatments for rheumatoid arthritis.

Step 6: Share the information on this form with your doctor

It will help your doctor understand what you think about this treatment.

Rheumatoid arthritis and DMARDs
Summaries and decision aid

How well does a combination of disease modifying antirheumatic drugs (DMARDs) work for treating rheumatoid arthritis and how safe is it?

To answer this question, scientists found and analysed 1 high quality review and 9 more studies. People with rheumatoid arthritis taking one DMARD on its own or a combination of DMARDs were tested. These studies and reviews provide the best evidence we have today.

What are DMARDs and why are they prescribed in combination?

Rheumatoid arthritis is a condition in which the body's immune system attacks its own healthy tissues. The attack happens mostly in the joints of the feet and hands and causes redness, pain, swelling, and heat around the joint. Disease modifying antirheumatic drugs or DMARDs are often prescribed to decrease pain and swelling and slow the progress of rheumatoid arthritis. Taking one DMARD sometimes does not work well for people and so a combination of two or more DMARDs may be prescribed. Therefore it is important to know how well a combination of DMARDs works and how safe it is.

How well did a combination of DMARDs work?

The review showed that many combinations of DMARDs are useful. Some of the studies in the review showed that more people receiving methotrexate combined with other DMARDs and people receiving a combination of different DMARDs improved more than people receiving methotrexate alone or another DMARD alone.

The studies and the review did not compare a specific combination of DMARDs to another combination to find out which combinations work better.

What side effects occurred with a combination of DMARDs?

The review showed that side effects with a combination of two or more DMARDs may occur more often due to the chance of more drug interactions. Side effects also depend on the drugs that are combined.

Two studies showed that people receiving combinations had side effects such as headache, rash, pneumonia, stomach and intestinal side effects, and changes in liver enzymes, and that the number of people who had side effects was the same for many combinations.

What is the bottom line?

There is "Gold" level evidence that combining disease modifying antirheumatic drugs works better than using a drug on its own to decrease pain and improve function. But the side effects must be balanced with the benefits of the combination.

Different combinations of DMARDs have not been compared.

Based on Suarez-Almazor M, Osiri M, Emery P, Ottawa Methods Group. Rheumatoid arthritis. In: *Evidence-based Rheumatology*. London: BMJ Books, 2003.

How well does a combination of disease modifying antirheumatic drugs (DMARDs) work for treating rheumatoid arthritis and how safe is it?

What are DMARDs and why are they prescribed in combination?

Rheumatoid arthritis is a condition in which the body's immune system attacks its own healthy tissues. The attack happens mostly in the joints of the feet and hands and causes redness, pain, swelling, and heat around the joint. There also can be damage to cartilage, bone, tendons, and ligaments. The pain and damage from rheumatoid arthritis limits people's ability to carry out daily activities at home and work and affects their wellbeing.

Disease modifying antirheumatic drugs or DMARDs are often prescribed to decrease pain and swelling and slow the progress of rheumatoid arthritis. Taking one DMARD sometimes does not work well for people and so a combination of two or more DMARDs may be prescribed. Therefore it is important to know how well a combination of DMARDs works and how safe it is.

How did the scientists find the information and analyse it?

The scientists searched for studies and reviews of the medical literature that tested patients who received a combination of DMARDs. Not all studies and reviews found were of a high quality and so only those studies that met high standards were selected.

Studies were randomised controlled trials – where a group of patients receiving a combination of DMARDs were compared to a group of patients receiving one DMARD. The reviews were done systematically and tested the results from randomised controlled trials.

Which high quality studies and reviews were examined in this summary?

One high quality review of the literature and 9 more studies were examined. Results from one of the high quality studies are included in this summary.

This study tested 102 patients receiving methotrexate alone, sulphasalazine and hydroxychloroquine (SSZ and HC) or a combination of all three.

How well did a combination of DMARDs work?

The review showed that many combinations of DMARDs are useful. Some of the studies in the review showed that more patients receiving methotrexate combined with other DMARDs and patients receiving a combination of different DMARDs improved more than people receiving methotrexate alone or a different DMARD alone.

Specifically, one of the studies in the review showed that after 2 years of treatments, at least a 50% improvement in pain, number of swollen and tender joints, and disease activity (or ACR 50 response) occurred in:

- 33 out of 100 patients with methotrexate alone
- 40 out of 100 patients with SSZ and HC
- 77 out of 100 patients with a combination of methotrexate, SSZ and HC.

The studies and the reviews did not compare a specific combination of DMARDs to another combination to find out which combination works better.

What side effects occurred with a combination of DMARDs?

The review showed that side effects with a combination of two or more DMARDs may occur more often due to the chance of more drug interactions. Side effects also depend on the drugs that are combined. One study showed that patients receiving combinations had side effects such as headache, rash, pneumonia, stomach and intestinal side effects, and changes in liver enzymes, and that the number of patients who had side effects was the same for many combinations.

One study in the review showed that the number of people who stopped taking the medications because of side effects was about equal:

- 19 out of 100 patients stopped taking methotrexate due to side effects
- 9 out of 100 patients stopped taking the combination of SSZ and HC due to side effects
- 10 out of 100 patients stopped taking the combination of methotrexate, SSZ, and HC due to side effects.

What is the bottom line?

There is "Gold" level evidence that combining disease modifying antirheumatic drugs works better than using a drug on its own to decrease pain and improve function. But the side effects must be balanced with the benefits of the combination.

Different combinations of DMARDs have not been compared.

Based on Suarez-Almazor M, Osiri M, Emery P, Ottawa Methods Group. Rheumatoid arthritis. In: *Evidence-based Rheumatology*. London: BMJ Books, 2003.

Information about rheumatoid arthritis and treatment

What is rheumatoid arthritis?

Rheumatoid arthritis is a disease in which the body's immune system attacks its own healthy tissues. The attack happens mostly in the joints of the feet and hands, causing redness, pain, swelling, and heat around the joint. There also can be damage to cartilage, bone, tendons, and ligaments. The pain and damage from rheumatoid arthritis limits people's ability to do daily activities at home and work and affects their well-being.

The pain and swelling sometimes gets worse and then gets better on its own. However, if the disease progresses or if it is moderate or severe rheumatoid arthritis and is not treated, it may result in:

- limited daily activities
- deformed joints
- permanent damage to joints
- need for surgery.

What can I do on my own to manage my disease?

✓ exercise ✓ hot/cold packs ✓ relaxation ✓ activity with less stress on joints

What treatments are used for rheumatoid arthritis?

Four kinds of treatment may be used alone or together. The common (generic) names of treatment are shown below:

1. *Pain medicine, aspirin, and non-steroidal anti-inflammatory drugs (NSAIDs)*
    - Acetylsalicylic acid
    - Acetaminophen
    - Celecoxib
    - Diclofenac
    - Etodolac
    - Ibuprofen
    - Indomethacin
    - Ketoprofen
    - Naproxen
    - Piroxicam
    - Rofecoxib
    - Sulindac
    - Tenoxicam
2. *Disease modifying antirheumatic drugs (DMARDs)*
    - Antimalarials
    - Auranofin
    - Azathioprine
    - Chloroquine
    - Cyclophosphamide
    - Ciclosporin
    - Leflunomide
    - Methotrexate
    - Minocycline
    - Parenteral gold
    - Penicillamine
    - Sulphasalazine
3. *Biologic agents*
    - Etanercept
    - Infliximab
    - Adalimimab
    - Anakinra
4. *Oral corticosteroids*
    - Prednisolone
    - Prednisone

What about other treatments I have heard about?

There is not enough evidence about the effects of some treatments. Other treatments do not work. For example:

- Acupuncture
- Electropuncture
- Ultrasound
- Thermotherapy
- Electrical stimulation

What are my choices? How can I decide?

Treatment for your disease will depend on your condition. You need to know the good points (pros) and the bad points (cons) about each treatment before you can decide.

Rheumatoid Arthritis (RA) decision aid

Should I take a combination of DMARDs?

This guide can help you make decisions about the treatment your doctor is asking you to consider.

It will help you to:

1. Clarify what you need to decide.
2. Consider the pros and cons of different choices.
3. Decide what role you want to have in choosing your treatment.
4. Identify what you need to help you make the decision.
5. Plan the next steps.
6. Share your thinking with your doctor.

Step 1: Clarify what you need to decide

What is the decision?

Should I start taking a combination of disease modifying antirheumatic drugs (DMARDs) when methotrexate alone is not working to control rheumatoid arthritis?

A combination of DMARDs may be taken as pills.

When does this decision have to be made? Check ✓ one

☐ within days ☐ within weeks ☐ within months

How far along are you with this decision? Check ✓ one

☐ I have not thought about it yet

☐ I am considering the choices

☐ I am close to making a choice

☐ I have already made a choice

Step 2: Consider the pros and cons of different choices

What does the research show?

A combination of DMARDs is classified as: Trade-off between benefits and harms

There is "Gold" level evidence about how well a comination of DMARDs work from 1 review and 9 more studies of people with rheumatoid arthritis. The studies lasted up to 2 years. These studies found pros and cons that are listed in the chart below.

What do I think of the pros and cons of a combination of DMARDs?

1. Review the common pros and cons.
2. Add any other pros and cons that are important to you.
3. Show how important each pro and con is to you by circling from one (*) star if it is a little important to you, to up to five (*****) stars if it is very important to you.

PROS AND CONS OF TREATMENT WITH A COMBINATION OF DMARDs

PROS (number of people affected)	How important is it to you?	CONS (number of people affected)	How important is it to you?
Improves pain and function 40 to 77 out of 100 people are helped a lot	* * * * *	Side effects: headache, rash, lung infections, stomach upset, diarrhoea 9 out of 100 people stopped taking the combination of DMARDs because of side effects	* * * * *
More effective than one DMARD on its own (such as methotrexate)	* * * * *	Extra clinic visits and blood tests needed	* * * * *
Other pros:	* * * * *	More pills to take each day	* * * * *
		Cost of medicine	* * * * *
		Other cons:	* * * * *

What do you think about taking a combination of DMARDs? *Check ✓ one*

☐ Willing to consider this treatment
Pros are more important to me than the Cons

☐ Unsure

☐ Not willing to consider this treatment
Cons are more important to me than the Pros

Step 3: Choose the role you want to have in choosing your treatment Check ✓ one

☐ I prefer to decide on my own after listening to the opinions of others

☐ I prefer to share the decision with: ____________________

☐ I prefer someone else to decide for me, namely: ______________

Step 4: Identify what you need to help you make the decision

What I know	Do you know enough about your condition to make a choice?	☐ Yes	☐ No	☐ Unsure
	Do you know which options are available to you?	☐ Yes	☐ No	☐ Unsure
	Do you know the good points (pros) of each option?	☐ Yes	☐ No	☐ Unsure
	Do you know the bad points (cons) of each option?	☐ Yes	☐ No	☐ Unsure
What's important	Are you clear about which **pros** are most *important to you?*	☐ Yes	☐ No	☐ Unsure
	Are you clear about which **cons** are most *important to you?*	☐ Yes	☐ No	☐ Unsure
How others help	Do you have enough support from others to make a choice?	☐ Yes	☐ No	☐ Unsure
	Are you choosing without pressure from others?	☐ Yes	☐ No	☐ Unsure
	Do you have enough advice to make a choice?	☐ Yes	☐ No	☐ Unsure
How sure I feel	Are you clear about the best choice for you?	☐ Yes	☐ No	☐ Unsure
	Do you feel sure about what to choose?	☐ Yes	☐ No	☐ Unsure

If you answered No or Unsure to many of these questions, you should talk to your doctor.

Step 5: Plan the next steps

What do you need to do before you make this decision?

For example – talk to your doctor, read more about this treatment or other treatments for rheumatoid arthritis.

Step 6: Share the information on this form with your doctor

It will help your doctor understand what you think about this treatment.

Rheumatoid arthritis and infliximab Summaries and decision aid

How well does infliximab (Remicade) work when methotrexate alone is not controlling rheumatoid arthritis and how safe is it?

To answer this question, scientists found and analyzed 2 high quality studies in a Cochrane Review. The studies tested over 400 people who had rheumatoid arthritis for 7 to 9 years. People had either injections of infliximab at 3 mg/kg or 10 mg/kg every 4 or 8 weeks plus methotrexate (MTX) or MTX plus placebo injections. This Cochrane Review provides the best evidence today.

What is infliximab (Remicade) and why is it prescribed?

Rheumatoid arthritis is a disease in which the body's immune system attacks its own healthy tissues. The attack happens mostly in the joints of the feet and hands and causes redness, pain, swelling, and heat around the joint. Infliximab (Remicade) is a "biologic" used to decrease pain and swelling and slow the progress of rheumatoid arthritis. It is usually prescribed when other DMARDs (disease modifying antirheumatic drugs) do not work well.

How well does it work?

After 1 year of treatment, more people who had infliximab plus MTX improved compared to people who had injections of MTX alone. These people showed a 20%, 50% or 70% improvement in the number of tender and swollen joints and improvement in pain, disease activity, ability to do everyday activities, physical check-ups or blood tests.

According to *x*-rays taken after 1 year of treatment, more people who had infliximab plus MTX improved and fewer worsened compared to people who had MTX alone.

How safe is it?

In these studies, common side effects were upper respiratory infections (colds), headache, diarrhoea, and stomach pain. Headache, nausea, and hives, occurred during or immediately after the injection of infliximab. The levels of anti-nuclear antibodies (ANA) and anti-double stranded DNA antibodies (ds-DNA) were higher in more people who received infliximab plus MTX than in people with MTX alone. But the number of people who stopped taking infliximab due to side effects was the same as the number of people who stopped taking a placebo. Other studies have found that tuberculosis and other serious infections that sometimes cause death have occurred in people taking infliximab.

What is the bottom line?

There is "Gold" level evidence that when methotrexate is not controlling rheumatoid arthritis, infliximab up to 1 year decreases pain and swelling and slows the progress of rheumatoid arthritis. Infliximab also works within weeks rather than months.

More cases of infections, such as tuberculosis, have occurred when receiving infliximab. More time is needed before rare and late side effects are known.

Based on Suarez-Almazor M, Osiri M, Emery P, Ottawa Methods Group. Rheumatoid arthritis. In: *Evidence-based Rheumatology*. London: BMJ Books, 2003.

How well does infliximab (Remicade) work when methotrexate alone is not controlling rheumatoid arthritis?

What is infliximab and how does it work?

Rheumatoid arthritis is a disease in which the body's immune system attacks its own healthy tissues. The attack happens mostly in the joints of the feet and hands and causes redness, pain, swelling, and heat around the joint. Medications known as DMARDs (disease modifying antirheumatic drugs) are often prescribed to decrease pain and swelling and slow the progress of rheumatoid arthritis. In some people, these drugs do not work well and they may even cause side effects that people cannot tolerate. In cases when DMARDs do not work well, new and more expensive agents called "biologics" are often prescribed.

Infliximab (Remicade) is one "biologic agent" or "biological response modifier" that was recently approved in Canada to treat rheumatoid arthritis. These new biologic agents are injected into the body and work by clamping onto a substance in the body called the tumour necrosis factor-alpha (TNF-alpha). TNF-alpha may start a chain reaction in the body that causes swelling, pain, and damage in the body's joints. When clamping onto TNF-alpha, the biologic agents stop the chain reaction, which may decrease the pain and swelling in the joints. And since biologics work in a different way than DMARDs, they may help people in whom DMARDs did not work. But there are concerns that infliximab may increase the chances of infections such as tuberculosis or the chances of cancer. Up to June 2001, approximately 170 000 patients have been treated worldwide with infliximab.

How did the scientists find the information and analyse it?

The scientists searched for studies testing infliximab. Not all studies found were of a high quality and so only those studies that met high standards were selected.

The studies selected to include in this summary were reported in a Cochrane Review and had to be randomised controlled trials or controlled clinical trials – where a group of patients receiving infliximab was compared to patients receiving a different treatment or a placebo (or sugar pill). The studies also had to show how well infliximab works and its safety by using internationally accepted measurements.

Which high quality studies were included in the summary?

One study and a report that was a follow-up of the study were included in a Cochrane Review. The study tested 428 rheumatoid arthritis patients, aged 16 years or more, who did not improve with methotrexate (MTX) after 3 or 6 months. Most of the patients were women and had rheumatoid arthritis for about 7 to 9 years. The study tested different doses of infliximab with MTX:

- a 30 week (7 month) study with 428 patients compared injections of infliximab at 3 mg/kg every 4 or 8 weeks or 10 mg/kg every 4 or 8 weeks to placebo every 4 weeks. Patients stayed on the same dose of MTX they were on before they started the study. This study was called the ATTRACT study; and,
- a 54 week (1 year) report that was a follow-up of the ATTRACT study above.

How well did infliximab work?

In both the 7 month and 1 year studies, more patients improved with all doses of infliximab than patients who had injections of MTX and placebo. In all of the studies improvement was measured by using ACR

20, ACR 50, and ACR 70 responses. These responses mean that patients experienced either a 20%, 50% or 70% improvement in the number and tenderness of inflamed joints. They also had either a 20%, 50% or 70% improvement in at least three of the following five measures: the level of pain they reported, the level of disease activity they described, their ability to do everyday activities, their physical check-up, and their results on blood tests.

After 1 year, the study showed:

ACR 20 response: 42 out of 100 patients with infliximab plus MTX had a 20% improvement compared to 17 out of 100 patients with MTX alone. *This means that after 1 year 25 more patients out of 100 benefited from receiving infliximab.*

ACR 50 response: 41 out of 100 patients with infliximab plus MTX had a 50% improvement compared to 8 out of 100 patients with MTX alone. *This means that after 1 year 13 more patients out of 100 benefited from receiving infliximab.*

ACR 70 response: 10 out of 100 patients with infliximab plus MTX had a 70% improvement compared to 2 out of 100 patients with MTX alone. *This means that after 1 year 9 more patients out of 100 benefited from receiving infliximab.*

The progress of the disease shown in *x*-rays was tested in the 1 year study. More patients improved and fewer patients worsened when they received infliximab compared to MTX and placebo injections:

- 47 out of 100 patients improved with infliximab plus MTX compared to 14 out of 100 patients with MTX injections alone. *This means that about 33 more patients out of 100 benefited from receiving infliximab*
- 11 out of 100 patients worsened with infliximab plus MTX compared to 31 out of 100 patients with MTX and placebo injections. *This means that about 20 more patients out of 100 benefited from receiving infliximab.*

What side effects occurred with infliximab?

Common side effects in these studies were upper respiratory infections (colds), headache diarrhoea, and stomach pain. Other side effects, such as headache, nausea and hives, occurred during or immediately after the injection of infliximab.

In these studies, people tested after receiving infliximab plus MTX for 6 months or 1 year had infections or developed cancer just as often as people who had MTX alone. And, the number of patients (5 out of 100) who stopped infliximab injections due to side effects was about equal to the number (7 out of 100) who stopped methotrexate.

At 1 year, blood tests that measure antibodies such as anti-nuclear antibodies (ANA) and anti-double stranded DNA antibodies (ds-DNA) were higher in more patients who received infliximab plus MTX than in patients who received MTX alone. These high levels may have occurred due to chance or they may mean a reaction in disease activity of rheumatoid arthritis. It is not known whether those patients with high levels will have health problems in the future. But it is known that patients with uncontrolled rheumatoid arthritis have a higher risk of death and disability than patients with controlled rheumatoid arthritis.

Other studies have found that serious harms such as tuberculosis and other infections occurred in patients receiving infliximab. Some of the infections have caused death. Before starting infliximab, patients should be tested for tuberculosis and patients who have tuberculosis should be treated.

What is the bottom line?

There is "Gold" level evidence that when methotrexate is not controlling rheumatoid arthritis, infliximab up to 1 year decreases pain and swelling and slows the progress of rheumatoid arthritis. Infliximab also works within weeks rather than months.

More cases of infections, such as tuberculosis, have occurred when receiving infliximab. More time is needed before rare and late side effects are known.

Based on Suarez-Almazor M, Osiri M, Emery P, Ottawa Methods Group. Rheumatoid arthritis. In: *Evidence-based Rheumatology.* London: BMJ Books, 2003.

Information about rheumatoid arthritis and treatment

What is rheumatoid arthritis?

Rheumatoid arthritis is a disease in which the body's immune system attacks its own healthy tissues. The attack happens mostly in the joints of the feet and hands, causing redness, pain, swelling, and heat around the joint. There also can be damage to cartilage, bone, tendons, and ligaments. The pain and damage from rheumatoid arthritis limits people's ability to do daily activities at home and work and affects their wellbeing.

The pain and swelling sometimes gets worse and then gets better on its own. However, if the disease progresses or if it is moderate or severe rheumatoid arthritis and is not treated, it may result in:

- limited daily activities
- deformed joints
- permanent damage to joints
- need for surgery.

What can I do on my own to manage my disease?

✓exercise ✓hot/cold packs ✓ relaxation ✓activity with less stress on joints

What treatments are used for rheumatoid arthritis?

Four kinds of treatment may be used alone or together. The common (generic) names of treatment are shown below:

1. *Pain medicine, aspirin, and non-steroidal anti-inflammatory drugs (NSAIDs)*
   - Acetylsalicylic acid
   - Acetaminophen
   - Celecoxib
   - Diclofenac
   - Etodolac
   - Ibuprofen
   - Indomethacin
   - Ketoprofen
   - Naproxen
   - Piroxicam
   - Rofecoxib
   - Sulindac
   - Tenoxicam
2. *Disease modifying antirheumatic drugs (DMARDs)*
   - Antimalarials
   - Auranofin
   - Azathioprine
   - Chloroquine
   - Cyclophosphamide
   - Ciclosporin
   - Leflunomide
   - Methotrexate
   - Minocycline
   - Parenteral gold
   - Penicillamine
   - Sulphasalazine
3. *Biologic agents*
   - Etanercept
   - Infliximab
   - Adalimimab
   - Anakinra
4. *Oral corticosteroids*
   - Prednisolone
   - Prednisone

What about other treatments I have heard about?

There is not enough evidence about the effects of some treatments. Other treatments do not work. For example:

- Acupuncture
- Electropuncture
- Ultrasound
- Electrical stimulation.
- Thermotherapy

What are my choices? How can I decide?

Treatment for your disease will depend on your condition. You need to know the good points (pros) and the bad points (cons) about each treatment before you can decide.

Rheumatoid arthritis (RA) decision aid

Should I take infliximab?

This guide can help you make decisions about the treatment your doctor is asking you to consider.

It will help you to:

1. Clarify what you need to decide.
2. Consider the pros and cons of different choices.
3. Decide what role you want to have in choosing your treatment.
4. Identify what you need to help you make the decision.
5. Plan the next steps.
6. Share your thinking with your doctor.

Step 1: Clarify what you need to decide

What is the decision?

Should I start taking infliximab when methotrexate alone is not working to control rheumatoid arthritis?

Infliximab is an intravenous (IV) injection given at set times every few weeks.

When does this decision have to be made? Check ✓one

☐ within days ☐ within weeks ☐ within months

How far along are you with this decision? Check ✓one

☐ I have not thought about it yet

☐ I am considering the choices

☐ I am close to making a choice

☐ I have already made a choice

Step 2: Consider the pros and cons of different choices

What does the research show?

Infliximab is classified as: Trade-off between benefits and harms

There is "Gold" level evidence from 2 studies of 428 people with rheumatoid arthritis. The studies tested infliximab and lasted 6 months to 1 year. These studies found pros and cons that are listed in the chart below.

What do I think of the pros and cons of infliximab?

1. Review the common pros and cons.
2. Add any other pros and cons that are important to you.
3. Show how important each pro and con is to you by circling from one (*) star if it is a little important to you, to up to five (*****) stars if it is very important to you.

PROS AND CONS OF INFLIXIMAB TREATMENT

PROS (number of people affected)	How important is it to you?
Improves pain and function 41 out of 100 people are helped at least a little 31 out of 100 people are helped a lot	* * * * *
Slows progress of disease *X*-rays are better in 47 out of 100 people	* * * * *
Works within weeks rather than months	* * * * *
Other pros:	* * * * *

CONS (number of people affected)	How important is it to you?
Side effects: colds, headache, diarrhoea, abdominal pain 5 out of 100 people stopped taking infliximab because of the side effects 7 out of 100 people stopped taking methotrexate because of side effects	* * * * *
Reactions during or immediately after the injection headache, nausea, and hives	* * * * *
Serious harms: tuberculosis and other serious infections (some have caused death)	* * * * *
Unsure if can travel with this medicine	* * * * *
Extra clinic visits and blood tests needed	* * * * *
Cost of medicine	* * * * *
Other cons:	* * * * *

What do you think about taking infliximab? Check✓ one

☐ Willing to consider this treatment
Pros are more important to me than the Cons

☐ Unsure

☐ Not willing to consider this treatment
Cons are more important to me than the Pros

Step 3: Choose the role you want to have in choosing your treatment Check ✓ one.

☐ I prefer to decide on my own after listening to the opinions of others

☐ I prefer to share the decision with: ______________________

☐ I prefer someone else to decide for me, namely: ______________

Step 4: Identify what you need to help you make the decision

What I know	Do you know enough about your condition to make a choice?	☐ Yes ☐ No ☐ Unsure
	Do you know which options are available to you?	☐ Yes ☐ No ☐ Unsure
	Do you know the good points (pros) of each option?	☐ Yes ☐ No ☐ Unsure
	Do you know the bad points (cons) of each option?	☐ Yes ☐ No ☐ Unsure
What's important	Are you clear about which **pros** are most *important to you?*	☐ Yes ☐ No ☐ Unsure
	Are you clear about which **cons** are most *important to you?*	☐ Yes ☐ No ☐ Unsure
How others help	Do you have enough support from others to make a choice?	☐ Yes ☐ No ☐ Unsure
	Are you choosing without pressure from others?	☐ Yes ☐ No ☐ Unsure
	Do you have enough advice to make a choice?	☐ Yes ☐ No ☐ Unsure
How sure I feel	Are you clear about the best choice for you?	☐ Yes ☐ No ☐ Unsure
	Do you feel sure about what to choose?	☐ Yes ☐ No ☐ Unsure

If you answered No or Unsure to many of these questions, you should talk to your doctor.

Step 5: Plan the next steps

What do you need to do before you make this decision?

For example – talk to your doctor, read more about this treatment or other treatments for rheumatoid arthritis.

Step 6: Share the information on this form with your doctor

It will help your doctor understand what you think about this treatment.

10
Shoulder and elbow pain

Shoulder pain

Rachelle Buchbinder, Sally Green, Ottawa Methods Group

Introduction

Shoulder pain is common, with a reported prevalence of 7 to 34% in the general population and 21% in those over 70 years of age.[1–5] Approximately 10% of the general adult population will experience an episode of shoulder pain in their lifetime.[6] Shoulder disorders account for 1·2% of all general practice encounters, being third only to back and neck complaints as musculoskeletal reasons for primary care consultation.[4]

There are many accepted standard forms of conservative therapy for shoulder disorders, including non-steroidal anti-inflammatory drugs, steroid injections, and physiotherapy interventions. However, evidence of their efficacy is not well established. Previous systematic reviews of randomised controlled trials investigating these treatments concluded that there was little evidence to either support or refute the efficacy of interventions commonly used to treat shoulder pain.[6–8] Furthermore, interpretation of the results of many studies was hampered by lack of a clear description of the study population, interventions, and outcome measures.[7–9]

Shoulder problems are labelled and defined in diverse and often conflicting ways. A methodological review of the selection criteria defining study populations with shoulder pain in one systematic review of randomised controlled trials determined that trial populations could be broadly categorised as adhesive capsulitis (including periarthritis and frozen shoulder), rotator cuff disease or tendonitis (including impingement, subacromial bursitis, partial rotator cuff tears) or unspecified or mixed populations of shoulder pain.[7] Inclusion and exclusion criteria varied between studies of the same disorder, there were no standard definitions, and conflicting criteria often defined the same condition in different trials. For the purposes of this evidence-based summary, rotator cuff disorders and adhesive capsulitis will be discussed separately.

Methodology

This chapter is based on a series of Cochrane Reviews of interventions for shoulder pain, which update our original Cochrane Review.[10] Eligibility criteria for including studies into the reviews were determined a priori and applied against retrieved trials by two independent reviewers. Eligibility criteria were as follows.

Types of studies

- Randomised or pseudo-randomised controlled trials. Studies where participants were not randomised into intervention groups were excluded from the review.
- Trials in which allocation to treatment or control group was not concealed from the outcome assessor were not excluded. A sensitivity analysis including and excluding these trials was planned, because

foreknowledge of treatment allocation may lead to biased assessment of outcome.
- Studies in all languages were translated into English and considered for inclusion in the review. A sensitivity analysis including and excluding non-English language trials was planned to test the effect of inclusion of these trials.

Types of participants

Inclusion in this review was restricted to trials with participants meeting the following criteria.

All studies which primarily concerned pain arising from the shoulder in adult populations (greater than 18 years of age) were included irrespective of diagnostic label. Studies that included various rheumatological disorders were considered if the results for shoulder pain were presented separately or if 90% or more of the study participants had shoulder pain. Specific exclusions were duration of shoulder pain less than 3 weeks, rheumatoid arthritis, polymyalgia rheumatica, and fracture.

Based upon our methodological review of the selection criteria used in the studies included in our previous review, we categorised the study populations as adhesive capsulitis, rotator cuff disease, full thickness rotator cuff tear or shoulder pain of mixed or unspecified diagnoses.

Types of interventions

- All randomised controlled comparisons of non-steroidal anti-inflammatory drugs (NSAIDs) versus placebo, or another modality, or of varying types and dosages of NSAID were included.
- All randomised controlled comparisons of glucocorticosteroid injections versus placebo, or another modality, or of varying types and dosages of injection were included.
- All randomised controlled comparisons of shoulder joint distension versus placebo or another intervention were included and comparisons established according to intervention.
- All randomised controlled comparisons of oral steroids versus placebo or another intervention were included and comparisons established according to intervention.
- All randomised controlled comparisons of physiotherapy modalities versus placebo, or another modality, or of varying modalities compared to each other were included.
- All randomised controlled comparisons of acupuncture versus placebo, or another modality, or of varying types and dosages of acupuncture were included.
- All randomised controlled comparisons of extracorporeal shock wave therapy (ESWT) versus placebo, or another modality, or of varying types and dosages of ESWT were included, and comparisons established according to intervention.
- All randomised controlled comparisons of suprascapular nerve block versus placebo or another intervention were included and comparisons established according to intervention.

Literature search

MEDLINE, EMBASE, CINAHL (includes all major physiotherapy and occupational therapy journals from USA, Canada, England, Australia, and New Zealand), and Science Citation Index (SCISEARCH) were searched 1966 to November 2002. The search strategy is outlined below. Keywords gained from previous reviews and all relevant articles were searched as text terms and any additional keyword identified from subsequent articles was searched again.

1 shoulder pain/
2. shoulder impingement syndrome/
3. rotator cuff/
4. exp bursitis/
5. (shoulder$ or rotator cuff) adj5 (bursitis or frozen or impinge$ or tendinitis or tendonitis or pain$)).mp.

6. rotator cuff.mp.
7. adhesive capsulitis.mp.
8. or/1–7
9. acupuncture*
10. analgesics*
11. anti-inflammatory drugs*
12. N.S.A.I.D.S.*
13. NSAID*
14. extra corporeal shock wave therapy*
15. shock wave therapy*
16. non steroidal anti-inflammatory*
17. orthopaedic surgery*
18. surgery*
19. exp rehabilitation/
20. exp physical therapy techniques/
21. exp musculoskeletal manipulations/
22. exp exercise movement techniques/
23. exp ultrasonography, interventional/
24. (rehabilitat$ or physiotherap$ or physical therap$ or manual therap$ or exercis$ or ultrasound or ultrasonograph$ or TNS or TENS or shockwave or electrotherap$ or mobili$). mp.
25. or/19–24
26. injection*
27. cortisone*
28. steroid*
29. prednis*
30. distension*
31. hydrodilatation*
32. nerve block*
33. or/10–18
34. or/25–32
35. 33 or 34
36. clinical trial.pt
37. random$.mp.
38. ((single or double) adj (blind$ or mask$)).mp.
39. placebo$.mp.
40. or/36-39
41. 8 and 35 and 40

Further electronic searches were made for key identified authors, and a record of these searches kept. Printouts of all search strategies were compiled and stored for future reproduction and review if required.

In addition, the Cochrane Controlled Trials Register (CCTR) Issue 2, 2002 was searched.

Following identification of potential trials for inclusion by the search strategy outlined, the methods sections of all identified trials were reviewed independently according to predetermined criteria (see selection criteria), by two of four investigators (RB, SG, Joanne Youd or Sarah Hetrick). All articles were coded and details of source, intervention, population, and funding recorded.

Trials meeting inclusion criteria were collated, and the methods and results sections were re-assessed by the same two of four reviewers (RB, SG, JY, SH) for assessment of validity.

Where the two reviewers disagreed, discussion was facilitated in order to reach consensus. If this failed, the trial was sent to a third reviewer for arbitration.

Data extraction and analysis

In order to assess efficacy, raw data for outcomes of interest (means and standard deviations for continuous outcomes and number of events and total population number for binary outcomes) were extracted, where available, from the published reports. All standard errors of the mean were converted to standard deviation. Wherever reported data was converted or imputed, this was recorded. For trials where the required data were not reported or able to be calculated, further details were requested of first authors. If no further details were provided, the trial was included in the review and fully described, but not included in the meta-analysis.

The following choices of statistic and 95% confidence intervals were presented for all outcomes.

Continuous outcomes

Weighted mean difference using a fixed effect model was selected when outcomes were measured on standard scales. When outcomes were reported on non-standard scales, using differing units and methods of assessment (for example disability scales), a standardised mean difference (SMD) was selected. Possible clinical reasons for heterogeneity were explored, and in the presence of significant heterogeneity, trial results were not combined. For the purpose of this summary, standardised mean differences are reported.

Dichotomous outcomes

Relative risk using a fixed effects model was selected for interpretation of dichotomous outcome measures in this review, as this is the most appropriate statistic for interpretation when the event is common. Reasons for heterogeneity were evaluated, and in the event of significant heterogeneity trial results were not pooled.

Sensitivity analysis

Three sensitivity analyses were planned.

1. Trials in which the outcome assessor was not blinded were to be excluded to assess the possible effect of detection bias.
2. Trials published in languages other than English were to be excluded to assess the possible effect of publication bias.
3. Trials for which allocation concealment was unclear were to be excluded to assess their effect upon the conclusion of the review.

Outcomes

No studies were excluded on the basis of outcome measure used. Reported outcomes included pain (at night, at rest, and on movement), range of motion (active and/or passive: flexion, abduction, external rotation, internal rotation and hand behind back), function, strength, and return to work or school.

Evaluating the evidence

This review included only randomised controlled trials.

Validity of included trials was assessed by comment on whether they met key criteria (appropriate randomisation, allocation concealment, blinding, number lost to follow up, and intention to treat analysis). These criteria were selected as they were thought to potentially bias the overall outcome of the included trial. The only quantitative scoring was given for allocation concealment, ranked as:

A adequate
B unclear, or
C inadequate.

Whether or not trials were appropriately randomised, included blinded participants, care providers and outcome assessor, had complete follow up and used an intention to treat analysis was recorded on a pre-piloted data extraction sheet and later transposed into the review. Validity of trials was assessed in this way as opposed to using a numerical or summary scale due to concerns regarding the validity of such scales and lack of information about whether all the criteria included in such scales impact on the overall outcome of the trial.

Summary

The following will present an evidence summary of recent systematic review and meta-analysis of interventions for shoulder pain including non-steroidal anti-inflammatory medication, corticosteroid injections, shoulder joint distension, oral steroids, physiotherapy interventions, acupuncture, suprascapular nerve block, and extracorporeal shock wave therapy. A more detailed assessment of the validity of the trials can be found in the individual Cochrane systematic reviews.

Interventions for rotator cuff disease (includes study populations described as rotator cuff tendinitis, bursitis, supraspinatus tendinitis, biceps tendinitis, subdeltoid bursitis, and full thickness rotator cuff tear) and adhesive capsulitis (includes study populations described as periarthritis, frozen shoulder) have been presented separately. Trials that included a study population of either unspecified or mixed diagnoses have not been included in this evidence summary. Case presentations will illustrate how different treatments may be selected depending on the desired outcome, risk profile, and preferences of the individual.

A systematic review of interventions for acute shoulder pain (defined as pain present for less than three months) has recently been performed as part of the development of Evidence-based Guidelines for the Management of Acute Musculoskeletal Pain, recently commissioned by the Commonwealth Department of Health and Ageing, Australia.[11] The Dutch College of General Practitioners have also published Practice Guidelines for shoulder complaints that provide guidance for the diagnosis and treatment of these complaints in the setting of Dutch general practice and these are now available in English.[12] Our results are consistent with the recommendations of both guidelines.

Rotator cuff disease

Case presentation 1

A 60-year-old right-handed man presents at your practice complaining of a four-month history of a painful right shoulder. The onset of pain seemed to relate to a particularly strenuous game of tennis. The pain is particularly noticeable at night and he is unable to sleep on the affected side. During the day the pain is less of a problem but is aggravated by use of the arm in certain directions, particularly overhead, and he has been unable to resume his regular weekly tennis game. Clinical examination reveals pain between 30 and 120 degrees of active abduction although range of motion is not restricted. There is pain on resisted abduction and external rotation but no weakness. He has normal radiographs. He is seeking your advice regarding treatment options.

Non-steroidal anti-inflammatory drugs (NSAIDs)

We found two systematic reviews of NSAIDs in shoulder pain that included four and three trials respectively.[10,13] The Cochrane review[10] has been updated into a series of separate reviews of interventions for shoulder disorders and includes 19 NSAID trials with a combined total of 1203 participants.[14] The number of participants per trial ranged from 13 to 147 (median 41 participants), with only 8 trials involving more than 50 participants

Eight trials were performed for rotator cuff disease, with a total of 417 participants, range 26–100, median of 60 participants.[15–22] One study compared NSAID to placebo NSAID,[15] one study compared two types of NSAID,[16] and one study compared slow-release NSAID with conventional NSAID.[17] One study compared indomethacin (and saline injection) to steroid injection.[18] Two studies were three-arm comparisons: one of NSAID versus laser therapy versus placebo[19] and another of NSAID plus a placebo injection of lidocaine (lignocaine) versus steroid injection versus placebo (lidocaine) injection alone.[20] One study was a four-arm comparison of NSAID and steroid injection versus NSAID and placebo (lidocaine) injection versus steroid injection versus placebo

Comparison: 01 NSAID *v* PLACEBO INJECTION
Outcome: 02 Pain at 4 weeks

Study	NSAID n	NSAID mean (sd)	placebo n	placebo mean (sd)	SMD (95% CI Fixed)	Weight %	SMD (95% CI Fixed)
01 Rotator cuff disease at 4 weeks							
Adebajo 1990	20	−3·60 (2·99)	20	−1·35 (0·74)		41·9	−1·01 [−1·67, 0·35]
Petri 1987	25	−1·76 (1·55)	25	−1·00 (1·60)		58·1	−0·47 [−1·04, 0·09]
Total (95%CI)	45		45			100·0	−0·70 [−1·13, 0·27]
Test for heterogeneity chi-square = 1·47 df = 1 p = 0·23							
Test for overall effect z = 3·20 p = 0·001							

−10 −5 0 5 10

Favours NSAID Favours placebo

Figure 10.1

(lidocaine) injection.[21] One study was a five-arm comparison of acupuncture versus steroid injection versus steroid injection and NSAID versus physiotherapy versus placebo.[22] Results are presented below for the trials that provided data suitable for pooling.

Outcomes

NSAID versus placebo (NSAID)

Benefits: One small trial of 37 participants reported no difference with respect to pain at 7 days (mean improvement in pain −1·58 (1·41) and −1·46 (1·42) in the NSAID and placebo groups respectively on a five-point categorical scale (1 very mild to 5 very severe), SMD = −0·08 (−0·74, 0·57).[15]

Adverse effects: There was no difference in the incidence of adverse effects between NSAID and placebo when the results of two trials (60 participants) were pooled (5/31 *v* 7/29 RR 0·70 (0·28, 1·78).[15,22]

Evidence summary: Silver

One small RCT found no evidence of benefit after 7 days. Limited data from one small RCT found no difference between NSAIDs and placebo with respect to adverse effects. However the potential adverse effects of NSAIDs are well described and should be considered, particularly in high risk groups.

NSAID versus placebo injection

The pooled results of two small studies (90 participants) found a small benefit of NSAID over placebo injection for improvement in pain (SMD −0·7 (−1·13, −0·27)(pain measured by 10 cm VAS in Adebajo *et al*[20] and linear scale 0 = worst, 5 = best in Petri *et al*[21]) (Figure 10.1) and range of abduction in degrees (SMD 0·7 (0·27, 1·13) (Figure 10.2) (Table 10.1) at 4 weeks but no difference with respect to function, patient-reported response to treatment or tenderness.[20,21]

Evidence summary: Silver

A systematic review including a meta-analysis of two small RCTs found a small improvement in pain but not function at 4 weeks for NSAID compared to a placebo injection.

Comparison of NSAIDs

One trial of 28 participants reported a benefit after one week of phenylbutazone compared to fentiazac for restriction in function reported by

Comparison: 01 NSAID v PLACEBO INJECTION
Outcome: 04 Range of abduction

Study	NSAID n	NSAID mean (sd)	placebo n	placebo mean (sd)	SMD (95% CI Fixed)	Weight %	SMD (95% CI Fixed)
01 Rotator cuff disease at 4 weeks							
Adebajo 1990	20	46·80 (25·22)	20	5·40 (46·82)		41·4	1·08, [−0·41, 1·75]
Petri 1987	25	1·39 (1·55)	25	0·77 (1·20)		58·6	0·44 [−0·12, 1·00]
Total (95%CI)	45		45			100·0	0·70 [0·27, 1·13]

Test for heterogeneity chi-square = 2·06 df = 1 p = 0·15
Test for overall effect z = 3·21 p = 0·001

−10 −5 0 5 10
Favours placebo Favours NSAID

Figure 10.2

Table 10·1 Number needed to treat for NSAID versus placebo injection (pooled results from two trials, Adebajo *et al*, 1990 and Petri *et al*, 1987)[20,21]

Outcome	Pooled standardised mean difference (95% CI)	% benefiting (95% CI) with NSAID	NNT (95% CI)
Pain at 4 weeks	−0·70 (−1·13, −0·27)	32% (13, 47)	4 (3, 8)
Range of abduction	0·70 (0·27, 1·13)	32% (13, 47)	4 (3, 8)

patients (mean improvement −2·80 (1·48) and 0·20 (1·22) in the phenylbutazone and fentiazac groups respectively on a VAS (0 better, 10 worse), SMD −2·16 (−3·16, −1·16); and change in patient-reported stiffness – mean improvement −0·80 (0·59) and 0·70 (1·10) in the phenylbutazone and fentiazac groups respectively on a VAS (0 better, 10 worse), SMD −1·61 (−2·51, −0·70)); but no differences were detected in other outcomes including failure rates reported by physicians and patients, range of motion, pain and tenderness at one week.[16]

Evidence summary: Silver

A small RCT found no consistent effects across endpoints of phenylbutazone compared to fentiazac at 4 weeks.

Slow release versus standard NSAID

There were no reported differences with respect to efficacy in one trial of 65 participants comparing slow release fentiazac (300 mg) to either 100 mg fentiazac four times daily or 200 mg fentiazac twice a day.[17]

Evidence summary: Silver

One RCT found no difference in efficacy between slow release and standard NSAID.

NSAID plus intra-articular steroid injection versus placebo

A small trial of 20 participants found no significant differences at 4 weeks between combination NSAID and intra-articular steroid injection versus placebo for pain (improvement in pain −9·9 (28·37) and −30·0 (29·98) in the NSAID/injection and placebo groups respectively on a 100 mm VAS, SMD 0·66 (−0·16, 1·49)); abduction (improvement in abduction 13·00 (24·06) and 29·00 (28·24) in the NSAID/ injection and placebo groups respectively in degrees, SMD −16·0 (−36·99, 4·99)); and

Comparison: 12 NSAID *v* SUBACROMIAL STEROID INJECTION
Outcome: 01 Pain score

Study	NSAID n	NSAID mean (sd)	Subacromial steroid n	Subacromial steroid mean (sd)	Weight %	SMD (95% CI Fixed)
01 Rotator cuff disease						
Adebajo 1990	20	−3·60 (2·99)	20	−4·95 (3·31)	32·9	0·42, [−0·21, 1·05]
Petri 1987	25	−1·71 (1·55)	25	−2·04 (1·55)	41·9	0·21 [−0·35, 0.77]
White 1986	15	−5·50 (8.30)	15	−4·30 (5·20)	25·2	−0·17 [0·89, 0·55]
Total (95% CI)	60		60		100·0	0·18 [−0·18, 0·54]

Test for heterogeneity chi-square = 1·48 df = 2 p = 0·48
Test for overall effect z = 1·00 p = 0·3

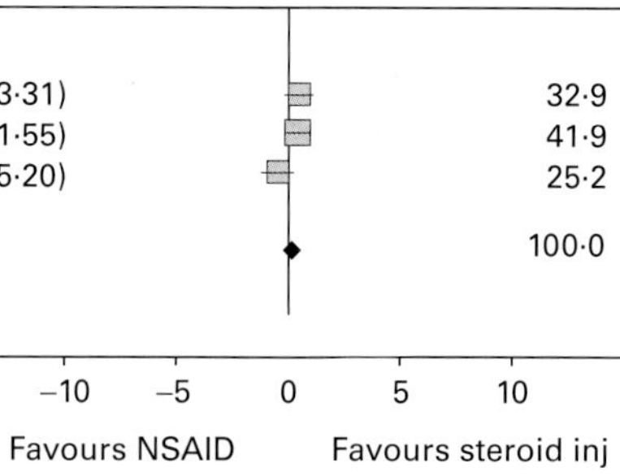

−10 −5 0 5 10
Favours NSAID Favours steroid inj

Figure 10.3

Comparison: 12 NSAID *v* SUBACROMIAL STEROID INJECTION
Outcome: 02 Range of shoulder abduction

Study	NSAID n	NSAID mean (sd)	Subacromial steroid n	Subacromial steroid mean (sd)	Weight %	SMD (95% CI Fixed)
01 Rotator cuff disease						
Adebajo 1990	20	46·80 (25·99)	20	50·40 (36·00)	33·5	−0·11 [−0·73, 0·51]
Petri 1987	25	1·39 (1·55)	25	1·56 (1·20)	41·8	−0·12 [−0·68, 0.43]
White 1986	15	16·00 (45·00)	15	30·00 (37·00)	24·7	−0·33 [−1·05, 0·39]
Total (95% CI)	60		60		100·0	−0·17 [−0·53, 0·19]

Test for heterogeneity chi-square = 0·25 df = 2 p = 0·88
Test for overall effect z = 0·93 p = 0·4

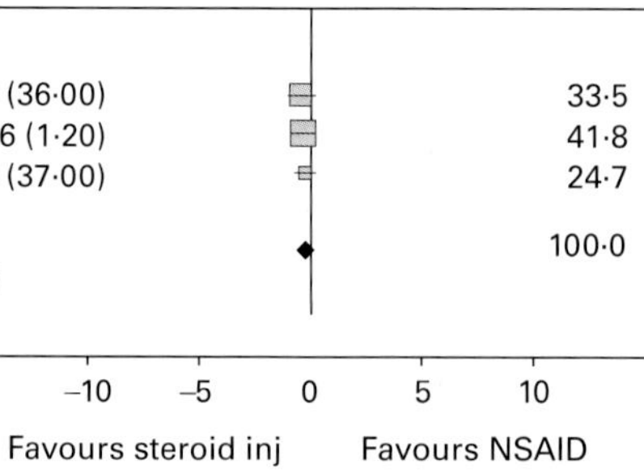

−10 −5 0 5 10
Favours steroid inj Favours NSAID

Figure 10.4

success rate (5/12 versus 9/12 in the NSAID/injection and placebo groups respectively, RR 0·50 (0·26, 1·17)).[22]

Evidence summary: Silver

One small RCT found no benefit of combination NSAID and steroid injection over placebo at 4 weeks.

NSAID versus subacromial steroid injection

The pooled results of three trials (100 participants) found no difference between NSAID and steroid injection with respect to pain (SMD 0·18 (−0·18, 0·54) (pain measured by 10 cm VAS in Adebajo *et al*;[20] linear scale 0 = worst, 5 = best in Petri *et al*,[21] and 9 cm VAS in White *et al*[18] (Figure 10.3)) or abduction in degrees (SMD −0·17 (−0.53, 0.19)) (Figure 10.4) at 4 weeks.[18,20,21]

Evidence summary: Silver

Systematic review of three small trials found no difference in benefit of NSAID compared with steroid injection at 4 weeks.

NSAID plus steroid injection versus steroid injection

One trial of 50 participants found no added benefit of NSAID and subacromial steroid injection compared to steroid injection alone with respect to pain, range of abduction, and function at 4 weeks.[21] Another trial of 24 participants found no added benefit of NSAID and intra-articular steroid compared to steroid injection alone with respect to pain, abduction, and success rate.[22]

Evidence summary: Silver

Systematic review of two small RCTs found no added benefit of NSAID over steroid injection alone.

NSAID versus laser therapy

One small trial of 20 participants reported range of flexion at 2 weeks was better in the laser therapy treated group (mean improvement in flexion, measured in degrees, 22·3 (16·06) and 5·0 (9·13)) in the laser and NSAID group respectively (SMD 1.27 (0·29, 2·25)).[19]

Evidence summary: Silver

Limited data from one small RCT showed better range of flexion with laser than NSAID at 2 weeks.

Conclusion

Based upon the results of studies for which data was available for pooling, there is conflicting data concerning the benefits of NSAID in rotator cuff disease. There is weak evidence from two trials of some short-term benefits of NSAID compared to placebo. There is weak evidence from three small trials that there is no difference in benefit between steroid injection and NSAID, and two trials have reported no added benefit of NSAID over steroid injection alone.

Recommendation for case presentation 1

NSAIDs may be of limited value for the patient described above with respect to short term pain relief. The small benefit of NSAIDs should be weighed up against the potential risks of NSAID, particularly in high risk patients.

Corticosteroid injection

Four systematic reviews of corticosteroid injection for shoulder pain were identified.[6,7,23,24] The review by van der Heijden *et al* did not differentiate between studies on the basis of the nature of the populations being studied and did not calculate effect sizes for the same reported outcome measures in different trials.[6] The review by Goupille and Sibilia included non-randomised studies, reported results of primary studies only as significant or not significant and made no attempt to quantify effect sizes or pool results.[23] The Cochrane Review by Buchbinder *et al* is the most up to date and includes 26 randomised controlled trials with a combined total of more than 1455 participants (one trial did not specify number of participants[25]).[24] Trial populations varied between 24 and 150 participants, median sample size was 52. We found one additional trial of 48 participants published in Spanish comparing up to three intra-articular steroid injections to transdermal nitroglycerin patches in rotator cuff tendinitis.[26]

Twelve trials were performed for rotator cuff tendonitis (including impingement, subacromial bursitis, partial rotator cuff tears, and one trial for full thickness rotator cuff tear) with a total of 650 participants, range 25–100, median of 51 participants.[18,20–22,26,27–33] There were seven trials that compared subacromial steroid injection to placebo[20,21,27–31] and one trial that compared supraspinatus tendon injection to placebo.[32] There were three trials that compared

Comparison: 02 SUBACROMIAL STEROID INJECTION *v* PLACEBO
Outcome: 01 Improvement in pain at 4 weeks

Study	Steroid injection n	Steroid injection mean (sd)	placebo n	placebo mean (sd)	SMD (95% CI Fixed)	Weight %	SMD (95% CI Fixed)
01 Rotator cuff disease							
Adebajo 1990	20	4·95 (3·31)	20	1·35 (3·31)		42·2	1·07 [0·40, 1·73]
Petri 1987	25	2·04 (1·55)	25	1·00 (1·60)		57·8	0·65 [0·08, 1.22]
Total (95% CI)	45		45			100·0	0·83 [0·39, 1·26]
Test for heterogeneity chi-square = 0·86 df = 1 p = 0·35							
Test for overall effect z = 3·73 p = 0·0002							

Figure 10.5

subacromial steroid injection to non-steroidal anti-inflammatory medication,[18,20,21] and one trial that compared combination subacromial steroid injection and anti-inflammatory medication to non-steroidal anti-inflammatory medication alone.[21] One trial compared crystalline versus lipoid subacromial steroid injection.[27] One five-arm trial compared intra-articular steroid injection to placebo, physiotherapy, and acupuncture and also compared intra-articular steroid injection and non-steroidal anti-inflammatory medication to placebo[22] and one trial compared up to three intra-articular steroid injections to transdermal nitroglycerin patches.[26]

There was a wide variation in the corticosteroid preparation used, the dosage, number of injections given and their timing. Six trials used triamcinolone: a single 80 mg triamcinolone hexacetomide injection;[20] a single 40 mg triamcinolone acetonide injection (three trials);[18,21,28] a single 20 mg triamcinolone hexacetomide injection;[31] and a single 10 mg triamcinolone acetonide injection.[27] Three trials used methylprednisolone: a single 40 mg injection of methylprednisolone acetate (two trials);[33,29] and a single 80 mg methylprednisolone injection.[32] Two trials used dexamethasone (7·7%): a single injection of 2·5 mg dexamethasone[27] (note: Plafki *et al* compared triamcinolone to dexamethasone); and up to five injections (at weekly intervals) of 2 mg dexamethasone.[33] One trial used a single injection of 6 mg betamethasone.[30] The total volume injected varied between 2 and 25 ml and the use of local anaesthetic also varied widely.

The anatomical site of steroid injection also varied. Injections were placed into the subacromial space (or bursa) in seven trials[18,20,21,27–30] and supraspinatus tendon in one trial;[32] into the glenohumeral joint via an anterior approach in one trial,[22] a superior approach in one trial,[31] and approach not described in one trial.[33] Only one study confirmed needle placement: Plafki *et al* used ultrasound to confirm needle placement in the subacromial space.[27]

Outcomes: benefits

Subacromial steroid injection versus placebo

Only the results of two of the seven trials of subacromial steroid injection versus placebo could be pooled.[20,21] The pooled results of these two small trials (90 participants) found a small benefit of subacromial steroid injection over placebo for improvement in pain (SMD 0·83 (0·39, 1·26; pain measured by 10 cm VAS in Adebajo *et al*[20] and linear scale 0 = worst, 5 = best in Petri *et al*[21]) (Figure 10.5), function (SMD = 0·63 (0·20, 1·06; function measured by

Comparison: 02 SUBACROMIAL STEROID INJECTION *v* PLACEBO
Outcome: 02 Improvement in function at 4 weeks

Study	Steroid injection n	Steroid injection mean (sd)	placebo n	placebo mean (sd)	SMD (95% CI Fixed)	Weight %	SMD (95% CI Fixed)
01 Rotator cuff disease							
Adebajo 1990	20	0·85 (0·67)	20	0·30 (0·44)		42·1	0·95 [0·29, 1·61]
Petri 1987	25	1·64 (1·30)	25	1·02 (1·75)		57·9	0·40 [−0·16, 0·96]
Total (95% CI)	45		45			100·0	0·63 [0·20, 1·06]
Test for heterogeneity chi-square = 1·59 df = 1 p = 0·21							
Test for overall effect z = 2·89 p = 0·004							

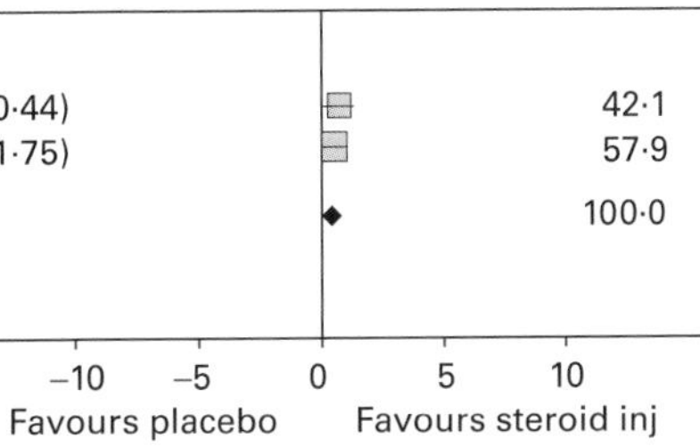

−10 −5 0 5 10
Favours placebo Favours steroid inj

Figure 10.6

Comparison: 02 SUBACROMIAL STEROID INJECTION *v* PLACEBO
Outcome: 03 Improvement in range of active abduction at 4 weeks

Study	Steroid injection n	Steroid injection mean (sd)	placebo n	placebo mean (sd)	SMD (95% CI Fixed)	Weight %	SMD (95% CI Fixed)
01 Rotator cuff disease							
Adebajo 1990	20	50·40 (36·00)	20	5·40 (46·82)		42·3	1·06 [0·39, 1·72]
Petri 1987	25	1·56 (1·20)	25	0·77 (1·20)		57·7	0·65 [0·08, 1·22]
Total (95% CI)	45		45			100·0	0·82 [0·39, 1·25]
Test for heterogeneity chi-square = 0·83 df = 1 p = 0·36							
Test for overall effect z = 0·93 p = 0·4							

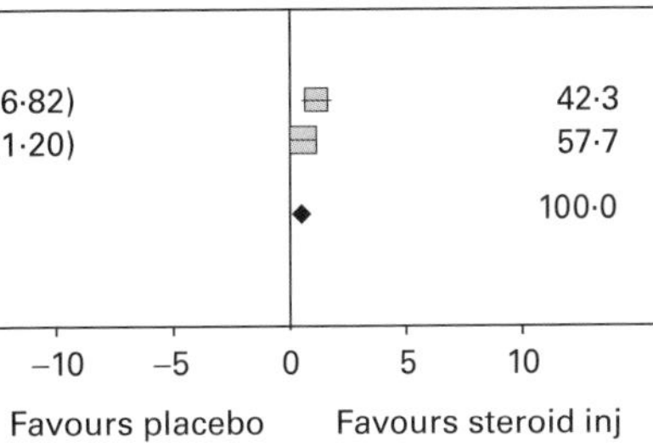

−10 −5 0 5 10
Favours placebo Favours steroid inj

Figure 10.7

four-point scale where 0 = no limitation of function and 3 = severe limitation of function, in Adebajo *et al*[20] and by six-point scale where 0 = worst function and 5 = best function in Petri *et al*[21] (Figure 10.6), and range of abduction in degrees (SMD = 0·82 (0·39, 1·25)) (Figure 10.7) (Table 10.2).[20,21]

The five trials that were unable to be pooled (239 participants) were of varying methodological quality.[27–31] They reported varying results – at least some benefit favouring steroid injection in two trials,[27,28] no difference in two trials,[29,30] and some benefit favouring placebo in one trial.[31]

Evidence summary: Silver

A systematic review of seven trials found a small improvement in pain, function and range of abduction at 4 weeks for subacromial steroid injection compared to placebo injection when the results of two studies were pooled. Results for the other five studies could not be pooled and reported varying results.

Supraspinatus tendon injection versus placebo

A single trial of 25 participants with "supraspinatus tendonitis" (defined as tenderness over the

Table 10·2 Number needed to treat for subacromial corticosteroid injection versus placebo (pooled results from two trials, Buchbinder, 2003)[24]

Outcome	Pooled standardised mean difference (95% CI)	% benefiting (95% CI) with corticosteroid injection	NNT (95% CI)
Improvement in pain at 4 weeks	0·83 (0·39, 1·26)	37% (19, 51)	3 (2, 6)
Improvement in function at 4 weeks	0·63 (0·20, 1·06)	29% (10, 45)	4 (3, 11)
Improvement in abduction at 4 weeks	0·82 (0·39, 1·25)	37% (19, 51)	3 (2, 6)

supraspinatus tendon and pain on resisted abduction of the glenohumeral joint in the presence a normal passive range of glenohumeral movement) comparing supraspinatus steroid injection to placebo reported no difference with respect to pain or analgesic consumption at 2 and 8 weeks' follow up.[32]

Evidence summary: Silver

One small trial found no benefit of supraspinatus injection versus placebo.

Intra-articular steroid injection versus placebo

A single trial of 24 participants with rotator cuff disease comparing intra-articular steroid injection to placebo reported no benefit of steroid injection over placebo at 4 weeks with respect to pain, range of abduction or success of therapy.[22]

Evidence summary: Silver

One small trial found no benefit of intra-articular steroid injection versus placebo.

Subacromial steroid injection versus NSAID

The pooled results of three trials (100 participants) found no difference between NSAID and steroid injection with respect to pain (SMD 0·18 (–0·18, 0·54); pain measured by 10 cm VAS in Adebajo *et al*,[20] linear scale 0 = worst, 5 = best in Petri *et al*,[21] and 9 cm VAS in White *et al*[18]; see Figure 10.3) or abduction in degrees (SMD –0.17 (–0.53, 0.19); see Figure 10.4) at 4 weeks.[18,20,21]

Evidence summary: Silver

Systematic review including meta-analysis of three small trials found no difference in benefit of NSAID compared with steroid injection at 4 weeks.

Intra-articular steroid injection versus ultrasound or acupuncture

No difference with respect to pain, range of abduction or success of therapy at 4 weeks was found in one trial of 60 participants comparing intra-articular steroid injection to ultrasound or acupuncture for rotator cuff disease (12 participants in each of 5 treatment groups).[22]

Evidence summary: Silver

One trial found no difference in efficacy between intra-articular steroid injection, ultrasound, and acupuncture.

Intra-articular steroid injection and NSAID versus placebo

A small trial of 20 participants found no significant differences at 4 weeks between combination

NSAID and intra-articular steroid injection versus placebo for pain (improvement in pain –9·9 (28·37) and –30·0 (29·98) in the NSAID/injection and placebo groups respectively on a 100 mm VAS, SMD 0·66 (–0·16, 1·49); abduction (improvement in abduction 13·00 (24·06) and 29·00 (28·24) in the NSAID/injection and placebo groups respectively in degrees, SMD –16·0 (–36·99, 4·99); and success rate (5/12 versus 9/12 in the NSAID/injection and placebo groups respectively; RR 0·50 (0·26, 1·17)).[22]

Evidence summary: Silver

One small RCT found no benefit of combination NSAID and steroid injection over placebo at 4 weeks.

Subacromial steroid injection and NSAID versus NSAID alone

There was no added benefit of subacromial steroid injection over NSAID alone in one trial of 50 participants with respect to improvement in pain, function, range of abduction and remission at 4 weeks.[21]

Evidence summary: Silver

One trial found no added benefit of subacromial steroid injection over NSAID alone.

Intra-articular steroid injection versus transdermal nitroglycerin patches

One trial reported that intra-articular steroid injections were superior to transdermal nitroglycerin patches at 4 weeks with respect to complete improvement (19/24 *v* 5/25, RR = 3·96 (1·76, 8·90).[26]

Evidence summary: Silver

One trial found intra-articular steroid injection more beneficial than transdermal nitroglycerin patches with respect to complete improvement at 4 weeks.

Intra-articular steroid injection versus hyaluronate injection

No difference with respect to satisfaction with treatment at 4 weeks was found in one trial of 78 participants comparing intra-articular steroid injection to hyaluronate injection for full thickness rotator cuff tears.[33]

Evidence summary: Silver

One trial found no differences between intra-articular steroid and hyaluronate injections for full thickness rotator cuff tears with respect to patient satisfaction with treatment at 4 weeks.

Outcome: adverse effects

The incidence of uncommon to rare adverse effects cannot be estimated from randomised controlled trials. Rare adverse effects that have been reported to be associated with steroid injection include infection (estimated risk 1/14 000 to 1/50 000 injections), subcutaneous fat necrosis and skin atrophy (<1 in 100 injections)[34,35] and painful reactions lasting 24–48 hours.[20,26,29] While rotator cuff tendon rupture has also been reported to occur following steroid injection, this may be due to detection bias and the strength of any association between steroid injection and tendon rupture has not been assessed in properly conducted studies. In diabetics blood glucose elevation occurs but is usually transient (24–48 hours).

Four of the 12 trials reviewed did not describe adverse effects of interventions[27,30–32] and three trials reported that there were no adverse effects of steroid injections.[22,28,33] Three trials reported that there was some degree of discomfort during the post-injection period in all or some participants,[20,29,26] while one trial specifically noted no worsening of pain in the injection group.[18] One trial reported no difference in the number of participants with adverse effects in the steroid injection versus NSAID group.[21] Petri *et al* reported change in skin pigmentation at injection site in one participant, postmenopausal bleeding in one participant, pityriasis rosea appearing two days after injection in one patient.[21]

Evidence summary: Silver

Few adverse effects of steroid injections have been reported in clinical trials of rotator cuff disorders.

Conclusion

There is limited evidence to support the use of subacromial corticosteroid injection for rotator cuff tendonitis although its effect may be small and not well maintained, and it may be no better than NSAID. Issues that need to be resolved include the importance of accurate placement of the injection in the subacromial and/or intra-articular space, and whether the frequency, dose and type of steroid influences treatment outcome.

Recommendations for case presentation 1

A subacromial steroid injection may be of limited value for the patient described above with respect to short term pain relief. Transient pain following the injection may occur and diabetics should be aware that steroid injection might elevate blood glucose

Physiotherapy interventions

The most recent review is a Cochrane systematic review of 26 randomised controlled trials, of variable methodological quality, in 1499 participants, investigating the effect of physiotherapy interventions for shoulder disorders.[36] Trial populations were generally small (median sample size = 48, range 14–180) with many trials underpowered to demonstrate a difference between groups if one was present. There were 13 trials in rotator cuff disease,[19,22,37–47] including three specifically for calcific tendinitis.[39,40,41] The physiotherapeutic modalities studied included low power laser therapy;[19,46,47] ultrasound;[22,39,41,42] acetic acid iontophoresis and ultrasound;[40] pulsed electromagnetic field;[43,44] supervised exercise and manual physical therapy.[37,38,45]

Outcomes: benefits

Laser therapy versus placebo

Data from the three trials that compared laser therapy to placebo could not be pooled.[19,46,47] One trial of 20 participants demonstrated a significant difference favouring laser therapy for reduction of pain (difference in median pain measured on a 10 cm VAS at 2 weeks = 2·5 cm (2, 3).[19] There was a trend favouring the laser therapy group in one trial of 24 participants that reported an excellent or good response in 10/12 participants in the laser therapy group compared to 5/12 in the placebo group (RR 2·00 (0·98, 4·09)).[46] No differences between groups were demonstrated for any of the reported outcome measures including pain, function or range of movement at 4 and 8 weeks in the third trial of 35 participants.[47]

Evidence summary: Silver

Systematic review of three trials found varying results. One trial reported no differences in outcome of laser therapy compared to placebo while two trials reported limited evidence of benefit of laser therapy.

Ultrasound +/- iontophoresis of acetic acid versus placebo

There were three trials of ultrasound compared to placebo for rotator cuff disease (24/60, 20

Table 10.3 Number needed to treat for pulsed electromagnetic field versus placebo (Dal Conte, 1990)[43]

Outcome	Benefit with placebo	Benefit with pulsed electromagnetic field	Relative risk with pulsed electromagnetic field (95% CI)	Absolute benefit increase (95% CI)	NNT (95% CI)
No pain at 6 days	0/30 (0%)	9/30 (30%)	19·0 (1·16, 12·43)	30% (13, 48)	4 (3, 9)
No pain at 4-6 weeks	0/30 (0%)	19/30 (63%)	39·0 (2·46, 617·84)	63% (42, 78)	2 (2, 3)

and 61 participants respectively),[22,41,42] one trial in calcific tendonitis (54 participants, 61 shoulders),[39] and one trial in calcific tendonitis comparing ultrasound plus iontophoresis of acetic acid (22 participants).[40] A pooled analysis of two trials (78 participants (84 shoulders)) assessing the effect of ultrasound on short-term recovery or substantial improvement demonstrated a very small but significant benefit over placebo (35/43 *v* 24/41; RR 1·39 (1·02,1·9)).[22,39] One of these trials reported no difference between groups (6/12 and 9/12 recovered or significant improvement in the ultrasound and placebo groups respectively)[22] while the other trial reported a significant benefit favouring the ultrasound group (29/31 and 15/29 recovered or significant improvement in the ultrasound and placebo groups respectively).[39] The same trial demonstrated a significant improvement in radiological appearance of calcific tendonitis in the short term (end of treatment) (15/32 *v* 3/29; RR 4·53 (1·46, 14·07)) and long term (9 month follow up) (20/31 *v.* 5/29; RR 3·74 (1·62, 8·66)). Two trials demonstrated no benefit of ultrasound over placebo[41,42] and one trial demonstrated no benefit of ultrasound plus iontophoresis of acetic acid compared to placebo.[40]

Evidence summary: Silver

Systematic review of five trials found limited evidence of benefit of ultrasound in one trial and no evidence of benefit in four trials.

Pulsed electromagnetic field versus placebo

Pulsed electromagnetic field has been shown in one trial to have a significantly beneficial effect on calcific tendonitis in both the short term (no pain at the end of 6 days 9/30 in pulsed electromagnetic field group versus 0/30 in placebo group; RR 19·0 (1·16, 12·43) and medium-term (no pain at 4–6 weeks 19/30 in pulsed electromagnetic field group and 0/30 placebo group; RR 39·0 (2·46, 617·84)) (Table 10.3).[43]

Evidence summary: Silver

One RCT found a significant benefit of pulsed electromagnetic field over placebo.

Exercise versus placebo

One trial demonstrated sustained significant benefit with respect to function after two and a half years for exercise compared to placebo (good or excellent function – Neer score) in 27/44 exercise groups and 7/28 placebo group; RR 2·45 (1·24, 4·86))[45] (Table 10.4). There was also a trend favouring the exercise group for no pain at rest (21/45 *v* 6/28, RR 2·18 (1·0, 4·73)), no pain on activity (19/45 and 6/28, RR1·97 (0·90, 4·33)), and no night pain (20/45 and 6/28, RR 2·07 (0·95, 4·53)).

Evidence summary: Silver

Evidence from at least one RCT found a significant and sustained benefit of exercise over placebo.

Exercise and mobilization versus exercise alone

Two small trials of 49 and 14 participants respectively demonstrated a significant

Table 10.4 Number needed to treat for exercise versus placebo (Brox, 1997)[45]

Outcome	Benefit with placebo	Benefit with exercise	Relative risk with exercise (95% CI)	Absolute benefit increase (95% CI)	NNT (95% CI)
Good to excellent function at 2½ years	7/28 (25%)	27/44 (61%)	2·45 (1·24, 4·86)	36% (13, 54)	3 (2, 8)

Comparison: 16 MOBILISATION PLUS EXERCISE *v* EXERCISE ALONE (RCD)
Outcome: 01 Pain at 3–4 weeks

Study	Mobilisation and Ex n	Mobilisation and Ex mean (sd)	Exercise alone n	Exercise alone mean (sd)	SMD (95% CI Fixed)	Weight %	SMD (95% CI Fixed)
Bang 2000	27	174·41 (183·06)	22	360·64 (272·32)		80·0	−0·81 [−1·39, −0·22]
Conroy 1998	7	12·02 (14·35)	7	44·09 (31·98)		20·0	−1·21 [−2·39, −0.04]
Total (95% CI)	34		29			100·0	−0·89 [−1·41, −0·36]

Test for heterogeneity chi-square = 0·37 df = 1 p = 0·55
Test for overall effect z = 3·31 p = 0·0009

−4 −2 0 2 4
Favours Mobils/Exer Favours Exercise

Figure 10.8

difference in reduction in pain (measured by pain score composite of several 100 mm scales in Bang *et al*[37] and 100 mm VAS in Conroy *et al*[38] at 3–4 weeks for exercise and mobilisation compared to exercise alone (pain at 3–4 weeks 174·41 (183·06) and 360·64 (272·32) in the exercise and mobilisation groups respectively in Bang *et al* and 12·02 (14·35) and 44·09 (31·98) in the exercise and mobilisation groups respectively in Conroy *et al*; SMD −0·89 (−1·41, −0·36) (Figure 10·8, Table 10.5).[37,38] Function at 3 weeks also favoured the mobilisation and exercise group in Bang *et al.*[37]

Evidence summary: Silver

Two small trials found a significant added benefit of mobilisation over exercise alone.

Ultrasound versus intra-articular steroid injection

No difference with respect to pain, range of abduction or success of therapy at 4 weeks was found in one trial of 60 participants comparing intra-articular steroid injection to ultrasound (12 participants in each of five treatment groups).[22]

Evidence summary: Silver

One trial found no difference in efficacy between ultrasound and intra-articular steroid injection.

Laser therapy versus NSAID

One small trial of 20 participants reported range of flexion at 2 weeks was better in the laser therapy treated group (mean improvement in flexion, measured in degrees 22·3 (16·06) and 5·0 (9·13) in the laser and NSAID group respectively; SMD 1·27 (0·29, 2·25)).[19]

Evidence summary: Silver

Limited data from one small RCT showed better range of flexion with laser than NSAID at 2 weeks.

Table 10.5 NNT for mobilisation plus exercise versus exercise alone (pooled results from Bang, 2000 and Conroy, 1998)[37,38]

Outcome	Pooled standardised mean difference (95% CI)	% benefiting (95% CI) with mobilisation plus exercise	NNT (95% CI)
Pain at 3–4 weeks	−0·89 (−1·41, −0·36)	39% (17, 55)	3 (2, 6)

Outcome: adverse effects

None of the reviewed trials assessed adverse effects of ultrasound or laser therapy. Pulsed electromagnetic field was reported to be associated with more post treatment pain than placebo.

Evidence summary: Silver

No serious adverse effects have been reported in the reviewed trials of physiotherapeutic interventions.

Conclusion

There is evidence from one trial of the benefit of a structured exercise programme for rotator cuff disease with evidence of additional benefit of mobilisation demonstrated from another two trials. There is limited evidence from two trials suggesting a short term benefit of laser therapy although results of a third trial were negative. Ultrasound is unlikely to be of benefit for rotator cuff disease based upon the results of four negative trials although a fifth trial reported limited benefit and one trial demonstrated improvement in the radiological appearance of calcific deposits. Based upon the results of a single trial, pulsed electromagnetic field may be of benefit for rotator cuff disease in the short term.

Recommendation for case presentation 1

A structured exercise programme and mobilization are likely to be helpful and laser therapy may confer some short term benefit for the patient described.

Acupuncture

One Cochrane Systematic Review identified five randomised controlled trials with a combined total of 328 participants.[48] Included studies were of varying methodological quality. Trial populations were on the whole small (median sample size 52, range 24 to 150). Two trials investigated the efficacy of acupuncture for rotator cuff disease.[22,49]

Outcomes

Acupuncture compared to placebo

Benefits: Berry *et al* demonstrated no significant difference between acupuncture and placebo for pain post intervention (24/60 participants).[22] One trial of 52 participants demonstrated acupuncture to be of benefit at 4 weeks compared to placebo according to the Constant Murley score (composite score for pain, function and range of motion measured out of a possible 100) (improvement 19·2 (16·1) and 8·37 (14·56) in the acupuncture and placebo groups respectively; SMD 0·70 (0·13, 1·26)), but clinical benefit was not sustained at 4 months.[49] Both trials assessed the overall success of acupuncture for rotator cuff disease, as rated yes or no by patients[49] or assessors.[22] Neither trial found any difference between success rates for acupuncture compared to placebo at 4 weeks (RR 1·01 (0·69–1·48)).

Adverse effects: Only one trial included adverse effects as an outcome.[49] There was no difference between acupuncture and sham acupuncture with respect to the incidence of fainting, headache, dizziness, inflammatory reactions or leg weakness.

Evidence summary: Silver
Systematic review of two RCTs found no significant benefit of acupuncture compared to placebo. One trial found no differences in adverse effects between acupuncture and sham acupuncture.

Acupuncture compared to steroid injection
No difference with respect to pain, range of abduction or success of therapy at 4 weeks was found in one trial of 60 participants comparing intra-articular steroid injection to acupuncture (12 participants in each of five treatment groups).[22]

Evidence summary: Silver
One trial found no difference in efficacy between intra-articular steroid injection and acupuncture.

Acupuncture compared to ultrasound
One trial comparing acupuncture to ultrasound (12 participants in each group) demonstrated no significant differences between groups 4 weeks following treatment with respect to pain or success rate (RR 0·83 (0·35, 2)).[22]

Evidence summary: Silver
One small trial found no difference in efficacy between acupuncture and ultrasound.

Conclusion
There is minimal evidence of benefit of acupuncture for rotator cuff disease.

> ***Recommendation for case presentation 1***
> Acupuncture is unlikely to be helpful for the case described above.

Suprascapular nerve block
We found no systematic reviews of suprascapular nerve block for shoulder pain. We found one published trial comparing suprascapular nerve block with placebo in 28 participants with either rotator cuff tendonitis or rotator cuff tears.[50]

Outcomes
Suprascapular nerve block versus placebo
Benefits: At 12 weeks there was a statistically significant benefit of suprascapular nerve block versus placebo with respect to night pain measured on a 10 cm VAS where 0 = no pain and 10 = maximal pain (improvement in night pain –3·9 (2·84) and 0·40 (2·23) in the nerve block and placebo groups respectively in the rotator cuff tendinitis group and –2·2 (4·02) and 1·0 (1·97) in the nerve block and placebo groups respectively in the rotator cuff tear group; SMD –1·27 (–2·14, –0·40)). Similar differences were detected for movement pain (SMD –1·08 (–2·00, –0·16)), active abduction (SMD 0·91 (0·09, 1·73)), flexion (SMD 1·21 (0·35, 2·07)), but not external rotation (SMD 0·72 (–0·09, 1·53))[50] (Table 10.6).

Adverse effects: One trial reported transient paraesthesia in 9 participants and mild aching in the area of the injection up to a week post procedure in 16 participants but the treatment group was not specified (suprascapular nerve block or placebo injection).[50]

Evidence summary: Silver
One small RCT reported evidence of benefit of suprascapular nerve block compared to placebo. No serious adverse effects of suprascapular nerve block were reported.

Conclusion
There is weak evidence from one small trial that suprascapular nerve block may be superior to placebo for rotator cuff disease at 12 weeks.

Table 10.6 Number needed to treat for suprascapular nerve block versus placebo (Vecchio, 1993)[50]

Outcome	Standardised mean difference (95% CI)	% benefiting (95% CI) suprascapular nerve block	NNT (95% CI)
Night pain	−1·27 (−2·14, −0·40)	51% (19, 65)	2 (2, 6)
Movement pain	−1·08 (−2·00, −0·16)	46% (8, 64)	3 (2, 13)
Active abduction	0·91 (0·09, 1·73)	40% (4, 61)	3 (2, 23)
Flexion	1·21 (0·35, 2·07)	50% (17, 65)	3 (2, 6)

Recommendation for case presentation 1

Suprascapular nerve block may be beneficial for the described patient.

Extracorporeal shock wave therapy (ESWT)

We found no systematic review of ESWT for shoulder pain. We found two trials performed in participants with calcific tendonitis[51,52] and two trials were performed in participants with non-calcific rotator cuff tendonitis[53,54] (total study population of 359 participants). The trial by Seil *et al* was published in German.[52]

One trial included a four-arm comparison of two sessions of high energy ESWT (2000 impulses of 0·32 mJ/mm^2 energy) versus one session of high energy ESWT versus 1 session with low energy ESWT (2000 impulses) versus no treatment (80 participants) and a separate two-arm comparison of either one or two sessions of high pulse energy (0·3 mJ/mm^2) (115 participants) in calcific tendonitis.[51] The second trial in calcific tendonitis compared low energy ESWT once per week for 3 weeks (5000 low dose impulses without anaesthesia) to single treatment of ESWT with 5000 high dose impulses with intravenous analgesia/sedation in 50 participants.[52]

One trial compared low energy shockwave therapy (2000 impulses of 0·11 mJ/mm^2 given weekly for three sessions) under local anaesthesia (10 ml mepivacaine to sham shockwave therapy in 40 participants with rotator cuff tendonitis but no calcification.[53] The second trial in non-calcific tendonitis compared moderate doses of ESWT (1500 pulses ESWT at 0·12 mJ/mm^2) monthly for 3 months to sham treatment in 74 participants.[54]

Outcomes: calcific tendonitis

ESWT versus no treatment

Benefits: One four-armed trial of 80 participants reported a significant benefit of two sessions of high energy ESWT compared to no treatment with respect to subjective improvement in pain at 3 months (14/20 and 1/20 respectively; RR 14·0 (2·01, 96·63)).[51] There was also a significant benefit for one session of high energy ESWT compared to no treatment (12/20 and 1/20 respectively; RR 12·0 (1·72, 83·81)). There was also a significant benefit for both high-energy ESWT groups compared to no treatment for Constant score (combined measure of pain and function) (mean (SD) Constant and Murley score for two sessions of high-energy ESWT and no treatment 68·5 (13·1) and 47·8 (11·40) respectively; SMD = 1·65 (0·92, 2·38); and for one session of high-energy ESWT and no treatment 63·7 (14·60) and 47·8 (11·40) respectively; SMD = 1·19 (0·51, 1·87)). There were also a significantly greater proportion of participants in the high-energy treatment groups who had disappearance of calcium deposits after 6 months compared to no treatment (two sessions of high-energy ESWT and no treatment 12/20 and 2/20 respectively; RR 6·0 (1·54, 23.44)); and one session of high-energy ESWT and no treatment 12/20 and 2/20 respectively; RR 5·50 (1·39, 21·72)).

The same trial reported non-significant differences for low energy ESWT compared to no treatment for number of participants reporting improvement in pain at 3 months (6/20 and 1/20 respectively; RR 6·0 (0·79, 45·42)); Constant and Murley score at 3 months (51·6 (20·10) and 47·8 (11·40); SMD = 0·23 (–0·39, 0·85)); and number of participants with disappearance of calcium deposits (4/20 and 2/20 respectively; RR = 2·0 (0·49, 9·71)).[51]

Evidence summary: Silver

One RCT found high energy but not low energy ESWT of benefit for calcific tendinitis.

High versus low dose ESWT

The authors of one trial of 50 participants concluded that at 6 weeks a 3 week course of weekly low dose ESWT and the single high dose ESWT with intravenous analgesia/sedation both significantly improve pain VAS and function as measured by the Constant Score at 6 weeks after treatment.[52] One trial of 80 participants found that two sessions of high energy ESWT was better than low energy ESWT for number of participants reporting improvement in pain at 3 months (14/20 and 6/20 respectively; RR 2·33 (1·13, 4·83)); Constant and Murley score at 3 months (68·5 (13·10) and 51·6 (20·10); SMD = 0·98 (0·32, 1·64)); and number of participants with disappearance of calcium deposits (12/20 and 4/20 respectively; RR = 3·0 (1.16, 7.73)).[51] The same trial also found that one session of high energy ESWT was better than low energy ESWT for number of participants reporting improvement in pain at 3 months (12/20 and 6/20 respectively; RR 2·0 (0·94, 2·47); Constant and Murley score at 3 months (63·7 (14·6) and 51·6 (20·10); SMD = 0·68 (0·04, 1·31)); and number of participants with disappearance of calcium deposits (11/20 and 4/20 respectively; RR = 2·75 (1·05, 7·20)).[51]

Adverse effects: Transient subcutaneous petechial bruising and haematomas were reported to occur in some participants who received high dose ESWT in two trials.[51,52]

Evidence summary: Silver

One RCT found no differences in outcome between high versus low dose ESWT although a second RCT found that high energy ESWT was superior to low energy ESWT for pain, function and disintegration of calcium deposits. No serious adverse effects of ESWT have been reported in the reviewed trials.

Rotator cuff tendonitis without calcification

ESWT versus placebo

Benefits: Data from two trials (40 and 74 participants respectively) could not be pooled because of different measures of outcome.[53,54] There were no significant differences between groups for any of the measured outcomes at 6 or 12 weeks in either trial.[53,54]

Adverse effects: Two trials in non-calcific rotator cuff tendonitis reported no adverse effects of ESWT.[53,54]

Evidence summary: Silver

Two trials found no benefit of ESWT over placebo for rotator cuff tendonitis without calcification. No serious adverse effects of ESWT have been reported in the reviewed trials.

Conclusion

Evidence from one trial suggests some benefits of ESWT for calcific tendonitis with respect to pain, function, and disintegration of calcific deposit. For non-calcific rotator cuff disease, evidence from two trials suggests that there is no benefit of ESWT compared to placebo. It is not clear whether the total dose, type of shock wave generation, method of administration (for example, repeated low dose versus single high dose) influences treatment outcome.

Recommendation for case presentation

For the patient described above, there is sufficient data to advise against recommending ESWT on the basis that it is unlikely to be beneficial.

Adhesive capsulitis

Case presentation 2

A 51-year-old right-handed woman presents at your practice complaining of gradual onset of right-sided shoulder and upper arm pain,which has been worsening over several months. She can recall no trauma. The pain is particularly noticeable at night and she is unable to sleep on the affected side. She also complains of pain and increasing stiffness during the day with inability to undo her bra or reach for things in the back seat of her car. Clinical examination reveals evidence of global restriction of passive and active shoulder movement in all planes by about 50%. She has normal radiographs. She has been taking analgesics but she is still waking with pain at night and is becoming sleep-deprived. She is seeking your advice regarding treatment options.

Non-steroidal anti-inflammatory drugs (NSAIDs)

We found two systematic reviews of NSAID in shoulder pain that included four and three trials respectively.[10,13] The Cochrane Review has been updated and now includes 19 trials with a combined total of 1203 participants.[14] There were seven studies performed in adhesive capsulitis, including 420 participants (median 41 participants, range 13–146 participants).[55–61] One study compared oral NSAID to placebo,[56] one study compared topical NSAID to placebo,[55] and five studies compared two types of oral NSAID.[57–61]

Outcomes

Oral NSAID versus placebo

Benefits: One small trial of 13 participants reported no significant differences between oral NSAID and placebo at 7 and 14 days (no data presented).[56]

Adverse effects: The single trial of oral NSAID versus placebo did not report adverse effects.[56]

Evidence summary: Silver

One small RCT found no benefit of oral NSAID over placebo. No data regarding adverse effects was available from this trial.

Topical NSAID versus placebo

Benefits: There were no statistically significant differences between groups for any variables at 7 and 14 days in one trial including 80 participants of topical NSAID compared to placebo.[55]

Adverse effects: There were no differences in tolerability between treatment groups in the trial of topical NSAID versus placebo (local effects of erythema were reported to occur in three participants in the topical flurbiprofen group versus one in the placebo group, and one participant in the flurbiprofen group reported furunculosis).[55]

Evidence summary: Silver

One trial found no significant difference in benefit between topical NSAID and placebo. One trial found no difference between topical NSAIDs and placebo with respect to adverse effects.

Comparison of NSAIDs

Benefits: Four of the five trials that were systematically reviewed reported no differences for any of the measured outcomes (naproxen versus indomethacin, 41 participants;[59] indomethacin versus piroxicam, 146 participants;[61] and two trials of ibuprofen versus diclofenac, 50 and 40 participants respectively).[57,58] One trial of 34 participants reported a benefit at 3 weeks of fentiazac compared to diclofenac with respect to pain at rest (SMD −1·12 (−1·85, −0·3951)) and pain on movement (SMD −0·75 (−1·45, −0·05)), but no difference in overall effect.[60]

Adverse effects: None of the five trials comparing oral NSAIDs reported significant differences between NSAIDs with respect to adverse effects.[57–61] One trial reported no difference between ibuprofen and diclofenac with respect to treatment tolerability according to a four-point patient and clinician scale (3 = very good, 0 = nil/slight).[57] Three participants in each treatment group discontinued therapy due to gastrointestinal adverse effects (ibuprofen group – nausea, constipation plus gastritis, and epigastric pain; diclofenac group – abdominal pain, constipation, and pyrosis).[57] One trial reported a similar high incidence of adverse effects with both naproxen to indomethacin – 14 participants in naproxen and 16 in indomethacin groups.[59] The most common adverse effects were nausea, headache, indigestion, bowel disturbance, and dizziness. Discontinuations of therapy due to adverse effects occurred in three participants in the naproxen group and five participants in the indomethacin group.[59] Thumb *et al* reported no differences in reported adverse effects – 5/19 (26·3%) fentiazac and 4/19 (21·1%) diclofenac (RR 1·25 (0·40, 3·95)).[60] The majority were gastrointestinal adverse effects although one participant in each group discontinued therapy due to skin rash and one participant in the diclofenac group discontinued therapy due to pruritis.[60] Yamamoto *et al* also reported no differences between groups with respect to reported adverse effects (piroxicam – 21 participants (14·3%); indomethacin – 27 participants (18.2%), mostly abdominal pain) or discontinuations due to adverse effects (piroxicam – 6 (4·1%); indomethacin – 14 (9·5%)).[61] Huskisson *et al* also reported similar incidence of reported adverse effects that were mostly gastrointestinal (diclofenac 7 participants; ibuprofen 4 participants).[58]

Evidence summary: Silver

Systematic review of five RCTs found no clinically significant differences in outcome or adverse effects between different oral NSAIDs. Gastrointestinal adverse effects were commonly reported.

Conclusion

There is no evidence that oral NSAID is of benefit for adhesive capsulitis but data is limited to one small trial of 13 participants. There is no evidence that topical NSAID is of benefit for adhesive capsulitis (data limited to one trial of 80 participants). There is considerable evidence of potential adverse effects, particularly gastrointestinal, of oral NSAIDs.

Recommendation for case presentation 2

Consideration of a short trial of oral NSAID for the patient described above should take into account their unknown effectiveness and the potential for adverse effects, particularly in patients at increased risk of gastrointestinal and cardio-renal toxicity.

Corticosteroid injections

Based upon the recent Cochrane Review,[24] 12 trials were conducted for adhesive capsulitis.[25,62–72] We found one additional trial including 30 participants of intra-articular steroid injection versus suprascapular nerve block.[73]

Intra-articular steroid injection was compared to placebo in one trial;[64] no treatment in one trial;[65] physiotherapy in one trial;[68] physiotherapy and non-steroidal anti-inflammatory drug in one trial;[70] capsular distension in two trials;[62,71] ice in one trial;[66] infrared irradiation in one trial;[65] stellate ganglion block in one trial;[25] and suprascapular nerve block in one trial.[73] One trial compared a combination of both intra-articular and subacromial steroid injection to no treatment and to physiotherapy;[66] one trial compared high versus low dose intra-articular steroid injection;[67] and the anterior and posterior intra-articular approach was compared in one trial.[63] Intra-articular steroid injection was compared to subacromial and intrabursal injections in one trial,[64] and bicipital injection in one trial.[65] One trial compared steroid injected "anteriorly around the shoulder joint" to physiotherapy[69] (this was included within the intra-articular steroid versus physiotherapy comparisons). There were three trials that studied intra-articular steroid injection combined with another intervention (with physiotherapy versus physiotherapy alone;[69] with capsular distension versus capsular distension alone;[71] with manipulation under anaesthesia versus manipulation under anaesthesia alone.[72] One trial also compared steroid injected into the synovial sheath surrounding the bicipital tendon with no treatment.[65]

Just as for rotator cuff disease, there was a wide variation in the corticosteroid preparation used, the dosage, number of injections given and their timing. Six trials used triamcinolone: a single 20 mg triamcinolone hexacetomide injection;[69] up to six injections (at weekly intervals) of 20 mg triamcinolone hexacetomide;[62] three injections (at six week intervals) of 40 mg triamcinolone acetonide;[71] up to three injections of 20 mg triamcinolone acetonide (interval between injections not reported);[73] three injections (at a one week then two week interval) of either 10 mg or 40 mg triamcinolone actonide;[67] and no more than three injections over six weeks of 40 mg triamcinolone acetonide.[68] Three trials used methylprednisolone: a single 40 mg injection of methylprednisolone acetate;[70] three injections (at weekly intervals) of 20 mg methylprednisolone;[66] and three injections (at weekly intervals) of 40 mg methylprednisolone.[64] Three trials used hydrocortisone: a single injection of 25 mg hydrocortisone acetate (two trials);[63,65] and three injections (at weekly intervals) of 50 mg hydrocortisone.[25] One trial (7·7%) used a single injection of 6 mg betamethasone.[72] The total volume injected varied between 2 and 25 ml and the use of local anaesthetic also varied widely.

Injections were placed into the glenohumeral joint via a posterior approach in seven trials;[62,63,67,68,70,71,73] an anterior approach in four trials;[63,64–66] and the approach was not specified in two trials.[25,72] Injections were placed into the subacromial space in one trial.[64] Other sites included anteriorly around the shoulder joint in one trial[70] and bicipital tendon sheath in one trial.[65] Most studies did not confirm the accurate placement of the injection. One study used ultrasound to confirm intra-articular needle placement.[62] White *et al* mixed urograffin with the corticosteroid preparation and took post-injection plain films.[63]

Outcomes: benefits

Intra-articular steroid injection versus placebo

One trial of 48 participants reported no differences between intra-articular steroid injection and placebo with respect to pain and range of movement up to 6 months.[64]

Evidence summary: Silver

One RCT found no benefit of intra-articular steroid injection versus placebo.

Intra-articular steroid injection versus no treatment

One trial with 80 participants reported significant benefit of injection over analgesia alone up to 6 weeks (unblinded, results only displayed graphically).[65] The same trial also reported significant benefit of bicipital tendon sheath injection over analgesia alone.

Evidence summary: Silver

One RCT reported benefit of intra-articular steroid injection versus no treatment.

Intra-articular and subacromial steroid injection versus no treatment

One trial of 42 participants comparing combination intra-articular and subacromial steroid injection to no treatment reported little difference with respect to long term outcome but some early benefit of injection with respect to pain and range of movement (only outcome assessment blinded, statistical analysis unclear).[66]

Evidence summary: Silver

One small RCT found small short term benefit of intra-articular and subacromial steroid injection versus no treatment.

Comparison of high and low dose steroid injection

One trial of 57 participants compared two doses of intra-articular steroid injection.[67] While a trend favouring higher dose intra-articular steroid injection was found with respect to improvement in pain at 6 weeks, no differences were found between the higher and lower dose steroid injection with respect to improvement in sleep disturbance, functional impairment or improvement in external rotation.

Evidence summary: Silver

One small RCT found no significant differences between high and low dose intra-articular steroid injection.

Comparison of anterior and posterior intra-articular steroid injection

The one trial (involving 40 participants) that compared anterior to posterior intra-articular steroid injection for adhesive capsulitis did not provide any comparative data, although reported a significantly higher level of injection accuracy with the anterior approach (19/20, 95% *v* 10/20 50%, $p < 0{\cdot}02$).[63] They also compared patients' response based upon whether the injection was intra-articular or not, irrespective of anatomical approach to injection used and reported no statistically significant difference. Good, moderate, and poor response, measured at 6 weeks, was reported in 5 (17·2%), 10 (34·5%), and 14 (48·3%) of 29 participants with intra-articular placement of injection compared to 0 (0%), 3 (27·3%), and 8 (72·7%) in the 11 participants with extra-articular injection (good response – no pain, no analgesia, and restoration of abduction to 160 degrees or above; moderate response – reduction in pain, reduction in analgesics (if previously taken) and 30 degrees increase in abduction; poor response – persistent nocturnal pain and abduction less than 100 degrees).

Evidence summary: Silver

One small RCT concluded that blind intra-articular steroid injection using the anterior approach is more accurate than the posterior approach. No difference in outcome was found between intra-articular and extra-articular placement of the injection.

Intra-articular steroid injection versus physiotherapy

Only one of four trials comparing intra-articular steroid injection to physiotherapy contained sufficient data for meta-analysis (109 participants).[68] Physiotherapy in this trial consisted of 12 30-minute sessions of passive mobilisation and exercises; and ice, hot packs or electrotherapy to reduce pain if required. At 7 weeks, treatment success favoured steroid injection (40/52 and 26/56 in the steroid injection and physiotherapy groups respectively; RR = 1·66, 95% CI 1·21, 2·28). At 3 and 7 weeks, all outcomes measured favoured steroid injection (including improvement in severity of main complaint (3 weeks: 32·00 (26·00) and 17·00 (21·00) in the steroid injection and physiotherapy groups respectively; SMD 0·63 (0·24, 1·02); 7 weeks: 58·00 (28·00) and 32·00 (29·00) in the steroid injection and physiotherapy groups respectively; SMD 0·91 (0·51, 1·30)), improvement in pain during the day (3 weeks: 22·00 (20·00) and 10·00 (15·00) in the steroid injection and physiotherapy groups respectively; SMD 0·68 (0·29, 1·07); 7 weeks: 58·00 (28·00) and 32·00 (29·00) in the steroid injection and physiotherapy groups respectively; SMD 0·91 (0·51, 1·30)), pain at night (3 weeks: 21·00 (26·00) and 9·00 (23·00) in the steroid injection and physiotherapy groups respectively; SMD 0·49 (0·10, 0·87); 7 weeks: 35·00 (20·00) and 23·00 (24·00) in the steroid injection and physiotherapy groups respectively; SMD 0·54 (0·15, 0·92)), functional disability (3 weeks: 19·00 (27·00) and 6·00 (22·00) in the steroid injection and physiotherapy groups respectively; SMD 0·53 (0·14, 0·91); 7 weeks: 39·00 (27·00) and 14·00 (27·00) in the steroid injection and physiotherapy groups respectively; SMD 0·92 (0·52, 1·32)), and abduction (3 weeks: 2·00 (12·00) and –3·00 (13·00) in the steroid injection and physiotherapy groups respectively; SMD 0·40 (0·01, 0·78); 7 weeks: 4·00 (110·00) and –1·00 (14·00) in the steroid injection and physiotherapy groups respectively; SMD 0·39 (0·01, 0·77)). By 13 weeks, benefit favouring steroid injection remained statistically significant only for improvement in severity of main complaint. No difference in outcome was demonstrated for any of the measured outcomes at 26 weeks and a small benefit favouring steroid injection was found for improvement in severity of main complaint at 52 weeks.

A second trial of 42 participants compared a combination of both intra-articular and subacromial steroid injection to physiotherapy (consisting of Maitland's mobilisation three times a week for 6 weeks) and reported little difference between groups with respect to long term outcome but some early benefit of the combined injections with respect to pain and range of movement.[66] The third trial of 66 participants compared steroid injection placed anteriorly around the shoulder joint to physiotherapy (mobilisation) and reported no significant differences between groups at 6 weeks and 6 months.[69] A fourth trial of 80 participants reported no significant group differences between injection and scheme of graduated active exercises compared to infrared irradiation and scheme of graduated active exercises at 6 weeks, but range of motion was the only outcome assessed.[65]

Adverse effects: One trial reported no difference in overall frequency of adverse reactions between steroid injection and physiotherapy, however facial flushing was more common in the steroid injection group (9/57 compared to 1/57 in the physiotherapy group; RR 9·0 (1·18, 68·74)).[68] Menstrual irregularities were also reported more frequently in the steroid injections group (6/57 *v* 0/57 in the physiotherapy group, RR = 13·0 (0·75, 225·50)).[68]

Evidence summary: Silver

Review of four RCTs found some early benefit of steroid injection versus physiotherapy in two trials. No serious adverse effects of steroid injection were reported in any of the reviewed trials.

Intra-articular steroid injection versus physiotherapy and non-steroidal anti-inflammatory medication (NSAID)

No difference with respect to pain was demonstrated between physiotherapy (consisting of hot pack application, ultrasonic therapy, passive glenohumeral joint stretching exercises, Codman exercises, and wall climbing) and NSAID versus intra-articular steroid injection at 2 and 12 weeks following treatment in one trial of 20 participants.[70]

Evidence summary: Silver

One small RCT found no difference between intra-articular steroid injection versus physiotherapy and NSAID.

Intra-articular steroid injection versus shoulder joint distension with steroid

None of the data from three trials could be pooled. Results from one trial of 45 participants found no significant difference between shoulder joint distension with steroid versus intra-articular steroid injection alone in terms of pain (rest pain at 3 months 2/25 versus 3/20, RR 0·53 (0·1, 2·89); night pain at 3 months 4/25 versus 4/20, RR = 0·8 (0·23, 2·81).[74]One trial of 33/47 participants found no significant difference between shoulder joint distension with steroid versus steroid injection alone for range of movement (SMD = 0·22 (–0·46, 0·91).[72] Results of the third trial of 22 participants were presented graphically.[62] There was a reported benefit favouring the capsular distension group with respect to range of movement and analgesic use, no difference with respect to pain at rest, but a trend favouring the distension group for pain with activity.

Evidence summary: Silver

A systematic review of three small RCTs found limited evidence of added benefit of joint distension over steroid injection alone.

Intra-articular steroid injection versus shoulder joint distension without steroid

Only one trial of 29/47 participants compared shoulder joint distension (with air and anaesthetic and without steroid) to steroid injection.[71] There was no difference between groups with respect to improvement in abduction, flexion or external rotation. Data regarding improvement in pain were not presented according to treatment group.

Evidence summary: Silver

One small RCT found no differences in range of shoulder movement between joint distension without steroid and steroid injection alone.

Intra-articular steroid injection versus suprascapular nerve block

One trial of 30 participants reported that both treatment groups improved over 12 weeks but nerve block was superior to intra-articular steroid injection with respect to pain ($p< 0·01$) and range of movement ($p< 0·05$), but this could not be verified from the data presented in the publication (only medians and p-values reported) and neither participants nor outcome assessors were blinded to treatment intervention.[73]

Evidence summary: Silver

One small RCT reported no differences in outcome between intra-articular steroid injection and suprascapular nerve block.

Intra-articular steroid injection and manipulation under anaesthesia versus manipulation under anaesthesia alone

One trial of 24 participants demonstrated no difference with respect to range of abduction at 4 months between participants who had received an intra-articular injection of steroid with manipulation under anaesthesia compared to those who had manipulation under anaesthesia alone.[72]

Evidence summary: Silver

One small RCT reported no differences in outcome between intra-articular steroid injection and manipulation under anaesthesia versus manipulation under anaesthesia alone.

Intra-articular steroid injection versus stellate ganglion block

The one trial (involving an unknown number of participants) that compared intra-articular steroid injection to stellate ganglion block for adhesive capsulitis reported no differences in outcome between treatment groups at 4 weeks and 3 months.[25]

Evidence summary: Silver

One small RCT reported no differences in outcome between intra-articular steroid injection and stellate ganglion block.

Conclusion

Intra-articular steroid injections are of unknown effectiveness in adhesive capsulitis although a small short-term benefit has been demonstrated in some trials. While most studies have failed to confirm the accurate placement of injection, one small trial found that intra-articular injection using an anterior approach was more accurate than a posterior approach. However, the same study reported no statistically significant difference in outcome between intra- and extra-articular placement of injection. Issues that still need to be resolved include whether the accurate intra-articular placement of the injection, as well as the frequency, dose and type of steroid, influences treatment outcome. Facial flushing and menstrual irregularities have been reported.

Recommendation for case presentation 2

Intra-articular steroid injection may be of value for the patient described above although pain relief may be short-lived. Transient pain following the injection may occur and diabetics should be aware that steroid injection might elevate blood glucose.

Shoulder joint distension

We found one systematic review of shoulder joint distension for adhesive capsulitis,[7] which included two trials of 47 and 45 participants respectively,[71,74] the latter published in French. We found one additional published trial of 22 participants[62] and one trial of 48 participants.[75]

One trial compared shoulder joint distension with steroid and saline to placebo[75] and three trials compared shoulder joint distension with or without steroid to intra-articular steroid injection alone.[62,71,74] Jacobs *et al* compared joint distension using 6 ml local anaesthesia and 3 ml air (total volume 9 ml) to intra-articular steroid injection alone and to combined distension and intra-articular steroid (total volume 10 ml).[71] Corbeil *et al* compared arthrogram and distension using local anaesthetic and corticosteroid to a volume of 20 ml or capsular rupture, to arthrogram and intra-articular steroid injection alone.[74] Gam *et al* compared distension with 19 ml of 2% lidocaine (lignocaine) and 20 mg triamcinolonhexacetonid to steroid injection alone, repeating treatment once a week for a maximum of 6 weeks or until there were no symptoms.[62] Buchbinder *et al* compared distension using 40 mg depomedrol (1 ml) and up to 82 ml normal saline (median volume 43·4 ml; range 21–80 ml) to placebo (arthrogram alone).[75] There were no trials of shoulder joint distension with saline alone versus placebo.

Outcomes

Shoulder joint distension with saline and steroid versus placebo

Benefits: One trial of 48 participants reported significant benefit of shoulder joint distension with steroid and saline over placebo at 3 weeks with respect to mean overall improvement in pain, measured on a 10 cm VAS where 0 = no pain and 10 = maximal pain (improvement in pain 2·5 (2·5) and 0·19 (1·7) in the active and placebo groups respectively; SMD –1·04 (–1·67, –0·42)); improvement in function, measured by the Shoulder Pain and Disability Index (SPADI) (scored out of 100 where a higher score indicates more pain/disability) was SPADI 21·8 (19·3) and 4·7 (19·8) in the active and placebo

Table 10.7 Number needed to treat for saline and steroids versus placebo (Buchbinder, 2000)[75]

Outcome	Standardised mean difference (95% CI)	% benefiting (95% CI) with saline and steroids	NNT (95% CI)
Pain	−1·04 (−1·67, −0·42)	45% (20, 60)	3 (2, 5)
Function (SPADI)	−0·86 (−1·47, −0·25)	28% (12, 56)	3 (2, 9)
Problem elicitation technique	−0·89 (−1·51, −0·28)	39% (14, 57)	3 (2, 8)
Total shoulder abduction	−0·74 (−1·34, −0·14)	34% (7, 53)	3 (2, 15)

groups respectively; SMD −0·86 (−1·47, −0·25)); Problem Elicitation Technique (PET) (higher score indicates more disability) (PET 62·5 (75·5) and 8·7 (29·0) in the active and placebo groups respectively; SMD −0·89 (−1·51, −0.28)); and improvement in shoulder movement (total shoulder abduction measured in degrees 20·2 (30·2) and −0·20 (22·5) in the active and placebo groups respectively; SMD −0·74 (−1·34, −0·14) (Table 10.7).[75] At 6 and 12 weeks, while the results of the intention to treat analysis favoured shoulder joint distension, the between group differences were only significant for improvement in the PET.[75]

Adverse effects: In one trial, more participants in the distension group had pain at or following the procedure compared to those in the placebo group (4/25 (8%) *v* 1/21 (2%)).[75]

Evidence summary: Silver

One RCT found a significant short term benefit in pain and function of arthrographic distension with saline and steroid compared to placebo. No serious adverse effects of join distension with steroid and saline were reported.

Shoulder joint distension with steroid versus steroid injection alone

Benefits: None of the data from three trials could be pooled. Results from one trial of 45 participants found no significant difference between shoulder joint distension with steroid versus intra-articular steroid injection alone in terms of pain (rest pain at 3 months 2/25 *v* 3/20 (RR 0·53 (0·1, 2·89) and night pain at 3 months 4/25 *v* 4/20 (RR = 0·8 (0·23, 2·81)).[74] One trial of 33/47 participants found no significant difference between shoulder joint distension with steroid versus steroid injection alone for range of movement (SMD = 0·22 (−0·46, 0·91)).[71] Results of the third trial of 22 participants were presented graphically.[62] There was a reported benefit favouring the capsular distension group with respect to range of movement and analgesic use, no difference with respect to pain at rest, but a trend favouring the distension group for pain with activity.

Adverse effects: One trial of distension with steroid versus steroid injection alone reported 2 cases of unacceptable pain after injection but the treatment group was not specified.[62]

Evidence summary: Silver

A systematic review of three small RCTs found mixed evidence of added benefit of joint distension over steroid injection alone. No serious adverse effects were reported.

Shoulder joint distension without steroid versus steroid injection

Only one trial of 29/47 participants compared shoulder joint distension (with air and anaesthetic and without steroid) to steroid injection.[71] There was no difference between groups with respect to improvement in abduction, flexion or external rotation. Data regarding improvement in pain were not presented according to treatment group.

Evidence summary: Silver

One small RCT found no differences in range of shoulder movement between joint distension without steroid and steroid injection alone.

Shoulder joint distension with steroid versus distension without steroid

Benefits: Only one trial of 32/47 participants compared shoulder joint distension with steroid to distension without steroid.[71] There was no statistically significant difference between groups with respect to improvement in abduction, flexion or external rotation. Data regarding improvement in pain were not presented according to treatment group.

Adverse effects: Two participants in one trial developed facial flushing after steroid injection.[71]

Evidence summary: Silver

One small trial found no differences in range of shoulder movement between joint distension with steroid and joint distension alone. No serious adverse effects of joint distension were reported.

Conclusion

There is evidence from one small trial that joint distension with saline and steroid is superior to placebo at 3 weeks for adhesive capsulitis but the effect appears to diminish over time. There is no evidence that joint distension with steroid is superior to steroid injection alone or distension alone but the observed lack of additional benefit may be due to the low volumes injected, Type 2 error due to small number of patients studied in all trials, and/or the lack of sensitive endpoints.

Recommendation for case presentation 2

Radiologically guided joint distension with steroid and saline may be of short term benefit to the patient described.

Oral corticosteroids

We found one systematic review of oral steroids for adhesive capsulitis.[7] It included two trials of 32 and 40 participants respectively.[76,77] One trial compared cortisone acetate (200 mg for the first 3 days, and 100 mg thereafter until the 14th day, then daily dose tapered off in decrements of 12·5 mg every 2 days, total dose = 2·5 g over 4 weeks) to placebo.[76] At the end of 4 weeks, the patients who had not progressed satisfactorily had their shoulders manipulated under general anaesthesia. This manipulation was followed by a second 4 week course of cortisone or placebo. The second trial compared a regime of prednisolone (10 mg daily for 4 weeks, then 5 mg daily for 2 weeks) to no treatment.[77] We found an additional published trial of oral steroids (15 mg daily for 4 weeks) and manipulation and intra-articular steroid injection (after 2 weeks oral steroids) versus manipulation and intra-articular steroid injection alone for adhesive capsulitis (32 participants).[78]

Outcomes

Oral steroid versus no treatment

Benefits: One trial of 40 participants found that the overall pattern of improvement in pain at night over 8 weeks showed a significant difference in favour of oral prednisolone ($p<0·05$) but the results were only presented graphically. It was characterised by a more rapid initial recovery but by 5 months the difference between the groups was negligible. Improvement in pain at rest and with movement, range of motion and a cumulative recovery curve were not significantly different between groups over 8 months.[77]

Adverse effects: One trial reported that upon cessation of oral steroids, two participants had a recurrence of severe pain and four had mild pain that settled spontaneously.[77] Mild indigestion was reported in two participants in the oral steroid group that resolved after the dosage was reduced.[77] No other serious adverse effects were reported.

Evidence summary: Silver

One small RCT suggested an early benefit of oral steroids compared to no treatment with respect to improvement in night pain but this could not be verified from the available reported data. No differences for any measured outcome were found at 8 months. No serious adverse effects of a short course of oral steroids were reported.

Oral steroid +/– manipulation versus placebo +/– manipulation

Benefits: One trial of 32 participants reported no statistically significant differences between groups for any of the measured outcomes at the end of the trial (18 weeks).[76] However, they noted an earlier, clinically important improvement in both pain and range of movement in the oral steroid group. No statistical analysis was performed to confirm this impression and no standard deviations were reported to enable analysis to be performed from the reported data. Pain was measured on a four-point categorical scale converted into an interval scale (none = 0, slight = 1, moderate = 2, severe = 3). At baseline, 1, 4, and 18 weeks the mean pain score was 1·4, 0·9, 0·5, and 0.6 in the oral steroid group and 1·4, 1·3, 0·8, and 0·5 in the control group. At baseline, 1, 4, and 18 weeks, total shoulder abduction in degrees was 82, 103, 125, and 153 in the oral steroid group and 75, 89, 106, and 154 in the control group. The number of patients requiring manipulation after 4 weeks was 6/15 (40%) and 11/16 (68·8%) in the oral steroid and placebo groups respectively (RR = 0·30 (0·05, 1·66)).

Adverse effects: One trial reported no adverse effects of a short course of oral steroids.[76] However, one participant died suddenly from coronary occlusion during the third week of treatment and one participant withdrew because of follicular dermatitis.[76] Neither of these events was attributed to oral steroids by the authors.

Evidence summary: Silver

One small RCT did not demonstrate any benefit of oral steroids +/– manipulation compared to placebo after 18 weeks but suggested that oral steroids may be associated with an earlier improvement in pain and range of movement. This could not be verified from the available reported data. No serious adverse effects of a short course of oral steroids were reported.

Oral steroid, manipulation and intra-articular steroid injection versus manipulation and intra-articular steroid injection

One trial reported "dramatic response" to manipulation in 7/12 (58·3%) participants taking oral steroid compared to 5/16 (31·25%) participants taking placebo (RR 1·87 (0·78, 4·46)).[78] The proportion of participants with external rotation better than ¾ normal movement as compared with the unaffected shoulder 6 weeks following manipulation favoured the oral steroid group (7/12 (60%) *v* 2/16 (12%), RR = 4·67 (1·17, 18·58)) (Table 10.8) but there were no statistically significant differences between treatment groups for flexion at 6 weeks, and both external rotation and flexion at 12 and 18 weeks following manipulation.

Evidence summary: Silver

One small RCT demonstrated a non-significant trend favouring oral steroid over placebo with respect to response to manipulation. It also

Table 10.8 NNT for oral steroid, manipulation and intra-articular steroid injection versus manipulation and intra-articular steroid injection (Kessel, 1981)[78]

Outcome	Benefit with manipulation and intra-articular steroid injection	Benefit with oral steroid, manipulation and intra-articular steroid injection	Relative risk for oral steroid, manipulation and intra-articular steroid injection (95% CI)	Absolute benefit increase (95% CI)	NNT (95% CI)
External rotation at 6 wk	2/16 (13%)	7/12 (58%)	4·67 (1·17, 18·58)	46% (11, 70)	3 (2, 10)

reported a benefit with respect to external rotation but not flexion at 6 weeks following manipulation and no difference between groups at 12 and 18 weeks. No serious adverse effects of a short course of oral steroids were reported.

Conclusion

Oral steroids are of unknown effectiveness for adhesive capsulitis but two studies have suggested a more rapid improvement in pain and one study has suggested a more rapid improvement in external rotation.

Recommendation for case presentation 2

A short course of oral corticosteroids may provide short term pain relief to the patient described.

Physiotherapy

The most recent review is a Cochrane systematic review of 26 randomised controlled trials, of variable methodological quality, in 1499 participants investigating the effect of physiotherapy interventions for shoulder disorders.[36] There were seven trials in adhesive capsulitis.[65,66,68,69,79,80,81] The physiotherapeutic modalities studied included infrared irradiation and a graduated exercise programme,[65] mobilisation or ice therapy;[66] passive mobilisation and exercise,[68] mobilisation;[69] mobilisation and exercise versus exercise alone;[79] electromagnetic therapy;[80] and laser therapy.[81] We found one additional trial of physiotherapy and NSAID versus intra-articular steroid injection.[70]

Outcomes

Mobilisation versus no treatment

One small trial of 42 participants assessed the effect of mobilisation compared to no treatment, ice or intra-articular corticosteroid injection.[66] The data from this trial was only presented graphically, but the authors concluded no significant differences between groups with respect to pain.

Evidence summary: Silver

One small RCT found no difference in outcome for mobilisation compared to no treatment, ice therapy or intra-articular steroid injection.

Mobilisation and exercise versus exercise alone

One trial of 20 participants found no difference in outcome between participants randomised to mobilisation and exercise compared to exercise alone.[79]

Evidence summary: Silver

One small RCT found no added benefit of mobilisation over exercise alone.

Laser therapy versus placebo

One trial of 40 participants reported a significant benefit of laser therapy with respect to a good or excellent result in the short term (16/20 *v* 2/20 in

Table 10.9 Number needed to treat for laser therapy versus placebo (Taverna, 1990)[81]

Outcome	Benefit with placebo	Benefit with laser therapy	Relative risk with laser therapy (95% CI)	Absolute benefit increase (95% CI)	NNT (95% CI)
Good or excellent short term results	2/20 (10%)	16/20 (80%)	8·0 (2·11, 30·34)	70% (41–84)	2 (2, 3)

the placebo group; RR 8·0 (2·11, 30·34)[81] (Table 10.9).

Evidence summary: Silver

One small RCT found a significant short term benefit of laser therapy compared to placebo.

Electromagnetic therapy versus physiotherapy alone

One trial of 47 participants demonstrated no additional benefit of electromagnetic therapy over physiotherapy alone.[80]

Evidence summary: Silver

One RCT found no added benefit of electromagnetic therapy over physiotherapy alone.

Physiotherapy versus intra-articular steroid injection

Benefits: Only one of four trials comparing intra-articular steroid injection to physiotherapy contained sufficient data for meta-analysis (109 participants).[68] Physiotherapy in this trial consisted of 12 30-minute sessions of passive mobilisation and exercises; and ice, hot packs or electrotherapy to reduce pain if required. At 7 weeks, treatment success favoured steroid injection (40/52 and 26/56 in the steroid injection and physiotherapy groups respectively; RR = 1·66, 95% CI 1·21, 2·28). At 3 and 7 weeks, all outcomes measured favoured steroid injection (including improvement in severity of main complaint (3 weeks: 32·00 (26·00) and 17·00 (21·00) in the steroid injection and physiotherapy groups respectively; SMD 0·63 (0·24, 1·02); 7 weeks: 58·00 (28·00) and 32·00 (29·00) in the steroid injection and physiotherapy groups respectively; SMD 0·91 (0·51, 1·30)), improvement in pain during the day (3 weeks: 22·00 (20·00) and 10·00 (15·00) in the steroid injection and physiotherapy groups respectively; SMD 0·68 (0·29, 1·07); 7 weeks: 58·00 (28·00) and 32.00 (29.00) in the steroid injection and physiotherapy groups respectively; SMD 0·91 (0·51, 1·30)), pain at night (3 weeks: 21·00 (26·00) and 9·00 (23·00) in the steroid injection and physiotherapy groups respectively; SMD 0·49 (0·10, 0·87); 7 weeks: 35·00 (20·00) and 23·00 (24·00) in the steroid injection and physiotherapy groups respectively; SMD 0·54 (0·15, 0·92)), functional disability (3 weeks: 19·00 (27·00) and 6·00 (22·00) in the steroid injection and physiotherapy groups respectively; SMD 0·53 (0·14, 0·91); 7 weeks: 39·00 (27·00) and 14·00 (27·00) in the steroid injection and physiotherapy groups respectively; SMD 0·92 (0·52, 1·32)) and abduction (3 weeks: 2·00 (12·00) and –3·00 (13·00) in the steroid injection and physiotherapy groups respectively; SMD 0·40 (0·01, 0·78); 7 weeks: 4·00 (110·00) and –1·00 (14·00) in the steroid injection and physiotherapy groups respectively; SMD 0·39 (0·01, 0·77)). By 13 weeks, benefit favouring steroid injection remained statistically significant only for improvement in severity of main complaint. No difference in outcome was demonstrated for any of the measured outcomes at 26 weeks and a small benefit favouring steroid injection was found for improvement in severity of main complaint at 52 weeks.

A second trial of 42 participants compared a combination of both intra-articular and subacromial steroid injection to physiotherapy (consisting of Maitland's mobilisation three times a week for 6 weeks) and reported little difference between groups with respect to long term outcome but some early benefit of the combined injections with respect to pain and range of movement.[66] The third trial of 66 participants compared steroid injection placed anteriorly around the shoulder joint to physiotherapy (mobilisation) and reported no significant differences between groups at 6 weeks and 6 months.[69] A fourth trial of 80 participants reported no significant between group differences between injection and scheme of graduated active exercises compared to infrared irradiation and scheme of graduated active exercises at 6 weeks, but range of motion was the only outcome assessed.[65]

Adverse effects: One trial reported no difference in overall frequency of adverse reactions between steroid injection and physiotherapy, however facial flushing was more common in the steroid injection group (RR 9·0 (1·18, 68·74). Menstrual irregularities were also reported more frequently in the steroid injections group (6/57 *v* 0/57 in the physiotherapy group, RR = 13·0 (0·75, 225·50)).[68]

Evidence summary: Silver

Review of four RCTs found some early benefit of steroid injection versus physiotherapy in two trials. No serious adverse effects of steroid injection were reported in any of the reviewed trials.

Physiotherapy and non-steroidal anti-inflammatory medication (NSAID) versus intra-articular steroid injection

No difference with respect to pain was demonstrated between physiotherapy (consisting of hot pack application, ultrasonic therapy, passive glenohumeral joint stretching exercises, Codman exercises, and wall climbing) and NSAID versus intra-articular steroid injection at 2 and 12 weeks following treatment in one trial of 20 participants.[70]

Evidence summary: Silver

One small RCT found no difference between physiotherapy and NSAID versus intra-articular steroid injection.

Adverse effects: No serious adverse effects were reported in any of the trials of physiotherapy interventions.

Evidence summary

No serious adverse effects of physiotherapy interventions were reported in the reviewed trials.

Conclusion

Based upon the results of a single trial, laser therapy may be of benefit for adhesive capsulitis in the short term. There is no evidence that other physiotherapy interventions are of benefit for adhesive capsulitis.

Recommendation for case presentation 2

For the patient described, laser therapy may be beneficial but other physiotherapy treatments are unlikely to be helpful based upon current data.

Acupuncture

We found no trials of acupuncture compared to placebo in adhesive capsulitis. We found one trial, published in Chinese, including 150 participants, that compared electroacupuncture to regional nerve block (anaesthesia of stellate ganglion and suprascapular nerve.[82]

Outcomes

Electroacupuncture compared to suprascapular nerve and stellate ganglion block

Benefits: There was a significant difference in pain favouring nerve block after 30 hours (mean pain 2·41 (0·35) and 1·08 (0·21) in the nerve block and electroacupuncture groups respectively; SMD 4·57 (3·82, 5·33) (pain was measured on a four-point scale, n = 50 in each group).[82] The time to achieve maximum pain relief (measured in minutes) was significantly shorter in the nerve block group (8·72 (5·09) *v* 73·68 (15·27) in the acupuncture group) (SMD 5·66 (4·77, 6·56)).

Adverse effects: No adverse effects were reported.

Evidence summary: Silver

One RCT found a small benefit of suprascapular nerve and stellate ganglion block compared to electroacupuncture with respect to pain relief after 30 hours and time to maximal pain relief. The same trial reported no adverse effects of suprascapular nerve and stellate ganglion block or electroacupuncture.

Conclusion

Acupuncture is of unknown effectiveness for adhesive capsulitis.

Recommendation for case presentation 2

Based upon the available data, acupuncture is unlikely to be helpful for the case described above.

Suprascapular nerve block

We found four published trials with a combined total study population of 255 participants.[73,82–84] One of these compared suprascapular nerve block to placebo injection (34 participants);[83] one compared suprascapular nerve block to intra-articular steroid injection (30 participants);[73] one compared two techniques for suprascapular nerve block: needle tip guided by superficial bony landmarks or near-nerve electromyography (41 participants);[84] and one trial (published in Chinese) compared regional nerve block (anaesthesia of stellate ganglion and suprascapular nerve) to electroacupuncture (150 participants).[82]

Outcomes

Suprascapular nerve block versus placebo

Benefits: Results from one trial of 34 participants indicated that at one month, there was a statistically significant benefit of suprascapular nerve block over placebo with respect to pain measured on a 100 mm VAS (improvement in pain –30·4 (9·3) and –21·20 (10·3) in the active and placebo groups respectively; SMD –0·91 (–1·72, –0·11)) (Table 10.10). This was accompanied by a statistically significant difference favouring suprascapular nerve block with respect to overall McGill–Melzack Pain Questionnaire (MPQ) multidimensional pain descriptors score (improvement –10·3 (2·5) and –2·1 (2·7) in the active and placebo groups respectively; SMD –3·07 (–4·24, –1·90); Present Pain Index (5-point categorical scale) (improvement in pain –1·5 (0·40) and –0·09 (0·50) in the active and placebo groups respectively; SMD –3·07 (–4·27, –1·88)); and functional capacity of the shoulder measured by the Simple Shoulder Test (improvement 15·8 (6·7) and 4·1 (7·4) in the active and placebo groups; SMD 1·62 (0·73, 2·51)).[83] There was no difference with respect to glenohumeral range of motion expressed as a composite score for active and passive shoulder motion (SMD 0·17 (–0·59, 0·93)).

Adverse effects: One trial reported transient vasovagal episodes and local injection site tenderness.[83]

Table 10.10 Number needed to treat for suprascapular nerve block versus placebo (Dahan, 2000)[83]

Outcome	Standardised mean difference (95% CI)	% Benefit (95% CI) suprascapular nerve block	NNT (95% CI)
Pain (VAS)	–0·91 (–1·72, –0·11)	40% (5, 61)	3 (2, 19)
Pain (MPQ)	–3·07 (–4·24, –1·90)	69% (63, 69)	2 (2, 2)
Pain (Present Pain Index)	–3·07 (–4·27, –1·88)	69% (63, 69)	2 (2, 2)
Functional capacity (simple shoulder test)	1·62 (0·73, 2·51)	59% (33, 68)	2 (2, 3)

Evidence summary: Silver

One small RCT found a small benefit of suprascapular nerve block compared to placebo with respect to pain and function at one month. No serious adverse effects of suprascapular nerve block were reported.

Suprascapular nerve block versus intra-articular steroid injection

One trial of 30 participants reported that both treatment groups improved over 12 weeks but nerve block was superior to intra-articular steroid injection with respect to pain ($p< 0·01$) and range of movement ($p< 0·05$) but this could not be verified from the data presented in the publication (only medians and p-values reported) and neither participants nor outcome assessors were blinded to treatment intervention.[73] No adverse effects were reported.

Evidence summary: Silver

One small trial reported no differences in outcome between intra-articular steroid injection and suprascapular nerve block.

Suprascapular nerve block guided by bony landmarks or near-nerve electromyography

One trial of 41 participants reported a significant benefit with respect to pain relief 10 and 60 minutes following suprascapular nerve block when guided by near-nerve electromyography compared to bony landmarks (SMD –0·76 (–1·40, –0·12) and SMD –0·99 (–1·64, –0·34) respectively) (pain measured by 100 mm VAS where 0 = no pain and 100 indicated severe pain.)[84] This was accompanied by a significant benefit in passive shoulder range of movement in all planes except for glenohumeral abduction (which may have been explained by a significant difference in baseline values in the two groups).[84] No adverse effects were reported.

Evidence summary: Silver

Suprascapular nerve block guided by near-nerve electromyography resulted in better pain relief at 10 and 60 minutes compared to suprascapular nerve block guided by bony landmarks.

Suprascapular nerve and stellate ganglion block versus electroacupuncture

There was a significant difference in pain favouring nerve block after 30 hours (mean pain 2·41 (0·35) and 1·08 (0·21) in the nerve block and electroacupuncture groups respectively; SMD 4·57 (3·82, 5·33) (pain was measured on a four-point scale, $n = 50$ in each group).[82] The time to achieve maximum pain relief (measured in minutes) was significantly shorter in the nerve block group (8·72 (5·09) *v* 73·68 (15·27) in the acupuncture group) (SMD 5·66 (4·77, 6·56)).

Adverse effects: No adverse effects were reported.

Evidence summary: Silver

One RCT found a small benefit of suprascapular nerve and stellate ganglion block compared to electroacupuncture with respect to pain relief after 30 hours and time to maximal pain relief.

Conclusion

There is weak evidence from one small trial that suprascapular nerve block may be superior to placebo for adhesive capsulitis at 4 weeks. Near-nerve electromyographically guided suprascapular nerve block may be superior to nerve block guided by bony landmark but outcomes have only been measured up to one hour following injection. No conclusions can be drawn regarding the comparative efficacy of suprascapular nerve block and intra-articular steroid injections for adhesive capsulitis. Suprascapular nerve and stellate ganglion block is superior to electroacupuncture.

Recommendation for case presentation 2

A suprascapular nerve block may provide short term (one month) pain relief and improvement in function for the patient described.

References

1 Chard MD, Hazleman R, Hazleman BL, King RH, Reiss BB. Shoulder disorders in the elderly: a community survey. *Arthritis Rheum* 1991;**34**:766–9.

2 Chakravarty K, Webley M. Disorders of the shoulder: an often unrecognised cause of disability in elderly people. *BMJ* 1990;**300**:848–9.

3 Badley E, Tennant A. Changing profile of joint disorders with age: findings from a postal survey of the population of Calderdale, West Yorkshire, United Kingdom. *Ann Rheum Dis* 1992;**51**:366–71.

4 Rekola K, Keinanen-Kiukaanniemi S, Takala J. Use of primary health services in sparsely populated country districts by patients with musculoskeletal symptoms: consultations with a physician. *J Epidemiol Comm Health* 1993;**47**:153–7.

5 Bridges-Webb C. Assessing health status in general practice. *Med J Aust* 1992;**157**:321–5.

6 van der Heijden GJ, van der Windt DA, Kleijnen J, Koes BW, Bouter LM. Steroid injections for shoulder disorders: a systematic review of randomised clinical trials. *Br J Gen Pract* 1996;**46**:309–16.

7 Green S, Buchbinder R, Glazier R, Forbes A. Systematic review of randomised controlled trials of interventions for painful shoulder: selection criteria, outcome assessment, and efficacy. *BMJ* 1998;**316**:354–60.

8 van der Heijden GJ, van der Windt DA, de Winter AF. Physiotherapy for patients with soft tissue shoulder disorders: a systematic review of randomised clinical trials. *BMJ* 1997;**315**:25–30.

9 Philadelphia panel evidence-based clinical practice guidelines on selected rehabilitation interventions for shoulder pain. *Phys Ther* 2001;**81**:1719–30.

10 Green S, Buchbinder R, Glazier R, Forbes A. Interventions for shoulder pain. *Cochrane Database of Systematic Reviews* 2000;**2**:CD001156.

11 National Health and Medical Research Council. 2003. Evidence-Based Management of Acute Musculoskeletal Pain.

12 Winters JC, de Jongh AC, van der Windt DAWM, *et al.* NHG Practice Guideline 'Shoulder complaints' (May 1999) http://www.artsennet.nl/nhg/guidelines/E08.htm

13 van der Windt DA, van der Heijden GJ, Scholten RJ, Koes BW, Bouter LM. The efficacy of non-steroidal anti-inflammatory drugs (NSAIDS) for shoulder complaints. A systematic review. *J Clin Epidemiol* 1995;**48**: 691–704.

14 Buchbinder R, Green S, Youd JM. Non steroidal anti-inflammatory drugs (NSAIDS) for shoulder pain. *Cochrane Database of Systematic Reviews* 2003 (in press).

15 Cohen A, Cohen RW. Short term treatment of acute bursitis of the shoulder. *Penn Med* 1968;**71**:66–70.

16 Wielandts L, Dequeker J. Double-blind trial comparing fentiazac with phenylbutazone in patients with tendinitis. *Curr Med Res Opin* 1979;**6**:85–9.

17 Ginsberg F, Famaey JP. A double-blind comparison of slow-release and standard tablet formulations of fentiazac in the treatment of patients with tendinitis and bursitis. *Curr Med Res Opin* 1985;**9**:442–8.

18 White RH, Paull DM, Fleming KW. Rotator cuff tendinitis: comparison of subacromial injection of a long acting

corticosteroid versus oral indomethacin therapy. *J Rheumatol* 1986;**13**:608–13.

19 England S, Farrell A, Coppock J, Struthers G, Bacon P. Low power laser therapy of shoulder tendonitis. *Scand J Rheumatol* 1989;**18**:427–31.

20 Adebajo AO, Nash P, Hazleman BL. A prospective double blind dummy placebo controlled study comparing triamcinolone hexacetonide injection with oral diclofenac 50 mg TDS in patients with rotator cuff tendinitis. *J Rheumatol* 1990;**17**:1207–10.

21 Petri M, Dobrow R, Neiman R, Whiting-O'Keefe Q, Seaman WE. Randomised, double-blind, placebo-controlled study of the treatment of the painful shoulder. *Arthritis Rheum* 1987;**30**:1040–5.

22 Berry H, Fernandes L, Bloom B, Clark RJ, Hamilton EB. Clinical study comparing acupuncture, physiotherapy, injection and oral anti-inflammatory therapy in shoulder-cuff lesions. *Curr Med Res Opin* 1980;**7**:121–6.

23 Goupille P, Sibilia J. Local corticosteroid injections in the treatment of rotator cuff tendinitis (except for frozen shoulder and calcific tendinitis). Groupe Rhumatologique Francais de l'Epaule (G.R.E.P.). *Clin Exp Rheumatol* 1996;**14**:561–6.

24 Buchbinder R, Green S, Youd JM. Corticosteroid injections for shoulder pain. *Cochrane Database of Systematic Review.* 2003;(1):CD004016.

25 Williams NE, Seifert MH, Cuddigan JH, Wise RA. Treatment of capsulitis of the shoulder. *Rheumatol Rehab* 1975;**14**:236.

26 Pons S, Gallardo C, Caballero JC, Martinez T. Transdermal nitroglycerin versus corticosteroid infiltration for rotator cuff tendinitis. *Aten Primaria* 2001;**28**:452–5.

27 Plafki C, Steffen R, Willburger RE, Wittenberg RH. Local anaesthetic injection with and without corticosteroids for subacromial impingement syndrome. *Int Orthop* 2000;**24**:40–2.

28 Blair B, Rokito AS, Cuomo F, Jarolem K, Zuckerman JD. Efficacy of injections of corticosteroids for subacromial impingement syndrome. *J Bone Joint Surg Am* 1996;**78**:1685–9.

29 Vecchio PC, Hazleman BL, King RH. A double-blind trial comparing subacromial methylprednisolone and lignocaine in acute rotator cuff tendinitis. *Br J Rheumatol* 1993;**32**:743–5.

30 Kirkley A, Litchfield R, Alvarez C, Herbert S, Griffin S. Prospective double blind randomised clinical trial of subacromial injection of betamethasone and xylocaine versus xylocaine alone in rotator cuff tendinosis. *J Bone Jt Surg [Br]* 1999;**81–B** (Suppl) I:107.

31 Strobel G. [Long-term therapeutic effect of different intra-articular injection treatments of the painful shoulder – effect on pain, mobility and work capacity]. *Rehabil* 1996;**35**:176–8.

32 Withrington R, Crirgis F, Seifert M. A placebo-controlled trial of steroid injections in the treatment of supraspinatus tendonitis. *Scand J Rheumatol* 1985;**14**:76–8.

33 Shibata Y, Midorikawa K, Emoto G, Naito M. Clinical evaluation of sodium hyaluronate for the treatment of patients with rotator cuff tear. *J Shoulder Elbow Surg* 2001;**10**:209–16.

34 Gray RG, Gottlieb NL. Intra-articular steroids. An updated assessment. *Clin Orthop* 1983;**177**:235–63.

35 Speed C, Hazleman B. Musculoskeletal disorders: shoulder pain. *Clin Evid* 2002;**7**:1122–39.

36 Green S, Buchbinder R, Hetrick S. Physiotherapy for shoulder pain. (Cochrane Review) In: The Cochrane Library, Issue 2, 2003. Oxford: Update Software.

37 Bang MD, Deyle GD. Comparison of supervised exercise with and without manual physical therapy for patients with shoulder impingement syndrome. *J Orthop Sports Phys Ther* 2000;**30**:126–37.

38 Conroy D, Hayes K. The effect of mobilization as a component of comprehensive treatment for primary shoulder impingement syndrome. *J Orthop Sports Phys Ther* 1998;**28**:3–14.

39 Ebenbichler GR, Erdogmus CB, Resch KL, *et al.* Ultrasound therapy for calcific tendinitis of the shoulder. *NEJM* 1999;**340**:1533–8.

40 Perron M, Malouin F. Acetic acid iontophoresis and ultrasound for the treatment of calcifying tendinitis of the shoulder: a randomised control trial. *Arch Phys Med Rehabil* 1997;**78**:379–84.

41 Downing DS, Weinstein A. Ultrasound therapy of subacromial bursitis. A double blind trial. *Phys Ther* 1986;**66**:194–9.

42 Nykanen M. Pulsed ultrasound treatment of the painful shoulder a randomised, double-blind, placebo-controlled study. *Scand J Rehabil Med* 1995;**27**:105–8.

43 Dal Conte G, Rivoltini P, Combi F. Trattamento della periartrite calcarea di spalla con campi magnetici pulsanti: studio controllato. *La Riabilitazione* 1990;**23**:27–33.

44 Binder A, Parr G, Hazleman B, Fitton-Jackson S. Pulsed electromagnetic field therapy of persistent rotator cuff tendinitis. A double-blind controlled assessment. *Lancet* 1984;**1**:695–8.

45 Brox JI, Roe C, Saugen E, Vollestad NK. Isometric abduction muscle activation in patients with rotator tendinosis of the shoulder. *Arch Phys Med Rehabil* 1997;**78**:1260–7.

46 Saunders L. The efficacy of low level laser therapy in supraspinatus tendinitis. *Clin Rehabil* 1995;**9**:126–34.

47 Vecchio P, Cave C, King V, *et al.* A double-blind study of the effectiveness of low level laser treatment of rotator cuff tendinitis. *Br J Rheumatol* 1993;**32**:740–2.

48 Green S, Buchbinder R, Hetrick S. Acupuncture for shoulder pain. *Cochrane Database of Systematic Reviews* (submitted), in press.

49 Kleinhenz J, Streitberger K, Windeler J, *et al.* Randomised clinical trial comparing the effects of acupuncture and a newly designed placebo needle in rotator cuff tendinitis. *Pain* 1999;**83**:235–41.

50 Vecchio PC, Adebajo AO, Hazleman BL. Suprascapular nerve block for persistent rotator cuff lesions. *J Rheumatol* 1993

51 Loew M, Daecke W, Kusnierczak D, Rahmanzadeh M, Ewerbeck V. Shock-wave therapy is effective for chronic calcifying tendinitis of the shoulder. *J Bone Joint Surg Br* 1999;**81**:863–7.

52 Seil R, Rupp S, Hammer D, *et al.* Extrakorporale stosswellentherapie bei der tendionosis calcarea der rotatorenmanschette: vergleich verschiedener behandlungsprotokolle (Extracorporeal shock wave therapy in the treatment of chronically painful calcifying tendinitis: comparison of two treatment protocols). *Z Orthop Ihre Grenzgeb* 1999;**137**:310–15.

53 Schmitt J, Haake M, Tosch A, *et al.* Low-energy extracorporeal shock-wave treatment (ESWT) for tendinitis of the supraspinatus: a prospective randomised study. *J Bone J Surg Br* 2001;**83B**:873–6.

54 Speed CA, Richards C, Nichols D, *et al.* Extracorporeal shock-wave therapy for tendonitis of the rotator cuff. A double-blind, randomised, controlled trial. *J Bone Joint Surg Br* 2002;**84**:509–12.

55 Mattara L, Trotta F, Biasi D, Cervetti R. Evaluation of the efficacy and tolerability of a new locally acting preparation of flurbiprofen in scapulohumeral periarthritis. *Eur J Rheumatol Inflamm* 1994;**14**:15–20.

56 Ward MC, Kirwan JR, Norris P, Murray N. Paracetamol and diclofenac in the painful shoulder syndrome. *Br J Rheumatol* 1986;**25**:412.

57 Famaey JP, Ginsberg F. Treatment of periarthritis of the shoulder: A comparison of ibuprofen and diclofenac. *J Int Med Res* 1984;**12**:238–43.

58 Huskisson EC, Bryans R. Diclofenac sodium in the treatment of painful stiff shoulder. *Curr Med Res Opin* 1983;**8**:350–3.

59 Rhind V, Downie WW, Bird HA, Wright V, Engler C. Naproxen and indomethacin in periarthritis of the shoulder. *Rheumatol Rehab* 1982;**21**:51–3.

60 Thumb N, Kolarz G, Scherak O, Mayrhofer F. The efficacy and safety of fentiazac and diclofenac sodium in peri-arthritis of the shoulder: a multi-centre, double-blind comparison. *J Int Med Res* 1987;**15**:327–34.

61 Yamamoto M, Sugano T, Kashiwazaki S, *et al.* Double-blind comparison of piroxicam and indomethacin in the treatment of cervicobrachial syndrome and periarthritis scapulohumeralis (stiff shoulder). *Eur J Rheumatol Inflamm* 1983;**6**:266–73.

62 Gam AN, Schydlowsky P, Rossel I, Remvig L, Jensen EM. Treatment of "frozen shoulder" with distension and glucorticoid compared with glucorticoid alone. A randomised controlled trial. *Scand J Rheumatol* 1998;**27**:425–30.

63 White A, Tuite J. The accuracy and efficacy of shoulder injections in restrictive capsulitis. *J OrthopRheumatol* 1996;**9**:37–40.

64 Rizk TE, Pinals RS, Talaiver AS. Corticosteroid injections in adhesive capsulitis: investigation of their value and site. *Arch Phys Med Rehabil* 1991;**72**:20–2.

65 Lee M, Haq AMMM, Wright V, Longton EB. Periarthritis of the shoulder: A controlled trial of physiotherapy. *Physiotherapy* 1973;**59**:312–15.

66 Bulgen DY, Binder A, Hazleman B, Dutton J, Roberts S. Frozen shoulder: prospective clinical study with and evaluation of three treatment regimens. *Ann Rheum Dis* 1984;**43**:353–60.

67 de Jong BA, Dahmen R, Hogeweg JA, Marti RK. Intra-articular triamcinolone acetonide injection in patients with capsulitis of the shoulder: a comparative study of two dose regimens. *Clin Rehabil* 1998;**12**:211–15.

68 van der Windt DA, Koes BW, Deville W, *et al.* Effectiveness of corticosteroid injections versus physiotherapy for treatment of painful stiff shoulder in primary care: randomised trial. *BMJ* 1998;**317**:1292–6.

69 Dacre JE, Beeney N, Scott DL. Injections and physiotherapy for the painful stiff shoulder. *Ann Rheum Dis* 1989;**48**:322–5.

70 Arslan S, Celiker R. Comparison of the efficacy of local corticosteroid injection and physical therapy for the treatment of adhesive capsulitis. *Rheumatol Int* 2001;**21**:20–3.

71 Jacobs LG, Barton MA, Wallace WA, *et al.* Intra-articular distension and steroids in the management of capsulitis of the shoulder. *BMJ* 1991;**302**:1498–501.

72 Kivimaki J, Pohjolainen T. Manipulation under anesthesia for frozen shoulder with and without steroid injection. *Arch Phys Med Rehab* 2001;**82**:1188–90.

73 Jones DS, Chattopadhyay C. Suprascapular nerve block for the treatment of frozen shoulder in primary care: a randomised trial. *Br J Gen Pract* 1999;**49**:39–41.

74 Corbeil V, Dussault RG, Leduc BE, Fleury J. [Adhesive capsulitis of the shoulder: a comparative study of arthrography with intra-articular corticotherapy and with or without capsular distension]. *Can Assoc Radiol J* 1992;**43**:127–30.

75 Buchbinder R, Green S, Forbes A, Hall S, Lawler G. Arthrographic joint distension with saline and steroid improves function and reduces pain in patients with painful stiff shoulder: results of a random double-blind placebo-controlled trial. *Ann Rheum* Dis (in press).

76 Blockey A, Wright J. Oral cortisone therapy in periarthritis of the shoulder. *BMJ* 1954;**1**:1455–7.

77 Binder A, Hazleman BL, Parr G, Roberts S. A controlled study of oral prednisolone in frozen shoulder. *Br J Rheumatol* 1986;**25**:288–92.

78 Kessel L, Bayley I, Young A. The upper limb: the frozen shoulder. *Br J Hosp Med* 1981;**25**:334, 336–7, 339.

79 Nicholson G. The effects of passive joint mobilization on pain and hypomobility associated with adhesive capsulitis of the shoulder (abstract). *J Orthop Sports Phys Ther* 1985;**6**:238–46.

80 Leclaire R, Bourgouin J. Electromagnetic treatment of shoulder periarthritis: a randomised controlled trial of the efficiency and tolerance of magnetotherapy. *Arch Phys Med Rehabil* 1991;**72**:284–7.

81 Taverna E, Parrini M, Cabitza P. Laserterapia IR versus placebo nel trattamento di alcune patologie a carcio dell'apparato locomotore [Laser therapy versus placebo in the treatment of some bone and joint pathology]. *Minerva Ortopedica Traumatologica* 1990;**41**:631–6.

82 Lin ML, Huang CT, Lin JG, Tsai SK. [A comparison between the pain relief effect of electroacupuncture, regional never block and electroacupuncture plus regional never block in frozen shoulder]. *Acta Anaesthesiol Sinica* 1994;**32**:237–42.

83 Dahan TH, Fortin L, Pelletier M, *et al.* Double blind randomised clinical trial examining the efficacy of bupivacaine suprascapular nerve blocks in frozen shoulder. *J Rheumatol* 2000;**27**:1464–9.

84 Karatas G, Meray J. Suprascapular nerve block for pain relief in adhesive capsulitis: Comparison of 2 different techniques. *Arch Phys Med Rehabil* 2002;**83**:593–7.

Elbow pain: lateral epicondylitis

Rachelle Buchbinder, Sally Green, Ottawa Methods Group

Introduction

"Tennis elbow" has many analogous terms, including lateral elbow pain, lateral epicondylitis, rowing elbow, tendonitis of the common extensor origin, and peritendonitis of the elbow. It is characterised by pain and tenderness over the lateral epicondyle of the humerus and pain on resisted dorsiflexion of the wrist and/or middle finger.

Tennis elbow is common (population prevalence 1–3%).[85] Peak incidence is 40–50 years, and for women between 42 and 46 years the incidence increases to10%.[86,87] The incidence of lateral elbow pain in general practice is 4–7 per 1000 patients per year.[88–90]

Tennis elbow is considered to be an overload injury, typically following minor and often unrecognised trauma of the extensor muscles of the forearm. Despite the title tennis elbow, tennis is a direct cause in only 5% of cases.[90]

Tennis elbow is generally self-limiting. In a trial of general practice patients with elbow pain of greater than 4 weeks duration, 80% following an expectantly awaiting policy were recovered after one year.[91] In some cases, however, symptoms persist for 18 months to two years,[92] and in a few, for much longer. The cost is therefore high, both in terms of loss of productivity, and health care utilisation.

Methodology

This work is based on a series of Cochrane systematic reviews of interventions for tennis elbow (lateral elbow pain), and two published systematic reviews not yet submitted to the Cochrane Library (corticosteroid injections and physiotherapy interventions). Eligibility criteria for including studies into the reviews were determined a priori and applied against retrieved trials by two independent reviewers.

Eligibility criteria were as follows.

Types of studies

- Randomised or pseudo-randomised controlled trials. Studies where participants were not randomised into intervention groups were excluded from the review.
- Studies in all languages were translated into English and considered for inclusion in the review. A sensitivity analysis including and excluding non-English language trials was conducted to test the effect of inclusion of these trials.

Types of participants

Inclusion in this review was restricted to trials with participants meeting the following criteria:

- Adults >16 years of age.
- Lateral elbow pain for greater than 3 weeks' duration.
- No history of significant trauma or systemic inflammatory conditions such as rheumatoid arthritis.
- Studies of various soft tissue diseases and pain due to tendonitis at all anatomical sites were included, provided that the lateral elbow pain results were presented separately or greater than 90% of participants in the study had lateral elbow pain.

Types of interventions

The following interventions were included:

- All randomised controlled comparisons of non-steroidal anti-inflammatory drugs (NSAIDs) versus placebo, or another modality, or of varying types and dosages of NSAID.

- All randomised controlled comparisons of glucocorticosteroid injections versus placebo, or another modality, or of varying types and dosages of injection.
- All randomised controlled comparisons of physiotherapy modalities versus placebo, or another modality, or of varying modalities compared to each other.
- All randomised controlled comparisons of acupuncture versus placebo, or another modality, or of varying types and dosages of acupuncture.
- All randomised controlled comparisons of extracorporeal shock wave therapy (ESWT) versus placebo, or another modality, or of varying types and dosages of ESWT.
- All randomised controlled comparisons of surgery versus placebo, or another modality, or of varying types of surgery.
- All randomised controlled comparisons of bracing, or another modality, or of varying types of bracing.

Literature search

Randomised trials were identified from searches of the Cochrane Controlled Trials Register (Cochrane Library Issue 2, 2002), MEDLINE, EMBASE, CINAHL, and Science Citation Index (SCISEARCH). Searches were conducted in June 2002 and were not restricted by date. The following search strategy was used to search MEDLINE, and was adapted for the remaining databases. It was decided not to include search terms for specific interventions, but simply to identify all possible trials related to tennis elbow.

1. exp tennis elbow/
2. exp tendinitis/
3. exp bursitis/
4. (tennis elbow or elbow pain or epicondylitis or tendonitis or tendinitis or common extensor origin).mp.
5. or/1–4
6. clinical trial.pt.
7. random$.mp.
8. ((singl$ or doubl$) adj (blind$ or mask$)).mp.
9. placebo$.mp.
10. or/6–9
11. 5 and 10

Following the identification of potential trials for inclusion by the search strategy two independent reviewers reviewed the methods sections of all identified trials independently according to the eligibility criteria. Where the two reviewers disagreed, discussion was facilitated in order to reach consensus. If this failed, the trial was sent to a third reviewer for arbitration.

Data extraction and analysis

In order to assess efficacy, raw data for outcomes of interest (means and standard deviations for continuous outcomes and number of events for binary (dichotomous) outcomes) were extracted where available from the published reports. All standard errors of the mean were converted to standard deviation. Wherever reported data was converted or imputed, this was recorded. For trials where the required data was not reported or able to be calculated, further details were requested of first authors. If no further details were provided, the trial was included in the review and fully described, but not included in the meta-analysis.

The following choices of statistic and 95% confidence intervals were presented for all outcomes.

Continuous outcomes

Standardised mean difference (SMD) using a fixed effect model with 95 % confidence intervals were used to present the between group differences for continuous outcomes. Possible clinical reasons for heterogeneity were explored, and in the presence of significant heterogeneity, trial results were not combined.

Dichotomous outcomes:
Relative risk using a fixed effects model was selected for interpretation of dichotomous outcome measures in this review as this is the most appropriate statistic for the interpretation when the event is common. Reasons for heterogeneity were evaluated and in the event of significant heterogeneity trial results were not pooled.

Outcomes

The clinically relevant outcomes of interest in lateral elbow pain are: pain, range of motion (active and passive), function/disability and quality of life, grip strength, return to work, patient's perception of overall effect, global preference, physician's preference, and adverse effects. All methods of measuring individual outcomes were included in the systematic reviews, but for the purposes of this summary, outcomes are presented as pain and global improvement (self-reported benefit or participant satisfaction).

Evaluating the evidence

This review included only randomised controlled trials. Validity of included trials was assessed by comment on whether they met key criteria (see Introduction).

Summary

The following will present a summary of recent systematic reviews and meta-analysis of interventions for tennis elbow including acupuncture, bracing, non-steroidal anti-inflammatory medication, corticosteroid injections, physiotherapy, extracorporeal shock wave therapy, and surgery.

We use the following case presentation to illustrate how different treatments may be selected depending on the desired outcome, risk profile and preferences of the individual.

Case presentation

A 48-year-old right-handed man presents to your practice complaining of right-sided lateral elbow pain, which he has had for several months. The pain is worsening and is now impacting on his ability to garden, play tennis, and his elbow is aching at the end of the day. He works as a designer, using a computer for most of the day. He has noticed lifting his briefcase, ironing, and grip worsens the pain. He has normal radiographs. He has been wearing a strap brace just distal to his elbow, but this does not appear to be helping and he is seeking your advice regarding his treatment options.

Acupuncture

One Cochrane Systematic Review[93] included four small randomised controlled trials with a combined total of 239 participants, all with tennis elbow defined as lateral elbow pain aggravated by wrist and finger dorsiflexion. The review found that due to problems with methodology of the trials included in the review (particularly small populations, uncertain allocation concealment, and substantial loss to follow up) and clinical differences between trials, data from trials could not be combined in a meta-analysis.

Outcomes

The results of the trials included in this systematic review are summarised in Table 10·11. Statistically significant results are marked with an asterisk (*).

Pain

One randomised controlled trial[94] found needle acupuncture brings about relief of pain for significantly longer than placebo (SMD = 1·2 (0·58, 1·82)). When expressed on a time scale this reflects an increase of pain-free time in the acupuncture group of 18 hours longer than placebo (WMD = 18·8 hours, 95%CI 10·1–27·5). The same trial demonstrated acupuncture to be more likely to result in a 50% or greater reduction in pain after 1 treatment (RR = 3 (1·45, 6·23)).

Overall effect

A second randomised controlled trial[95] demonstrated that needle acupuncture was more likely to result in overall improvement as reported by the participant (RR = 15·36, 95% CI 1·86, 126·68) after 10 treatments. No significant differences were found in the longer term (after 3–12 months).

A randomised controlled trial of laser acupuncture versus placebo demonstrated no differences between laser acupuncture and placebo with respect to overall benefit.[96] A fourth trial published in Chinese demonstrated no difference between vitamin B12 injection plus acupuncture and vitamin B12 injection alone with respect to cure (cure not defined) (RR 0·44, 95% CI 0·15–1·29).[97] No trial assessed the effect of acupuncture on function, quality of life, strength, or return to work and no adverse effects were recorded in any of the four included trials.

Evidence summary: Silver

A systematic review of four small randomised controlled trials suggested short-term benefit from needle acupuncture with respect to pain relief, but this benefit is not maintained in the longer term.

Case presentation

Acupuncture may provide some relief of your patient's pain for a short period of time after treatment, but is unlikely to last for a long period of time. Given your patient's duration of symptoms of pain for several months, acupuncture may be of limited benefit.

Bracing

Two systematic reviews were identified,[98,99] the most recent one[99] focusing on effectiveness of bracing only.

Five RCTs have been published. Two studies compared bracing to corticosteroid injection,[100,101] one study compared bracing to anti-inflammatory cream,[102] and one study compared bracing to physiotherapy (details of treatment not specified).[103] Three studies investigated the additive value of bracing combined with other interventions.[100,102,104] The validity of the trials was variable.[99] Statistical pooling was not possible due to large heterogeneity amongst trials.

Outcomes

The trial results are summarised in Table 10.12. Statistically significant results are marked with an*.

Pain

Comparing bracing to corticosteroid injections, Erturk failed to demonstrate any difference between treatments in terms of short term reduction in pain (SMD) = 0·70; 95% CI –0·33; 1·73).[100] A study comparing an elbow-support with physiotherapy[103] failed to demonstrate a difference between groups with respect to short term patient satisfaction (RR= 1·03; 95% CI 0·6; 1·6) or decrease in pain. This study had a dropout rate of 30%. The results of a study comparing anti-inflammatory cream with an elbow strap failed to demonstrate any difference for pain reduction in the short-term (SMD = 0·96 (–0·06, 1·98).[102]

Overall effect

Haker *et al*[101] showed significantly better short term results with respect to global measure of improvement favouring corticosteroid injection to bracing (RR = 2·91; 95% CI 1·49; 5·68), but this difference was not maintained in the longer term.

Three studies[100–102] investigated the additive value of a brace when used in conjunction with corticosteroid injections,[100] manipulation,[102] anti-inflammatory cream[102] or ultrasound.[104] All three studies reported only short term results. In these studies there was insufficient data or too low power to indicate the added value of braces.

Evidence summary: Silver

RCTs of bracing compared to other interventions showed no benefit of bracing compared to anti-inflammatory cream or physiotherapy, and corticosteroid injection was more effective than bracing. There are no randomised controlled trials comparing bracing to placebo.

Case presentation

Your patient has reported that he has been using a brace and that it is not helping. This is consistent with the evidence that other interventions are more likely to be of benefit than bracing.

Corticosteroid injection

Three systematic reviews were identified,[98,105,106] which included 5, 11, and 13 studies respectively. The most recent review is the systematic review by Smidt *et al*,[106] which forms the basis of this section.

In general, the methodological quality of the trials was poor to modest.

Outcomes

Short term effect

Nine randomised controlled trials (eight with quantitative results) assessing the short term effects (≤ 6 weeks) of corticosteroid injections are summarised in Table 10.13 (see also Visual Rx Faces 10.1). Statistically significant results are marked with an *.

There were statistically significant and clinically relevant short term results in favour of corticosteroid injections (only one small study did not have positive results).[108] Corticosteroid injection appears to be superior to placebo, local anaesthetic injection, NSAID, bracing, and physiotherapy interventions in the short term.

Long term effect

Only six studies performed an intermediate (6 weeks to 6 months) or long term (≥ 6 months) outcome assessment. These studies are summarised in Table 10.14. Statistically significant results are marked with an *.

None of the studies found statistically significant results in favour of corticosteroid injections. In contrast, the only study reporting significant differences[112] compared corticosteroid injections to non-steroidal anti-inflammatory drugs and found statistically significant and clinically relevant results for some outcome measures in favour of non-steroidal anti-inflammatory drugs at 6 months of follow up. Corticosteroid injections therefore do not appear to be better than local anaesthetic injections, bracing, NSAID or physiotherapy interventions in the longer term.

Adverse effects

Eight studies provided information on the adverse effects of corticosteroid injections, such as facial flushes, post injection pain, and local skin atrophy.[106] Although these adverse effects are often mentioned in the literature, in the RCTs there was no difference in incidence of adverse effects between the corticosteroid injections and control interventions.

Table 10.11 Summary of results of RCTs of acupuncture for tennis elbow

Trial	Sample size	Effect in acupuncture group	Effect in control group	SMD	RR	% benefit (95% CI)	NNT (95% CI)
Duration of pain relief (hours)							
Molsberger[94] Acupuncture *v* placebo	48	20·2 (21·54)	1·4 (3·5)	1·2 (0·58, 1·82)*		49% (27, 62)	3 (2, 4)
50% or greater pain relief after one treatment							
Molsberger[94] Acupuncture *v* placebo	48	18/24 (75%)	6/24 (25%)		3 (1·45, 6·23)*	50% (22, 68)	2 (2, 5)
Overall improvement (number of patients improved)							
Haker[95] Needle acupuncture *v* placebo *After 10 treatments*	82	43/44 (98%)	28/38 (74%)		15·36 (1·86,126·68)*	24% (9, 40)	5 (3, 11)
Haker[95] Needle acupuncture *v* placebo *At 3 months*	82	39/43 (91%)	32/35 (91%)		0·91 (0·19, 4·39)		136
Haker[96] Needle acupuncture *v* placebo *At 12 months*	82	37/40 (93%)	30/33 (91%)		1·23 (0·23, 6·56)		63
Haker[96] Laser acupuncture *v* placebo *After 10 treatments*	49	17/23 (74%)	21/26 (76%)		0·67 (0·18, 2·60)		15
Haker[95] Laser acupuncture *v* placebo *At 3 months*	49	20/22 (91%)	19/25 (76%)		3·16 (0·57, 17·62)		7
Haker[96] Laser acupuncture v placebo *At 12 months*	49	17/18 (94%)	21/21 (100%)		0·27 (0·01, 7·08) Favours placebo		18
Cure							
Wang[97] Acupuncture plus Vitamin B injection compared to Vitamin B injection alone	60	4/30 (13%)	9/30 (30%)		0·44 (0·15, 1·29)		6

*Statistically significant result.

Table 10.12 Summary of results of RCTs of bracing for tennis elbow

Trial	Sample size	Effect in braced group	Effect in control group	SMD (95% CI)	RR (95% CI)	% benefit (95% CI)	NNT (95% CI)
Pain							
Burton[102] Brace *v* anti-inflammatory cream *Short term follow up*	17	−1·62 (0·42)	−2 (0·33)	0·96 (−0·06, 1·98)			
Erturk[100] Brace *v* corticosteroid injection *Short term follow up*	16	−13·62 (18·76)	−27·11 (17·81)	0·70 (−0·33, 1·73)			
Erturk[100] Brace plus corticosteroid injection *v* corticosteroid injection *Short term follow up*	19	40·9 (22·18)	27·11 (17·81)	0·65 (−0·28, 1·58)			
Burton[100] Brace plus anti-inflammatory cream *v* anti-inflammatory cream *Short term follow up*	17	−2·13 (1·55)	−2 (1)	−0·1 (−1·05, 0·86)			
Burton[102] Brace plus manipulation *v* manipulation *Short term follow up*	16	−1·62 (1·19)	−1·75 (1·91)	0·13 (−1·43, 1·69)			
Global improvement							
Dwars[103] Brace *v* physiotherapy *Short term follow up*	84	23/49 (47%)	16/35 (46%)		1·03 (0·6, 1·6)		82

(*Continued*)

Table 10.12 (*Continued*)

Trial	Sample size	Effect in braced group	Effect in control group	SMD (95% CI)	RR (95% CI)	% benefit (95% CI)	NNT (95% CI)
Haker[101] Brace *v* corticosteroid injection *Short term follow up*	56	34/37 (92%)	6/19 (32%)		2·91 (1·49, 5·68)* *Favours injection*	60% (34, 77)	2 (2, 3)
Haker[101] Brace *v* corticosteroid injection *Medium term follow up*	56	19/37 (51%)	14/19 (74%)		0·70 (0·46, 1·05)		
Haker[101] Brace *v* corticosteroid injection *Long term follow up*	56	22/37 (59%)	13/19 (68%)		0·87 (0·58, 1·30)		
Holdsworth[104] Brace plus ultrasound and hydrocortisone coupling medium *v* ultrasound and hydrocortisone coupling medium *Short term follow up*	17	55·9 (16·1)	49·6 (12·4)	0·41 (–0·57, 1·38)			
Holdsworth[104] Brace plus ultrasound and aquasonic coupling medium *v* ultrasound and aquasonic coupling *Short term follow up*	17	62·6 (11·3)	63 (12·2)	–0·03 (–0·98, 0·92)			

*Statistically significant result.

Table 10.13 NNT for short term results of corticosteroid injection for tennis elbow[107]

Trial	Outcome	Sample size	Effect in treatment group	Effect in control group	SMD	RR(RR < 1 favours treatment)	% benefit (95% CI)	NNT (95% CI)
Corticosteroid injection *v* placebo								
Day[107]	Global improvement Number improved: Placebo: 7/29 Injection: 33/36	65	33/36 (92%)	7/29 (24%)		0·11 (0·04, 0·33)*	68% (45, 81)	2 (2, 3)
Saartook[108]	Pain	10			0·04 (–0·82, 0·90)			
	Global improvement	10				1·21 (0·65, 2·26)		
Corticosteroid plus local anaesthetic injection *v* local anaesthetic injection								
Price†[109]	Pain	29			–0·62 (–1·15, –0·1)*		29% (5, 48)	4 (3, 21)
Price‡[109]	Pain	29			–1·04 (–1·59, –0·5)*		45% (24, 58)	3 (2, 5)
Corticosteroid injection *v* local anaesthetic injection								
Murley[110]	Global improvement	37	14/19 (74%)	7/18 (39%)		0·32 (0·10, 0·98)*	35% (3, 58)	3 (2, 34)
Day[107]	Global improvement	35	33/36 (92%)	7/35 (20%)		0·10 (0·03, 0·31)*	72% (51, 83)	2 (2, 2)
Corticosteroid injection *v* brace								
Haker[111]	Global improvement	18	13/19 (68%)	2/17 (12%)		0·36 (0·18, 0·71)*	57% (25, 75)	2 (2, 5)
Corticosteroid injection *v* NSAID								
Hay[112]	Pain					0·57 (0·43, 0·76)*		
	Global improvement					0·62 (0·49, 0·79)*		
Corticosteroid injections *v* physiotherapy								
Verhaar[113]	Pain	53				0·61 (0·48, 0·78)*		
	Global improvement	53				0·45 (0·29, 0·69)*		
Halle[114]	*Results not reported numerically*							

*Statistically significant result.

†Hydrocortisone versus local anaesthetic.

‡Triamcinolone versus local anaesthetic.

Visual Rx Faces 10.1 NNT for Corticosteroid injection versus placebo

Global improvement

No Treatment

Key

Good Outcome

Bad Outcome

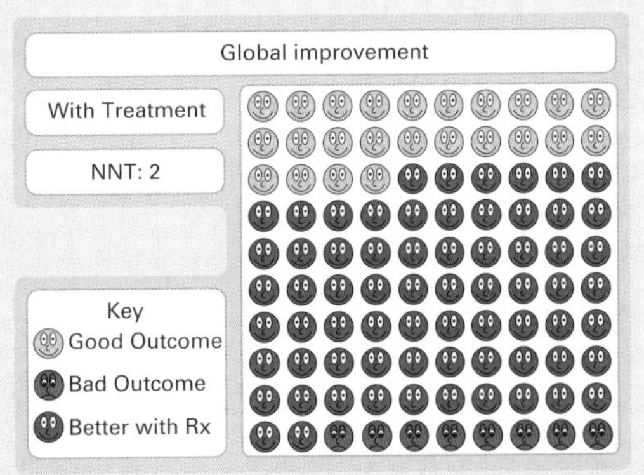

Evidence summary: Silver

A systematic review of 13 randomised controlled trials demonstrates corticosteroid injection to be of short term clinical benefit in eight of nine relevant trials. None of the six RCTS looking at outcomes in the longer term showed that this benefit lasted.

Case presentation

Your patient is likely to benefit in the shorter term from a corticosteroid injection, but these benefits are not likely to last beyond a few weeks.

Non-steroidal anti-inflammatory drugs (NSAIDs)

A Cochrane systematic review specifically of NSAIDs[117] and two systematic reviews of varying interventions[92,98] have been published discussing NSAIDs for tennis elbow. The Cochrane review is the most current and includes 14 randomised controlled trials. All trials in the other systematic reviews are included in the Cochrane Review. Few of the trials included used intention to treat analysis, and the sample size of most was small (populations range from 18 to 128 participants for trials included in the meta-analysis).

Outcomes

The results of the individual trials included in the systematic review are summarised in Table 10.18. Statistically significant results are marked with an *.

Topical NSAID

Pain: There is evidence from meta-analysis of three trials (combined population of 130) that topical NSAIDs are significantly more effective than placebo with respect to pain (pooled SMD = –0·93 (–1·29 to –0·56)). Topical NSAIDs used in these trials were diclofenac (two trials) and Amuno gel (one trial).

Global improvement: There is evidence from two trials that topical NSAIDs offer significant benefit compared to placebo with respect to global improvement (RR 1·87 (1·33, 2·62)).

Adverse effects: Two trials reported adverse effects of topical NSAID with the risk of adverse effect greater than placebo in one trial (RR = 2·26 (1·04, 4·94)).[121] Adverse effects were mild and

Table 10.14 Summary of longer term results of RCTs of corticosteroid injection for tennis elbow[108]

Trial	Outcome	Sample size	SMD	RR
Corticosteroid plus local anaesthetic injection *v* local anaesthetic injection				
Price[109†]	Pain	29	−0·15 (−0·69, 0·38)	
Price[109‡]	Pain	29	−0·48 (−1·02, 0·06)	
Baily[115]	Global improvement	20		0·67 (0·40, 1·11)
Corticosteroid injection *v* local anaesthetic injection				
Freeland[116]	Global improvement	7		0·97 (0·41, 2·32)
Corticosteroid injection *v* brace				
Haker[111]	Global improvement	18		0·76 (0·32, 1·80)
Corticosteroid injection *v* NSAID				
Hay[112]	Pain	106		1·71 (1·17, 2·51)*
Corticosteroid injections *v* physiotherapy				
Verhaar[113]	Pain	53		1·20 (0·96, 1·51)
	Global improvement	53		1·24 (0·81, 1·90)
Halle[114]	*Results not reported numerically*			

*Statistically significant result.

†Hydrocortisone versus local anaesthetic.

‡Triamcinolone versus local anaesthetic.

did not stop use of the drug. Adverse effects reported in the published trials are foul breath and minor skin irritation.

Oral NSAID

There is some evidence from one trial for short term benefit of oral NSAIDs with respect to pain and function (SMD = −0·51, 95%CI −0·87 to −0·16), but this benefit was not sustained.[98] In this trial the intervention was diclofenac. A second trial demonstrated no significant benefit with respect to pain (median (range) pain score at 4 weeks in NSAID (naproxen) group 4 (2–6), in placebo group 3·5 (2–6)).[112]

Adverse effects: Based on one gold trial in tennis elbow, oral NSAIDs were associated with an increased risk of abdominal pain (RR = 3·17 (1·35 to 7·41)) and diarrhoea (RR = 1·92 (1·08 to 3·14)). A systematic review of 12 randomised controlled trials of NSAID in a variety of disorders[122] demonstrated the overall relative risk of complications from oral NSAIDs to range from 3·0 to 5·0. Adverse effects were predominantly gastrointestinal.

Oral NSAID versus corticosteroid injection

While four studies investigated NSAID compared to injection, only two could be included in meta-analysis due to incomplete reporting of results. These studies compared 20 mg methoprednisolone and lidocaine (lignocaine) with 500 mg naproxen and betamethasone and prilocaine with 500 mg naproxen. Pooled short

Table 10.15 Summary of results of RCTs of NSAIDs for tennis elbow

Trial	Sample size	Effect in NSAID group	Effect in control group	SMD (95% CI)	RR (95% CI)	% benefit (95% CI)	NNT (95% CI)
Topical NSAID:							
Pain							
Burnham[118]	28	2·1 (2·1)	3·6 (2·1)	–0·69 (–1·46, 0·07)			
Jenoure[119]	85	1·73 (1·84)	3·83 (1·89)	–·12 (–1·58, –0·66)		47% (31, 58)	3 (2, 4)
Burton[102]	17	2 (1·6)	3 (2·6)	–1 (–1·4, –0·61)*		43% (28, 54)	3 (2, 4)
Global improvement (number improved)							
Jenoure[119]	85	32/44 (73%)	20/41 (49%)		2·8 (1·14, 6·91)*	24% (3, 42)	5 (3, 42)
Primbs[120]	34	14/16 (88%)	4/18 (22%)		24·5 (3·84, 156·13)*	65% (32, 81)	2 (2, 4)
Oral NSAID:							
Pain							
Labelle[98]	128	–29·9 (26·3)	–16 (27·4)	–0·51 (–0·87, –0·16)*		24% (8, 39)	5 (3, 13)
Oral NSAID *v* corticosteroid injections:							
Global improvement (number improved)							
Hay[112]	105	29/52 (56%)	48/52 (92%)		0·11 (0·03, 0·33)*	37% (20, 51)	3 (2, 5)
Saartook[108]	21	6/10 (60%)	6/11 (55%)		1·25 (0·22, 7·08)		18

*Statistically significant result.

term global improvement demonstrated a significant difference in favour of injection (RR 3·06 (1·55, 6·06)). When the results of the two trials not able to be included in the meta-analysis are considered, a result of increased benefit from injection is consistent with the differences demonstrated in pain and function by one trial. The other trial, however, demonstrated no significant differences in pain following injection as compared to NSAID.

Evidence summary: Silver

A Cochrane Systematic Review including 14 RCTs demonstrated short term benefit from topical and oral NSAIDS. Topical NSAIDs have fewer gastrointestinal adverse effects. The short term benefit of injection may be greater than that of oral NSAID.

Case presentation

There is likely to be short term benefit to your patient from use of topical or oral NSAIDs. Given fewer adverse effects from topical NSAID, this may be an appropriate first line of treatment.

Physiotherapy (including ultrasound, laser therapy, electrotherapy, and exercises

Four systematic reviews were identified.[91,98,123,124] The following section is based on the most recent of these reviews.[91] Because of clinical heterogeneity the results of most interventions, except ultrasound, were not pooled.

Table 10.16 Summary of results of RCTs of therapeutic ultrasound for tennis elbow

Trial	Outcome	Sample size	SMD	RR	% benefit	NNT
Ultrasound *v* placebo						
Haker[125]	Global improvement	21		1·13 (0·68, 1·89)		
Lundeberg[126]	Global improvement	33		0·79 (0·49, 1·27)		
Lundeberg[126]	Pain	33	−1·33 (−1·87, −0·80)*		53% (8, 63)	2 (2, 13)
Binder[127]	Pain	38	−0·66 (−1·13, −0·20)*		31% (10, 47)	4 (3, 11)
Binder[128]	Global improvement	38		0·52 (0·33, 0·82)*		
Ultrasound *v* no treatment						
Lundeberg[126]	Pain	33	−1·70 (−2·26, 0·74)			
Lundeberg[126]	Global improvement	33		0·44 (0·26, 0·74)*		
US + friction massage *v* exercises						
Pienimäki[128]	Pain	19	0·95 (0·26, 1·64)*	42% (13, 59)		3 (2, 8) (Favours exercise)
US + friction massage versus laser						
Vasseljen[129]	Pain	15	−0·84 (−1·58, −0·09)*		38% (4, 58)	3 (2, 23)
Vasseljen[129]	Global improvement	15		0·63 (0·26, 1·47)		

*Statistically significant results.

Outcomes

Ultrasound (US)

Nine RCTs examined the effectiveness of ultrasound therapy, using various comparators. Three compared US to placebo and are summarised in Table 10.16 above. Statistically significant results are marked with an asterisk (*).

Pooling of these three studies resulted in a large effect size for pain in favour of ultrasound (SMD −0·98 (−1·64, −0·33), indicating there is evidence for the effectiveness of US in comparison with placebo.

Seven studies compared US with other physiotherapy modalities or with other conservative treatments, like laser and exercises. Not all presented data that could be summarised. Those presenting quantitative results are included in Table 10.16 and show contradictory results. Consequently, there appears to be insufficient evidence to determine the effect of US when compared to other active interventions.

Evidence summary: Silver

Ultrasound appears to be effective for reducing pain when compared to placebo, but there are conflicting results when it is compared to other interventions.

Case presentation

Therapeutic ultrasound is likely to be of benefit with respect to pain in the short term and would be an appropriate treatment to try.

Laser therapy

Eight RCTs (five presenting results numerically) comparing the effects of laser with placebo are presented in Table 10.17. Statistically significant results are marked with an *.

Short term follow up (≤6 weeks) showed no statistically significant effects on pain. Contradictory results were reported for intermediate (6 weeks to 6 months) and long term follow up (≥6 months) assessments, and for comparisons with other physiotherapeutic modalities. Therefore, there is insufficient evidence to either demonstrate benefit or lack of effect.

Evidence summary: Silver

There are eight small RCTs investigating laser therapy for tennis elbow, but they show conflicting results. Hence the effect of treating tennis elbow with laser remains unknown.

> ***Case presentation***
> As the effects of laser therapy for tennis elbow are unknown, and there is evidence to support the use of other interventions (needle acupuncture, topical and oral NSAID, corticosteroid injection, and therapeutic ultrasound) for short term benefit, laser therapy is unlikely to be recommended as a treatment option for your patient.

Electrotherapy

Only one of four RCTs evaluating the effectiveness of electrotherapy (electromagnetic field therapy, transcutaneous electrical nerve stimulation) was of adequate methodological quality, but this study provided insufficient data on important outcomes to calculate an effect size. No conclusions can be drawn regarding the effectiveness of electrotherapy for lateral epicondylitis due to insufficient evidence.

Evidence summary

No conclusions can be drawn regarding the effectiveness of electrotherapy for lateral epicondylitis due to insufficient evidence.

> ***Case presentation***
> Electrotherapy is not recommended as a treatment option for your patient.

Exercises and mobilisation techniques

One RCT with acceptable validity, but only 19 participants, demonstrated a large beneficial effect on pain of exercises compared to ultrasound plus friction massage (SMD (95% CI) 0·95 (−1·64, −0·26). Four other studies were either of poor validity or provided insufficient data on relevant outcome measures. The evidence is therefore inconclusive.

Evidence summary: Silver

One RCT has demonstrated that exercises and mobilisation produce more benefit than ultrasound plus friction massage.

> ***Case presentation***
> Exercises and mobilisation are an option in the management of your patient, but the evidence for other interventions (topical NSAID, corticosteroid injection) is stronger.

Adverse effects

No adverse effects of physiotherapy were described in any of the trials.

> ***Case presentation***
> In summary, physiotherapy in the form of ultrasound and exercise and mobilization techniques may benefit your patient and has no documented harms. There is little evidence to guide you in recommending combinations of treatment (for example NSAIDs and physiotherapy).

Table 10.17 Summary of RCTs of laser therapy for tennis elbow

Trial	Outcome	Sample size	SMD	RR	% benefit	NNT
Laser *v* placebo						
Vasseljen[130]	Pain: <6 weeks follow up	15	–0·25 (–0·96, 0·47)			
	Global improvement	15		0·81 (0·61, 1·06)		
Haker[131]	Global improvement	23		0·95 (0·51, 1·75)		
Haker[132]	Global improvement	29		0·87 (0·65, 1·16)		
Krasheninnikoff[133]	Global improvement	8		1·07 (0·82, 1·39)		
Lundeberg[134]	Pain	19	–2 (–2·8, –1·2)*		64% (49, 68)	2 (2, 3)
Gudmundsen[135]	Global improvement			0·72 (0·6, 0·87)		
Laser *v* friction massage						
Vasseljen[139]	Pain	15	0·92 (0·17, 1·67)*		40% (8, 60)	3 (2, 13)
	Global improvement	15		1·09 (0·73, 1·62)		

*Statistically significant result.

Extracorporeal shock wave therapy (ESWT)

We found one Cochrane Review of ESWT for lateral elbow pain,[136] which included one published RCT of ESWT versus placebo (115 participants)[137] and one unpublished RCT of ESWT versus placebo (271 participants).[138] A systematic review of ESWT for lateral epicondylitis has also been published in the German language.[139] This included the same published RCT.[137] Methodological concerns raised about this RCT include uncertain allocation concealment and failure to analyse 15/115 (13%) early dropouts. Both RCTs included similar study populations (mean age 41·9 to 46·9 years, slightly more women) with chronic symptoms (mean duration 21·9 to 27·6 months) who had failed at least 6 months of conservative therapy including NSAIDs, injections, brace or taping, casting, and physiotherapy. The frequency, doses, and technique of ESWT application were similar in both trials. The active treatment consisted of 1000 impulses of 0·08 mJ/mm^2 of ESWT at weekly intervals for 3 weeks in one RCT[137] and "low-energy" ESWT with 2000 pulses under local anaesthesia (3 ml mepivacaine 1%) at weekly intervals for 3 weeks using device-dependent energy flux density ED+ between 0·07 and 0·09 mJ/mm^2 in the other RCT.[138]

Outcomes

Pain

One RCT demonstrated highly significant differences in favour of ESWT,[137] although the other RCT found no benefits of ESWT over placebo.[138] When the data from the two trials were pooled, the benefits observed in the first trial were no longer statistically significant. The relative risk for treatment failure of ESWT over placebo was 0·40 (95% CI, 0·08 to 1·91) at 6 weeks and 0·44 (95% CI, 0·09 to 2·17) at one year.

After 6 weeks, there was no statistically significant improvement in pain at rest (SMD = – 0·59 (–1.48 to 0·30), pain with resisted wrist extension (SMD –1·12 (–3·33 to 1·09)) or pain with resisted middle finger extension (SMD = –1·49 (–4·32 to 1·33)). Likewise, after 12 or 24 weeks, there was no significant difference between groups in improvement of pain at rest (SMD = – 0·97 (–2·6 to 0·65), pain with resisted wrist extension (SMD –0·86 (–2·57 to 0·85)) and pain with resisted middle finger extension (SMD = –1·43 (–4·13 to 1·27)).

Adverse effects

One RCT did not report adverse effects.[137] The other RCT reported significantly more adverse effects in the EWST group compared to placebo (OR 4·3, 95% CI 2·9 to 6·3).[138] However, there were no treatment discontinuations or dosage adjustments related to adverse effects. The most frequently reported adverse effects in the ESWT-treated group were transitory reddening of the skin (21·1%), pain (4·8%), and small haematomas (3·0%). Migraine occurred in four patients and syncope in three patients following ESWT.

Evidence summary: Silver

Two trials have reported conflicting results.

> ***Case presentation***
> As there is conflicting evidence for the use of EWST, and there may be some minor adverse effects, the use of ESWT should be considered only after other treatment options (corticosteroid injection, topical NSAID or physiotherapy) have been tried.

Surgery

Numerous surgical procedures have been described for lateral elbow pain but none has been evaluated in the context of an RCT. Case series have usually reported good outcomes with respect to alleviation of pain. However, in the absence of a control group, it is not possible to draw any conclusions about the benefits or risks associated with surgical interventions for lateral elbow pain.

Adverse effects

Case series have usually reported few adverse effects but there is no data from clinical trials.

Evidence summary: Bronze

No RCTs have been reported of surgery for tennis elbow.

> ***Case presentation***
> Surgery is not recommended unless all other conservative treatments have been exhausted and the duration of symptoms is at least 12 months.

References

85 Allander E. Prevalence, incidence and remission rates of some common rheumatic diseases and syndromes. *Scand J Rheumatol* 1974;**3**:145–53.

86 Chard MD, Hazleman BL. Tennis elbow – a reappraisal. *Br J Rheumatol* 1989;**28**(3):186–90.

87 Verhaar J. Tennis elbow: anatomical, epidemiological, and therapeutic aspects. *Int Orthopaedics* 1994; **18**:263–7.

88 Hamilton P. The prevalence of humeral epicondylitis: a survey in general practice. *J R Coll Gen Pract* 1986;**36**:464–5.

89 Kivi P. The etiology and conservative treatment of lateral epicondylitis. *Scand J Rehabil Med* 1983;**15**:37–41.

90 Murtagh J. Tennis elbow. *Aust Family Physician* 1988;**17**:90, 91, 94–5.

91 Smidt N, Assendelft WJJ, Arola H, *et al.* Effectiveness of physiotherapy for lateral epicondylitis: a systematic review. *Ann Med* 2003; **35**:51–62.

92 Hudak P, Cole D, Haines T. Understanding prognosis to improve rehabilitation: the example of lateral elbow pain. *Arch Phys Rehabil* 1996;**77**:568–93.

93 Green S, Buchbinder R, Hall S, *et al.* Acupuncture for lateral elbow pain (Cochrane Review). In: Cochrane Collaboration. *Cochrane Library.* Issue 4. Oxford: Update Software, 2001.

94 Molsberger A, Hille E. The analgesic effect of acupuncture in chronic tennis elbow pain. *Br J Rheumatol* **33**:1162–5.

95 Haker E, Lundberg T. Acupuncture treatment in epicondylalgia: a comparative study of two acupuncture techniques. *Clin J Pain* 1990;**6**:221–6.

96 Haker E, Lundeberg T. Laser treatment applied to acupuncture points in lateral humeral epicondylalgia. A double-blind study. *Pain* 1990;**43**:243–7.

97 Wang, L. 30 cases of tennis elbow treated by moxibustion. *Shanghai J Acupuncture Moxibustion* 1997;**16**(6):20.

98 Labelle H, Guibert R, Joncas J *et al.* Lack of scientific evidence for the treatment of lateral epicondylitis of the elbow. *J Bone Joint Surg* 1992;**74**:646–51.

99 Struijs P, Smidt N, Arola H *et al.* Orthotic devices for tennis elbow (Cochrane Review). In: Cochrane Collaboration. *Cochrane Library.* Issue 4. Oxford: Update Software, 2001.

100 Erturk H. Celiker R, Sivri A, Cetin A, Cindas A. Tenisci dirseginde sik kullanilan farkli tedavi yaklasimlarinin etkinligi [The efficacy of different treatment regimens that are commonly used in tennis elbow]. *J Rheum Med Rehab* 1997;**8**:298–301.

101 Haker E, Lundberg T. Elbow-band, splintage and steroids in lateral epicondylalgia (tennis elbow). *Pain Clinic* 1993;**6**:103–12.

102 Burton A. A comparative trial of forearm strap and topical anti-inflammatory as adjuncts to manipulative therapy in tennis elbow. *Man Med* 1988;**3**:141–3.

103 Dwars B, Feiter P, Patka P and Haarman H. Functional treatment of tennis elbow. A comparative study between an elbow support and physical therapy. *Sports Med Hlth* 1990:237–41.

104 Holdsworth L, Anderson D. Effectiveness of ultrasound used with a hydrocortisone coupling medium or epicondylitis clasp to treat lateral epicondylitis: pilot study. *Physiotherapy* 1993;**79**:19–25.

105 Assendelft W, Hay E, Adshead R, Bouter L. Corticosteriod injections for lateral epicondylitits: a systematic overview. *Br J Gen Pract* 1996;**46**:209–216.

106 Smidt N, Assendelft WJ Windt D v D, Hay EM, Buchbinder R, Bouter L. Corticosteroid injections for lateral epicondylitis: a systematic review. *Pain* 2002;**96**:23–40.

107 Day BH, Godvindasamy N, Patnaik R. Corticosteroid injections in the treatment of tennis elbow. *Practitioner* 1978;**220**:459–62.

108 Saartok T, Eriksson E. Randomised trial of oral naproxen or local injection of betamethasone in lateral epicondylitis of the humerus. *Orthopaedics* 1986; **9**:191–4.

109 Price R, Sinclair H, Henrich I, Gibson T. Local injection treatment of tennis elbow: hydrocortisone, triamcinolone and lignocaine compared. *Br J Rheumatol* 1991;**30**:39–44.

110 Murley AH, Lond MB. Tennis elbow: treated with hydrocortisone acetate. *Lancet* 1954;**2**:223–5.

111 Haker E, Lundeberg T. Elbow band, splintage and steroids in lateral epicondylalgia (tennis elbow). *Pain Clin* 1993;**6**:103–12.

112 Hay E, Paterson S, Lewis M, Hosie M, Croft P. Pragmatic randomised controlled trial of local cortico-steroid injection and naproxen for the treatment of lateral epicondylitis of the elbow in primary care. *BMJ* 1999; **319**:964–8.

113 Verhaar JA, Walenkamp GH, van Mameren H, Kester AD, van der Linden AJ. Local corticosteroid injection versus Cyriax-type physiotherapy for tennis elbow. *J Bone Joint Surg [Br]* 1996;**78**:128–32.

114 Halle J. Comparison of four treatment approaches for lateral epicondylitis of the elbow. *J Orthop Sports Phys Therapy* 1986;**8**:62–9.

115 Baily RAJ, Brock BH. Hydrocortisone in tennis elbow: a controlled series. *J R Soc Med* 1957;**50**:389–90.

116 Freeland DE, Gribble MG. Hydrocortisone in tennis elbow. *Lancet* 1954;**2**:225

117 Green S, Buchbinder R, Hall S *et al.* Non-steroidal anti-inflammatory drugs (NSAIDs) for lateral elbow pain.In: Cochrane Collaboration. *Cochrane Library.* Issue 4. Oxford: Update Software, 2001.

118 Burnham R, Gregg R, Healy P, Steadward R. The effectiveness of topical diclofenac for lateral epicondylitis. *Clin J Sports Med* 1998;**8**:78—81.

119 Jenoure P, Rostan A, Gremion G *et al.* Multi-centre, double-blind, controlled clinical study on the efficacy of diclofenac epolamine tissugel plaster in patients with epicondylitis. *Medicina Dello Sport* 1997;**50**:285–92.

120 Primbs P, Tomasi M. Results of a double-blind study with Amuno gelo versus placebo. *Fortschr Med* 1983;**101**:242–4.

121 Percy E, Carson P. The use of DMSO in Tennis Elbow and Rotator Cuff Tendonitis: A double Blind Study. *Med Sci Sports Exercise* 1981;**13**(4):215–19.

122 Rodriguez G. Non-steroidal anti-inflammatory drugs, ulcers and risk: a collaborative meta-analysis. *Semin Arthritis Rheum* 1997;**26**(6):Suppl.

123 Ernst E. Use a new treatment while it still works: ultrasound for epicondylitis. *Eur J Phys Med* 1994;**4**:50–1.

124 Windt DVD, Heijden GVD, Berg SVD, Riet GT, Winter AD, Bouter L. Ultrasound therapy for musculoskeletal disorders: a systematic review. *Pain* 1999;**81**(3):257–71.

125 Haker E, Lundeberg T. Pulsed ultrasound treatment in lateral epicondylalgia. *Scand J Rehabil Med* 1991;**23**: 115–18.

126 Lundeberg T, Abrahamsson P, Haker E. A comparative study of continuous ultrasound, placebo ultrasound and rest in epicondylalgia. *Scand J Rehabil Med* 1988;**20**:99–101.

127 Binder A, Hodge G, Greenwood AM, Hazleman BL, Page Thomas DP. Is therapeutic ultrasound effective in treating soft tissue lesions? *BMJ (Res. ed.)* 1985;**290**: 512–14.

128 Pienimaki T. Tarvainen T, Siira P, Vanharanta H. Progressive strengthening and stretching exercises and ultrasound for chronic lateral epicondylitis. *Physiotherapy* 1996;**82**:522–30.

129 Vasseljen O. Low-level laser versus traditional physiotherapy in the treatment of tennis elbow. *Physiotherapy* 1992;**78**:329–34.

130 Vasseljen O, Hoeg N, Kjeldstad B, Johnsson A, Larsen S. Low level laser versus placebo in the treatment of tennis elbow. *Scand J Rehabil Med* 1992;**24**:37–42.

131 Haker E, Lundeberg T. Is low-energy laser treatment effective in lateral epicondylalgia? *J Pain Sympt Management* 1991;**6**:241–6.

132 Haker EH, Lundeberg TC. Lateral epicondylalgia: report of noneffective midlaser treatment. *Arch Phys Med Rehabil* 1991;**72**:984–8.

133 Krasheninnikoff M, Ellitsgaard N, Rogvi-Hansen B, *et al.* No effect of low power laser in lateral epicondylitis. *Scand J Rheumatol* 1994;**23**:260–3.

134 Lundeberg T, Haker E, Thomas M. Effect of laser versus placebo in tennis elbow. *Scand J Rehabil Med* 1987;**19**:135–8.

135 Gudmundsen J, Vikne J. Laserbehandling av epicondylitis humeri og rotatorcuffsyndrom. *Nor Tidskr Idrettsmed* 1987;**2**:6–15.

136 Buchbinder R, Green S, White M, Barnsley L, Smidt N, Assendelft W. Shockwave therapy for lateral elbow pain. In: Cochrane Collaboration. *Cochrane Library.* Issue 1. Oxford: Update Software, 2001.

137 Rompe J, Hopf C, Kullmer K, Heine J, Burger R, Nafe B. Low-energy extracorporal shock-wave therapy for persistent tennis elbow. *Int Orthopaedics* 1996;**20**:23–7.

138 Haake M, Konig I, Decker T, *et al.* No effectiveness of Extracorporeal Shock Wave Therapy in the treatment of tennis elbow – results from a prospective randomised placebo-controlled multicenter trial (in press).

139 Boddeker I, Haake M. Extracorporeal shock-wave therapy as a treatment for radiohumeral epicondylitis. Current overview. *Orthopade* 2000;**29**(5):463–9.

Shoulder pain and tennis elbow Summaries and decision aids

Shoulder pain in rotator cuff disease and steroid injections Summaries and decision aid

How well do steroid injections work for treating shoulder pain in rotator cuff disease and how safe are they?

To answer this question, scientists found and analysed 12 studies (included in a Cochrane Systematic Review) testing 650 people who had rotator cuff disease. People received either injections of steroids or placebo, or pain relief medicines. These studies provide the best evidence we have today.

What is rotator cuff disease and how can steroid injections help?

The rotator cuff is a group of tendons that surrounds the shoulder joint. In some people, the muscles and tendons pinch when they move their shoulder over and over again. The pinching can cause the rotator cuff to swell, break down, and it may tear away from the bone – this is called rotator cuff disease or tendonitis. In a lot of people, it is a normal part of ageing and they may not have symptoms. But many people with rotator cuff disease do have pain in their shoulder at some time, that may go away on its own. Steroids injections may help decrease the pain and are injected into a specific area of the shoulder. They can be injected into the "subacromial" space or into the shoulder joint itself – an "intra-articular" injection. It is not clear whether it is worth having a steroid injection for quicker and short term relief or just simply waiting for the pain to go away.

How well do steroid injections work?

Two small studies of high quality showed that "subacromial" steroid injections improve pain, function, and movement in the shoulder more than a placebo did 4 weeks after injection.

Three studies showed no difference in improvement between "subacromial" steroid injection and non-steroidal anti-inflammatory drugs (NSAIDs), 4 or 6 weeks after injection.

What side effects occurred with steroid injections?

Facial flushing. Pain where the injection may occur. People with diabetes may have a temporary rise in blood sugar.

What is the bottom line?

There is "Silver" level evidence that subacromial steroid injections may improve pain and function in rotator cuff disease. But the improvement may be small and pain relief may not last long. It also may not be better than taking non-steroidal anti-inflammatory drugs (NSAIDs).

Based on Buchbinder R, Green S, Ottawa Methods Group. Shoulder Pain. In *Evidence-Based Rheumatology.* London: BMJ Books, 2003.

How well do steroid injections work for treating shoulder pain in rotator cuff disease and how safe are they?

What is rotator cuff disease and how can steroid injections help?

The rotator cuff is a group of tendons that surrounds the shoulder joint and attaches to muscles that move the shoulder. In some people, the muscles and tendons are pinched when they move their shoulder over and over again. The pinching (or impingement) can cause the rotator cuff to swell, break down, and it may tear away from the bone – this is called rotator cuff disease or tendonitis. In a lot of people this may occur as part of normal ageing and they will not have any symptoms. But many people with rotator cuff disease have pain or aching in the shoulder which may be worse at night or when lifting the arm up. The pain will eventually go away, but can affect a person's ability to carry out daily activities at home and at work while waiting for the pain to go away.

Pain relief medicines, such as acetaminophen, or non-steroidal anti-inflammatory drugs, such as ibuprofen, are taken by mouth and may help decrease the pain and swelling. Steroids injections may also help and are injected into a specific area of the shoulder. They can be injected into the "subacromial" space or into the shoulder joint itself – an "intra-articular" injection. It is not clear whether it is worth having a steroid injection for quicker and short term relief or just simply waiting for the pain to go away.

How did the scientists find the information and analyse it?

A Cochrane Review was done in which the scientists searched for studies testing steroid injections in patients with rotator cuff disease. Not all studies found were of a high quality and so only those studies that met the high standards were selected.

- Studies had to be randomised controlled trials – studies where one group of patients who received steroid injections was compared to another group of patients who received a placebo injection, non-steroidal anti-inflammatory drugs, physiotherapy or some other treatment.

Which high quality studies were included in the summary?

The Cochrane Review included 12 studies that tested a total of 650 patients with rotator cuff disease or tendonitis. Patients received 1 steroid injection (and some received another injection if the first one did not work). Pain and function were measured after 4 weeks to 1 year.

How well do steroid injections work?

Two small studies of high quality showed that "subacromial" steroid injections decreased pain and improved function and movement in the shoulder more than a placebo injection 4 weeks after injection.

Pain: 37 out of 100 more patients benefited from receiving "subacromial" steroid injections than a placebo.

Function: 30 out of 100 more patients benefited from receiving "subacromial" steroid injections than a placebo.

Shoulder movement: 37 out of 100 more patients benefited from receiving "subacromial" steroid injections than a placebo.

There were five other studies that compared "subacromial" steroid injections to a placebo injection but were not as high in quality as the two above. Two showed improvement with "subacromial" steroid injections, 2 showed no difference between the steroid injections or placebo, and 1 showed more improvement with placebo.

Three studies showed no difference in improvement between "subacromial" steroid injection and non-steroidal anti-inflammatory drugs (NSAIDs), 4 or 6 weeks after injection. There was also one study that showed no difference in improvement (after 4 weeks) between those receiving NSAIDs alone or receiving NSAIDs and having a "subacromial" steroid injection as well.

One study showed no difference in improvement between "intra-articular" steroid injections compared to ultrasound or acupuncture after 4 weeks. One study showed no difference in improvement between corticosteroid injections alongside the "supraspinatus tendon" (one of the tendons of the rotator cuff) and placebo injection after 2 and 8 weeks. One study showed no difference between "intra-articular" steroid injections plus an NSAID compared to a placebo after 4 weeks. One study showed improved pain and function with "intra-articular" steroid injections compared to nitroglycerin patches after 4 weeks.

What side effects occurred with steroid injections?

Although side effects were not reported in many of the studies, side effects may include pain where the injection occurred. Some studies have found that between 18 and 28 out of 100 people had mild pain where the "intra-articular" steroid injection occurred. Some studies have found that between 10 and 20 out of 100 people had facial flushing after "intra-articular" steroid injection. In people with diabetes, a temporary rise in blood sugar occurs.

What is the bottom line?

There is "Silver" level evidence that subacromial steroid injections may improve pain and function in rotator cuff disease. But the improvement may be small and pain relief may not last long. It also may not be better than taking non-steroidal anti-inflammatory drugs (NSAIDs).

Based on Buchbinder R, Green S, Ottawa Methods Group. Shoulder Pain. In: *Evidence-based Rheumatology.* London: BMJ Books, 2003.

Information about shoulder pain in rotator cuff disease and treatment

What is rotator cuff disease?

The rotator cuff is a group of tendons that surrounds the shoulder joint and attaches to muscles that move the shoulder. In some people, the muscles and tendons are pinched when they move their shoulder over and over again. The pinching (or impingement) can cause the rotator cuff to swell, break down, and it may tear away from the bone – this is called rotator cuff disease or tendonitis. In a lot of people this may occur as part of normal ageing and they will not have any symptoms. But many people with rotator cuff disease have pain or aching in the shoulder which may be worse at night or when lifting the arm up.

The pain will often eventually go away. Not receiving treatment and waiting for the pain and swelling to go away is an option. But while waiting for it to go away, a person may not be able to or find it hard to:

- move or lift their arms
- do usual daily activities
- play sports
- work well.

What can I do on my own to manage my disease?

✓ hot or cold packs ✓ rest and relaxation ✓ activity that puts less stress on the shoulder

What treatments are used for rotator cuff disease?

Many kinds of treatment may be used alone or together. The common (generic) names of treatment are shown below:

1. *Pain medicines and non-steroidal anti-inflammatory drugs (NSAIDs)*
   - Acetaminophen
   - Acetylsalicylic acid
   - Celecoxib
   - Diclofenac
   - Etodolac
   - Ibuprofen
   - Indomethacin
   - Meloxicam
   - Naproxen
   - Piroxicam
   - Rofecoxib
   - Sulindac
2. *Steroid injections*
3. *Physical therapy options*
   - Structured exercise programme
   - Pulsed electromagnetic field
   - Mobilisation
4. *Suprascapular nerve block*
5. *Extracorporeal shock wave therapy*

What about other treatments I have heard about?

There is not enough evidence about the effects of some treatments. For example:

- Laser therapy
- Shock wave therapy (may work if have calcium deposits around the shoulder).
- Ultrasound
- Acupuncture

What are my choices? How can I decide?

Treatment for your disease will depend on your condition. You need to know the good points (pros) and the bad points (cons) about each treatment before you can decide.

Shoulder pain in rotator cuff disease decision aid

Should I have a steroid injection?

This guide can help you make decisions about the treatment your doctor is asking you to consider.

It will help you to:

1. Clarify what you need to decide.
2. Consider the pros and cons of different choices.
3. Decide what role you want to have in choosing your treatment.
4. Identify what you need to help you make the decision.
5. Plan the next steps.
6. Share your thinking with your doctor.

Step 1: Clarify what you need to decide

What is the decision?

Should I have a steroid injection when pain is bad and anti-inflammatory drugs are not working to decrease the pain in rotator cuff disease?

Steroid injections are injected into a specific area of the shoulder.

When does this decision have to be made? Check ✓ one

☐ within days ☐ within weeks ☐ within months

How far along are you with this decision? Check ✓ one

☐ I have not thought about it yet

☐ I am considering the choices

☐ I am close to making a choice

☐ I have already made a choice

Step 2: Consider the pros and cons of different choices

What does the research show?

Steroid injections are classified as: Likely beneficial

There is "Silver" level evidence from 12 studies (in a Cochrane Review) of 650 people that tested steroid injections. The studies lasted up to 1 year. These studies found pros and cons that are listed in the chart below.

What do I think of the pros and cons of steroid injections?

1. Review the common pros and cons.
2. Add any other pros and cons that are important to you.
3. Show how important each pro and con is to you by circling from one (*) star if it is a little important to you, to up to five (*****) stars if it is very important to you.

PROS AND CONS OF STEROID INJECTIONS

PROS (number of people affected)	How important is it to you?	CONS (number of people affected)	How important is it to you?
Improves pain and movement – 4 weeks after a "subacromial" corticosteroid injection 37 out of 100 more people improve with steroid injections than with a placebo (no treatment)	* * * * *	Side effects: facial flushing (between 10 and 20 out of 100 people), pain (between 16 and 28 out of 100 people where injection occurred), temporary rise in blood sugar in people with diabetes	* * * * *
Improves function – 4 weeks after a subacromial corticosteroid injection 30 out of 100 more people improve	* * * * *	Improved pain and function may not last long and pain may go away without treatment	* * * * *
Quicker relief compared to waiting	* * * * *	May not be better than non-steroidal anti-inflammatory drugs (NSAIDs)	* * * * *
Avoid risk of serious stomach side effects if NSAIDs are not taken	* * * * *	Personal cost of medicine and injection	* * * * *
Other pros:	* * * * *	Other cons:	* * * * *

What do you think of having a steroid injection? *Check ✓ one*

☐ Willing to consider this treatment
Pros are more important to me than the Cons

☐ Unsure

☐ Not willing to consider this treatment
Cons are more important to me than the Pros

Step 3: Choose the role you want to have in choosing your treatment Check ✓one

☐ I prefer to decide on my own after listening to the opinions of others

☐ I prefer to share the decision with: ____________________

☐ I prefer someone else to decide for me, namely: ____________

Step 4: Identify what you need to help you make the decision

What I know	Do you know enough about your condition to make a choice?	☐ Yes	☐ No	☐ Unsure
	Do you know which options are available to you?	☐ Yes	☐ No	☐ Unsure
	Do you know the good points (pros) of each option?	☐ Yes	☐ No	☐ Unsure
	Do you know the bad points (cons) of each option?	☐ Yes	☐ No	☐ Unsure
What's important	Are you clear about which **pros** are most *important to you?*	☐ Yes	☐ No	☐ Unsure
	Are you clear about which **cons** are most *important to you?*	☐ Yes	☐ No	☐ Unsure
How others help	Do you have enough support from others to make a choice?	☐ Yes	☐ No	☐ Unsure
	Are you choosing without pressure from others?	☐ Yes	☐ No	☐ Unsure
	Do you have enough advice to make a choice?	☐ Yes	☐ No	☐ Unsure
How sure I feel	Are you clear about the best choice for you?	☐ Yes	☐ No	☐ Unsure
	Do you feel sure about what to choose?	☐ Yes	☐ No	☐ Unsure

If you answered No or Unsure to many of these questions, you should talk to your doctor.

Step 5: Plan the next steps
What do you need to do before you make this decision?

For example – talk to your doctor, read more about this treatment or other treatments for shoulder pain in rotator cuff disease

Step 6: Share the information on this form with your doctor

It will help your doctor understand what you think about this treatment.

Tennis elbow and steroid injections
Summaries and decision aid

How well do steroid injections work for treating tennis elbow and how safe are they?

To answer this question, scientists found and analysed 13 studies testing over 1000 people who had tennis elbow. People received either injections of steroids or placebo, an anaesthetic (pain numbing medication), pain pills or physiotherapy. These studies provide the best evidence we have today.

What is tennis elbow and how can steroid injections help?

Tennis elbow or lateral epicondylitis (elbow pain) is a "repetitive stress injury" caused by too much stress on the tendon at the elbow. Putting too much stress on the tendon by moving the wrist backwards over and over again or from an injury can cause the tendon to tear, become painful and swollen or tear away from the bone. This can cause the outside of the elbow and the upper forearm to become painful and tender to touch. The pain and swelling can last for 6 months to 2 years, and most times will eventually get better on its own. Steroids that are injected into the painful and swollen area may help stop the pain. But, it is not clear whether it is worth having a steroid injection or just simply waiting for the pain to go away.

How well do steroid injections work?

Nine of the 13 studies showed that up to 6 weeks after steroid injections, more people had less pain and had improved overall than people who received either a placebo injection, injection of anaesthetic, pain medications, braces or physiotherapy.

Six studies showed that **after** 6 weeks there was no difference in pain or overall improvement between people who received steroid injections and people who received an injection of anaesthetic, pain medications, braces or physiotherapy. The only difference that was found occurred in one study and it showed that more people had more improvement with pain medications than with steroid injections after 6 months.

What side effects occurred with steroid injections?

Side effects such as pain after injection, facial flushing and hardening of the skin where the injection was given occurred. But these side effects occurred in about the same number of patients who received steroid injections as those receiving a placebo injection.

What is the bottom line?

There is "Silver" level evidence that steroid injections improve pain and function in tennis elbow more than other treatments or no treatment over the short term (up to 6 weeks). It does not appear that the improvement will last beyond a few weeks.

Based on Buchbinder R, Green S, Ottawa Methods Group. Elbow pain. In: *Evidence-based Rheumatology*. London: BMJ Books, 2003.

How well do steroid injections work for treating tennis elbow and how safe are they?

What is tennis elbow and how can steroid injections help?

Tennis elbow or lateral epicondylitis (elbow pain) is a "repetitive stress injury" caused by too much stress on the tendon at the elbow. The tendon attaches the muscles of the forearm to the elbow and these muscles move the wrist backwards. Putting too much stress on the tendon by moving the wrist backwards over and over again or from an injury can cause the tendon to tear, become painful and swollen or tear away from the bone. This can cause the outside of the elbow and the upper forearm to become painful and tender to touch. Tennis elbow can affect a person's ability to do daily activities at home and at work.

The pain and swelling can last for 6 months to 2 years, and most times will eventually get better on its own. Pain medicines or non-steroidal anti-inflammatory drugs, such as acetaminophen or ibuprofen, are taken by mouth and may help decrease the pain and swelling. Steroids may also help and are injected into the painful and swollen area. But, it is not clear whether it is worth having a steroid injection or just simply waiting for the pain to go away.

How did the scientists find the information and analyse it?

The scientists searched for studies testing steroid injections in patients with tennis elbow. Not all studies found were of a high quality and so only those studies that met the high standards were selected:

- studies had to be randomised controlled trials – studies where a group of patients who received steroid injections was compared to patients who received a placebo, no treatment or a different treatment such as another type of steroid injection, injection of anaesthetic (to numb pain), braces or physiotherapy
- studies had to show how well steroid injections work by measuring pain, overall improvement, and elbow function.

Which studies were included in the summary?

There were 13 studies that tested a total of 1028 patients with tennis elbow. Patients received 1 steroid injection (and some received another injection if the first one did not work). Pain and function were measured after a short or long time period . Short term effects of steroid injections (effects up to 6 weeks) were measured in the 13 studies. But intermediate effects (6 weeks to 6 months) and long term effects (6 months or longer) were measured in only 6 studies. The quality of the studies was poor to modest.

How well do steroid injections work?

Nine of the 13 short term studies showed that up to 6 weeks after steroid injections that more patients had less pain and had improved better overall than patients who received either a placebo injection, injection of anaesthetic, pain medications, braces or physiotherapy.

Results taken from one study showed overall improvement was seen in:

- 92 out of 100 patients who had a steroid injections
- 24 out of 100 patients who had a placebo injection (no treatment).

Six long term studies showed that 6 weeks to 4 years after steroid injections, there was no difference in pain or overall improvement between patients who received steroid injections and patients who received an injection of anaesthetic, pain medications, braces or physiotherapy. The only difference that was found occurred in one study and it showed that more patients had more improvement with pain medications than with steroid injections 6 months after the injections.

What side effects occurred with steroid injections?

Eight studies gave information about side effects. Side effects such as pain after injection, facial flushing, and hardening of the skin where the injection was given occurred. But these side effects occurred in about the same number of patients who received steroid injections as those receiving a placebo injection.

What is the bottom line?

There is "Silver" level evidence that steroid injections improve pain and function in tennis elbow more than other treatments or no treatment over the short term (up to 6 weeks). It does not appear that the improvement will last beyond a few weeks.

Based on Buchbinder R, Green S, Ottawa Methods Group. Elbow pain. In: *Evidence-based Rheumatology.* London: BMJ Books, 2003.

Information about tennis elbow and treatment

What is tennis elbow?

Tennis elbow or lateral epicondylitis (elbow pain) is a "repetitive stress injury" caused by too much stress on the tendon at the elbow. The tendon attaches the muscles of the forearm to the elbow and these muscles move the wrist backwards. Putting too much stress on the tendon by moving the wrist backwards over and over again or from an injury can cause the tendon to tear, become painful and swollen or tear away from the bone. This can cause the outside of the elbow and the upper forearm to become painful and tender to touch.

The pain and swelling can last for 6 months to 2 years, and most times will eventually get better on its own. Not receiving treatment and waiting for the pain and swelling to go away is an option. But while waiting for it to go away, a person may not be able to or find it hard:

- to grip or lift things
- do usual daily activities
- play sports using the wrist and elbow
- function well at work.

What can I do on my own to manage my condition?

✓ cold packs ✓ relaxation ✓ activity that puts less stress on joints

What treatments are used for tennis elbow?

Three kinds of treatment may be used alone or together. The common (generic) names of treatment are shown below:

1. *Pain medicines and non-steroidal anti-inflammatory drugs (NSAIDs)*
   - Acetaminophen
   - Acetylsalicylic acid
   - Celecoxib
   - Diclofenac
   - Etodolac
   - Ibuprofen
   - Indomethacin
   - Naproxen
   - Piroxicam
   - Rofecoxib
   - Sulindac
2. *Steroid injections* (in the short term)
3. *Physical therapy options*
   - Needle acupuncture (in the short term)
   - Physiotherapy (ultrasound, exercise and mobilisation)

What about other treatments I have heard about?

There is not enough evidence about the effects of some treatments. Other treatments do not work. For example:

- Wearing a brace
- Shock wave therapy
- Surgery

What are my choices? How can I decide?

Treatment for your disease will depend on your condition. You need to know the good points (pros) and the bad points (cons) about each treatment before you can decide.

Tennis elbow decision aid

Should I have a steroid injection?

This guide can help you make decisions about the treatment your doctor is asking you to consider.

It will help you to:

1. Clarify what you need to decide.
2. Consider the pros and cons of different choices.
3. Decide what role you want to have in choosing your treatment.
4. Identify what you need to help you make the decision.
5. Plan the next steps.
6. Share your thinking with your doctor.

Step 1: Clarify what you need to decide

What is the decision?

Should I have a steroid injection when pain or anti-inflammatory drugs are not working to control the pain in tennis elbow?

Steroid injections are usually given one time.

When does this decision have to be made? Check ✓one

☐ within days ☐ within weeks ☐ within months

How far along are you with this decision? Check ✓one

☐ I have not thought about it yet

☐ I am considering the choices

☐ I am close to making a choice

☐ I have already made a choice

Step 2: Consider the pros and cons of different choices

What does the research show?

Steroid injections are classified as: Likely beneficial

There is "Silver" level evidence from 13 studies of 1028 people that tested steroid injections. The studies lasted up to 4 years. These studies found pros and cons that are listed in the chart below.

What do I think of the pros and cons of steroid injections?

1. Review the common pros and cons.
2. Add any other pros and cons that are important to you.
3. Show how important each pro and con is to you by circling from one (*) star if it is a little important to you, to up to five (*****) stars if it is very important to you.

PROS AND CONS OF STEROID INJECTIONS

PROS (number of people affected)	How important is it to you?	CONS (number of people affected)	How important is it to you?
Improves pain and overall wellbeing – up to 6 weeks after injection 92 out of 100 more people improved with steroid injections 24 out of 100 people improved with a placebo (no treatment)	* * * * *	Side effects: facial flushing pain after injection, and hardening of the skin where injected	* * * * *
Quick recovery from elbow pain	* * * * *	Tennis elbow can heal on its own without treatment	* * * * *
Avoid chances of serious stomach side effects if NSAIDs are not taken	* * * * *	Personal cost of medicine	* * * * *
Other pros:	* * * * *	Other cons:	* * * * *

What do you think of having a steroid injection? *Check ✓ one*

☐ Willing to consider this treatment
Pros are more important to me than the Cons

☐ Unsure

☐ Not willing to consider this treatment
Cons are more important to me than the Pros

Step 3: Choose the role you want to have in choosing your treatment Check ✓ one

☐ I prefer to decide on my own after listening to the opinions of others

☐ I prefer to share the decision with: ____________________

☐ I prefer someone else to decide for me, namely: ____________

Step 4: Identify what you need to help you make the decision

What I know	Do you know enough about your condition to make a choice?	☐ Yes ☐ No ☐ Unsure
	Do you know which options are available to you?	☐ Yes ☐ No ☐ Unsure
	Do you know the good points (pros) of each option?	☐ Yes ☐ No ☐ Unsure
	Do you know the bad points (cons) of each option?	☐ Yes ☐ No ☐ Unsure
What's important	Are you clear about which **pros** are most *important to you?*	☐ Yes ☐ No ☐ Unsure
	Are you clear about which **cons** are most *important to you?*	☐ Yes ☐ No ☐ Unsure
How others help	Do you have enough support from others to make a choice?	☐ Yes ☐ No ☐ Unsure
	Are you choosing without pressure from others?	☐ Yes ☐ No ☐ Unsure
	Do you have enough advice to make a choice?	☐ Yes ☐ No ☐ Unsure
How sure I feel	Are you clear about the best choice for you?	☐ Yes ☐ No ☐ Unsure
	Do you feel sure about what to choose?	☐ Yes ☐ No ☐ Unsure

If you answered No or Unsure to many of these questions, you should talk to your doctor.

Step 5: Plan the next steps

What do you need to do before you make this decision?

For example – talk to your doctor, read more about this treatment or other treatments for tennis elbow.

Step 6: Share the information on this form with your doctor

It will help your doctor understand what you think about this treatment.

11
Spondyloarthropathies

Annelies Boonen, Astrid van Tubergen, Sjef van der Linden, Carina Mihai, Ottawa Methods Group

Introduction

The group of disorders collectively labelled as spondyloarthritides (or spondyloarthropathies) constitutes a *family* of interrelated, but heterogeneous conditions with similarities but also differences in clinical manifestations. Members of this group are ankylosing spondylitis (AS), psoriatic arthritis, and reactive arthritis (ReA) (or Reiter's disease), but also arthritis associated with chronic inflammatory bowel disease (IBD) (Crohn's disease or ulcerative colitis) and undifferentiated spondyloarthritis. This last condition is not dealt with in this chapter. The group of the spondyloarthritides share several features, the most important of which are the frequent occurrence of clinical or radiological sacroiliitis and peripheral arthritis, which is usually an oligoarthritis of the lower limbs. Further, they share negative testing for rheumatoid factor, absence of subcutaneous rheumatoid nodules and finally a strong association with the HLA-B27 antigen. Classification criteria for the whole group of the spondyloarthritides and for AS are generally accepted and applied in clinical studies. This contrasts with criteria for the other subtypes of spondyloarthritides, such as reactive arthritis.

In the adult Caucasian population, the estimated prevalence of AS ranges from 0·1 to 1·4% and the prevalence of the disease parallels the prevalence of the HLA-B27 in the population. A recent German study suggested that AS is among the most frequent rheumatic diseases in Germany, with a prevalence of 0·86%.[1] Approximately 90% of white patients with AS are HLA-B27 positive. In the general population AS is likely to develop in up to 6 % of HLA-B27-positive adults.

Prevalence rates for psoriatic arthritis and reactive arthritis are not well known, but likely below 0·5 %. The prevalence of the whole group of spondyloarthritides equals almost the prevalence of rheumatoid arthritis, that is, about 1·9 % in recent studies.[1,2]

In this chapter we present the existing evidence for ten clinical questions that patients with AS, psoriatic arthritis, arthritis associated with IBD, or reactive arthritis may encounter (see Box below). We provide the best available evidence for these questions from high quality meta-analyses (Platinum), high quality randomised trials (Gold), meta-analyses or randomised control trials not fitting the high quality criterion (Silver) and case series or very poor quality trials (Bronze). See Grading in Introduction.

Ten clinical questions that patients with spondyloarthritides might raise

Question 1: What is the evidence that the so-called DMARDs (such as sulphasalazine or methotrexate) or biologics are really effective regarding maintenance of structure and function of spinal and peripheral joint manifestations of AS?

Question 2: Does sulphasalazine prevent eye disease (acute anterior uveitis) in patients with AS?

Question 3: Is there evidence that (pulse) therapy with steroids is useful?

Question 4: Have COX_2 inhibitors advantages in AS (less adverse effects) compared to on-selective COX inhibitors?

Question 5: Is physical therapy effective in AS?

Question 6: Is spa ("kur") therapy effective in AS?

Question 7: What is the evidence that so-called DMARD therapy (gold salts, sulphasalazine, methotrexate, ciclosporin, etc) or biologics are effective in psoriatic arthritis?

Question 8: In patients with reactive arthritis, does treatment with antibiotics improve arthritis by shortening the duration of the joint symptoms? If so, does response to antibiotic treatment differ between enteric and urogenital reactive arthritis?

Question 9: Are there any effective DMARDs for the treatment of chronic reactive arthritis?

Question 10: In patients with CIBD-associated arthritis of peripheral joints does treatment of the bowel disease cause remission of the joint disease?

Methodology

To answer each of the ten questions we searched MEDLINE from 1966 until November 2001 and Embase from 1984 until November 2001 (unless indicated otherwise). Since randomised controlled trials are often scarce in the literature on the spondyloarthritides, the search terms "controlled", "trial", "randomisation" etc have not been entered in each search strategy, with a few exceptions (explicitly stated in the search strategy of the specific question). The same holds true for cost-effectiveness studies. In addition, we checked the Cochrane Library and the references from the articles retrieved by electronic search. Finally, we hand searched for the years 2000 and 2001 the supplements of the *Annals of the Rheumatic Diseases* and of *Arthritis and Rheumatism*, presenting the abstracts from, respectively, the annual EULAR and ACR congress meetings.

Case reports, retrospective studies or chart reviews were discarded unless no prospective trials were identified. Also excluded were studies presenting results twice in different journals and abstracts presenting results that have subsequently been published as a full paper. Studies presenting results for spondyloarthritides as an aggregated group of diseases were only considered if the results were also presented separately for the subgroup of interest for the question reviewed. We have summarised the results using the strongest evidence available and did not include papers of lower methodological hierarchy.

Outcomes

One should keep in mind that the course of these inflammatory diseases can vary widely and that the end-result or the outcome is multidimensional (including pain and physical, psychological or social functional limitations). We report as much as possible to patient-oriented endpoints. Standardisation of outcomes of these disorders has currently only been established for AS, where separate core sets of domains and instruments are now available to assess outcome of symptom modifying treatments (including physical therapies), disease controlling agents, and observational studies. Validated improvement/response criteria have recently been published for symptom modifying drugs. Current work is on criteria sets for disease modifying drugs. In addition, research is in hand to validate instruments to measure structural damage. The majority of this work is done by a group of international experts in AS, the Assessment in Ankylosing Spondylitis (ASAS) Working Group (http://www.ASAS-group.org)

Ankylosing spondylitis (AS)

Case presentation

A 27-year-old male has had AS since he was 21 years old. One year ago he had a severe acute iridocyclitis of the right eye. Despite treatment with conventional NSAIDs, which caused upper gastrointestinal upset, he has persistent inflammatory low back pain and recent onset of neck complaints. On clinical examination both knee joints are swollen. Radiographically, there is bilateral sacroiliitis and a few syndesmophytes at the lumbar spine. The erythrocyte sedimentation rate and the C-reactive protein (CRP) are markedly elevated. He is too busy to attend regular physiotherapeutic sessions or group physical exercises. (Questions 1 to 6 apply to this patient.)

Introduction

Axial pain and stiffness are predominant complaints in AS, but about 30 % of the patients may also experience involvement of the peripheral joints and up to 40% may have one or more sudden attacks of anterior uveitis in the course of the disease. Non-steroidal anti-inflammatory drugs may well control symptoms, but probably do not modify the course of the diseases or prevent damage and ossification (ankylosis). In rheumatoid arthritis the efficacy of disease modifying (DMARD) or disease controlling (DCART) antirheumatic drugs or therapy is nowadays well established (see Chapter 9). What do we know about disease modifying and disease controlling drugs in AS? How promising is anti-TNF-α therapy in this disease?

Question 1

What is the evidence that DMARDs or biologics are effective in AS?

Can these treatments control the disease: control symptoms, maintain or improve function, improve peripheral joint disease, and prevent or lessen radiographic damage?

Literature search

Sulphasalazine: terms used for the electronic search were:

- ankylosing spondylitis
- sulfasalazine or sulphasalazine
- random*/controlled/trial/placebo

Result of the complete search: one meta-analysis including five RCTs,[2] five additional RCTs,[3–7] of which in one study in patients with different types of spondyloarthropathies, only the subgroup of patients with AS was considered,[4] one placebo-controlled study for which it was unclear whether the study was randomised.[5] In addition, we found one study comparing sulphasalazine with sulphapyridine and 5-ASA in AS[8] and one abstract with unclear randomisation procedure which reported a comparison between sulphasalazine and azathioprine.[9]

Methotrexate: terms used for the electronic search were:

- ankylosing spondylitis
- methotrexate

Result of the complete search: three open studies,[10–12] one comparative study (AS, rheumatoid arthritis, and psoriatic arthritis).[33]

Bisphosphonates: terms used for the electronic search were:

- ankylosing spondylitis
- bisphosphonate

Result of the complete search: one RCT (the abstract found during the search was published as a full article when preparing the manuscript)[13] and two open studies.[14,15]

D-penicillamine/thalidomide: terms used for the electronic search were:

- ankylosing spondylitis
- penicillamine/D-penicillamine, thalidomide

Result of the complete search: for D-penicillamine – one RCT[16] , two open studies,[17,18] and one additional study, which could not be retrieved by our library;[19] for thalidomide – one open study.[20]

Anti-TNF-alpha: the electronic search was extended until 1 July 2002. Terms used for the electronic search were:

- ankylosing spondylitis
- TNF, tumour/tumour necrosis factor
- etanercept, infliximab

Result of the complete search: for infliximab – one RCT,[21] (one in spondyloarthropathies, of which only the subgroup with AS is considered)[22] and three open studies[23–25]; for etanercept – one RCT.[26]

Evaluating the evidence

Sulphasalazine

Benefits: One meta-analysis[2] was identified including 272 patients from five RCTs.[27–31] All original studies compared sulphasalazine (SSZ) (2 or 3 g per day) with placebo in patients with active AS and follow up varied from 12 to 48 weeks. A pooled estimate of benefit was assessed for eight clinical measures and two laboratory outcome parameters. Measures of thoracolumbar flexion and erythrocyte sedimentation rate (ERS) or C-reactive protein (CRP) did not improve significantly but benefit was seen for duration of morning stiffness (–28%; 95%CI: –55% to –1·8%), severity of morning stiffness (–31%; 95%CI: –53% to –8·7%) and severity of pain (–27%; 95%CI: –44% to –9·1%). Due to small numbers of patients, subgroup analyses for isolated axial disease compared with axial and peripheral disease could not be done. Table 11.1 provides the number of patients benefiting from SSZ as derived from the data of this meta-analysis. Five other RCTs compared sulphasalazine 2 or 3 g per day with placebo in a follow up varying from 6 months to 3 years. In the largest of these RCTs, 264 patients with active AS were included.[3] The intention to treat (ITT) analysis of this study showed no difference in responders primary outcome (decrease in at least one category (on a five-point scale) of at least two of four outcome measures, one of which should be morning stiffness or back pain, comprising: patient global, physician global, duration of morning stiffness, severity of back pain, primary outcome) (38·2% in SSZ and 36% in the placebo group), nor in the secondary clinical outcome measures at the end of the study. There was no evidence of effect on axial disease in the subgroup with isolated axial disease (n = 187). In the longitudinal analyses a beneficial treatment response in favour of SSZ was noted (p = 0·04). The remaining four studies showed in the ITT analyses only some marginal benefit in one or two of many clinical variables tested.[4–7] One study compared SSZ (2 g per day), sulphapyridine (SP), and 5-ASA (800 mg/day).[8] After 6 months, patient and physician global were significantly better in the SSZ and SP group compared to the 5-ASA group but there was no difference among the SSZ and SP group. Finally, an abstract reported the comparison of

Table 11.1 Number of patients with active AS benefiting from sulphasalazine (pooled data from Ferraz *et al.*,1990)[2]

Outcome	Pooled standardised mean difference**	% benefiting*	NNT*
Duration of morning stiffness (3 studies)	−0·317	15%	7
Severity of morning stiffness (4 studies)	−0·407	19%	6
Severity of pain (5 studies)	−0·403	19%	6

*The meta-analysis reports effect sizes but no SD and therefore the CI can not be calculated.

**No differences were noted in the physical measures of spinal mobility.

6 months' SSZ (n = 14) and azathioprine (n = 18). It was not mentioned whether patients were randomised. No difference between groups was noted.[9]

Adverse effects: In the meta-analysis,[2] the odds ratio for adverse effects was 1·55 (p = 0·66) in the SSZ group. For one of the patients in the SSZ group the adverse event was judged to be severe. Higher withdrawal rates due to adverse events were reported in the treatment groups in three of the five other RCTs.[3–5] In the largest of these RCTs, 11 patients (n = 11) withdrew from the SSZ group because of adverse effects compared with 6 in the placebo group,[3] mainly due to gastrointestinal symptoms. In the meta-analysis the specific adverse events were not analysed due to small numbers.

Evidence summary: Silver

A systematic review of five RCTs (n = 272) and a further four RCTs found that sulphasalazine (SSZ) has a beneficial effect on morning stiffness and pain but not on spinal mobility.[5–7,27] However, one other large RCT (n = 264) failed to confirm the benefits of SSZ. It remains unclear if the observed benefits of SSZ apply equally for patients with isolated axial disease compared with those having axial and peripheral disease. Treatment with SSZ, however, causes more patients to discontinue due to adverse effects.

Case presentation

The patient in this case has active AS with axial (spinal) and peripheral joint involvement, extra-articular disease (acute anterior uveitis), and raised blood sedimentation rate. Sulphasalazine, if given for at least 2 months, may improve arthritic symptoms and may possibly prevent new attacks of uveitis (see question 2). If such spinal features prevail, if symptoms do not respond favourably to sulphasalazine or if side effects provide more harm than benefit, anti-TNF-α treatment should seriously be considered for patients with active AS.

Methotrexate

Benefits: The effectiveness of methotrexate (MTX) in AS has only been evaluated in four rather small, open, non-randomised studies which all included patients with active disease.[10–12,33] One of these was a comparison among patients with AS, psoriatic arthitis, and rheumatoid arthritis (RA).[33] In a trial that reported on the treatment of 11 patients with MTX 7·5 to 15 mg per week during 24 weeks, good effects were observed in 5 of 11 patients at the end of the study but no detailed information was provided.[11] Another trial of 24 patients reported that 56% of patients responded (improvement of 25% in morning stiffness, spinal pain, reduced need for NSAIDs, and ESR) after one year of 12·5 mg MTX per week IM.[10] A third study among 17 patients showed large beneficial effects of methotrexate 7·5 to 10 mg per week, starting at 6 months and continuing after 36 months with improvement in night pain (100%), patient global (94%), Schöber (145%), occiput–wall distance (57%), finger–floor distance (78%), ESR (68%), CRP (89%), reduction NSAIDs (85%). However, no improvement was seen in number of tender and swollen joints.[12] In the comparative study, no effect was seen of MTX in AS, while patients with psoriatic arthritis and rheumatoid arthritis showed significant improvement.[33]

Adverse effects: Overall, adverse effects were mild and transitory.

Evidence summary: Bronze

One cohort study and three case series found mixed results with methotrexate.

Case presentation

The likelihood that the patient described in the case scenario will experience substantial improvement if given methotrexate is low. This judgement includes experts' opinion.

Bisphosphonates

Benefits: In a double blind RCT 84 patients with active AS despite NSAIDs were randomised to pamidronate 60 mg intravenous (IV) once monthly or 10 mg IV once monthly each for a period of 6 months.[13] In the intention to treat analyses at 6 months significant differences between the groups were reported. Improvement in disease activity measured by the Bath Ankylosing Spondylitis Disease Activity Index (BASDAI; range 0–10) was –2·22 and –0·93 ($p = 0·002$), in physical function measured by the Bath Ankylosing Spondylitis Functional Index (BASFI; range 0–10) was –1·69 and –0·15 ($p<0·001$), in patient global as measured by the Bath Ankylosing Spondylitis Global Assessment (BASG; range 0–10) was –2·2 and –1·2 ($p = 0·01$) and in the spinal mobility measured by the Bath Ankylosing Spondylitis Disease Metrology Index (BASMI; range 0–10) was –0·4 and +0·1 ($p = 0·03$), in the high and low dose respectively. In addition, the proportions of patients with more than 25% improvement in disease activity (BASDAI) were 63% and 30% ($p = 0·004$), and with more than 25% improvement of physical function was 63% and 21% ($p < 0·01$), in the high and low dose respectively. There were four withdrawals in the low dose group compared to one in the high dose group due to lack of effectiveness. The number of patients benefiting from the treatment is presented in Table 11.2.

Adverse effects: Transient myalgia after the first infusion was noticed in 68% of patients in the high dose and in 47% in the low dose group ($p = ns$). The number of patients to treat to encounter one experiencing such infusion reaction because of treatment is shown in Table 11.3. In addition, in the high dose group one patient withdrew because of persisting post-transfusion adverse effects, and one was lost to follow up. In the low dose group, two withdrew because of persisting post-infusion adverse effects, one had major surgery at 5 months, and one had an intramuscular injection with corticosteroids because of Crohn's disease.

Evidence summary: Silver

One RCT found that intravenous pamidronate 60 mg monthly has a beneficial effect over pamidronate 10 mg monthly on disease activity

Table 11.2 Number needed to treat for pamidronate 60 mg versus 10 mg (Maksymowych *et al*, 2002)[13]

Outcome	Improved with 10 mg pamidronate	Improved with 60 mg pamidronate	Relative risk of improvement with high dose treatment (95% CI)	Absolute benefit increase (95% CI)	NNT (60 mg) (95% CI)
>25% improvement in disease activity	13/43 (30%)	26/41 (63%)	2·10 (1·26–3·49)	33% (12, 51)	4 (2, 9)
>25% improvement in physical function	9/43 (21%)	26/41 (63%)	3·03 (1·62–5·66)	42% (22, 59)	3 (2, 5)

*The endpoint in the table is secondary endpoint. In addition, the primary endpoint (improvement in BASDAI) was significantly different between treatment groups (see text).

Table 11.3 Number needed to harm of pamidronate 60 mg versus 10 mg (Maksymowych *et al*, 2002)[13]

Outcome	With 10 mg pamidronate	With 60 mg pamidronate	Relative risk with high dose treatment (95% CI)	Absolute risk increase (95% CI)	NNH (60 mg) (95% CI)
Transient arthralgia and myalgia after Ist infusion	20/43 (46·5%)	28/41 (68·3%)	1·47 (1·00, 2·05)	22% (1, 40)	4 (2, 149)

and physical function but not on spinal mobility. Many patients experience transient infusion reactions during the infusion.

Case presentation

Based upon (1) the results from literature, (2) our own limited (six patients) experience with pamidronate infusions for patients resembling the case scenario, and (3) the frequency of adverse effects, we consider the likelihood of clinical meaningful benefit low, and therefore do not recommend this treatment as long as other options (anti-TNF-α treatment) are available and affordable.

D-penicillamine

Benefits: One RCT compared D-penicillamine (dose up to 750 mg per day) with placebo in 17 patients.[16] At 6 months follow-up there was no improvement in any of the clinical variables nor in the measures of spinal mobility.

Adverse effects: Adverse effects were frequent and caused two patients in the treatment group to withdraw.

Evidence summary: Silver

A small RCT found that D-penicillamine has no beneficial effect in AS. Moreover, this therapy caused frequent adverse effects.

Case presentation

We do not recommend D-penicillamine for treatment of AS at any time.

Thalidomide

One abstract reported an open study of thalidomide (200–300 mg per day) in 30 patients.[20] After one year, 80% of patients had improved more than 20% in 4 of 7 clinical

Table 11.4 Number needed to treat for etanercept versus placebo (Gorman, 2002)[26]

Outcome	Improved with placebo	Improved with etanercept	Relative risk of improvement with entanercept (95% CI)	Absolute benefit increase (95% CI)	NNT (95% CI)
> 20% improvement in 3 of 5 clinical measures	6/20 (30%)	16/20 (80%)	2·67 (1·32–5·39)	50% (20, 70)	2 (2, 6)

*The endpoint reported in this table is the primary endpoint of the study. Also most secondary endpoints were significantly different between treatment groups.

Visual Rx Faces 11.1 NNT for etanercept versus placebo

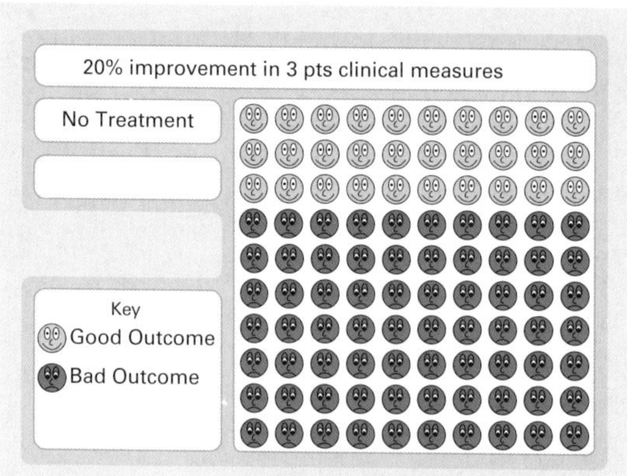

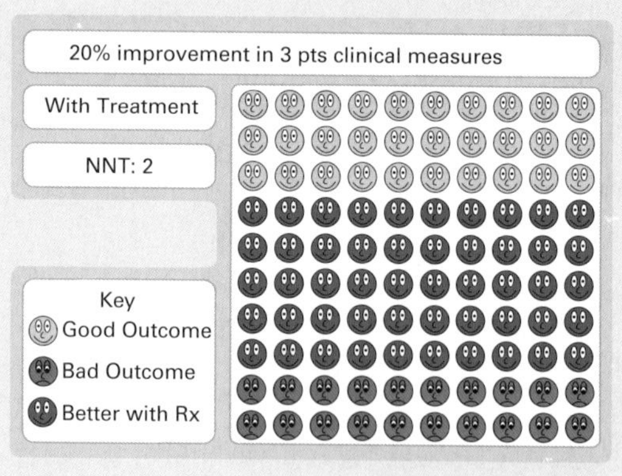

outcome measures (BASFI, BASDAI, early morning stiffness, total body pain score, spinal pain, patient global, and physician global) and 50% improved more than 50% in 4 of 7 clinical outcome measures. The effect on spinal mobility was not reported. Adverse effects were mild and were no reason for drug discontinuation.

Evidence summary: Bronze

A small open case series found that patients improved with thalidomide without causing adverse effects.

Case presentation

The evidence in favour of treatment with thalidomide is not yet strong enough to counterbalance possible cutaneous and neurological adverse effect as long as other options (anti-TNF-α treatment) are available and affordable.

Anti-TNF-α blockade

One RCT compared the effect of twice weekly etanercept ($n = 20$) subcutaneously with placebo ($n = 20$) in patients with longstanding NSAID-resistant AS. After 4 months, 37 patients were

Table 11.5 Number needed to treat for infliximab versus placebo (Braun *et al*, 2002)[21]

Outcome	Improved with placebo	Improved with infliximab	Relative risk of improvement with infliximab (95% CI)	Absolute benefit increase (95% CI)	NNT (95% CI)
>50% improvement in disease activity (BASDAI)	3/35 (9%)	18/34 (53%)	6·18 (2·00–19·07)	44% (23, 61)	3 (2, 5)

*The endpoint reported in this table is the primary endpoint of the study. Also most secondary endpoints were significantly different between treatment groups.

Visual Rx Faces 11.2 NNT for infliximab versus placebo

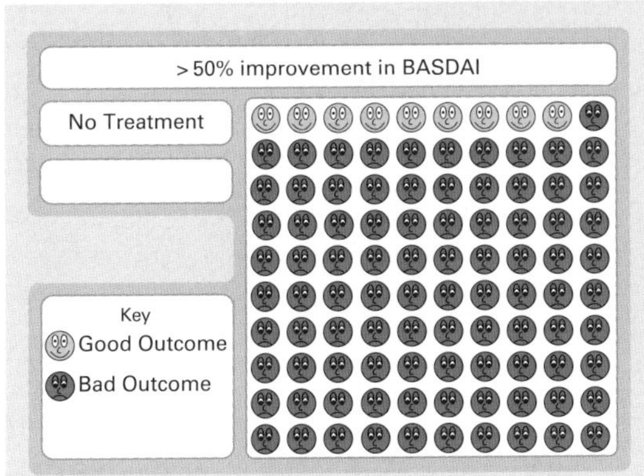

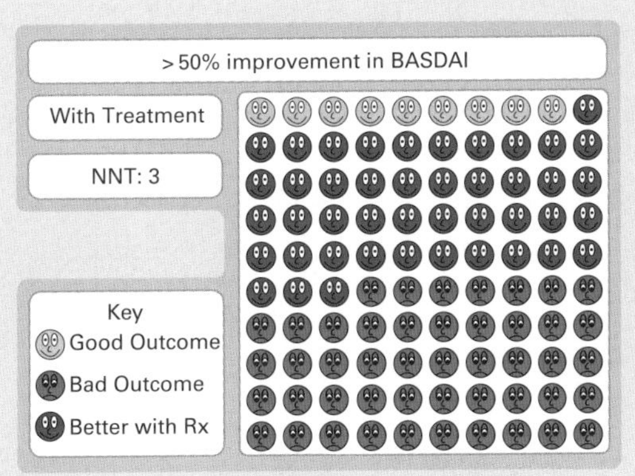

included in the 6 months open label extension study.[26] Primary outcome was defined as 20% improvement in three of five clinical measures: morning stiffness, nocturnal spinal pain, physical function (BASFI), patient global, and score for joint swelling. Improvement in morning stiffness or nocturnal pain was required and worsening in the variables without 20% improvement was not allowed. In the intention to treat (ITT) analyses at 4 months, 80% of patients responded in the treatment group compared with 30% in the placebo group ($p = 0{\cdot}004$). Table 11.4 presents the NNT to have one patient improved (also see Visual Rx Faces 11.1). In the secondary outcome measures significant improvements were noted in physician global (–11.5 *v* + 7·5; $p < 0{\cdot}001$), chest expansion (0·9 *v* –0·2; $p = 0{\cdot}006$), enthesitis index (–4·5 *v* –1·5; $p = 0{\cdot}001$), ESR (–26 *v* –3·5; $p<0{\cdot}001$) and CRP (–1·3 *v* + 0·5; $p = 0{\cdot}003$), but not Schöber ($p = 0{\cdot}26$), occiput–wall distance ($p = 0{\cdot}11$) or peripheral joint tenderness ($p = 0{\cdot}07$). Treatment response was rapid. In the open label extension study ($n = 37$) the patients who had previously received placebo responded rapidly to etanercept and response was sustained in the former treatment group. At 10 months response in the entire group was about 80%.

A second RCT described the effect of IV infliximab 5 mg/kg at 0·2 and 6 weeks ($n = 35$) compared to placebo ($n = 35$) in patients with longstanding active AS.[21] Primary outcome measure at week 12 was 50% improvement of disease activity (BASDAI). In the intention to treat

(ITT) analysis response was 53% in the treatment group compared to 9% in the placebo group ($p < 0{\cdot}0001$). The NNT to achieve this response are presented in Table 11.5 and Visual Rx Faces 11.2. Notably, response was already significantly higher than in the placebo group at week 2, before the second infusion was scheduled. Also, in the treatment group ASAS 20% response was observed in 70% of patients in the active treatment group compared with 30% in the placebo group ($p = 0{\cdot}0007$). The ASAS (ASessments in Ankylosing Spondylitis) response criteria were proposed for therapy with symptom modifying drugs in AS and require a 20% and at least 10 points improvement in three of four domains without worsening in the remaining domain, comprising (a) patient global, (b) pain, (c) function and (d) inflammation each measured on a scale from 0 to 100. For the other secondary outcome measures there was significant improvement in patient global (–3.6 *v* –0·3; $p < 0{\cdot}0001$), physician global (–3·5 *v* –0·5; $p < 0{\cdot}0001$), BASMI ($p = 0{\cdot}0023$), number enthesitic sites (–1.0 *v* –0·4; $p = 0{\cdot}05$), ESR (–23 *v* –4; $p < 0{\cdot}0001$), CRP (–18 *v* –3; $p < 0{\cdot}0001$), the physical component of the SF-37 (+15% *v* –1·6%; $p < 0{\cdot}0001$), and the mental component of the SF-23 (+14% *v* +5·3%; $p = 0{\cdot}063$), but not in number of swollen joints ($p = 0{\cdot}07$).

A third RCT among different types of spondyloarthropathies included 21 patients with AS; (infliximab: 9; placebo:12).[22] After the 12 weeks, significant improvements were noted for duration of morning stifness (–60% *v* +33%; between group p value at 12 weeks = 0·006), spinal pain (–53% *v* +-7%; between group p value at 12 weeks = 0·002), disease activity (BASDAI) (–55% *v* –8%; between group p value at 12 weeks = 0·006), physical function (BASFI) (–41% *v* + 13%; between group p value at 12 weeks = 0·041), but not for a composite index of spinal mobility (BASMI) (–20% *v* 0%; between group p value at 12 weeks not significant).

Adverse effects: In the etanercept study[26] only minor adverse effects were noted, not necessitating withdrawal from the study. In the infliximab study among patients with AS only,[21] 3 withdrawals due to adverse events were reported, one because of active tuberculosis, one because of allergic granulomatosis of the lung and one because of mild leucopenia. In the infliximab study including patients with different types of spondyloarthropathies,[22] two withdrawals in the entire (n = 40) group were reported, one because of pulmonary tuberculosis and one because of suspicion of septic arthritis after synovial biopsy.

Comments

Especially for the biological treatments, it needs to be assessed whether the long term structural damage (ankylosis) can be prevented. The criteria and instruments that are currently under development and validation will help assessing such an outcome (ASAS working group). In addition, insight into predictors of outcome in AS are needed as well as long term safety data of these drugs. Finally, future cost-effectiveness analyses may contribute to the decision as to in which patient groups costly therapies are preferable. International recommendations for the treatment of AS with anti-TNF-α directed therapies have recently been published.[34]

Evidence summary: Silver

In three RCTs it was found that TNF-α blockade has strong effects on clinical outcome measures and (smaller) effects on spinal mobility. Adverse effects with infliximab may be more frequent than with etanercept. More data on this issue are needed, especially on the risk to reactivate tuberculosis and need for screening and prophylaxis.

> ***Case presentation***
> This patient with AS experiencing active axial and peripheral disease might benefit from TNF-alpha inhibitors if this treatment is available and affordable (reimbursed), and if coexisting infectious disease, in particular tuberculosis, was screened and treated, then we strongly favour therapy with anti-TNF-α directed drugs. This judgement is based upon our knowledge of the literature complemented with our ample experience with this therapy for patients with active AS. Therapeutic responses tend to be quick and substantial. The choice between regular intravenous therapy (infliximab) and twice weekly self-administered subcutaneous injection (etanercept) may largely be based on patient's preference. However, if coexisting inflammatory bowel disease is present, then infliximab is the most rational choice as this drug has beneficial effects on gastrointestinal symptoms while the efficacy of etanercept for the bowel disease is currently debated. It should be kept in mind that currently anti-TNF-α directed therapies have proved to ameliorate signs and symptoms of active AS, but there is no proof yet that such therapy can really control the disease by preventing structural damage or ossification. Such evidence requires more data from patients followed for longer periods of time.

Question 2

Does sulphasalazine prevent eye disease (acute anterior uveitis) in AS?

Literature search

Sulphasalazine: terms used for the electronic search were:

- spondylitis, ankylosing (Bechterew disease; ankylosing spondylitis; Marie-Struempell disease; rheumatoid spondylitis; spondylarthritis ankylopoetica)
- sulphasalazine, sulfasalazime, salicylazo-sulfapyridine, asulfidine, azulfagine, salazopyrin, salazosulfapyridine
- eye disease, anterior uveitis, iridocyclitis

Result of the complete search: one small RCT.[35]

Evaluating the evidence

Benefits: Altogether 22 patients with anterior uveitis associated with AS were randomised and followed for 3 years: 10 received oral sulphasalazine (SSZ) and 12, no treatment. Those who had received treatment developed significantly less often recurrences of acute uveitis than those who had received no treatment. Table 11.6 shows the number needed to treat to prevent one attack.

Adverse effects: All 10 patients on sulphasalazine completed treatment. No adverse reactions were reported or observed.

Comments

Recurrences of uveitis in one person are not independent events. A small RCT is liable to several sources of bias. The results of this study need to be confirmed by larger, well developed RCTs. Also the effects of anti-TNF-α therapy on the occurrence of acute anterior uveitis should be studied thoroughly. Current findings in this respect are anecdotally, of weak design and therefore inconclusive.[36]

Evidence summary: Silver

From one small RCT there is some evidence that sulphasalazine can to some degree prevent attacks of acute anterior uveitis in patients with AS.

Case presentation

If a patient with AS has *recurrent* acute anterior uveitis we favour treatment with sulphasalazine for at least one year to assess whether the incidence of new attacks seems to decrease (as long as the patients does not experience relevant adverse effects, such as gastrointestinal symptoms, liver function abnormalities, or blood dyscrasias). If the patient would have joint involvement – as in the case scenario here – then some improvement of these manifestations might also be expected from sulphasalazine therapy.

Table 11.6 Number needed to treat for sulphasalazine (Benitez-Del-Castillo *et al*, 2000)[35]

Outcome	Placebo arm	Sulphasalazine	ARR	NNT
Mean number of cuveitis attacks per patient per year	1·05	0·47	0·58	1·7

*The endpoint reported in this table is one of the secondary endpoints.

Question 3

Is there evidence that (pulse) therapy with steroids is useful in AS?

Literature search

Terms used for the electronic search were:

- ankylosing spondylitis
- steroid/cortico*/prednisolone/methyl prednisolone

Result of the complete search: one RCT,[37] three open studies.

Evaluating the evidence

Benefits: One small double blind RCT was available, randomising 17 AS patients with active disease to methylprednisolone 1 g or to 375 mg intravenously during three consecutive days.[37] In both groups a rapid improvement for morning stiffness, patient global, Schöber, chin–manubrium distance, finger–floor distance, and thorax excursion was reported, but not quantified. Also, after 6 months, improvements compared with baseline were observed except for morning stiffness and pain. There were no between group differences except for the effect on chest expansion. However, baseline differences between the groups compromise interpretation of the between group results. Reinstitution of NSAID therapy was required after a mean of 8 days in the low dose group compared to 25 days in the high dose group.

Adverse effects: In both treatment arms all patients experienced flushing during the infusion. Further, in the first 4 days of the treatment, in the high dose group two patients reported dizziness, one a bitter taste, one insomnia, one tachycardia for 5 minutes, and one a dry mouth. In the low dose group, one patient reported dizziness, one irritability, one increase in weight, and one a dry mouth in the first 4 days of the treatment. In the 6 months following the infusions, one patient in the low dose group reported sexual dysfunction and another patient experienced symptomatic tachycardia for 30 minutes on day 5.

Comments

Randomised placebo controlled trials comparing different (oral and intravenous) doses of steroids and assessing short and long term (structural) effects using recognised outcome measures are necessary.

Table 11.7 Number needed to treat for celecoxib versus placebo (Dougados *et al*, 2001)[38]

Outcome	Improved with placebo	Improved with celecoxib	Relative risk of improvement with celecoxib (95% CI)	Absolute benefit increase (95% CI)	NNT (95% CI)
Response (> 50% improvement in pain)	15/76 (20%)	38/80 (48%)	2·41 (1·45–4·00)	28% (13, 41)	4 (3, 8)

*The endpoint reported in this table was one of two of the primary endpoints of the study.

Table 11.8 Numbers benefiting from celecoxib versus placebo (Dougados *et al*, 2001)[38]

Outcome	Standardised mean difference (95% CI)	% benefiting (95% CI)	NNT (95% CI)
BASFI	–0.66 (–0.98, –0·33)	30% (16, 43)	4 (3, 7)

*The endpoint reported in this table is one of the secondary endpoints.

Evidence summary: Bronze

There are no placebo controlled RCTs. In one RCT, when comparing high with low dose steroid pulse therapy, both groups improved equally except for longer time before restarting NSAIDs in the low dose group.

Case presentation

If the symptoms of a patient such as described in the case scenario are likely to be due to a *flare* of the disease, then we support a trial with high doses of methylprednisolone intravenously. We admit that the evidence in favour is not very strong, but consider the risk of such a trial as acceptable in light of the improvement that can be gained.

Question 4

Have COX_2 inhibitors advantages in AS (less adverse effects) compared to non-selective COX inhibitors?

Literature search

Terms used for the electronic search were:

- ankylosing spondylitis
- COX
- Celecoxib, rofecoxib

Result of the complete search: one RCT.[38]

Evaluating the evidence

Benefits: One RCT randomised 246 patients into three treatment groups, one receiving ketoprofen (100 mg twice per day), a second receiving celecoxib 100 mg twice per day, and a last group receiving placebo.[38] In the intention to treat (ITT) analysis after 6 weeks there were significant improvements in pain for celecoxib (change –38%; p = 0·007) and ketoprofen (change –31%; p = 0·05) compared with placebo (change –19%) as well as in physical function (BASFI) for celecoxib (change –25%; p = 0·0006) and ketoprofen (change –15%; p = 0·04) compared with placebo (change –3%). Response (more than 50% improvement in pain) was most frequently seen in both treatment groups (celecoxib 48%, ketoprofen 36%, and placebo 20%). No improvements in measures of spinal mobility were observed. Tables 11.7 and 11.8 present number needed to treat to have a response, or percentage benefiting in BASFI for celecoxib compared to placebo and Tables 11.9 and 11.10 the NNT to have response and the percentage benefiting in BASFI for ketoprofen compared to placebo.

Adverse effects: Adverse effects occurred more often in both active treatment groups compared to

Table 11.9 Number needed to treat for ketoprofen versus placebo (Dougados *et al*, 2001)[38]

Outcome	Improved with placebo	Improved with ketoprofen	Relative risk of improvement with ketoprofen (95% CI)	Absolute benefit increase (95% CI)	NNT (95% CI)
Response (> 50% improvement in pain)	15/76 (20%)	32/90 (36%)	1·80 (1·06–3·07)	16% (2, 29)	7 (4, 49)

* The endpoint reported in this table was one of two of the primary endpoints of the study.

Table 11.10 Number of patients benefiting from ketoprofen versus placebo (Dougados *et al*, 2001)[38]

Outcome	Standardised mean difference (95% CI)	% benefiting (95% CI)	NNT (95% CI)
BASFI	–0.37 (–0.68, –0·07)	18% (3,31)	6 (4, 30)

placebo (42%, 69%, and 68%) ketoprofen, and celecoxib groups respectively. Also withdrawal due to adverse effects occurred more often in the treatment groups. Epigastric pain occurred in 7·9%, 14·4%, and 12·5% in placebo, ketoprofen, and celecoxib groups respectively ($p = 0{\cdot}42$), a difference that was not significant ($p = 0{\cdot}42$). In the ketoprofen group one gastric ulcer was diagnosed and one other patient had a marked fall in haemoglobin level. Tables 11.11 and 11.12 present the NNH for adverse events and withdrawals due to adverse events for celecoxib versus placebo and ketoprofen compared with placebo respectively.

Evidence summary: Silver

From one RCT there is evidence of efficacy for celecoxib, a COX_2 selective NSAID, over placebo for improvement in pain, function, and patient global but not for spinal mobility. There is evidence that celecoxib has no additional efficacy over conventional NSAIDs. Adverse effects occurred more often in all NSAID groups (mainly gastrointestinal). The study was not powered to prove a relevant difference in serious gastrointestinal complications (perforation, obstruction, bleeding) between the newer selective and the traditional aselective COX inhibitors (NSAIDs).

Case presentation

As the patient in the case has experienced gastrointestinal adverse effects, we recommend taking a COX_2 selective NSAID. The same clinical efficacy might be expected in the absence of GI adverse effects. Other adverse effects might still occur.

Question 5

Is physical therapy in AS effective?

The targets of therapeutic interventions in patients with AS are: (1) to reduce pain and stiffness, (2) to maintain or improve physical function. Drug therapy aims at reaching these goals by reducing inflammation and (hopefully) preventing structural damage. Such expectations would be unrealistic for physiotherapy. Therefore, what is the evidence that physiotherapy really can improve symptoms and improve functioning?

Literature search

Terms used for the electronic search were:

- ankylosing spondylitis
- physical therapy
- physiotherapy
- hydrotherapy

Table 11.11 Number needed to harm for celecoxib versus placebo (Dougados *et al*, 2001)[38]

Outcome	With placebo	With celecoxib	Relative risk adverse effect celecoxib (95% CI)	Absolute risk increase (95% CI)	NNH (95% CI)
Withdrawal due to adverse effects*	0/76 (0%)	5/80 (6%)	Not calculated	6% (0·3, 14)	16 (7, 370)
Incidence of adverse effects†	32/76 (42%)	54/80 (68%)	1·60 (1·18–2·17)	25% (10, 39)	3 (2, 10)

*Not all considered to be drug related.

†most common: upper GI complaints, diarrhoea, headache, upper respiratory tract infection, pruritius.

Table 11.12 Number needed to harm for ketoprofen versus placebo (Dougados *et al*, 2001)[38]

Outcome	With placebo	With ketoprofen	Relative risk adverse effect ketoprofen (95% CI)	Absolute risk increase (95% CI)	NNH (95% CI)
Incidence of adverse effects*	32/76 (42%)	54/90 (60%)	1·42 (1·04–1·95)	18% (3, 32)	5 (3, 37)

* Most common: Upper GI complaints, diarrhoea, headache, upper respiratory tract infection, pruritius.

- exercise
- cost-effectiveness

Results of the complete search included, one Cochrane Review, one non-randomised controlled trial, and nine open studies. The Cochrane Review[39] included three RCTs, which are discussed below.[40–42]

Evaluating the evidence

Benefits: One systematic review included randomised and quasi-randomised studies where at least one of the comparison groups received some kind of physiotherapy. The main outcomes were spinal mobility, pain, stiffness, physical function, and global assessment of change. Altogether 21 stud ies were considered for inclusion in the review; 16 were excluded, while of the five remaining studies two were crossover or follow up studies of patients included in one of the three other studies – together comprising 241 patients with AS – which finally were included in this Cochrane Review. All three randomised controlled studies were assessed to have moderate to high risk of bias. Two trials compared the effects of supervised group physical therapy with an individualised home exercise programme, and reported differences in favour of the supervised group. For pain and stiffness, the relative difference in change from baseline for the supervised group compared to the home exercise group was 50% after treatment. One of these studies reported also on the direct costs. One trial compared an individual programme of exercises and disease education with no intervention, and found differences in favour of the exercise group. The reviewers indicate that there is a tendency toward positive effects of physiotherapy, in the management of AS. They also state that the only treatment alternatives investigated are exercises applied in different settings, that the total number of participants is small, and that the quality of data reporting is insufficient. Finally, it is concluded that there is evidence for short term effects of physiotherapy on pain, stiffness, patient-rated assessment, and spinal mobility when interventions such as exercises including hydrotherapy, performed in groups as compared to home exercises are applied. There is also some evidence to support the view that an individual programme is better than no intervention.

Adverse effects: Adverse effects were not assessed in any of these studies.

Evidence summary: Silver

Three RCTs found that physiotherapy provided as *exercises* is effective in the short term (up to 6 months) in particular to *groups* of patients with AS. Scientific evidence for long term effectiveness is not yet available.

Case presentation

Although this patient states he has no time to practise exercises, we strongly recommend all patients with AS, in particular if they have active disease, to set aside enough time to perform regular exercises, preferably in groups. AS patient societies often provide facilities for such therapy. Membership of such organisations should in our view also strongly be considered.

Question 6

Is spa ("kur") therapy effective in AS?

Literature search

Terms used for the electronic search were:

- ankylosing spondylitis
- spa therapy
- balneotherapy
- cost-effectiveness

Result of the complete search: one RCT.[39]

Evaluating the evidence

Benefits: The studies retrieved have been performed by authors of this chapter. The randomised study evaluated the efficacy of 3 weeks of combined spa-exercise therapy as an adjunct to standard treatment with drugs and weekly group physical therapy in patients with AS[43] (Table 11.13). Two groups of 40 patients each were randomly allocated to treatment at two different spas (one in Austria, the other in the Netherlands). A control group of 40 patients stayed at home and received weekly group therapy for 40 weeks. The "spa" patients followed a regimen of combined spa/group physical exercises for 3 weeks, followed by weekly group physical therapy for an additional 37 weeks. The improvements in function and global wellbeing in the spa-exercise therapy groups were greatest early in the study. At 4 weeks after the start of spa-exercise therapy, significant improvements were seen in the pooled index of change (which was an aggregate of the following primary outcomes: BASFI, patient global wellbeing, pain, and duration of morning stiffness) in the "spa" group, compared to the control group. Benefit was maintained over the 40 week study period in patients receiving spa-exercise therapy, although at 40 weeks the improvement in the pooled index of change had lost statistical significance, as compared to controls. During the 9 months follow up period use of analgesics and sick leave declined in those who had received spa-exercise treatment. Since the authors of this chapter were involved in this study, the additional incremental cost-effectiveness and cost-utility analysis (accepted

Table 11.13 Number needed to treat for spa therapy versus control (van Tubergen *et al*, 2001)[43]

Outcome	Standardised mean difference (95% CI) spa therapy *v* control at 16 wk	% benefiting (95% CI) with spa therapy	NNT (95% CI)
BASFI	0·57 (0·13, 1·02)	27% (6, 44)	4 (3, 16)
Global wellbeing	0·62 (0·17, 1·07)	29% (8, 46)	4 (2, 13)
BASDAI	0·64 (0·19, 1·09)	30% (9, 46)	4 (3, 11)

for publication at the time the chapter was written) can be presented.[44] Direct (health care and non-health care) as well as productivity costs were included. The incremental cost-effectiveness ratio per unit effect gained in functional ability on a 0–10 scale (based on the BASFI) was €1269 and €2477 for the Austrian and Dutch group respectively. The incremental costs per QALY (quality adjusted life year) gained (assessed by EuroQol) were €7465 (spa therapy in Bad Gastein, Austria) and €18 575 (spa therapy in Arcen, The Netherlands) for the respective groups. No substantial changes in the cost ratios were found in sensitivity analyses for a whole range of variables.

Adverse effects: Adverse effects were not assessed in this study.

Evidence summary: Silver

An RCT of a 3 week course of combined spa-exercise therapy found improvement in function and global wellbeing for 9 months after completion of the therapeutic course. It is unclear which components of such interventions contribute most to reported effect. Health resource utilization may decrease following combined spa-exercise treatment.

Case presentation

If affordable (reimbursement) and the time required (a 3 week period) can be freed, we strongly recommend participation in an intensive spa-exercise therapy programme.

Guidelines and recommendations:

The ASAS international working group on outcome assessment in AS aims at developing recommendations for outcome measurement and helps to set guidelines to identify patients benefiting from treatment with biologics. These guidelines are also available through the internet (http://www.ASAS-group.org). These recommendations will be updated regularly.

Psoriatic arthritis

Case presentation

A 35-year-old female attorney with psoriatic arthritis since the age of 3 has persistent swelling of the finger joint and sausage-like toes. Treatment with NSAIDs had strikingly reduced pain. However, her physical ability deteriorated. She likes to play the piano, but is experiencing increasing difficulties. She asked for a second opinion from a rheumatologist, who ordered radiographs of hands and feet and told the patient that damage to the joint had increased considerably. The rheumatologist advised second-line drugs. After reading about possible adverse effects of these drugs the patient wanted to be convinced that the so-called disease modifying drugs, if applied to patients with psoriatic arthritis, really are able to control the disease and restrict further progression of damage and loss of function. Both searched the medical literature. In other words, they addressed Question 7.

Introduction

Psoriatic arthritis (PSA) is a heterogeneous condition belonging to the spondyloarthritides. Classically five subtypes are distinguished, among which are the sausage-like digits that are strongly associated with HLA-B27. Methotrexate, nowadays well established as a disease controlling agent in rheumatoid arthritis, is widely used in the treatment of psoriatic arthritis with the intention to improve both skin and joint disease. Other drugs applied to this purpose include sulphasalazine (SSZ) and ciclosporin (CsA).

Question 7

What is the evidence that DMARD therapy (gold salts, sulphasalazine, methotrexate, ciclosporin, etc.) or biologics are effective in psoriatic arthritis?

Literature search

- General search
- psoriatic arthritis/arthropathy
- Cochrane Review

Result of the complete search: one Cochrane Review in which different DMARDs were included and compared with placebo and with each other.[45]

Sulphasalazine (SSZ): terms used for the electronic search were:

- psoriatic arthritis/arthropathy
- sulfasalazine
- sulphasalazine

Result of the complete search: five RCTs,[46–50]one comparative RCT (comparing SSZ with CsA and symptomatic therapy),[51] three open studies.[52–54]

Methotrexate (MTX): terms used for the electronic search were:

- psoriatic arthritis/arthropathy
- methotrexate

Result of the complete search: two RCTs,[55,56] one comparative RCT (comparing MTX with CsA)[57], five open studies.[58–62]

Ciclosporin (cyclosporin) A (CsA): terms used for the electronic search were:

- psoriatic arthritis/arthropathy
- cyclosporine
- cyclosporin

Results of the complete search: two comparative RCTs (one comparing CsA with MTX,[57] one comparing CsA with SSZ and symptomatic therapy[51]), 12 open studies.[63–74]

Gold: terms used for the electronic search were:

- psoriatic arthritis/arthropathy
- gold
- auranofin

Result of the complete search: two RCT[75,76] one controlled trial,[77] one case–control study,[78] three open studies.[79–81]

Colchicine: terms used for the electronic search were:

- psoriatic arthritis/arthropathy
- colchicine

Result of the complete search: two RCTs with crossover design.[82,83]

Etretinate: terms used for the electronic search were:

- psoriatic arthritis/arthropathy
- etretinate
- tigason

Result of the complete search: one RCT,[84] three open studies,[85–87] one comparative study (comparing etretinate with gold).[88]

D-penicillamine: terms used for the electronic search were:

- psoriatic arthritis/arthropathy
- penicillamine

Result of the complete search: one RCT.[89]

Fumaric acid: terms used for the electronic search were:

- psoriatic arthritis/arthropathy
- fumaric acid
- fumarate

Result of the complete search: one RCT.[90]

Azathioprine: terms used for the electronic search were:

- psoriatic arthritis/arthropathy
- azathioprine

Results: one RCT,[91] one open study,[92] one case–control study.[93]

Antimalarials: terms used for the electronic search were:

- psoriatic arthritis/arthropathy
- chloroquine
- hydroxychloroquine
- antimalarial

Result of the complete search: one case–control study.[94]

Vitamin D: terms used for the electronic search were:

- psoriatic arthritis/arthropathy
- vitamin D

Result of the complete search: one open study.[95]

Leflunomide: terms used for the electronic search were:

- psoriatic arthritis/arthropathy
- leflunomide

Result of the complete search: two open studies (abstracts).[96,97]

Anti-TNF-α: terms used for the electronic search were:

- psoriatic arthritis/arthropathy
- TNF, tumour/tumour necrosis factor
- etanercept
- thalidomide
- infliximab

Result of the complete search: etanercept: two RCTs,[98,99] two open studies.[100,101] Infliximab: four open studies.[102–105] Alefacept: one open study.[106] Thalidomide: none.

Evaluating the evidence

Benefits: The Cochrane Review identified 20 RCTs published until February 2000; 13 of these were included in the quantitative analysis, comprising data of 1022 patients.[1] The main outcome variables measured were acute phase reactants, disability, pain, patient global, physician global, swollen joint count, tender joint count, and radiographic changes of joints in any trial of duration of 1 year or longer and the change in pooled index of disease activity. The study provided the first comprehensive overview of RCTs in PsA. Based upon a global index of disease activity it demonstrated efficacy for sulphasalazine (SSZ) and parenteral high dose methotrexate and suggestive evidence for azathioprine, etretinate, and low dose methotrexate. The trial sizes were generally small with insufficient statistical power and of short duration (with a mean duration of 6 months). There are no hard data on either the prevention of structural damage or the exact relationship between improvement of the arthritis and skin manifestations. The evidence for individual DMARDs is presented below.

Case presentation

For patients who experience at the same time both active and persisting PsA and also disturbing skin involvement, we think weekly treatment with oral methotrexate is the most logical choice as this therapy probably will also ameliorate skin disease. If skin manifestations are well controlled otherwise or if they are just minimal, then patient preference may guide the choice between methotrexate (once a week) and twice daily sulphasalazine tablets. Monitoring of blood (erythrocytes, leucocytes, thrombocytes, renal function, and liver tests) should be done regularly with both drugs, which share the occurrence of rather frequent gastrointestinal complaints. Sulphasalazine may give raise to skin rashes. Either treatment should be followed for at least 2 months to allow any firm conclusions about efficacy.

Note: It should also be mentioned that for patients with psoriatic arthritis none of the so-called DMARDs has proven to possess disease-controlling properties. That means, there is no evidence yet that these drugs can really stop progression of structural damage in this disease.

Sulphasalazine

Benefits: Several randomised controlled trials have studied the efficacy of SSZ in PsA.[46–50]. Three small studies, with less than 40 patients in each, and in which the patient groups were not well defined, all suggested beneficial effects of SSZ with respect to morning stiffness, global wellbeing, pain, ESR, number of painful joints, and skin involvement (Table 11.14).[48–50] Two large multicentre randomised controlled trials confirmed these observations (Table 11.14).[46,47] Both trials studied the efficacy of SSZ 2·0 g/day versus placebo in patients with PsA. In the first study (including 117 patients; mean duration of arthritis 8 years), pain significantly decreased in the SSZ group, with 41% compared with 24% in the placebo group.[46] Morning stiffness, joint pain/tenderness index, and ESR showed a trend favouring SSZ. In the second study (including 221 patients; mean duration of arthritis 12 years), a treatment response (including improvements in patient and physician global, joint pain/tenderness, and joint swelling) of 58% was found in the SSZ group versus 45% in the placebo group ($p = 0·05$) after 36 weeks.[47] In the longitudinal analysis, only the difference in patients' global wellbeing and ESR reached statistical significance, and a trend favouring SSZ over placebo with respect to physician's global and skin involvement was found. The benefits of SSZ over placebo were greatest at 36 weeks, suggesting that the full effects of SSZ may take some time to become apparent.

One study reported a multicentre randomised open trial comparing a group with CsA 3 mg/kg/day, a group with SSZ 2 g/day, and a group with symptomatic treatment only (NSAIDs, analgesics, and/or prednisone <5 mg/day) in 99 patients with active PsA.[51] The primary endpoint was the 6 month change in pain. The CsA group showed significantly more improvement in pain (44%) compared with both the SSZ group (33%) and the symptomatic treatment group (21%). The difference between SSZ and symptomatic therapy was not significant. Using the American College of Rheumatology (ACR) criteria for defining improvement in patients with RA, the number of patients meeting an ACR20 response was similar for both active treatment groups (CsA 44%, SSZ 44%) and not significant versus symptomatic treatment (36%). The ACR70 response (almost similar to clinical remission) was higher in the CsA group (14%) compared with SSZ (0%) ($p = 0·05$), and symptomatic treatment (0%) ($p = 0·05$).

Adverse effects: Adverse effects were often reported, and led to withdrawal in 13–30% for the

Table 11.14 Number needed to treat for sulphasalazine versus placebo (Jones, 2001)[45]

Outcome	Standardised mean difference (95% CI) sulphasalazine *v* placebo	% benefiting (95% CI)	NNT (95% CI)
Change in pooled index of disease activity (n = 564), 6 studies: Clegg,[47] Combe,[46] Dougados,[4] Farr,[49] Fraser[50], Gupta[48]	0·36 (0·20, 0·53)	17% (10, 25)	6 (5, 11)
Pain (n = 320), 4 studies: Combe,[46] Dougados,[4] Farr,[49] Fraser[50]	–0·37 (–0·59, –0·15)	18% (7, 28)	6 (4, 14)
Patient global assessment (n = 159), 2 studies: Dougados,[4] Gupta[48]	–0·71 (–1·03, –0·38)	32% (18, 44)	4 (3, 6)
Physician global assessment (n = 159) 2 studies: Dougados,[4] Gupta[48]	–0·41 (–0·73, –0·09)	20% (4, 33)	6 (4, 23)

SSZ group, and 5–23% for the placebo group. Gastrointestinal side effects and skin reactions were most often reported.

Evidence summary: Silver

Six RCTs found a moderate benefit. Mild adverse effects are found in up to 30% of patients.

Methotrexate

Benefits: Although MTX is currently considered as the preferred second-line drug treatment in PsA, only two small RCTs on the efficacy of respectively high dose MTX (n = 21, mean disease duration of arthritis 8 years)[55] and low dose MTX (n = 37, mean disease duration of arthritis 11 years)[56] in PsA have been published. Both studies showed significant improvements in skin involvement. In the high dose MTX study significant improvement in joint involvement and ESR were reported.[55] In the low dose MTX study, only the between-group difference with respect to physician's assessment of disease severity reached statistical significance (p = 0·001)[56] (Table 11.15). There was, however, a trend favouring MTX with respect to morning stiffness and patients' assessment of disease severity.

One study compared in a RCT the efficacy of CsA 3–5 mg/kg/day (n = 17) with MTX 7·5–15 mg/week (n = 18) in PsA patients with active peripheral joint involvement.[57] After 1 year, significant improvements in all clinical parameters were observed in both groups. No significant differences between the two treatment groups were found, but more patients from the CsA group had withdrawn because of adverse effects.

Adverse effects: Adverse effects that led to withdrawal from the study were reported in 0–22% of the patients in the MTX group and in one of the patients in the placebo group. The adverse effects most often reported were gastrointestinal symptoms.

Evidence summary: Silver

Two RCTs found moderate symptomatic benefit. Adverse effects resulted in discontinuation of therapy in up to 30% of patients.

Table 11.15 Number needed to treat for low dose methotrexate versus placebo (Jones, 2001)[45]

Outcome	Standardised mean difference (95% CI) (methotrexate *v* placebo)	% benefiting (95% CI)	NNT (95% CI)
Patient global assessment (*n* = 36), 1 study: Willkens[56]	−0·70 (−1·38, −0·03)	32% (1, 54)	4 (2, 69)
Physician global assessment (*n* = 36), 1 study: Willkens[56]	−1·56 (−2·31, −0·80)	58% (36, 67)	2 (2, 3)

Ciclosporin (cyclosporin) A

Benefits: No randomised controlled trials have been conducted assessing the efficacy of CsA over placebo treatment. In two RCTs, both described above, the effects of CsA were compared with other treatments.[51,57] In the first study,[57] CsA 3–5 mg/kg/day was compared with MTX 7·5–15 mg/week. After 1 year, significant improvements compared with baseline in all clinical parameters were observed in both groups, but no significant differences between the two treatment groups were found. More patients from the CsA group had withdrawn because of adverse effects (not significant). In the second study,[51] CsA 3 mg/kg/day showed favourable effects over SSZ 2 g/day and symptomatic treatment only (NSAIDs, analgesics, and/or prednisone < 5 mg/day) with respect to 6 month change in pain. The ACR70 response (clinical remission) was higher in the CsA group (14%) compared with SSZ (0%) ($p = 0{\cdot}05$), and symptomatic treatment (0%) ($p = 0{\cdot}05$).

Several uncontrolled studies have been conducted.[63–74] In these open studies the results of 6–55 patients with PsA treated with CsA 1·5–7 mg/kg/day for 2 months to 2 years were described. Significant improvements of 46–57% in number of painful joints, 49–72% in the Ritchie index, 30–81% in number of swollen joints, 35–61% in pain, and 37–95% in morning stiffness were found. Also, clinically relevant reductions in skin involvement were observed. One study reported that CsA was able to control radiological progression after 2 years in 60% of the patients.[65]

Adverse effects: Adverse effects leading to discontinuation were found in up to 41% of the patients.

> ***Case presentation***
> This drug can be considered for this patient if methotrexate and sulphasalazine have failed. Renal function and blood pressure should be monitored closely.

Evidence summary: Silver

Two RCTs against methotrexate and sulphasalazine found that ciclosporin resulted in the same moderate symptomatic improvement as with the comparators. Adverse effects resulted in therapy discontinuation in over 40% of patients.

Gold salts

Benefits: The efficacy of gold salts in patients with PsA has been studied in two double blind controlled multicentre trials[75,76] (Table 11.16). In the first study, auranofin was compared with placebo in 238 patients (mean duration of arthritis 7 years).[75] Treatment with auranofin was significantly better compared with placebo with respect to physician global and functioning. In the second study, the effects of auranofin, thiomalate, and placebo treatment were assessed in 82 patients (mean duration of arthritis 8 years).[76] No significant clinical changes were found after treatment with oral

Table 11.16 Number needed to treat for auranofin versus placebo (Jones, 2001)[45]

Outcome	Standardised mean difference (95% CI) (auranofin *v* placebo)	% benefiting (95% CI)	NNT (95% CI)
Pain (*n* = 230), 2 studies: Carette,[75] Palit[76]	−2·05 (−2·43, −1·67)	65% (60, 67)	2 (2, 2)
Swollen joint score: (*n* = 188), 1 study: Carette[75]	−0·33 (−0·62, −0·04)	16% (2, 29)	7 (4, 54)

Table 11.17 Number needed to treat for IM gold thiomalite versus placebo (Jones, 2001)[45]

Outcome	Standardised mean difference (95% CI) (gold *v* placebo)	% benefiting (95% CI)	NNT (95% CI)
Tender Joint Score (Ritchie) (*n* = 39), one study: Palit[76]	−0·75 (−1·40, −0·09)	34% (4, 54)	3 (2, 23)

gold (auranofin). Treatment with intramuscular gold (thiomalate) showed significant improvements in pain and Ritchie index compared with baseline, but no comparison with the placebo group was made (Table 11.17).

One multicentre, double blind trial compared the effects of auranofin with thiomalate in 42 patients (mean duration of arthritis 7 years), but it was unclear whether this study was randomised.[77] Both groups showed improvements in disease activity, and number of swollen and tender joints, but the magnitude of improvement was slightly higher in the thiomalate group.

One case–control study assessed whether gold therapy prevents radiological progression of PsA in 18 patients (mean duration of arthritis 6 years) and 36 matched controls, who were on other DMARD treatments.[78] After 2 years, no difference between the groups was found, suggesting that gold therapy is not superior to other DMARDs in preventing radiological progression.

Adverse effects: Serious adverse effects that led to withdrawal from the study were reported in 12–20% of the patients in the auranofin group, 24–43% in the IM thiomalate group, and 0–7% of the patients in the placebo group. The adverse effects most often reported were gastrointestinal symptoms and skin reactions.

Case presentation

Based upon our experiences in clinical practice, oral gold compounds (auranofin) are not strongly advised due to lack of meaningful effectiveness in this setting. Intramuscular gold may be an alternative in this patient if sulphasalazine and methotrexate have failed.

Evidence summary: Silver

One RCT of auranofin against placebo and two RCTs against methotrexate and sulphasalazine found that ciclosporin resulted in the same moderate symptomatic improvement as with the comparators. Adverse effects resulted in therapy discontinuation in over 40% of patients.

Other DMARDs for psoriatic arthritis

The efficacy of several other, less frequently used DMARDs has also been assessed in

Table 11.18 Number needed to treat for etretinate versus placebo (Jones, 2001)[45]

Outcome	Standardised mean difference (95% CI) (etretinate *v* placebo)	% benefiting (95% CI)	NNT (95% CI)
Change in pooled index of disease activity (n = 29), 1 study: Hopkins[84]	0·82 (0·03, 1·60)	37% (2, 59)	3 (2, 69)

relatively small RCTs and/or open studies. A brief description of these studies is given below.

Colchicine

Benefits: The administration of colchicine, frequently used as an anti-inflammatory agent in gout, has also been investigated in patients with PsA in two RCTs with a crossover design, in 25 and 15 patients, respectively.[82,83] Patients received either colchicine or placebo and switched to the other treatment after 2 months. The first study found significant improvements in Ritchie index, joint pain, joint size, and overall assessment in patients taking colchicine, but no changes in psoriatic skin lesions and laboratory values.[83] The second study failed to find significant changes in any of the outcome measures.[82]

Adverse effects: Adverse effects that led to withdrawal from the study were reported for colchicine in 13–16% (mainly gastrointestinal symptoms).

Evidence summary: Silver

Two small RCTs found mixed results.

Etretinate

Benefit: The efficacy of etretinate, a vitamin A derivate that has been shown to reduce psoriatic skin involvement, was also investigated for PsA in a double blind randomised trial[84] (Table 11.18). Patients received either etretinate (n = 20) or ibuprofen (n = 20). Due to lack of efficacy, all but one patient from the ibuprofen group had discontinued at 24 weeks. No statistically significant differences were found between groups in the clinical parameters at any time point. However, ESR and CRP both decreased significantly in the etretinate group compared with the ibuprofen group. In addition, less skin involvement was observed in the etretinate group. One study compared efficacy and adverse effects of etretinate with those of thiomalate in 27 patients.[88] Both groups showed significant improvements in joint pain, swelling, and stiffness. The etretinate group showed more improvement in skin involvement.

Adverse effects: Adverse effects that led to withdrawal from the study were reported for etretinate in 11–35% of patients (sore lips and mouth).

Evidence summary: Silver

A small RCT showed no advantage of etretinate over ibuprofen on musculoskeletal symptoms. Adverse effects resulted in discontinuation of therapy in up to 35% of patients.

D-Penicillamine

One RCT reported effects of D-penicillamine in 11 patients with PsA[89] versus placebo crossover. No significantly better results were found for the D-penicillamine group.

Evidence summary: Silver

One very small RCT found no benefit of D-penicillamine on the musculoskeletal symptoms.

Table 11.19 Number needed to treat for azathioprine versus placebo (Jones, 2001)[45]

Outcome	Standardised mean difference (95% CI) (azathioprine *v* placebo)	% benefiting (95% CI)	NNT (95% CI)
Change in pooled index of disease activity ($n = 12$), 1 study: Levy[91]	2·03 (0·53, 3·54)	64% (25, 69)	2 (2, 5)
Tender joint score (Ritchie) ($n = 6$), 1 study: Levy[91]	−2·26 (−3·86, −0·86)	66% (38, 69)	2 (2, 3)

Fumaric acid

One RCT comparing fumaric acid with placebo in 27 patients did not show significantly better results with respect to joint involvement, pain, and functioning.[90] However, significant results favouring fumaric acid were clearly found regarding skin involvement.

Evidence summary: Silver

One small RCT found no benefit of fumaric acid on musculoskeletal symptoms.

Azathioprine

One RCT with crossover design compared azathioprine with placebo in 6 patients with PsA and 18 patients with rheumatoid arthritis.[91] In patients with PsA, significant improvements were found in morning stiffness, and skin and joint involvement during azathioprine treatment over placebo (Table 11.19). One case–control study assessed long term tolerability and clinical response to azathioprine in 28 patients compared with 36 matched controls on other treatments.[93] After 2 years, significantly more patients on azathioprine showed deterioration in clinically damaged joints compared with matched controls (83% *v* 64%, $p < 0.05$).

Adverse effects: Adverse effects were not clearly reported in the azathioprine studies.

Evidence summary: Silver

One small crossover RCT of patients with a majority of RA patients and 6 patients with psoriatic arthritis found benefit in these patients.

Antimalarials

Benefits: Antimalarials have been assessed in a case–control study in 24 patients versus 24 matched controls. A trend towards more improvement in the number of inflamed joints in the active treatment group was seen, but failed to reach statistical significance.

Adverse effects: More exacerbations of psoriasis were observed in patients on antimalarials compared with matched controls.

Evidence summary: Bronze

A small case control study found a trend towards benefit but more exacerbations of the psoriatic skin lesions.

Vitamin D

Benefits: Vitamin D produced significant improvements of tender joint count, global wellbeing, and ESR in a pilot study in 10 patients, but no RCTs have been performed.[95]

Adverse effects: Adverse effects (hypercalciuria) that led to withdrawal from the study were reported in 20% of patients.

Evidence summary: Bronze

A small case series found improvement in tender joint counts and global wellbeing.

Leflunomide

Benefits: Two abstracts reported effects of leflunomide in an open study.[96,97] Significant

Table 11.20 Number needed to treat for etanercept versus placebo (Mease, 2000)[98]

Outcome	Improved with placebo	Improved with anti-TNF-α	Relative risk of improvement with anti-TNF-α (95% CI)	Absolute benefit increase (95% CI)	NNT (95% CI)
ACR 20	4/30 (13%)	22/30 (73%)	5·50 (2·15–14·04)	60% (36, 75)	2 (2, 3)
Skin lesions (75% improvement in PASI)	0/19 (0%)	5/19 (26%)	Not calculated	26% (4, 49)	4 (3, 25)

* It should be noted that this is one of the four studies on sulphasalazine in ReA and in only two studies could some benefit of sulphasalazine be seen. The number of remissions (primary endpoint) was indeed significantly different among treatment groups at 2 months but not at the end of the study. All other variables were not different between groups (see text).

improvements in joint involvement and pain were noted, but not in skin involvement. No RCTs have yet been performed.

Adverse effects: Adverse effects (miscellaneous) that led to withdrawal from the study were reported in 25% of patients.

Evidence summary: Bronze

One case series found improvement. Adverse effects resulted in discontinuation of therapy in up to 25% of patients.

Case presentation

For patients such as the one described in the case, we do not recommend the use of other DMARDs if these patients fail on methotrexate, sulphasalazine, ciclosporin or gold. Nowadays, we favour the use of anti-TNF-α therapy, in particular etanercept, for such patients.

Anti-TNF-α blockade

Benefits: The efficacy of anti-TNF-α therapy was assessed in a 12 week randomised, placebo-controlled study among 60 patients with PsA and psoriasis[98] (Table 11.20). Response to treatment (based on improvements in patient and physician global, joint tenderness, and joint swelling) was observed in 87% of the etanercept group, and in 23% of the placebo group. An improvement of 20% (ACR20) in musculoskeletal manifestations was achieved by 73% of etanercept-treated patients as compared with 13% of placebo-treated patients. Skin involvement only improved in the etanercept group. Preliminary results of a larger RCT with 205 patients confirmed these findings.[99]

Adverse effects: There were insufficient data to examine toxicity. Etanercept was in general well tolerated.

Evidence summary: Silver

One RCT found moderate benefit

Case presentation

We favour the use of anti-TNF-α therapy, in particular etanercept, for patients with psoriatic arthritis, if methotrexate and sulphasalazine cannot control their disease. This treatment may be expected to ameliorate both the articular manifestations and the skin disease. Contraindications for etanercept should be considered.

Reactive arthritis/Reiter's syndrome

Case presentation

A 35-year-old nurse practitioner recently developed an acute arthritis of the left knee, right wrist, and both ankles, 2 weeks after a Salmonella enteric infection following a barbecue. She discusses this with a colleague who confides that several years ago he suffered a Chlamydia-triggered arthritis that disappeared after a long term course of antibiotics. Therefore, the patient wonders if she should return to her general practitioner and ask him if antibiotics are useful to shorten the duration of her rheumatologic manifestations. Also, she wants to question him about possible treatment options if the arthritis should become chronic. (Questions 8 and 9)

Introduction

For this member of the group of spondyloarthritides there is considerable variation in the use and meaning of the terms reactive arthritis and Reiter's syndrome. In this overview we address the clinical syndrome of predominantly asymmetrical oligoarthritis of (mostly) the lower limbs following a recent gastrointestinal or urogenital infection.[107] Recognised causative micro-organisms include Shigella, Salmonella, Yersinia, Campylobacter, and Chlamydia species. Especially HLA-B27 positive individuals are at risk for this condition, which occasionally may persist as chronic reactive arthritis. If the classical clinical features such as arthritis, urethritis, and conjunctivitis are present the term (complete) Reiter's syndrome is often used. The incidence of reactive arthritis after an enteric infection is estimated at between 2 and 15%. Estimates on the incidence of arthritis after a urogenital infection are not available.

Question 8

In patients with reactive arthritis, does treatment with antibiotics improve arthritis by shortening the duration of the joint symptoms? If so, does response to antibiotic treatment differ between enteric and urogenital ReA?

Literature search

Terms used for the electronic search were:

- reactive arthritis or Reiter or Reiter's
- antibiotic*
- fluoroquinolone
- ciprofloxacin
- tetracycline
- doxycycline

Results of the complete search: 10 RCTs[108–117] (two published as abstracts,[109,110] two open studies.

Evaluating the evidence

Benefits: Nine RCTs compared effectiveness of different antibiotics (doxycycline,[8,114] ofloxacin plus roxithromycin,[109] ciprofloxacin,[110–112,114,115] lymecycline,[116] or various types[117]) with placebo and one compares short term with long term antibiotic treatment.[114] Some studies included both enterogenic and urogenital ReA,[108–110,112,113,115,116] while others selected only enteric ReA patients (Yersinia,[111] early enteric ReA,[117] or urogenital ReA patients (Chlamydia-induced[114]). One study included patients with reactive arthritis and undifferentiated arthritis but from this study only the reactive arthritis group was considered for this review.[113] There was a large heterogeneity between trials, especially with regard to inclusion criteria (clinical signs of previous enteritis or urethritis or combinations of clinical signs with culture and serology), disease duration, (chronic compared with early[109,110,112,117]) treatment duration (10 days[117] to 12 months,[112] but most frequently 3 months,[108–111,113–116] duration of follow up (3–24 months), and endpoints assessed. Most studies showed no beneficial effect of antibiotics over placebo. One RCT reported a beneficial treatment effect of lymecycline 300 mg twice daily for 3 months in early Chlamydia-induced ReA ($n = 21$ lymecyline 12 and placebo 9).[116] The active treated patients had significantly shorter duration of arthralgia ($p = 0{\cdot}02$) and a faster decrease of CRP ($p = 0{\cdot}008$). Also, the time point at which 50% of patients had recovered was significantly shorter 15·0 weeks (95%CI: 13·5–30) in the treatment compared to 39·5 weeks (95%CI 29–50) in the placebo group ($p = 0{\cdot}017$). A large placebo effect was noted. Adverse effects due to the treatment were mild but four patients were lost to follow up. A second RCT reported a clinically important but statistically non-significant trend towards a higher proportion of responders at 3 months (37·5% *v* 0%), 6 months (66·7% *v* 20%) and 12 months of follow up (66·7% *v* 50%) in a trial comparing ciprofloxacine 300 mg per day during 3 months with placebo in the subgroup of patients with Clamydia-induced reactive arthritis ($n = 13$).[113] Moreover, this result was not confirmed in other, usually smaller, trials studying the effect of ciprofloxaxine.[110,112,115]

Adverse effects: Seven RCTs mention mild adverse reactions in both study arms. Relative risk for harm for ciprofloxacin compared with placebo was 1·13 (95% CI: 0·76–1·49) but 4 patients were lost to follow up in one study[110] and 1·26 (95%CI: 0·83–1·69) in another study,[113] confirming a mild but significant risk of adverse events with active treatment.

Comment

There is an urgent need for uniform classification criteria for ReA and insight into the prognostic variables of the course of the disease. Large randomised trials with stratification for prognostic subgroups (type of infectious trigger; HLA-B27 status; early or chronic disease) using well-defined outcome measures have to provide better evidence on the role of antibiotics in the treatment of the rheumatological manifestations of ReA. The authors wish to issue a reminder that urogenital Chlamydia infections need to be treated. It should be noted that this overview did not address the issue of prevention of ReA in outbreaks of infectious enteritis or prevention of recurrence of ReA in patients with Chlamydia reinfection.

Evidence summary: Silver

A review of nine RCTs showed mixed results. Further trials are needed to assess whether the positive trends in the small trials with ciprofloxacin or lymecycline are confirmed.

Case presentation

Although strong evidence in favour is lacking, we support a course of treatment with one of these antibiotics for this patient with early disease. This support is more based upon the likelihood of the absence of adverse effects from such treatments then on our belief in the efficacy of antibiotics in such clinical situations.

Question 9

Are there any effective DMARDs for the treatment of (chronic) reactive arthritis?

Literature search

Sulphasalazine: terms used for the electronic search were:

- reactive arthritis or Reiter or Reiter's
- sulphasalazine or sulfasalazine

Result of the complete search: four RCTs,[4,118–120] of which one was published only as an abstract,[120] and four open studies with a low number of patients.

Other DMARDs: terms used for the electronic search were:

- reactive arthritis or Reiter or Reiter's
- methotrexate
- azathioprine
- cyclosporine/ciclosporene
- gold
- penicillamine/d-penicillamine
- anti-TNF/infliximab/etanercept/biologic agent
- DMARD

Result of the complete search: one review of 21 case reports for methotrexate,[121] one crossover placebo-controlled study for azathioprine,[122] and two case reports on ciclosporin. The patients described in these two case reports of ciclosporin had arthralgia, but no arthritis and were therefore not considered.

Sulphasalazine

Benefits: Four RCTs[4,118–120] compared the effect of sulphasalazine (SSZ) (2–3 g per day) with placebo. Among the studies there was considerable heterogeneity in inclusion criteria. One study also included patients with oligoarthritis and those who were positive for HLA-B27 without any other evidence (clinical or serological) for ReA, who would be classified at present as having undifferentiated spondyloarthritis.[119] Another RCT included patients with different types of spondyloarthritides (n = 365) but stratified for the subtypes. From this study only this subgroup (n =88) was considered in this review.[4] None of the studies distinguished enterogenic and urogenital ReA. Mean disease duration varied from 3·9 months[118] to 10·4 years.[119] Study duration was 6 months in 3 publications[4,118,119] but is not defined in the abstract.[120] Two RCTs[4,118] reported no benefit in the intention to treat (ITT) analysis of the clinical outcome measures at the end of the study, although one trial[118] (n = 79) reported a statistically significant benefit in the active treatment group for remission at 2 months (23% compared to 0%, p = 0·013) and for the number of sick leave days at 6 months ($p < 0·01$), but more patients had a paid job at study entry in the treatment group. Table 11.21 provides the NNT for improvement for a beneficial short term (at 2 months) response. A third RCT (n = 134) did not find a significant treatment effect in the intention to treat (ITT) analysis between the groups for the primary endpoint (response) at 6 months, but the Spondylitis Articular Index and the ESR were significantly different between the two groups in favour of the intervention. The NNT for such positive response is presented in Table 11.22. In addition, longitudinal analysis showed significant differences in favour of the sulphasalazine (SSZ) group, from the fourth week onwards, for several endpoints including response ($p = 0·02$), joint scores ($p < 0·001$), physician global ($p = 0·05$), and ESR ($p = 0·002$).[119] At the end of the study, the RCT reported as an abstract (n = 50), showed significant difference between the groups in joint pain ($p < 0·001$), back pain ($p < 0·02$), patient and physician global ($p < 0·004$), and ESR ($p < 0.04$) in favour of the intervention.[120] It might be noted that this abstract dated from 1990 but was never published as a full paper. All three fully published papers reported a large placebo effect and a higher withdrawal rate in the treatment group. In one study the higher withdrawal was due to adverse events ($p = 0·002$).[118] One other RCT also showed more adverse events in the treatment group ($p = 0·23$) but these were not the reason for withdrawal.[4]

Adverse effects: Two of the three published papers noted no increase in adverse events (RR: 3·42; CI 95%: 1·17 to 5·68,[118] RR: 1·24; CI 95%: –0·34 to 2·88[114] and p = 0·23[4]. However, in one study the adverse events were significantly more often the cause of withdrawal from treatment compared to the placebo group ($p = 0.002$) (Table 11.23).[118]

Table 11.21 Number needed to treat for sulphasalazine versus placebo (Egsmose, 1997)[118]

Outcome	Improved with placebo	% Improved with SSZ	Absolute benefit increase (95% CI)	NNT (95% CI)
Remission at 2 months	0/34 (0%)	5/22 (23%)	23% (7, 43)	5 (3, 16)

*This is one of the four studies on sulphasalazine in ReA and in only two studies some benefit of sulphasalazine could be seen. The endpoint reported in this table was a secondary outcome and the only one significantly different between the two treatment groups. The analysis was efficacy. ITT for this outcome at 2 months was not reported.

Table 11.22 Number needed to treat for sulphasalazine versus placebo (Clegg, 1996)[119]

Outcome	Standardised mean difference (95% CI) (sulphasalazine *v* placebo)	% benefiting (95% CI)	NNT (95% CI)
Spondylitis articular index	−0·35 (−0·69, −0·01)	17% (0·5, 32)	6 (4, 206)

*The endpoint reported in this table was a secondary endpoint.

Evidence summary: Silver

Four RCTs found that sulphasalazine has only marginal effects in chronic reactive arthritis by accelerating clinical improvement. Since two of the three RCTs that reported adverse events showed significant (although mild) side effects, it is questionable whether the benefits outweigh these effects.

Case presentation

The patient presented has disease of recent onset. In such a case we prefer to observe the natural history of disease as many cases resolve spontaneously within 3–6 months. If no improvement occurs within this period we favour treatment of joint manifestations with twice daily sulphasalazine while closely monitoring the blood (erythrocytes, leucocytes, thrombocytes, renal function, and liver tests) and any subjective complaints (in particular skin rashes and gastrointestinal upset).

Methotrexate

One article reviewed 21 case reports of methotrexate treatment for Reiter's syndrome (RS) with arthritis and/or mucocutaneous lesions refractory to non-steroidal and steroidal anti-inflammatory drugs.[121] There was significant improvement of arthritis in 15 (75%) of 20 patients and the treatment was usually well tolerated. In three patients methotrexate needed to be stopped because of adverse effects.

Evidence summary: Bronze

A case series found improvement in arthritis in patients with Reiter's syndrome.

Case presentation

If the disease in this patient becomes chronic, we would advocate sulphasalazine, not methotrexate, based upon evidence from the literature.

Azathioprine

Benefits: A placebo controlled, double blind, crossover study of azathioprine in Reiter's syndrome was performed in 8 patients with RS for 16 weeks.[122] Two patients were withdrawn, one due to adverse effects (nausea) and the other because of lack of efficacy (placebo). At the end of the study, 5 of 6 completers preferred azothioprine to placebo and azothioprine-related improvement was noticed in joint score, morning stiffness, and global score.

Table 11.23 Number needed to harm for sulphasalazine versus placebo (Egsmose, 1997)[118]

Outcome	Placebo	Sulphasalazine	Relative risk adverse effect sulphasalazine (95% CI)	Absolute risk increase (95%)	NNH (95% CI)
Withdrawal due to adverse event	3/42 (7%)	9/37 (24%)	3·42 (1·17–5·68)	17% (1, 34)	5 (2, 97)

Adverse effects: One patient mentioned nausea during active treatment

Comments: The currently available evidence is not strong enough to prove the efficacy of azathioprine in chronic ReA. Randomised controlled trials are required to better assess the efficacy of DMARDs in chronic refractory ReA.

General comment: Question 9

Clear classification criteria and a core set of outcome measures for ReA would be helpful to design further studies and to evaluate the effectiveness of DMARDs.

Evidence summary: Silver

Out of four RCTs, only one small RCT showed some benefit of treatment by a DMARD in ReA.

Case presentation

If the disease in this patient becomes chronic, we would prefer sulphasalazine, not azathioprine, as a possible choice as second-line drug in addition to NSAIDs.

Arthritis associated with chronic inflammatory bowel disease

Case presentation

A 40-year-old teacher with severe Crohn's disease experiences frequent flares of peripheral arthritis, mainly of the lower limbs, that coincide with the inflammatory activity of his bowel disease. His gastroenterologist proposes treatment with anti-TNF-α therapy (infliximab infusions). The patient asks whether this will also alleviate his joint symptoms. (Question 10 applies to this patient.)

Introduction

Crohn's disease and ulcerative colitis are associated with spondyloarthritides. Both peripheral arthritis as well as axial manifestations may be seen. Among patients with chronic inflammatory bowel disease (IBD) AS occurs more often than expected compared to the general population, whereas IBD is also more often seen among patients with AS. The activity of the peripheral arthritis usually reflects the activity of the bowel disease, whereas axial involvement might follow an independent course.

Question 10

In patients with chronic IBD-associated arthritis of peripheral joints, does treatment of the bowel disease cause remission of the joint disease?

Literature search

Terms included in the search were:

- inflammatory bowel disease, Crohn's disease, ulcerative colitis

Table 11.24 Number needed to treat for budesonide versus placebo (Florin, 2000)[124]

Outcome	Improved with placebo	Improved with budesonide CIR 9 mg	Relative risk of improvement with treatment (95% CI)	Absolute benefit increase (95% CI)	NNT (95% CI)
Joint pain resolved	15/37 (41%)	96/129 (74%)	1·84 (1·23–2·75)	34% (16, 50)	3 (2, 7)

- spondylitis ankylosing, Bechterew disease, ankylosing spondylitis, rheumatoid spondylitis, spondyloarthritis ankylopoetica, arthritis, joints
- clinical trial, randomised controlled trial, meta-analysis, review (quantitative, methodologic, systemic)

Result of the complete search: no true RCT was available targeted to this question. One open study on TNF-α inhibitors[123] and one secondary analysis on budenoside in Crohn's disease[124] offered the best fit.

Budenoside

Benefits: A secondary analysis of 611 patients with Crohn's disease who had participated in prospective double blind controlled trials showed that 291 of them had either inflamed joints (arthritis) or painful joints (arthralgia) at entry to one of three large studies.[124] The outcome was nearly twice as good in those treated with daily oral budesonide (9 mg) as compared to those who had received placebo. In the budesonide group 74% (95% confidence interval 67–82%) experienced remission of joint pain, whereas this was also seen in 41% (95% confidence interval 34–57%) in the placebo group (Table 11.24).

Adverse effects: No harm was reported.

Evidence summary: Silver

Surprisingly, there is no Gold level evidence to support this view that daily oral budesonide benefits both the gastrointestinal and rheumatological manifestations of Crohn's disease.

> ***Case presentation***
>
> For the patient presented here we favour a trial with budesonide. If this treatment failed we would strongly recommend therapy with infliximab, which has shown itself to be efficacious in both AS and Crohn's disease. This drug has been approved for use for each of these indications.

Anti-TNF

Benefits: A small observational study was conducted among 4 patients with Crohn's disease and spondyloarthritis who were treated with anti-TNF-α therapy (infliximab) for treatment-resistant gut inflammation.[123] A substantial improvement in gastrointestinal manifestations was associated with clear-cut improvement of both axial manifestations and/or peripheral arthritis related to the spondyloarthritides.

Adverse effects: No harm was reported for this small group of 4 patients.

Comment

The near future will provide more and better data on the effectiveness of anti-TNF-α treatment on rheumatological manifestations of patients with Crohn's disease. Ongoing trials and follow up studies of such trials will include a considerable number of patients with AS, peripheral joint involvement, and associated chronic inflammatory bowel diseases, in particular Crohn's disease. Such studies will provide better insight into the efficacy of anti-TNF-α-directed therapies for these patients and will also give an answer to the question whether or not infliximab in more efficacious among this subset of patients than etanercept.

Evidence summary: Bronze

An RCT is needed to assess validity of the very small positive case series of 4 patients.

> ***Case presentation***
>
> Evidence from this small clinical trial is complemented with experiences from daily clinical practice. Based upon this combined evidence, we strongly recommend treatment with infliximab for a patient such as the one presented here who has active Crohn's disease together with therapy-resistant inflammation of peripheral joints.

References

1 Braun J, Bollow M, Remilinger G, *et al.* Prevalence of spondyloarthropathies in HLA-B27 positive and negative blood donors. *Arthritis Rheum* 1998;**41**(1):58–67.

2 Ferraz MB, Tugwell P, Goldsmith CH, Atra E. Meta-analysis of sulfasalazine in ankylosing spondylitis. J Rheumatol 1990;**17**(11):1482–6.

3 Clegg DO, Reda DJ, Weisman MH, *et al.* Comparison of sulfasalazine and placebo in the treatment of ankylosing spondylitis. A Department of Veterans Affairs Cooperative Study. *Arthritis Rheum* 1996;**39**(12):2004–12.

4 Dougados M, van der Linden S, Leirisalo Repo M, *et al.* Sulfasalazine in the treatment of spondylarthropathy. A randomised, multicenter, double-blind, placebo-controlled study. *Arthritis Rheum* 1995;**38**(5):618–27.

5 Kirwan J, Edwards A, Huitfeldt B, Thompson P, Currey H. The course of established ankylosing spondylitis and the effects of sulphasalazine over 3 years. *Br J Rheumatol* 1993;**32**(8):729–33.

6 Taylor H, Beswick E, Dawe P. Sulphasalazine in ankylosing spondylitis. A radiological, clinical and laboratory assessment. *Clin Rheumatol* 1991;**10**:43–8.

7 Winkler V. Sulphasalazine treatment in ankylosing Spondylitis: a comparison of sulphasalazine with placebo. *Magy-Rheumatol* 1989;**30**(Suppl):29–37.

8 Taggart A, Gardiner P, McEvoy F, Hopkins R, Bird H. Which is the active moiety of sulfasalazine in ankylosing spondylitis? A randomised, controlled study. *Arthritis Rheum* 1996;**39**(8):1400–5.

9 Brandt J, Buss B, Sieper J, Braun J. Treatment with sulfasalazine vs azathioprine of ankylosing spondylitis patients with a disease duration <10 years. *Arthritis Rheum* 2001;**43** (Suppl):S103.

10 Sampaio Barros PD, Costallat LT, Bertolo MB, Neto JF, Samara AM. Methotrexate in the treatment of ankylosing spondylitis. *Scand J Rheumatol* 2000;**29**(3):160–2.

11 Creemers MC, Franssen MJ, van de Putte LB, Gribnau FW, van Riel PL. Methotrexate in severe ankylosing spondylitis: an open study. *J Rheumatol* 1995;**22**(6):1104–7.

12 Biasi D, Carletto A, Caramaschi P, Pacor ML, Maleknia T, Bambara LM. Efficacy of methotrexate in the treatment of ankylosing spondylitis: a three-year open study. *Clin Rheumatol* 2000;**19**(2):114–17.

13 Maksymowych WP, Jhangri GS, Fitzgerald AA, *et al.* A six-month randomised, controlled, double-blind, dose-response comparison of intravenous pamidronate (60 mg versus 10 mg) in the treatment of nonsteroidal antiinflammatory drug-refractory ankylosing spondylitis. *Arthritis Rheum* 2002;**46**(3):766–73.

14 Haibel H, Brandt J, Rudwaleit M, Soerensen H, Sieper J, Braun J. Therapy of active ankylosing spondylitis with pamidronate. *Arthritis Rheum* 2001;**44**(9)(Supplement): S92.

15 Maksymowych WP, Jhangri GS, Leclercq S, Skeith K, Yan A, Russell AS. An open study of pamidronate in the treatment of refractory ankylosing spondylitis. *J Rheumatol* 1998;**25**(4):714–17.

16 Steven MM, Morrison M, Sturrock RD. Penicillamine in ankylosing spondylitis: a double blind placebo controlled trial. *J Rheumatol* 1985;**12**(4):735–7.

17 Bernacka K, Tytman K, Sierakowski S. Clinical application of D-penicillamine in ankylosing spondylitis: a 9-month study. *Med Interne* 1989;**27**(4):295–301.

18 Bird HA, Dixon AS. Failure of D-penicillamine to affect peripheral joint involvement in ankylosing spondylitis or HLA B27-associated arthropathy. *Ann Rheum Dis* 1977;**36**(3):289.

19 Golding DN. D-penicillamine in ankylosing spondylitis and polymyositis. *Postgrad Med J* 1974;**50**(Suppl): 262–5.

20 Huang F, Gu J, Zhao W, Zhu J, Zjang J, Yu Bejing DTY. Therapeutic effects and molecular targets of thalidomide in refractory ankylosing spondylitis. *Arthritis Rheumatism* 2001;**44**(9)(Suppl):S275.

21 Braun J, Brandt J, Listing J, *et al.* Treatment of active ankylosing spondylitis with infliximab: a randomised controlled multicentre trial. *Lancet* 2002;**359**:1187–93.

22 Van Den Bosch F, Kruithof E, Baeten D, *et al.* Randomised double-blind comparison of chimeric monoclonal antibody to tumor necrosis factor alpha (infliximab) versus placebo in active spondylarthropathy. *Arthritis Rheum* 2002;**46**(3):755–65.

23 Brandt J, Haibel H, Cornely D, *et al.* Successful treatment of active ankylosing spondylitis with the anti-tumor necrosis factor alpha monoclonal antibody infliximab. *Arthritis Rheum* 2000;**43**(6):1346–52.

24 Brandt J, Haibel H, Sieper J, Reddig J, Braun J. Infliximab treatment of severe ankylosing spondylitis: one-year followup. *Arthritis Rheum* 2001;**44**(12):2936–7.

25 Stone M, Salonen D, Lax M, Payne U, Lapp V, Inman R. Clinical and imaging correlates of response to treatment with infliximab in patients with ankylosing spondylitis. *J Rheumatol* 2001;**28**(7):1605–14.

26 Gorman JD, Sack KE, Davis JC, Jr. Treatment of ankylosing spondylitis by inhibition of tumor necrosis factor alpha. *NEJM* 2002;**346**(18):1349–56.

27 Dougados M, Boumier P, Amor B. Sulphasalazine in ankylosing spondylitis: a double blind controlled study in 60 patients. *Br Med J (Clin Res Ed)* 1986;**293**(6552): 911–14.

28 Feltelius N, Hallgren R. Sulphasalazine in ankylosing spondylitis. *Ann Rheum Dis* 1986;**45**(5):396–9.

29 Nissila M, Lehtinen K, Leirisalo Repo M, Luukkainen R, Mutru O, Yli Kerttula U. Sulfasalazine in the treatment of ankylosing spondylitis. A twenty-six-week, placebo-controlled clinical trial. *Arthritis Rheum* 1988;**31**(9): 1111–16.

30 Davis MJ, Dawes PT, Beswick E, Lewin IV, Stanworth DR. Sulphasalazine therapy in ankylosing spondylitis: its effect on disease activity, immunoglobulin A and the complex immunoglobulin A-alpha-1-antitrypsin. *Br J Rheumatol* 1989;**28**(5):410–13.

31 Corkill MM, Jobanputra P, Gibson T, Macfarlane DG. A controlled trial of sulphasalazine treatment of chronic ankylosing spondylitis: failure to demonstrate a clinical effect. *Br J Rheumatol* 1990;**29**(1):41–5.

32 Taylor HG, Beswick EJ, Dawes PT. Sulphasalazine in ankylosing spondylitis. A radiological, clinical and laboratory assessment. *Clin Rheumatol* 1991;**10**(1):43–8.

33 Ostendorf B, Specker C, Schneider M. Methotrexate lacks efficacy in the treatment of severe ankylosing spondylitis compared to rheumatoid and psoriatic arthritis. *J Clin Rheumatol* 1998;**4**(3):129–36.

34 Braun J, Pham T, Sieper J, *et al.* for the ASAS working group. International ASAS consensus statement for the use of biologic agents in patients with ankylosing spondylitis. *Ann Rheum Dis* 2003;**62:** (in press).

35 Benitez Del Castillo JM, Garcia Sanchez J, Iradier T, Banares A. Sulfasalazine in the prevention of anterior uveitis associated with ankylosing spondylitis. *Eye* 2000;**14**(Pt 3a):340–3.

36 Smith JR, Levinson RD, Holland GN, *et al.* Differential efficacy of tumor necrosis factor inhibition in the management of inflammatory eye disease and associated rheumatic disease. *Arthritis Rheum* 2001;**45**(3):252–7.

37 Peters ND, Ejstrup L. Intravenous methylprednisolone pulse therapy in ankylosing spondylitis. *Scand J Rheumatol* 1992;**21**(3):134–8.

38 Dougados M, Behier JM, Jolchine I, *et al.* Efficacy of celecoxib, a cyclooxygenase 2-specific inhibitor, in the treatment of ankylosing spondylitis: a six-week controlled study with comparison against placebo and against a conventional nonsteroidal antiinflammatory drug. *Arthritis Rheum* 2001;**44**(1):180–5.

39 Dagfinder H, Hagen K. Physiotherapy interventions for ankylosing spondylitis (Cochrane Review). In: Cochrane Collaboration. *Cochrane Library.* Oxford: Update Software, 2001.

40 Helliwell PS, Abbott CA, Chamberlain MA. A randomised trial of three different physiotherapy regimens in ankylosing spondylitis. *Physiotherapy* 1996;**82**:85–90.

41 Kraag G, Stokes B, Groh J, Helewa A, Goldsmith C. The effects of comprehensive home physiotherapy and supervision on patients with ankylosing spondylitis – a randomised controlled trial. *J Rheumatol* 1990;**17**(2): 228–33.

42 Hidding A, van der Linden S, Boers M, *et al.* Is group physical therapy superior to individualized therapy in ankylosing spondylitis? A randomised controlled trial. *Arthritis Care Res* 1993;**6**(3):117–25.

43 van Tubergen A, Landewe R, van der Heijde D, *et al.* Combined spa-exercise therapy is effective in patients with ankylosing spondylitis: a randomised controlled trial. *Arthritis Rheumatism [Arthritis Care Res]* 2001;**45**(5): 430–8.

44 van Tubergen A, Boonen A, Landewé R, *et al.* Cost-effectiveness of combined spa-exercise therapy in ankylosing spondylitis: a randomised controlled trial. *Arthritis Rheum [Arthritis Care Res]* 2002;**47**:459–67.

45 Jones G, Crotty M, Brooks P. Interventions for treating psoriatic arthritis (Systematic Review).In: Cochrane Collaboration. *Cochrane Library* . Issue 4. Oxford: Update Software, 2001.

46 Combe B, Goupille P, Kuntz JL, Tebib J, Liote F, Bregeon C. Sulphasalazine in psoriatic arthritis: a randomised, multicentre, placebo-controlled study. *Br J Rheumatol* 1996;**35**(7):664–8.

47 Clegg DO, Reda DJ, Mejias E, *et al.* Comparison of sulfasalazine and placebo in the treatment of psoriatic arthritis. A Department of Veterans Affairs Cooperative Study. *Arthritis Rheum* 1996;**39**(12):2013–20.

48 Gupta AK, Grober JS, Hamilton TA, *et al.* Sulfasalazine therapy for psoriatic arthritis: a double blind, placebo controlled trial. *J Rheumatol* 1995;**22**(5):894–8.

49 Farr M, Kitas GD, Waterhouse L, Jubb R, Felix Davies D, Bacon PA. Sulphasalazine in psoriatic arthritis: a double-blind placebo-controlled study. *Br J Rheumatol* 1990; **29**(1):46–9.

50 Fraser SM, Hopkins R, Hunter JA, Neumann V, Capell HA, Bird HA. Sulphasalazine in the management of psoriatic arthritis. *Br J Rheumatol* 1993;**32**(10):923–5.

51 Salvarani C, Macchioni P, Olivieri I, *et al.* A comparison of cyclosporine, sulfasalazine, and symptomatic therapy in the treatment of psoriatic arthritis. *J Rheumatol* 2001;**28**(10):2274–82.

52 Rahman P, Gladman DD, Cook RJ, Zhou Y, Young G. The use of sulfasalazine in psoriatic arthritis: a clinic experience. *J Rheumatol* 1998;**25**(10):1957–61.

53 Newman ED, Perruquet JL, Harrington TM. Sulfasalazine therapy in psoriatic arthritis: clinical and immunologic response. *J Rheumatol* 1991;**18**(9):1379–82.

54 Farr M, Kitas GD, Waterhouse L, Jubb R, Felix Davies D, Bacon PA. Treatment of psoriatic arthritis with sulphasalazine: a one year open study. *Clin Rheumatol* 1988;**7**(3):372–7.

55 Black RL, O'Brien WM, Van Scott EJ, Auerbach R, Eisen AZ, Bunim JJ. Methotrexate therapy in psoriatic arthritis. *JAMA* 1964;**189**(10):743–7.

56 Willkens RF, Williams HJ, Ward JR, *et al.* Randomised, double-blind, placebo controlled trial of low-dose pulse methotrexate in psoriatic arthritis. *Arthritis Rheum* 1984;**27**(4):376–81.

57 Spadaro A, Riccieri V, Sili Scavalli A, Sensi F, Taccari E, Zoppini A. Comparison of cyclosporin A and methotrexate in the treatment of psoriatic arthritis: a one-year prospective study. *Clin Exp Rheumatol* 1995;**13**(5): 589–93.

58 Abu Shakra M, Gladman DD, Thorne JC, Long J, Gough J, Farewell VT. Longterm methotrexate therapy in psoriatic arthritis: clinical and radiological outcome. *J Rheumatol* 1995;**22**(2):241–5.

59 Espinoza LR, Zakraoui L, Espinoza CG, *et al.* Psoriatic arthritis: clinical response and side effects to methotrexate therapy. *J Rheumatol* 1992;**19**(6):872–7.

60 Pigatto PD, Gibelli E, Ranza R, Rossetti A. Methotrexate in psoriatic polyarthritis. *Acta Derm Venereol (Stockh)* 1994;**186** (suppl):114–15.

61 Ranza R, Marchesoni A, Rossetti A, Tosi S, Gibelli E. Methotrexate in psoriatic polyarthritis. *J Rheumatol* 1993;**20**(10):1804–5.

62 Zachariae H, Zachariae E. Methotrexate treatment of psoriatic arthritis. *Acta Derm Venereol (Stockh)* 1987;**67**(3):270–3.

63 Cannavo SP, Bartolone S, Guarneri F. Low-dose cyclosporin A in severe psoriatic arthritis: Clinical results of a long-term study. *Dermatol Clin* 1996;**16**(1):58–62.

64 Gupta AK, Matteson EL, Ellis CN, *et al.* Cyclosporine in the treatment of psoriatic arthritis. *Arch Dermatol* 1989;**125**(4):507–10.

65 Macchioni P, Boiardi L, Cremonesi T, *et al.* The relationship between serum-soluble interleukin-2 receptor and radiological evolution in psoriatic arthritis patients treated with cyclosporin-A. *Rheumatol Int* 1998;**18**(1): 27–33.

66 Mahrle G, Schulze HJ, Brautigam M, *et al.* Anti-inflammatory efficacy of low-dose cyclosporin A in

psoriatic arthritis. A prospective multicentre study. *Br J Dermatol* 1996;**135**(5):752–7.

67 Mazzanti G, Coloni L, De Sabbata G, Paladini G. Methotrexate and cyclosporin combined therapy in severe psoriatic arthritis. A pilot study. *Acta Derm Venereol (Stockh)* 1994;**186** (Suppl):116–17.

68 Porzio F, Antonelli M, Antonelli S, *et al.* Cyclosporin A in the long-term treatment of psoriatic arthritis [letter]. *Br J Rheumatol* 1996;**35**(12):1331.

69 Prelog I, Krajnc I, Lukanovic K. Treatment of psoriatic arthritis with cyclosporin A. *Acta Dermatovenerol Alp Panonica Adriat* 2000;**9**(3):110–12.

70 Raffayova H, Rovensky J, Malis F. Treatment with cyclosporin in patients with psoriatic arthritis: results of clinical assessment. *Int J Clin Pharmacol Res* 2000; **20**(1–2):1–11.

71 Riccieri V, Sili Scavalli A, Spadaro A, Bracci M, Taccari E, Zoppini A. Short-term "cyclosporin A" therapy for psoriatic arthritis. *Acta Derm Venereol (Stockh)* 1994;**186** (Suppl):94–5.

72 Salvarani C, Macchioni P, Boiardi L, *et al.* Low dose cyclosporine A in psoriatic arthritis: relation between soluble interleukin 2 receptors and response to therapy. *J Rheumatol* 1992;**19**(1):74–9.

73 Steinsson K, Jonsdottir I, Valdimarsson H. Cyclosporin A in psoriatic arthritis: an open study. *Ann Rheum Dis* 1990;**49**(8):603–6.

74 Wagner SA, Peter RU, Adam O, Ruzicka T. Therapeutic efficacy of oral low-dose cyclosporin A in severe psoriatic arthritis. *Dermatology* 1993;**186**(1):62–7.

75 Carette S, Calin A, McCafferty JP, Wallin BA. A double-blind placebo-controlled study of auranofin in patients with psoriatic arthritis. *Arthritis Rheum* 1989;**32**(2):158–65.

76 Palit J, Hill J, Capell HA, *et al.* A multicentre double-blind comparison of auranofin, intramuscular gold thiomalate and placebo in patients with psoriatic arthritis. *Br J Rheumatol* 1990;**29**(4):280–3.

77 Brückle W, Dexel T, Grasedyck K, Schattenkirchner M. Treatment of psoriatic arthritis with auranofin and gold sodium thiomalate. *Clin Rheumatol* 1994;**13**(2):209–16.

78 Mader R, Gladman DD, Long J, Gough J, Farewell VT. Does injectable gold retard radiologic evidence of joint damage in psoriatic arthritis? *Clin Invest Med* 1995;**18**(2): 139–43.

79 Salvarani C, Zizzi F, Macchioni P, *et al.* Clinical responses to auranofin in patients with psoriatic arthritis. *Clin Rheumatol* 1989;**8**(1):54–7.

80 Tumiati B, Baricchi R, Bellelli A. Psoriatic arthritis. Long term treatment with auranofin. *Clin Rheumatol* 1986;**5**(1):124–5.

81 Barbieri P, Ciompi ML, Bini C, Pasero G. Long term experience with oral gold in psoriatic arthritis. *Clin Rheumatol* 1986;**5**(2):274–5.

82 McKendry RJ, Kraag G, Seigel S, al Awadhi A. Therapeutic value of colchicine in the treatment of patients with psoriatic arthritis. *Ann Rheum Dis* 1993;**52**(11):826–8.

83 Seideman P, Fjellner B, Johannesson A. Psoriatic arthritis treated with oral colchicine. *J Rheumatol* 1987;**14**(4): 777–9.

84 Hopkins R, Bird HA, Jones H, *et al.* A double-blind controlled trial of etretinate (Tigason) and ibuprofen in psoriatic arthritis. *Ann Rheum Dis* 1985;**44**(3):189–93.

85 Ciompi ML, Bazzichi L, Marotta G, Pasero G. Tigason (etretinate) treatment in psoriatic arthritis. *Int J Tiss Reac* 1988;**10**(1):25–8.

86 Chieregato GC, Leoni A. Treatment of psoriatic arthropathy with etretinate: a two-year follow-up. *Acta Derm Venereol (Stockh)* 1986;**66**:321–4.

87 Klinkhoff AV, Gertner E, Chalmers A, *et al.* Pilot study of etretinate in psoriatic arthritis. *J Rheumatol* 1989;**16**(6): 789–91.

88 Seppala J, Laulainen M, Reunala T. Comparison of etretinate (Tigason) and parental gold in the treatment of psoriatic arthropathy. *Clin Rheumatol* 1988;**7**(4):498–503.

89 Price R, Gibson T. D-penicillamine and psoriatic arthropathy [letter]. *Br J Rheumatol* 1986;**25**(2):228.

90 Peeters AJ, Dijkmans BA, van der Schroeff JG. Fumaric acid therapy for psoriatic arthritis. A randomised, double-blind, placebo-controlled study [letter]. *Br J Rheumatol* 1992;**31**(7):502–4.

91 Levy J, Paulus HE, Barnett EV, Sokoloff M, Bangert R, Pearson CM. A double-blind controlled evaluation of azathioprine treatment in rheumatoid arthritis and psoriatic arthritis [abstract]. *Arthritis Rheum* 1972;**15**(1): 116–17.

92 Feldges DH, Barnes CG. Treatment of psoriatic arthropathy with either azathioprine or methotrexate. *Rheumatol Rehab* 1974;**13**:120–4.

93 Lee JCT, Gladman DD, Schentag CT, Cook RJ. The long-term use of azathioprine in patients with psoriathic arthritis. *J Clin Rheumatol* 2001;**7**(3):160–5.

94 Gladman DD, Blake R, Brubacher B, Farewell VT. Chloroquine therapy in psoriatic arthritis. *J Rheumatol* 1992;**19**(11):1724–6.

95 Huckins D, Felson DT, Holick M. Treatment of psoriatic arthritis with oral 1,25-dihydroxyvitamin D3: a pilot study. *Arthritis Rheum* 1990;**33**(11):1723–7.

96 Liang GC, Barr WG. Long term follow-up of the use of leflunomide (LF) in recalcitrant psoriatic arthritis (PA) and psoriasis (PS) [abstract]. *Arthritis Rheum* 2001;**44** (Suppl):S121.

97 Scarpa R, Manguso F, Oriente A, Peluso R, Oriente P. Leflunomide in psoriatic polyarthritis: an italian pilot study [abstract]. *Arthritis Rheum* 2001;**44** (Suppl):S92.

98 Mease PJ, Goffe BS, Metz J, VanderStoep A, Finck B, Burge DJ. Etanercept in the treatment of psoriatic arthritis and psoriasis: a randomised trial. *Lancet* 2000;**356**:385–90.

99 Mease P, Goffe B, Metz J, Vanderstoep A. A phase II trial of etanercept (Enbrel) in patients with psoriatic arthritis (PsA) and psoriasis [abstract]. *Ann Rheum Dis* 2000;**59** (Suppl 1):199.

100 Cuellar ML, Mendez E, Deaver Collins R, Espinoza LR. Efficacy of etanercept in refractory psoriatric arthritis (PsA). *Arthritis Rheum* 2000;43:S106.

101 Yazici Y, Erkan D, Lockshin MD. A preliminary study of etanercept in the treatment of severe, resistant psoriatic arthritis. *Clin Exp Rheumatol* 2000;**18**(6):732–4.

102 Ogilvie AL, Antoni C, Dechant C, *et al.* Treatment of psoriatic arthritis with antitumour necrosis factor-alpha antibody clears skin lesions of psoriasis resistant to treatment with methotrexate. *Br J Dermatol* 2001;**144**(3):587–9.

103 Antoni C, Dechant C, Lorenz H-M, *et al.* Successful treatment of psoriatic arthritis with infliximab in a MRI controlled study [abstract]. *Ann Rheum Dis* 2000;**59** (Suppl 1):200.

104 Cauza EE, Spak MS, Cauza KC, Hanusch-Enserer UH, Dunky AD, Wagner EW. Treatment of psoriathric arthritis and psoriasis vulgaris with the tumor necrosis factor blocker infliximab. *Ann Rheum Dis* 2001;**60**(Suppl 1):217–18 [abstract].

105 Bray VJ, Huffstutter JE. Schwartzman S. Emerging role of infliximab (Remicade) in psoriatic arthritis patients resistant to disease modifying anti-rheumatic drugs: case studies [abstract]. *Arthritis Rheum* 2001;**44** (Suppl):S121.

106 Dinant HJ, van Kuijk AWR, Goedkoop AY, Kraan MC, de Bie MA. Alefacept (LFA 3-IgG1 Fusion protein, LFA3TIP) reduces synovial inflammatory infiltrate and improves outcome in psoriatic arthritis [abstract]. *Arthritis Rheum* 2001;**44** (Suppl):S91.

107 Braun J, Kingsley G, van der Heijde D, Sieper J. On the difficulties of establishing a consensus on the definition of and diagnostic investigations for reactive arthritis. Results and discussion of a questionnaire prepared for the 4th International Workshop on Reactive Arthritis, Berlin, Germany, 3–6 July 1999. *J Rheumatol* 2000;**27**:2185–92.

108 Smieja M, MacPherson DW, Kean W, *et al.* Randomised, blinded, placebo controlled trial of doxycycline for chronic seronegative arthritis. *Ann Rheum Dis* 2001; **60**(12):1088–94.

109 Leirisalo-Repo M, Paimela L, Julkunen H, *et al.* A 3-month randomised, placebo-controlled study with combination antimicrobial therapy in acute reactive arthritis. *Arthritis Rheum* 2001;**22**:S91.

110 Yli Kerttula T, Luukkainen R, Yli Kerttula U, *et al.* Effect of a three month course of ciprofloxacin on the outcome of reactive arthritis. *Ann Rheum Dis* 2000; **59**(7):565–70.

111 Hoogkamp Korstanje JA, Moesker H, Bruyn GA. Ciprofloxacin v placebo for treatment of Yersinia enterocolitica triggered reactive arthritis. *Ann Rheum Dis* 2000;**59**(11):914–17.

112 Wakefield D, McCluskey P, Verma M, Aziz K, Gatus B, Carr G. Ciprofloxacin treatment does not influence course or relapse rate of reactive arthritis and anterior uveitis. *Arthritis Rheum* 1999;**42**(9):1894–7.

113 Sieper J, Fendler C, Laitko S, *et al.* No benefit of long-term ciprofloxacin treatment in patients with reactive arthritis and undifferentiated oligoarthritis: a three-month, multicenter, double-blind, randomised, placebo-controlled study. *Arthritis Rheum* 1999;**42**(7):1386–96.

114 Wollenhaupt J, Homer M, Pott HG, *et al.* A double-blind placebo controlled comparison of 2 weeks versus 4 months treatment with doxycycline in Chlamydia induced reactive arthritis. *Arthritis Rheum* 1997;**42**:S143.

115 Toivanen A, Yli Kerttula T, Luukkainen R, *et al.* Effect of antimicrobial treatment on chronic reactive arthritis. *Clin Exp Rheumatol* 1993;**11**(3):301–7.

116 Lauhio A, Leirisalo Repo M, Lahdevirta J, Saikku P, Repo H. Double-blind, placebo-controlled study of three-month treatment with lymecycline in reactive arthritis, with special reference to Chlamydia arthritis. *Arthritis Rheum* 1991;**34**(1):6–14.

117 Fryden A, Bengtsson A, Foberg U, *et al.* Early antibiotic treatment of reactive arthritis associated with enteric infections: clinical and serological study. *BMJ* 1990;**301**(6764):1299–302.

118 Egsmose C, Hansen TM, Andersen LS, *et al.* Limited effect of sulphasalazine treatment in reactive arthritis. A randomised double blind placebo controlled trial. *Ann Rheum Dis* 1997;**56**(1):32–6.

119 Clegg DO, Reda DJ, Weisman MH, *et al.* Comparison of sulfasalazine and placebo in the treatment of reactive arthritis (Reiter's syndrome). A Department of Veterans Affairs Cooperative Study. *Arthritis Rheum* 1996;**39**(12):2021–7.

120 Peliskova Z, Pavelka KJ, Trnavsky K. A palcebo-controlled, double-blind study of salazopyrin-EN (SASP) in refractory reactive arthritis. *Scand J Rheumatol* 1990;**85**(Suppl):45.

121 Lally EV, Ho G, Jr. A review of methotrexate therapy in Reiter syndrome. *Semin Arthritis Rheum* 1985;**15**(2):139–45.

122 Calin A. A placebo controlled, crossover study of azathioprine in Reiter's syndrome. *Ann Rheum Dis* 1986;**45**(8):653–5.

123 Van den Bosch F, Kruithof E, De Vos M, De Keyser F, Mielants H. Crohn's disease associated with spondyloarthropathy: effect of TNF-alpha blockade with infliximab on articular symptoms. *Lancet* 2000; **356**:1821–2.

124 Florin TH, Graffner H, Nilsson LG, Persson T. Treatment of joint pain in Crohn's patients with budesonide controlled ileal release. *Clin Exp Pharmacol Physiol* 2000;**27**(4):295–8.

Spondyloarthropathies
Summaries and decision aids

Ankylosing spondylitis and biologic agents
Summaries and decision aid

How well do biologic agents, such as infliximab or etanercept, work for treating ankylosing spondylitis and are they safe?

To answer this question, scientists found and analysed 3 high quality studies testing over 130 people who had ankylosing spondylitis. People received either injections of infliximab, etanercept or placebo (water) injections. These studies provide the best evidence we have today.

What is ankylosing spondylitis and how can biologic agents help?

Ankylosing spondylitis (AS) is a type of arthritis, usually in the joints and ligaments of the spine. It may also affect the shoulders, hips, or other joints and cause tendinitis. Pain and stiffness occurs and limits movement in the back and affected joints. It can come and go, last for long periods, and be quite severe. Infliximab (Remicade) and etanercept (Enbrel) are "biologic agents" that are injected into the body under the skin or infused into veins (IV). In the body they block chemicals that cause pain and swelling and may control AS, slow its progress and stop damage.

How well did infliximab or etanercept work?

Two different studies showed that more people receiving etanercept (for 4 or 10 months) or infliximab (for 12 weeks) improved by 20% compared to people receiving a placebo. People had, for example, less pain, morning stiffness, swelling, back pain or disease activity; better ability to function; or felt better overall. Another study showed that infliximab for 12 weeks improved morning stiffness and disease activity, but not ability to function.

What side effects occurred with the biologic agents?

Minor side effects, such as the common cold, diarrhoea, and headache occurred. Reactions where etanercept was injected and flu-like symptoms when infliximab is infused can occur. Rare side effects such as tuberculosis (TB) and low white blood cells occurred in a small number of people and they stopped taking the medication. Other studies that tested biologic agents in other conditions found that TB, fungal infections, and other serious infections (which may cause death) occurred in people taking biologic agents.

What is the bottom line?

There is "Silver" level evidence that in patients with ankylosing spondylitis, biologic agents, such as infliximab and etanercept, improve pain, stiffness, function and well-being. It is not known if biologic agents stop long term damage in the spine or improve the ability to move the spine.

Side effects such as common colds, diarrhoea, and headache can occur. Side effects that cause people to stop the treatment may occur more often with infliximab than with etanercept. Longer studies are needed before rare and late side effects are known. Tuberculosis (TB) has been reported in some studies and it is important to test for TB before starting a biologic.

Based on Van der Linden S, van Tubergen A, Boonen A, Mihai C, Ottawa Methods Group. Spondyloarthropathies. In *Evidence-based Rheumatology.* London: BMJ Books, 2003.

How well do biologic agents, such as infliximab or etanercept, work for treating ankylosing spondylitis and are they safe?

What is ankylosing spondylitis and how can biologic agents help?

Ankylosing spondylitis (AS) is a type of arthritis, usually in the joints and ligaments of the spine. In some people the disease also affects the shoulders, hips, or other joints and can cause tendonitis. AS causes pain and stiffness, and limits movement in the back and affected joints. The pain and stiffness can come and go, last for long periods, and be quite severe. Over time the joints and vertebrae of the back may fuse together and lead to bent posture and reduced mobility. The pain and damage from AS can limit a person's ability to carry out daily activities at home and work and affects their wellbeing.

Infliximab (Remicade) and etanercept (Enbrel) are "biologic agents" or "biological response modifiers". These new biologic agents are injected into the body under the skin or infused into veins (IV). In the body, biologic agents clamp onto a chemical in the body called tumour necrosis factor alpha (TNF-alpha). TNF-alpha is thought to start a chain reaction in the body that causes swelling, pain, and damage in the body's joints. When clamping onto TNF-alpha, the biologic agents stop the chain reaction, which may decrease pain and swelling in the joints. Blocking TNF-alpha from working may control ankylosing spondylitis, slow the progress of the disease and stop permanent damage.

How did the scientists find the information and analyse it?

The scientists searched for studies testing infliximab or etanercept in patients with ankylosing spondylitis. Not all studies found were of a high quality and so only those studies that met high standards were selected.

The high quality studies had to be randomised controlled trials – where a group of patients receiving infliximab or etanercept were compared to a group of patients receiving a placebo (water injection). The studies also had to measure pain, function, stiffness, well-being, and joint swelling using agreed upon scales.

Which studies were included in the summary?

There were 3 studies included in this summary. The studies examined 131 patients with ankylosing spondylitis for 6 weeks to 10 months:

- a 4 month study tested 40 patients (20 received etanercept injections and 20 received a placebo injection); 37 of these patients were followed for another 6 months (all patients received etanercept for the next 6 months)
- a 12 week study tested 70 patients (35 received IV infliximab and 35 received IV placebo)
- another 12 week study tested 40 patients, 21 of whom had ankylosing spondylitis (9 received IV infliximab and 12 received IV placebo).

Infliximab is given by IV for about 2 hours. After the first dose, it is given 2 weeks later, then another 4 weeks later, and then every 6 weeks. Etanercept is given as an injection two times per week and can be given at home by the patient.

How well did infliximab or etanercept work to treat ankylosing spondylitis?

Etanercept: After 4 and 10 months, 80 out of 100 patients receiving etanercept improved by 20% compared to 30 out of 100 patients receiving placebo. A 20% improvement in this study meant that patients improved in at least three of the following five measures: pain, function, morning stiffness, swelling, overall wellbeing. This improvement happened quickly. But the improvement in movement of the spine was small.

Infliximab: After 12 weeks, the one study testing 70 patients showed that 53 out of 100 patients receiving infliximab improved by 50% in disease activity (pain and stiffness) compared to 9 out of 100 patients receiving placebo. The differences in improvement between the two groups of patients occurred after 2 weeks. The study also noted that the effect of infliximab on movement of the spine was good.

After 12 weeks, the other study showed that more patients receiving infliximab had less stiffness, back pain, and disease activity and better function than patients receiving a placebo. But receiving infliximab or a placebo did not make a difference in their ability to move their spine. Improvements with infliximab occurred within 2 weeks.

What side effects occurred with the biologic agents?

Etanercept: After 4, 6, and 10 months minor side effects occurred just as often in patients receiving etanercept as placebo. Minor side effects were:

- lung infections (in 50 out of 100 patients receiving etanercept and 60 out of 100 receiving placebo)
- diarrhoea (in 15 out of 100 receiving etanercept and 5 out of 100 receiving a placebo)
- reactions and redness where the injection was (in 20 out of 100 patients receiving etanercept and in 5 out of 100 patients receiving placebo)
- headaches (in 10 out of 100 patients receiving etanercept).

Infliximab: In the 12 week study with 70 patients:

- common colds and respiratory tract (lung) infections occurred about equally in patients receiving infliximab or a placebo (51 out of 100 patients receiving infliximab and 35 out of 100 receiving placebo)
- diarrhoea occurred in 15 out of 100 receiving infliximab and 5 out of 100 receiving a placebo
- 3 out of the 35 patients (or 9 out of 100) stopped receiving infliximab because 1 had tuberculosis, 1 had an allergic reaction that affected the lungs and 1 had low white blood cells.

In the other 12 week study, side effects such as the common cold, itching, fatigue, and headache occurred in about the same number of patients receiving infliximab as placebo. Two out of the 40 patients receiving infliximab stopped taking infliximab because 1 had tuberculosis and 1 may have had an infection.

Other studies that tested biologic agents in other conditions found that tuberculosis (TB), fungal infections, and other serious infections occurred in people taking biologic agents. Some of these infections caused death. Patients are now tested for previous contact with TB before they start a biologic and are told to call their doctor if they think they have an infection.

What is the bottom line?

There is "Silver" level evidence that in patients with ankylosing spondylitis, biologic agents, such as infliximab and etanercept, improve pain, stiffness, function, and well-being . It is not known if biologic agents stop long term damage in the spine or improve the ability to move the spine.

Side effects such as common colds, diarrhoea, and headache can occur. Side effects that cause people to stop taking the treatment may occur more often with infliximab than with etanercept.

Longer studies are needed before rare and late side effects are known. Tuberculosis (TB) has been reported in some studies, and it is important to test for TB before starting a biologic.

Based on Van der Linden S, van Tubergen A, Boonen A, Mihai C, Ottawa Methods Group. Spondyloarthropathies. In: *Evidence-based Rheumatology.* London: BMJ Books, 2003.

Information about ankylosing spondylitis treatment

What is ankylosing spondylitis (AS)?

Ankylosing spondylitis (AS) is a type of arthritis, usually in the joints and ligaments of the spine. AS also affects the shoulders, hips, or other joints and can cause tendonitis. AS causes pain and stiffness, and can limit movement in the back and affected joints. Over time the joints of the back may fuse together and lead to bent posture and reduced mobility. The pain and damage from AS can limit a person's ability to carry out daily activities at home and work and affects their well-being.

The pain and stiffness can come and go, last for long periods, and be quite severe. If it is not treated, it may result in:

- limited daily activities
- bent posture
- fused joints
- need for surgery

What can I do on my own to manage my disease?

✓ Relaxation and regular rest
✓ Hot/cold packs
✓ Regular daily exercise
✓ Activity that puts less stress on joints (such as swimming or walking)
✓ Spa therapy (available at a spa-resort)

What treatments are used for ankylosing spondylitis?

Four kinds of treatment may be used alone or together. The common (generic) names of treatment are shown below.

Treatments to control short-term symptoms (pain and stiffness):

1. *Pain medicines*
   - Acetaminophen
2. *Non-steroidal anti-inflammatory drugs (NSAIDs), some of which are listed below*
   - Acetylsalicylic acid
   - Celecoxib
   - Diclofenac
   - Ibuprofen
   - Indomethacin
   - Meloxicam
   - Nabumetone
   - Naproxen
   - Piroxicam
   - Rofecoxib
   - Sulindac

Treatments to limit the long term symptoms and the damage

3. *Disease modifying anti-rheumatic drugs (DMARDs)*
   - Methotrexate
   - Pamidronate
   - Sulphasalazine
4. *Biologic agents*
   - Etanercept
   - Infliximab

What about other treatments I have heard about?

There is not enough evidence about the effects of some treatments. Other treatments do not work. For example:

- Azathioprine
- Thalidomide
- D-penicillamine
- Prednisone

What are my choices? How can I decide?

Treatment for your disease will depend on your condition. You need to know the good points (pros) and bad points (cons) about each treatment before you can decide.

Ankylosing spondylitis decision aid

Should I take biologic agents, such as infliximab or etanercept?

This guide can help you make decisions about the treatment your doctor is asking you to consider.

It will help you to:

1. Clarify what you need to decide.
2. Consider the pros and cons of different choices.
3. Decide what role you want to have in choosing your treatment.
4. Identify what you need to help you make the decision.
5. Plan the next steps.
6. Share your thinking with your doctor.

Step 1. Clarify what you need to decide

What is the decision?

Should I start taking biologic agents when non-steroidal anti-inflammatory drugs (NSAIDS, see some examples on previous page) are not working enough to control ankylosing spondylitis?

Biologic agents are injections (given under the skin or intravenously) at pre-set times (at home or infusion center).

When does this decision have to be made? Check ✓ one

☐ within days ☐ within weeks ☐ within months

How far along are you with this decision? Check ✓one

☐ I have not thought about it yet

☐ I am considering the choices

☐ I am close to making a choice

☐ I have already made a choice

Step 2: Consider the pros and cons of different choices

What does the research show?

Biologic agents are classified as: Trade-off between benefits and harms

There is "Silver" level evidence from 3 studies of biologic agents in 131 people. The studies lasted up to 10 months. These studies found pros and cons that are listed in the chart below.

What do I think of the pros and cons of biologic agents?

1. Review the common pros and cons.
2. Add any other pros and cons that are important to you.
3. Show how important each pro and con is to you by circling from one (*) star if it is a little important to you, to up to five (*****) stars if it is very important to you.

PROS AND CONS OF BIOLOGIC AGENTS, SUCH AS INFLIXIMAB AND ETANERCEPT

PROS (number of people affected)	How important is it to you?	CONS (number of people affected)	How important is it to you?
Improves my pain and stiffness 80 out of 100 people receiving a biologic improve at least a little compared to 30 out of 100 patients receiving a placebo. 53 out of 100 people receiving a biologic improve a lot compared to 9 out 100 patients receiving placebo	* * * * *	Side effects: colds, headache, diarrhoea, abdominal pain	* * * * *
		Reactions during or immediately after the injection include headache, nausea, and hives	* * * * *
Improves my ability to do daily activities	* * * * *	Serious harms: tuberculosis (TB) and other serious infections Some of these infections have been fatal	* * * * *
Works within days/weeks rather than months	* * * * *	Unsure of what effect it will have if we still want to have children	* * * * *
Might improve long term damage to my spine	* * * * *	Personal cost of medicine	* * * * *
Other pros:	* * * * *	Unsure how easy it is to travel with this medicine Need needles and kept in the fridge	* * * * *
		Other cons:	* * * * *

***What do you think of biologic agents?* Check ✓ one**

☐ Willing to consider this treatment
Pros are more important to me than the Cons

☐ Unsure

☐ Not willing to consider this treatment
Cons are more important to me than the Pros

Step 3: Choose the role you want to have in choosing your treatment Check ✓ one

☐ I prefer to decide on my own after listening to the opinions of others

☐ I prefer to share the decision with: ______________________

☐ I prefer someone else to decide for me, namely: ______________

Step 4: Identify what you need to help you make the decision

What I know	Do you know enough about your condition to make a choice?	☐ Yes	☐ No	☐ Unsure
	Do you know which options are available to you?	☐ Yes	☐ No	☐ Unsure
	Do you know the good points (pros) of each option?	☐ Yes	☐ No	☐ Unsure
	Do you know the bad points (cons) of each option?	☐ Yes	☐ No	☐ Unsure
What's important	Are you clear about which **pros** are most *important to you?*	☐ Yes	☐ No	☐ Unsure
	Are you clear about which **cons** are most *important to you?*	☐ Yes	☐ No	☐ Unsure
How others help	Do you have enough support from others to make a choice?	☐ Yes	☐ No	☐ Unsure
	Are you choosing without pressure from others?	☐ Yes	☐ No	☐ Unsure
	Do you have enough advice to make a choice?	☐ Yes	☐ No	☐ Unsure
How sure I feel	Are you clear about the best choice for you?	☐ Yes	☐ No	☐ Unsure
	Do you feel sure about what to choose?	☐ Yes	☐ No	☐ Unsure

If you answered No or Unsure to many of these questions, you should talk to your doctor.

Step 5: Plan the next steps

What do you need to do before you make this decision?

For example – talk to your doctor, read more about this treatment or other treatments for ankylosing spondylitis.

Step 6: Share the information on this form with your doctor

It will help your doctor understand what you think about this treatment.

12 Systemic sclerosis

Daniel E Furst, Janet Pope, Phil Clements, Ottawa Methods Group

Disease modifying antirheumatic drug therapy

Introduction

This chapter deals with the treatment of systemic sclerosis. Systemic sclerosis (SSc) is a multifaceted, autoimmune disease whose pathogenesis is only partially understood.[1] Vascular abnormalities occur early in the disease and are heavily influenced by immunological phenomena. These, together, result in fibroblast proliferation, collagen formation, and the clinical manifestations of disease.

While there is no proven therapy for the disease as a whole, continued attempts have been made to develop such treatment. The initial portion of this chapter reviews the evidence for a rational approach to such therapy and includes those outcomes most likely to yield positive results, such as changes in the skin or lungs, two organ systems relatively easily measured. The second portion of the chapter concerns itself with the treatment of Raynaud's phenomenon (RP), which occurs in 95% of patients with systemic sclerosis. Here there has been more success and the various therapeutic options to treat Raynaud's phenomenon in association with systemic sclerosis are reviewed and analysed.

There are a number of articles in the literature which included patients with systemic sclerosis but did not separate them in the publication nor analyse the results specifically for those SSC patients. These articles are appropriate to include in this review but are separated from the other articles under a category called "Excluded".

Literature search

Randomised trials were identified from searches of the Cochrane Controlled Trials Register (Cochrane Library Issue 2, 2002), MEDLINE, EMBASE, CINAHL, and Science Citation Index (SCISEARCH). Searches were conducted in June 2002 and were not restricted by date. The search strategy included examining systemic sclerosis or scleroderma versus human trials, for both randomised clinical trials and cohort studies. The following key words were included: (1) scleroderma, (2) connective tissue disease, (3) Raynaud's, (4) randomised controlled trial, (5) calcium channel blockers, and (6) other specific drug classes. The bibliographies from the articles that were reviewed were also examined for further articles, as were chapters from books on systemic sclerosis.

Systemic Sclerosis

1 randomised-controlled trial in pt
2 randomised-controlled-trials
3 random-allocation
4 double-blind-method
5 single-blind-method
6 clinical-trial in pt
7 explode clinical-trials
8 (clin* near trial*) in ti
9 (clin* near trial*) in ab
10 (singl* or doubl* or trebl* or tripl*) near (blind* or mask*)
11 (#10 in ti) or (#10 in ab)
12 placebos
13 placebo * in ti

14 placebo in ab
15 random * in ti
16 random * in ab
17 research design
18 #1 #2 #3 #4 #5 #6 #7 #8 #9 #10 #11 #12 #13 #14 #15 #16 #17
19 explode raynauds or vasospasm
20 explode sclerderma
21 explode connective tissue disease
22 text words for all synonyms or/
23 #19 or #20 or #21 or #22
24 #18 and # 23
25 tg = animal not (tg = human and tg = animal)
26 #24 not 25

Following the identification of potential trials for inclusion by the search strategy two independent reviewers reviewed the methods sections of all identified trials independently, according to the eligibility criteria. Where the two reviewers disagreed, discussion was facilitated in order to reach consensus. If this failed, the trial was sent to a third reviewer for arbitration.

Evaluating the evidence

Suppressing autoimmunity and inflammation

Case presentation

A 35-year-old woman develops diffuse systemic sclerosis with a rapid and explosive onset. She has skin involvement which includes her face, chest, upper and lower arms as well as her feet and legs. Over 18 months, she develops pain in her left knee, both wrists, and both shoulders. The skin is so tight over the joints that it is not possible to tell whether there is active inflammation of the joints. She has dyspepsia, which is easily controlled with a proton pump inhibitor. She denies shortness of breath, her FVC is 75%, and her DLCO is 72% of predicted. The echocardiogram reveals an ejection fraction of 68% and PA. Systolic pressure is approximately 22 mmHg.

Question 1

Is there evidence that immunosuppression can improve the cutaneous or pulmonary manifestations of systemic sclerosis?

Chlorambucil

Benefits: Chlorambucil is an alkylating agent with immunosuppressive effects. Its use in SSc is predicated upon the presence of immunologically active T cells which are found in early SSc skin and other organs. A 3 year, randomised, double blind trial of chlorambucil versus placebo in 65 patients with SSc was negative.[2] Among the 33 chlorambucil-treated patients, the skin index (a combination of ulcers, calcinosis, skin score, and sclerodactyly) improved by 70·8%, compared to 84·4% improvement in the 32 placebo-treated patients. The skin score, *per se*, improved by 12·4% among the chlorambucil-treated group and 4·5% in the placebo-treated patients. This trial was limited by low numbers of patients (that is, low statistical power), late disease (average disease duration: 7·9 years), and a mixed group of patients with diffuse and limited disease. However, its failings led to improved study design thereafter.

Adverse effects: Leucopenia (< 3000 per mm^3), thrombocytopenia, gastrointestinal symptoms and infections were more common in the chlorambucil-treated patients, although none was statistically different.

Evidence summary: Silver

One small randomised, double-blind, placebo-controlled trial showed no benefit.

Cyclophosphamide

Benefits: Cyclophosphamide is a prototypic alkylating agent which has been used in the treatment of SSc. Unfortunately, the studies using cyclophosphamide are open and non-randomised. The study by Silver *et al* exemplifies one of the earlier open trials.[3] In patients with BAL proven alveolitis, a mean of 100 mg daily cyclophosphamide plus low dose prednisolone induced improvement of disease or stabilisation of

Table 12.1 Number needed to treat for 5-FU versus placebo (Casas *et al*, 1990)[5]

Outcome	Pooled standardized mean difference (95% CI)	% Benefiting with 5-FU (95% CI)	NNT (95% CI)
Total skin score	−1·63 (−2·31, −0·95)	59% (42, 67)	2 (2, 3)
Extension index (mm)	−3·98 (−5·01, −2·95)	69% (69, 69)	2 (2, 2)
Global assessment	0·17 (0·11, 1·31)	33% (5, 52)	4 (2, 19)
Raynaud's score	−3·13 (−4·02, −2·24)	69% (66, 69)	2 (2, 2)

pulmonary function in 15 of 17 patients. In contrast, the 11 patients who were not treated with cyclophosphamide demonstrated worsening in 4 and stabilisation in 7; no patients improved. The larger open, non randomised controlled trial by White *et al* compared 39 cyclophosphamide-treated patients with alveolitis by BAL versus 30 patients with alveolitis given no cyclophosphamide, and compared both of these groups to 34 SSc patients without alveolitis and also not treated with cyclophosphamide.[4] The patients with alveolitis receiving cyclophosphamide (median dose of 100 mg q.d.) did as well as the patients without alveolitis and better than the group with alveolitis but not given cyclophosphamide. In the alveolitis groups 7 patients died while on cyclophosphamide versus 14 who died without the drug ($p < 0·05$). There was a 4·3% improvement in forced vital capacity in the cyclophosphamide-treated patients with alveolitis versus a 1·5% improvement in patients without alveolitis and a 7·1% decrement in untreated alveolitis patients ($p < 0·05$). These changes in forced vital capacity did not exceed the coefficient of variation of the test, despite their statistical difference. A large, NIH funded, randomised, double blind, placebo controlled trial is presently ongoing to either corroborate or disprove these uncontrolled results.

Adverse effects: Leucopenia (10–15%), infections (7–10%), haemorrhagic cystitis (5–15%), and alopecia (3%) were noted in these trials.

Evidence summary: Silver

Cohort studies showed a small improvement in forced vital capacity in patients with alveolitis.

Recommendation for case presentation

Cyclophosphamide is used very frequently in the rheumatologic community for the treatment of systemic sclerosis at present, despite the lack of a well controlled trial. It would not be justified as the initial therapy in this patient, given the weight of evidence published thus far.

5-Fluorouracil (5-FU)

Benefits: Casas *et al* completed this randomised, double blind, placebo controlled international trial in 1990[5] (Table 12.1). This alkylating agent used to treat systemic sclerosis employed the skin score as its primary endpoint. With 20 patients in the 5-FU group and 26 patients in the placebo group, a 6·9 point improvement in skin score for the 5-FU-treated group occurred, compared to only a 1·8 point improvement in the placebo group ($p < 0·05$). Global estimates also differentiated 5-FU from placebo. Although 80% of the patients had the pulmonary involvement, the number who had alveolitis was unknown and there were no significant improvements in pulmonary function.

Adverse effects: Common adverse reactions associated with 5-FU include gastrointestinal toxicities such as nausea and vomiting in over 90% of patients and myelosuppression (decreased WBC) in 42% of patients (Table 12.2). Other rare but serious adverse effects, such as cerebellar ataxia and myocardial ischaemia, also occurred. The adverse effects noted in this study led the investigators to argue that the harms outweigh the benefits of the drug. With the availability of improved methods to administer this medication and treat its side effects such as nausea, another

Table 12.2 Number needed to harm for 5-FU versus placebo (Casas *et al*, 1990)[5]

Outcome	% with placebo	% with 5-FU	Relative risk of harm with 5-FU (95% CI)	Absolute risk increase (95% CI)	NNH (95% CI)
Side effects – any (most frequent haemocytopenia, GI)	10/20 (50%)	25/26 (96%)	1·92 (1·23, 3·00)	46% (21, 67)	2 (1, 4)

Table 12.3 Number needed to treat for methotrexate versus placebo (van den Hoogen *et al*,1996)[6]

Outcome	% with placebo	% with methotrexate	Relative risk with methotrexate (95% CI)	Absolute benefit increase (95% CI)	NNT (95% CI)
Favourable response (TSS or VAS improved by 30%+ or CMDC improved by 15%+. If digital ulcers persisted or CMDC decreased 15%+ response was unfavourable despite improvement of TSS or VAS)	1/10 (10%)	8/15 (53%)	5·33 (0·78, 36·33) p = 0·04	43% (5, 67)	3 (2, 20)

controlled randomised trial of this medication is justifiable.

Evidence summary: Silver

One small, randomised, placebo controlled trial showed improvement in the skin store and global rating.

Recommendation for case presentation

In this case, the patient had relatively aggressive disease which could justify the use of 5-FU. However, since the method of infusion in the trial led to so many adverse effects, this would not be a therapy to use initially in this patient.

Methotrexate

Benefits: There have been two randomised, controlled trials of methotrexate for the treatment of systemic sclerosis.[6,7] Van den Hoogen *et al* completed a small 12 month crossover study of methotrexate versus placebo[6] (Table 12.3 and Visual Rx Faces 12.1). Using a logical, but complex, definition of improvement, this trial showed an improvement in 53% of 15 methotrexate-treated patients compared to 10% of 12 placebo-treated patients ($p < 0·05$). Thirty-eight per cent of the 29 patients had diffuse systemic sclerosis with an average duration of disease of 38 months, making this a trial of mixed groups of patients with moderate disease duration.

In contrast, Pope *et al* examined 71 patients, all with diffuse disease, with a mean disease duration of 6·9 months.[7] The modified Rodnan Skin Score improved by 4·3 units on methotrexate, compared with worsening by 1·8 units on placebo ($p < 0·09$), while the UCLA skin score, which measured tethering, reached statistical significance comparing methotrexate to placebo ($p < 0·04$) (Table 12.4). Physician global assessment of disease activity also favoured methotrexate ($p < 0·035$), as did Carbon Monoxide Diffusion Capacity (CMDC) (%) ($p < 0·03$). Unfortunately,

Visual Rx Faces 12.1 NNT for MTX versus placebo

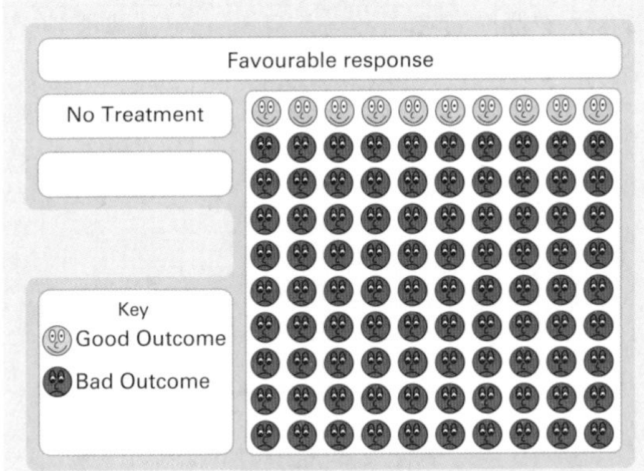

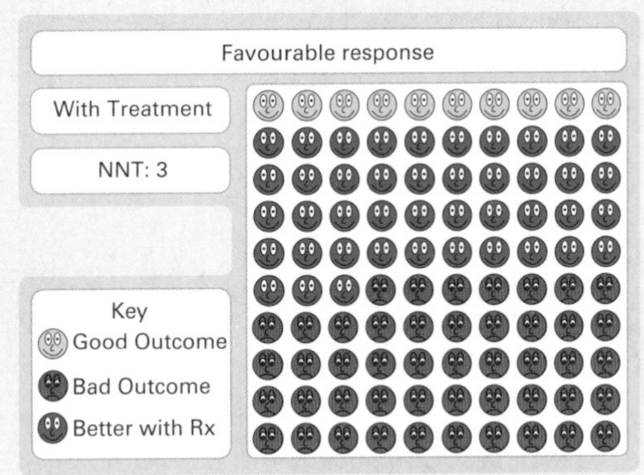

Table 12.4 Number needed to treat for methotrexate versus placebo (Pope *et al*, 2001)[7]

Outcome	Pooled standardized mean difference (95% CI)	% Benefiting with methotrexate (95% CI)	NNT (95% CI)
UCLA skin score (ITT)	–0·50 (–0·97, –0·03)	24% (1, 42)	5 (3, 69)
DLCO % predicted (ITT)	0·52 (0·05, 0·99)	24% (2, 43)	5 (3, 69)

Table 12.5 Number needed to harm for methotrexate versus placebo (van den Hoogen *et al*, 1996)[6]

Outcome	% with placebo	% with methotrexate	Relative risk with methotrexate (95% CI)	Absolute risk increase (95% CI)	NNH (95% CI)
Adverse reactions, (most frequent liver) withdrawals and deaths (2 MTX, 1 placebo)	2/12 (17%)	11/17 (65%)	3·88 (1·04, 14·03)	48% (11, 70)	2 (1, 8)

comparison between methotrexate and placebo for other measures such as patient and physician global assessment tests did not reach statistical significance in a consistent manner (Table 12.6 and Table 12.7). An analysis statistically combining the individual data from these two trials is underway.

Adverse effects: In the above trial, oral ulcers was the only adverse events of significance noted. However, dyspepsia, liver function test abnormalities, rashes, hair loss, teratogenicity, and pulmonary allergic reactions may occur (Table 12.5).

Evidence summary: Silver

Two RCTs showed some evidence for clinically important improvement in clinical endpoints and in one study for diffusing capacity.

Table 12.6 Primary outcome measures at 12 months for completers (Pope *et al*, 2001)[7]

Differences	Placebo	MTX	p-value
Modified Rodnan skin score (0–78)	−1·1	−6·3	< 0·17
UCLA skin score (0–30)	−0·3	−2·1	< 0·15
MD global (0–10)	−0·3	−0·9	< 0·035

Recommendation for case presentation
The patient in the case presented had early disease and one could safely assume that there would be some immunologically mediated effects ongoing. Methotrexate might be a good choice to use in this patient, with appropriate cautions regarding the potential adverse pulmonary effects of methotrexate.

Stem cell transplantation

Stem cell transplantation (SCT) has been done in more than 70 patients with the most severe, progressive form of systemic sclerosis (unpublished). This procedure uses high dose cyclophosphamide (120–200 mg/kg) plus anti-thymocyte globulin with or without total body irradiation and represents extremely aggressive immunosuppressive therapy. Among these patients there was some response in 69% of a published 41 patient cohort derived from the European Bone Marrow Transplant Registry while worsening occurred in 7% and there was a 17% transplant-related mortality.[8]

Among 19 patients in an open pilot study by McSweeney *et al*, patients who survived SCT had an impressive nearly 90% improvement in the Health Assessment Questionnaire Disability Index, which measures functions and activities of daily living.[9] There was also a 39% improvement in skin score.

Adverse effects: The mortality of SCT in SSC is 10–15% secondary to the profound immunosuppression associated with this treatment. Infections, direct treatment-related toxicity such as pulmonary fibrosis, or secondary effects such as myelodysplasia or post-transplant lymphoproliferative disorder have been documented.

Table 12.7 Secondary outcome measures at 12 months using I-T-T and *LOCF* (Pope *et al*, 2001)[7]

Differences	Placebo	MTX	p-value
Modified Rodnan skin score (0–78)	+1·8	−4·1	< 0·09
UCLA skin score (0–30)	+1·3	−1·3	< 0·04
MD global (0–10)	−0·2	−0·2	< 0·28
Patient global (0–10)	−0·4	0·0	< 0·58
DLCO (%)	−7·7	−3·7	< 0·03

Evidence summary: Bronze

Two case series (total 60 patients) found 39–69% improved.

Recommendation for case presentation
The patient presented had not been tried on other medications and, given the potential toxicities of this therapy and the lack of a controlled trial, stem cell transplantation would be an inappropriate therapy to choose.

Bovine type I collagen:

Benefits: Oral bovine type I collagen is being used as a toleragen, attempting to downregulate the immune response against collagen. McKown *et al* gave 500 mg daily oral bovine type I collagen to 19 SSc patients (15 with diffuse disease, 4 with limited disease) in an open, pilot study.[10] Both interferon-gamma and soluble IL-2R decreased over 12 months while the modified Rodnan Skin Score improved by 22·9% ($p < 0.005$) and diffusing capacity improved by nearly 10% ($p < 0.01$). These biologic and clinical responses in the open study have led to an ongoing, double blind, placebo controlled,

Table 12.8 Number needed to harm for dexamethasone versus placebo (Sharada, 1994)[11]

Outcome	% with placebo	% with dexamethasone	Relative risk with dexamethasone (95% CI)	Absolute risk increase (95% CI)	NNH (95% CI)
Patients with infection	6/18 (33%)	12/17 (71%)	2·12 (1·03, 4·36)	38% (4, 61)	2 (1, 23)

multicentre trial which should be completed by early 2004.

Adverse effects: No specific toxicities were mentioned in the published article.

Evidence summary: Bronze

Open study of 19 patients found improvement in skin score and diffusing capacity.

Recommendation for case presentation

This therapy is experimental and unproven in well controlled trials, making it inappropriate for use in our patient at this time.

Dexamethasone

Benefits: Corticosteroids are potent anti-inflammatory medications and Sharada *et al* compared 100 mg dexamethasone IV pulses to placebo, monthly for six months.[11] Seventeen patients with diffuse SSc received dexamethasone compared to 18 patients receiving placebo. Total skin score decreased from 32·9 to 28·4 ($p < 0·05$) in the dexamethasone group and increased from 30·6 to 34·7 in the placebo-treated patients ($p = 0·003$). A number of other measures changed in both groups but no direct comparisons were made between the dexamethasone-treated and placebo-treated patients, making the study uninterpretable. Other trials using dexamethasone in selected patients with systemic sclerosis may be justified.

Adverse effects: Dexamethasone's side effects and the possibility that corticosteroids might increase the incidence of scleroderma renal crisis must make one cautious (Table 12.8).

Evidence summary: Bronze

Although this study was a double-blind, placebo controlled randomised study, the only comparisons that were made were within groups. General perusal of the data indicated that it is unlikely that there were differences between the two groups, although it was not formally tested. The study's quality is hampered by the low number of patients, poor patient description and analysis only within patient groups, thus not allowing a true between group comparison.

Recommendation for case presentation

The data does not support the use of dexamethasone in our patient.

Preventing vascular damage

Case presentation

This 55-year-old woman has had limited systemic sclerosis (affecting her fingers, hands, forearm, and face) for 15 years. Her principal problem has been Raynaud's phenomenon, with occasional finger ulcerations but no gangrene. Gastrointestinal symptoms have included ongoing dyspepsia and mild dysphagia, reasonably controlled with proton pump inhibitors. Over the last 6 months she has had a dry cough and has felt mildly short of breath, although she can still climb three flight of stairs before she has to stop secondary to dyspnoea on exertion. Her haemoglobin is 13·0. Her FVC is 65% of predicted, the DLCO is 55% of predicted. Echocardiogram reveals a peak systolic pulmonary artery pressure of 35 mmHg with an ejection fraction of 62%. A VQ lung scan reveals low probability for pulmonary emboli.

What therapy is appropriate for the patient's pulmonary disease?

Epoprostenol (prostacyclin)

Benefits: Wax *et al*'s open study of 16 patients with primary pulmonary hypertension demonstrated a 23% improvement in the 6 minute walking test over 27 months. There were no deaths, implying improved survival, although no specifics were given and no comparison was made to a control population.[13] Badesch *et al*'s randomised study supported these findings in a group of patients with SSc. Six minute walking distance improved by 17% among the 55 epoprostenol treated patients and declined by 29% among the placebo treated group ($p < 0{\cdot}001$)[12] (Tables 12.9 and 12.10).

This therapy is appropriate for patients with severe pulmonary hypertension, as severe pulmonary hypertension has a very poor prognosis. Our patient has borderline pulmonary hypertension by echocardiogram. It would be appropriate to ask the patient to undergo a right heart catheterisation to prove whether or not she does, in fact, have pulmonary hypertension. Epoprostenol, with its need for continuous monitoring and intravenous infusion, would not be appropriate for this patient at this point. However, the prognosis for pulmonary hypertension in systemic sclerosis is poor, requiring very close follow up and keeping the option of epoprostenol in mind.

Adverse effects: The toxicity of continuous epoprostenol given as an IV infusion includes headache, jaw pain, nausea, abdominal cramps, and vomiting as well as pump malfunction, thrombosis or sepsis, while sudden discontinuation can result in pulmonary oedema within several hours.[14]

Evidence summary:

Silver

An RCT of 111 patients found improvement in walking distance.

Bronze

An open study in 16 patients showed better survival than predicted for patients with pulmonary hypertension receiving continuous intravenous prostacyclin. Toxicity is a concern.

The next two studies are included in this review, but are placed in the "Excluded" category because they do not separate the SSc patients from their overall analysis.

Treprostinil (Excluded)

Benefits: Treprostinil is a more stable prostacyclin analogue with a longer half-life than epoprostenol; it is administered as a subcutaneous infusion rather than as an intravenous infusion. Simonneau *et al* followed 470 patients with primary pulmonary hypertension or pulmonary hypertension secondary to connective tissue disease (58%), congenital heart disease with pulmonary shunts (22–25%) or pulmonary hypertension secondary to connective tissue disease (17–20% but not subgrouped by SSC) in a randomised, placebo controlled, double blind study.[15] After 12 weeks, the 6 minute walking distance was increased by a median of 10 metres in the treprostinil group compared with a decrease of six meters in the placebo group, a statistically significant but not very impressive change ($p < 0{\cdot}006$). On the other hand, this study demonstrated a significant improvement in the Borg dyspnoea index over 12 weeks and there was significant improvement in mean pulmonary artery pressure and pulmonary vascular resistance.

Table 12.9 Number needed to treat for epoprostenol versus placebo (Badesch, 2000)[12]

Outcome	% with placebo	% with epoprostenol	Relative risk with epoprostenol (95% CI)	Absolute benefit increase (95% CI)	NNT (95% CI)
Improved NYHA functional class	0/55 0%	21/56 38%	Not calculated	38% (24, 51)	3 (2, 5)
Pallor	29/55 53%	18/56 32%	0·61 (0·18, 0·98)	21% (2, 37)	5 (3, 45)

Table 12.10 Number needed to harm for epoprostenol versus placebo (Badesch, 2000)[12]

Outcome	% with placebo	% with epoprostenol	Relative risk of harm with epoprostenol (95% CI)	Absolute risk increase (95% CI)	NNH (95% CI)
Anorexia	26/55 47%	37/56 66%	1·40 (1·00, 1·96)	19% (0·4, 36)	5 (2, 24)
Nausea	9/55 16%	23/56 41%	2·51 (1·28, 4·93)	25% (8, 40)	4 (2, 12)
Diarrhoea	3/55 5%	28/56 50%	9·17 (2·96, 28·41)	45% (29, 58)	2 (1, 4)
Jaw pain	0/55 0%	42/56 75%	Not calculated	75% (60, 85)	1 (1, 1)

Adverse effects: Infusion site pain occurred in 85% of patients and led to discontinuation in 8%. Rare gastrointestinal haemorrhage was noted.

Evidence summary: Silver

This large study found improvement in walking distance, dyspnoea index, mean pulmonary pressure, and pulmonary vascular resistance in patients with pulmonary hypertension. Because it was not possible to examine patients who had SSc *per se*, it is not possible to say whether this therapy is effective in SSc patients.

Recommendation for case presentation

Like epoprostenol, this therapy should not be used in the patient described without further workup. This treatment, furthermore, has not been analysed in the SSc subset of patients, making it a less desirable alternative to epoprostenol at this time, based on the principle of evidence-based medicine.

Bosentan (Excluded)

Benefits: Endothelin-1 is a potent endogenous vasoconstrictor and smooth muscle nitrogen and bosentan is an oral endothelin antagonist, blocking endothelin-1 receptors[16,17] in primary pulmonary hypertension. A published case series demonstrated a 70 m increase in the 6 minute walking time in the bosentan group versus a 6 m decrease in the control group ($p = 0{\cdot}021$). Significant decreases in pulmonary artery pressure and pulmonary vascular resistance were shown in the bosentan versus placebo groups. Five of 27 patients (16%) had systemic sclerosis (one in the control group and four in the bosentan group).

A randomised, double blind, placebo controlled study of pulmonary hypertension, among which 20% of the patients had SSc, was published by Rubin *et al* in 2002.[18] Bosentan 125 or 250 mg orally twice daily was used in 144 patients and was compared to placebo in 69 patients, over 16 weeks. The 6 minute walking time remained stable in the scleroderma patients treated with bosentan (+3 m) and declined by 40 m in the group given placebo (no p value stated). At 28 weeks, 89% of the mixed group of patients given bosentan remained stable compared to 63% in the placebo treated patients ($p = 0{\cdot}002$).

Adverse effects: Liver function test abnormalities were found in approximately 30% of patients but were easily reversible, making it important to appropriately follow patients treated with this medication.

Recommendation for case presentation
While this therapy has only been approved in severe pulmonary hypertension, should our patient have even moderate pulmonary hypertension, given the poor prognosis of this complication of SSc (and despite the liver toxicity associated with this drug), one would be tempted to use this medication.

Evidence summary: Silver
Two RCTs with a total of 171 patients with pulmonary hypertension, of whom 16–20% had SSC, show improved walking time and, in the smaller RCT, improved pulmonary artery pressure and pulmonary vascular resistance.

Angiotensin-converting enzyme inhibitors (ACE inhibitors)

Benefits: Scleroderma renal crisis (SRC) was a leading cause of death in systemic sclerosis before ACE inhibitors were widely used. Early case reports and patient series of ACE inhibitor use in SRC in the 1980s documented improved survival.[19–21] A large prospective, observational cohort study done by Steen *et al* between 1972 and 1987 in 108 SRC patients showed a very impressive one-year cumulative survival difference of 61% (15% of 53 SSc patients not receiving ACE inhibitors survived and 76% of 58 patients using ACE inhibitors). During follow up of 145 SSc patients who developed renal crisis (which was defined as the new onset of severe hypertension associated with an increased serum creatinine >2 mg/dl, microangiopathic haemolytic anaemia or both), 90% of the group who did not require dialysis were alive after 5 years and 80–85% were still surviving after 8 years.[22] Fifty-five per cent of 62 patients who initially required dialysis were able to discontinue dialysis permanently while taking ACE inhibitors, although discontinuation required up to 18 months. Unfortunately, no randomised controlled studies have been done with this compound and it is unlikely that they will be done, for ethical reasons.

Adverse effects: The incidence of adverse effects was not detailed in the articles. In general, ACE inhibitors may be associated with headaches, postural changes, fatigue, sleepiness, nausea, and cough.

Evidence summary: Silver
A cohort study of 108 patients found improved survival and 55% of patients on dialysis were able to discontinue dialysis permanently while taking ACE inhibitors.

Recommendation for case presentation
There is no data that prophylactic ACE inhibitors prevent the occurrence of scleroderma renal crisis. Despite this, some rheumatologists use inhibitors in a "prophylactic" manner. This patient has no evidence of incipient renal disease and no hypertension so that it would not be appropriate to use inhibitors prophylactically.

Antiplatelet medications

Benefits: Aspirin and dipyridamole were originally aimed at preventing vascular damage associated with thromboses in SSc. A 1984, small, double blind trial did not show any positive results in SSc, perhaps due to the small number of patients analysed and to possible patient selection bias.[23]

Adverse effects: No adverse events were reported in the small trial described above.

Evidence summary: Silver

A small RCT showed no benefit.

Inhibition of fibrosis

N-acetylcysteine

Benefits: One of the earlier, double blind, randomised, placebo controlled trials in systemic sclerosis was published in 1979. It used N-acetylcysteine versus placebo in 22 systemic sclerosis patients.[24] The outcome variables remained unchanged after one year, possibly because patients had long disease duration (mean disease duration of approximately 9 years); the patients were a mixed group of limited and diffuse SSc patients and the study was statistically underpowered, with only 22 patients. This trial taught the rheumatology community that it was possible to do placebo controlled trials in systemic sclerosis disease.

Adverse effects: None have been described.

Evidence summary: Silver

A small RCT showed no benefit.

Gamma-interferon

Gamma-interferon is produced by activated T cells and activates macrophages as well as being a potent inhibitor of collagen synthesis. Grasseger *et al* published a small randomised, underpowered, controlled trial using gamma-interferon in 1998.[25] Despite 2 years of trying to recruit SSc patients with disease duration < 3 years, only 63% of the required patients were entered into the study. Among the 27 patients treated with gamma-interferon (100 micrograms three times per weeks), skin score decreased by 0·17 out of a maximum change in skin score of 3·0, compared to a decrease of 0·03 among the 17 control patients (not statistically different). The treatment group had a higher baseline skin score than the control group and numbers were too small, so the results must be considered as inconclusive, rather than definitively negative. Ziesche *et al* completed a pilot study in 18 patients who had idiopathic pulmonary fibrosis.[26] In this open study nine patients received oral prednisolone alone (7·5 mg daily, which could be increased to 15 mg daily) and nine received 200 micrograms interferon gamma weekly plus 7·5 mg prednisolone daily. Total lung capacity increased by 9% after 12 months in the gamma-interferon plus prednisolone group and decreased 4% in the control group ($p < 0·001$).

Adverse effects: Cytokine reactions occurred to varying degrees in nearly 85% of the patients in the Grasseger *et al* study and were also common in the Ziesche *et al* study.[25,26] Overall, this compound should be further studied, although its toxicity profile does not bode well for its success as a DMARD in SSc.

Evidence summary: Silver

One small RCT showed inconclusive results.

Alpha-interferon

Alpha-interferon has also been tried in systemic sclerosis. In a placebo controlled, 1 year study by Black *et al* ($n = 35$) usual doses of interferon-alpha (13·5 million units weekly) did less well than placebo at 6–12 months.[27] Skin score improved by 4·5 units in the placebo group versus 1·70 units in the interferon-alpha group while forced vital capacity worsened by 1·3% in the placebo group versus worsening by 8·2% in the interferon-alpha treated patients ($p < 0{\cdot}001$). Interferon-alpha seems to have little value for the treatment of systemic sclerosis.

Adverse effects: There was no discussion of adverse events.

Evidence summary: Silver

A small RCT showed no benefit.

D-penicillamine

D-penicillamine, at least *in vitro*, has both antifibrotic and immunosuppressive properties. A randomised, double blind, multicentre study of D-penicillamine in 134 patients with early diffuse SSc compared 62·5 mg daily D-penicillamine ($n = 68$) to 750 mg ($n = 68$).daily D-penicillamine.[28] Only 32 high dose and 36 low dose patients completed the 24 month trial, and there were no differences found in skin score, incidence of real crisis or mortality. Although not placebo controlled, this trial makes it very unlikely that D-penicillamine is effective in systemic sclerosis.

Adverse effects: Rash, thrombocytopenia, leucopenia, proteinuria, stomatitis, loss of sense of taste, dyspepsia, and one case of myesthenia gravis were documented. The incidence was so low that no statistics were generated.

Evidence summary: Silver

One RCT showed no benefit.

Relaxin

Relaxin is a protein secreted by the corpus luteum and placenta during pregnancy; it probably has an important role in loosening pelvic structures prior to delivery. It may enhance collagen degradation and inhibit collagen synthesis. These properties seemed to make it an ideal substance to treat systemic sclerosis. A phase II multicentre, randomised, placebo controlled trial in 64 patients showed a significant reduction in skin score at 24 weeks in the group taking 25 micrograms per kilogram relaxin ($p < 0{\cdot}04$), but results were not dose-related, as 100 micrograms per kilogram did not separate from placebo.[29] Unfortunately, a phase III trial, involving 239 patients followed over 10 months, did not show any benefit from relaxin (unpublished). Consequently, it is no longer being developed for the treatment of systemic sclerosis.

Adverse effects: Menorrhagia (19–35% *v* 11% (placebo)) was increased in the treatment groups. Local injection reactions, rash, infection, MI, and tachyarrhythmia each occurred in a very few instances.

Evidence summary: Silver

Two RCTs showed either mixed results or no benefit.

Cyclofenil

This diphenylethylene derivative, related to stilboestrol, may interfere with connective tissue metabolism.[30] Two small trials showed conflicting results.[31,32] Blom-Bulow *et al* tested 27 patients with SSc using cyclofenil versus placebo for one year. They found significant improvement in joint symptoms and possibly oesophageal peristalsis.[32] Another study by Gibson and Graham examined 11 scleroderma patients and failed to show any clinical benefits after a very short 4 month period.[31]

Adverse effects: Both studies suggested that this substance was associated with a more than 30% incidence of abnormally elevated liver enzymes, making cyclofenil too toxic to use at the doses given in the studies.

Evidence summary: Silver

Two RCTs showed conflicting results. Liver toxicity is a concern.

Anti-transforming growth factor beta (anti-TGF-β)

Transforming growth factor beta is probably a central protein in the pathogenesis of systemic sclerosis as it can increase fibroblast proliferation, increase fibrosis, and decrease angiogenesis.[33] Anti-TGF-β IgG4 has been tested in fibrosis, which can occur after glaucoma surgery. In a 3 month, double blind, placebo controlled trial, anti-TGF-β decreased the need for medical treatment after glaucoma surgery.[34] Seventy-five per cent of placebo-treated patients required medication to decrease fibrosis compared to 31% of the anti-TGF-β-treated patients ($p < 0{\cdot}05$). An anti-TGF-β trial in SSc has recently been completed and publication of results is eagerly awaited.[35]

Evidence summary: Silver

An RCT is completed and the results are awaited.

Miscellaneous agents

Potassium aminobenzoate (POTABA)

The mechanism of action by which POTABA was supposed to be associated with skin softening is unknown. While a retrospective study of 224 scleroderma patients reported skin softening, a multicentre, randomised, placebo controlled, double blind trial of 32 SSc patients taking POTABA versus 44 SSc patients taking placebo did not show any change in skin score after 48 weeks.[36,37] Interestingly, a recent reanalysis of the double blind study, published as an abstract in 2002, indicated decreased mortality in the POTABA-treated patients.[38] The full report should make interesting reading.

Evidence summary: Silver

One RCT showed no benefit in skin score.

Ketotifen

Ketotifen was tested because it is an oral mast cell stabilising agent and could possibly prevent activation of fibroblasts due to inhibition of inflammatory mediators. Gruber *et al* published a randomised, placebo controlled, double blind trial in 24 patients with diffuse SSc.[39] The patients in the ketotifen group had a mean disease duration of 28 months while those in the placebo group had a mean disease duration of 50 months, indicating possible confounding by disease duration. After conclusion of the 6 month study using 3 mg oral ketotifen b.d. versus placebo, there was no significant change in the total skin score (the primary outcome), pulmonary function or global assessment (secondary outcomes), although pruritus was improved.

Evidence summary: Silver

One small RCT showed no benefit in skin score, pulmonary function or gobal assessment; but showed improvement in pruritus.

Antioxidant therapy

Herrick *et al* evaluated a combination of micronutrient antioxidants (selenium, beta-carotene, vitamin C, vitamin E, and methionine) plus allopurinol in patients with limited cutaneous systemic sclerosis.[40] Although designed as a placebo controlled, double blind, crossover study, a carryover effect was detected during analysis and so the data was analysed as a between group comparison of the first 10 week treatment period plus a within group comparison of the first and second 10 week periods in those who received placebo treatment first. Of the 33 patients in this study, no clinical benefits could be demonstrated from active treatment, whether examining von Willebrand's factor, rewarming curve or patient's symptoms. Circulating oxidant levels increased, although there was no fall in free-radical mediated injury, indicating sufficient drug for a biologic effect. This study rules against this mechanism in SSc, although it is possible that an inappropriate dose was selected or that patients with earlier disease were necessary.

Evidence summary: Silver

One RCT showed no benefit.

References

1 Clements PJ, Furst DE. Pathogenesis, Fusion (Summary). *Systemic Sclerosis*. Baltimore: Williams and Wilkins, 1996:274–85.

2 Furst DE, Clements PJ, Hillis S, *et al.* Immunosuppression with chlorambucil, versus placebo, for scleroderma. *Arthritis Rheum* 1989;**32**:584–93.

3 Silver RM, Warrick JH, Kinsella MB, *et al.* Cyclophosphamide and low-dose prednisone therapy in patients with systemic sclerosis (scleroderma) with interstitial lung disease. *J Rheumatol* 1993;**20**:838–44.

4 White B, Moore W, Wigley F, *et al.* Cyclophosphamide is associated with pulmonary function and survival benefit in patients with scleroderma and alveolitis. *Ann Intern Med* 2000;**132**:947–54.

5 Casas JA, Saway PA, Villarreal I, *et al.* 5-Fluorouracil in the treatment of scleroderma: A randomised, double-blind, placebo-controlled international collaborative study. *Ann Rheum Dis* 1990;**49**:926–8.

6 Van den Hoogen FH, Boerbooms AM, Swaak AJ, *et al.* Comparison of methotrexate with placebo in the treatment of systemic sclerosis: a 24 week randomised double-blind trial, followed by a 24 week observational trial. *Br J Rheumatol* 1996;**35**(4):364–72.

7 Pope J, Bellamy N, Seibold J, *et al.* A randomised controlled trial of methotrexate versus placebo in early diffuse scleroderma. *Arthritis Rheum* 2001;**44**:1351–8.

8 Binks M; Passweg JR; Furst D; McSweeney P, *et al.* Phase I/II trial of autologous stem cell transplantation in systemic sclerosis: procedure related mortality and impact on skin disease. *Ann Rheum Dis* 2001;**60**(6):577–84.

9 McSweeney PA, Nash RA, Sullivan KM, *et al.* High-dose immunosuppressive therapy for severe systemic sclerosis: initial outcomes. *Blood* 2002;**100**(5):1602–10.

10 McKown KM, Carbone LD, Bustillo J, *et al.* Induction of immune tolerance to human type I collagen in patients with systemic sclerosis by oral administration of bovine type I collagen. *Arthritis Rheum* 2000;**43**(5):1054–61.

11 A.Sharada, A Kumar, R Kakkar, *et al.* Intravenous dexamethasone pulse therapy in diffuse systemic sclerosis: a randomised placebo-controlled trial. *Rheumatol Int* 1994;**14**:91–4.

12 Badesch DB, Tapson VF, McGoon MD, *et al.* Continuous intravenous epoprostenol for pulmonary hypertension due to the scleroderma spectrum of disease. A randomised, controlled trial. *Ann Intern Med* 2000;**132**(6): 425–34.

13 Wax D, Garofano R, Barst RJ. Effects of long-term infusion of prostacyclin on exercise performance in patients with primary pulmonary hypertension. *Chest* 1999;**116**:914–20.

14 Galie N, Manes A, Branzi A. Medical therapy of pulmonary hypertension. The prostacyclins. *Clin Chest Med* 2001;**22**(3):529–37.

15 Simonneau G, Barst RJ, Galie N, *et al.* Continuous subcutaneous infusion of treprostinil, a prostacyclin analogue, in patients with pulmonary arterial hypertension: a double-blind, randomised, placebo-controlled trial. *Am J Respir Crit Care Med* 2002;**165**(6): 800–4.

16 Rubens C, Ewert R, Halank M, *et al.* Big endothelin-1 and endothelin-1 plasma levels are correlated with the severity of primary pulmonary hypertension. *Chest* 2001;**120**(5):1562–9.

17 Iwabuchi H, Kasama T, Hanaoka R: Downregulation of intercellular adhesion molecule-1 expression on human synovial fibroblasts by endothelin-1. *J Rheumatol* 1999;**26**(3):522–31.

18 Rubin LF, Badesch DB, Barst RJ. Bosentan therapy for pulmonary arterial hypertension. *NEJM* 2002;**346**:896–903.

19 Zawada ET Jr, Clements PJ, Furst DE, *et al.* Clinical course of patients with scleroderma renal crisis treated with captopril. *Nephron* 1981;**27**:74–8.

20 Thurm RH, Alexander JC. Captopril in the treatment of scleroderma renal crisis. *Arch Intern Med* 1984;**144**: 733–55.

21 Beckett VL, Donadio JV, Brennan LA Jr, *et al.* Use of captopril as early therapy for renal scleroderma: A prospective study. *Mayo Clin Proc* 1985;**60**:763.

22 Steen VD, Medsger TA Jr. Long-term outcomes of scleroderma renal crisis. *Ann Intern Med* 2000;**17**:600–3.

23 Beckett VL, Conn DL, Ruster V, *et al.* Trial of platelet-inhibiting drug in scleroderma. Double-blind study with dipyridamole and aspirin. *Arthritis Rheum* 1984;**27**: 1137–43.

24 Furst DE, Clements PJ, Harris R, *et al.* Measurement of clinical change in progressive systemic sclerosis: a 1 year double-blind placebo-controlled trial of N-acetylcysteine. *Ann Rheum Dis* 1979;**38**:356–61.

25 Grassegger A, Schuler G, Hessenberger G, *et al.* Interferon-gamma in the treatment of systemic sclerosis: a randomised controlled multicentre trial. *Br J Dermatol* 1998;**139**:639–48.

26 Ziesche R, Hofbauer E, Wittman K, *et al.* A preliminary study of long-term treatment with interferon gamma-1b and low-dose prednisolone in patients with idiopathic pulmonary fibrosis. *NEJM* 1999;**341**:264–9.

27 Black{incomplete} Interferon-alpha does not improve outcome at one year in patients with diffuse cutaneous scleroderma: results of a randomised, double-blind, placebo-controlled trial. *Arthritis Rheum* 1999;**42**:299–305.

28 Clements PJ, Furst DE, Wong WK, *et al.* High-dose versus low-dose D-penicillamine in early diffuse systemic sclerosis: analysis of a two year, double-blind, randomised, controlled clinical trial. *Arthritis Rheum* 1999;**42**(6):1194–203.

29 Seibold JR, Korn JH, Simms R, *et al.* Recombinant Human Relaxin in the Treatment of Scleroderma; a randomised, double-blind, placebo controlled trial. *Ann Intern Med* 2000;**32**:871–9.

30 Williams HJ, Furst DE, Dahl SL, *et al.* Double-blind, multi-center controlled trial comparing topical dimethyl sulfoxide and normal saline for treatment of hand ulcers in patients with systemic sclerosis. *Arthritis Rheum* 1985,**28**:308–14.

31 Gibson T, Graham R. Cyclofenil treatment of scleroderma – a controlled study. *Br J Rheumatol* 1983;**22**:218–23.

32 Blom-Bulow B, Berg K, Wilhelm RA, *et al.* Cyclofenil versus placebo in progressive systemic sclerosis. A one-year double-blind crossover study of 27 patients. *Acta Med Scand* 1981;**210**:419–28.

33 Denton CP, Abraham DJ. Transforming growth factor-beta and connective tissue growth factor: key cytokines in scleroderma pathogenesis. *Curr Opin* 2001;**13**(6): 505–11.

34 Siriwardena D, Khaw PT, King AJ, *et al.* Human antitransforming growth factor beta(2) monoclonal antibody – a new modulator of wound healing in trabeculectomy: a randomised placebo controlled clinical study. *Ophthalmology* 2002;**109**:427–31.

35 Furst D. Personal communication, 2003.

36 Zarafonetis CJD, Dubach L, Skovronski JJ, *et al.* Retrospective studies in scleroderma: skin response to para-aminobenzoate therapy. *Clin Exp Rheumatol* 1988;**6**:261–8.

37 Clegg DO, Reading JC, Mayes MD, *et al.* Comparison of aminobenzoate potassium and placebo in the treatment of scleroderma. *J Rheumatol* 1994;**21**:105–10. 1994.

38 Cannella AC, Reading JC, Clegg DO. Aminobenzoate potassium improves mortality in patients with scleroderma. *Arth Rheum* 2003;**46**(Suppl):s358.

39 Gruber BL, Kaufman LD: A double-blind randomised controlled trial of ketotifen versus placebo in early diffuse scleroderma. *Arthritis Rheum* 1991;**34**:362–5.

40 Herrick AL, Hollis S, Schofield D, *et al.* A double-blind, placebo-controlled trial of antioxidant therapy in limited cutaneous sclerosis. *Clin Exper Rheum* 2000;**18**:349–56.

Raynaud's phenomenon in systemic sclerosis

Introduction

Scleroderma is a rare connective tissue disease with abnormal blood vessels, autoimmunity, and fibrosis. Raynaud's phenomenon (RP) is a common feature in scleroderma. It occurs in more than 90% of patients.[41] Raynaud's is defined by a vasospastic disorder with pallor and then cyanosis and/or rubor upon rewarming. RP associated with a connective tissue disease is called secondary. It is not associated with any other illness, it is called primary Raynaud's phenomenon or Raynaud's syndrome. The data in this chapter will deal only with Raynaud's phenomenon associated with scleroderma.

The complications of RP include pain, ischaemic damage, and injury, including digital tuft reabsorption and digital ulcers. In worst case scenarios gangrene and auto-amputation or surgical amputation can occur. The questions are do non-pharmacological interventions help in Raynaud's? Is there data to support treatments such as calcium channel blockers and other vasodilators in the treatment of scleroderma-associated RP?

We searched the Cochrane database and the published literature for randomised controlled trials of subjects with scleroderma studying specific outcomes with respect to Raynaud's phenomenon. The strongest evidence was obtained from randomised controlled trials, and pooled randomised controlled trials (such as meta-analyses) yielded even higher ranking evidence. Non-randomised, observational or uncontrolled trials were not included in this analysis. Trials were included if the majority of patients had scleroderma-associated RP (>75%) or if patients with secondary RP (associated with other disease) and primary RP were combined within one trial but the data on the scleroderma subjects could be extracted. The trials had to be at least one-day duration with a drop-out rate of < 30%. The trials did not have to be blinded but did have to be randomised and controlled by placebo or another intervention. In general the trials were small and without proper methodology (that is, crossover designs with no attempt to determine whether carry over occurred, thus biasing the results of the second treatment).

Outcomes

The outcome measurements included: decreased frequency of Raynaud's attacks; decreased severity of attacks; the prevention and healing of digital ulcers; global indices; and other parameters, such as skin temperature and digital artery pressure.

Evaluating the evidence

The data presented include meta-analyses and randomised controlled trials of the treatment of RP in scleroderma. A case presentation is provided to demonstrate how the information could be clinically used within an individual patient with scleroderma.

Case presentation

A 48-year-old woman with 8 years of limited systemic scleroderma (CREST syndrome) has at least four Raynaud's attacks per week. They are rated as very painful. She currently has a digital ulcer on her fingertip and last year required surgical intervention with an amputation on a different finger due to a severe digital ulcer that was not healing and became gangrenous. She is a smoker.

Question 3

What is the evidence of healing or preventing digital ulcers in scleroderma-associated Raynaud's phenomenon?

Question 4

What would be the best treatment in this woman?

There is evidence that many vasodilators, in particular the calcium channel blockers, can decrease the frequency and severity of Raynaud's attacks. In addition, prostacyclins may enhance digital ulcer healing or prevent new digital ulcers. There are no randomised controlled trials on surgical interventions such as sympathectomies. There is no evidence from randomised controlled trials for smoking cessation. Emerging therapies with endothelin receptor blockers may prevent the occurrence of new digital ulcers.

Non-pharmacological interventions

There are no randomised controlled trials of smoking cessation in Raynaud's phenomenon associated with scleroderma. Therefore, the evidence was not evaluated for the purposes of this chapter.

Evidence summary

No Gold or Platinum evidence was found.

Biofeedback

One RCT of biofeedback in subjects with RP secondary to scleroderma was conducted, in which two men and 22 women with scleroderma and RP were randomised to one of three treatment groups: (1) finger temperature biofeedback; (2) autogenic training; and (3) EMG feedback (to control for the effects of receiving any physiological feedback and to assess relaxation). Results indicated that only subjects in the temperature feedback group demonstrated a temperature feedback (the mean increase was 0·50°C, $p < 0{\cdot}05$). There was no significant clinical improvement in finger temperature, vasospastic attack frequency, and stress ratings in any of the treatment groups.[42]

Evidence summary: Silver

One RCT did not find that biofeedback was a successful intervention to control Raynaud's attacks.

Calcium channel blockers

Calcium channel blockers (CCBs) are the most studied treatments of scleroderma-associated RP, especially nifedipine.

Dimethyl sulfoxide (DMSO)

DMSO was tested in systemic sclerosis because it was said to solubilise collagen. It was tested in 84 SSc patients for its ability to heal digital skin ulcers in a double blind, randomised trial comparing 0·85% normal saline, 2% DMSO and 70% DMSO.[30] Although pain from digital ulcers was improved in a subset of patients, there were no statistically significant changes found in other parameters, such as ulcer healing.

Adverse effects: More than 25% of the patients treated with the high dose DMSO were withdrawn secondary to significant, local skin toxicity.

Evidence summary: Silver

One RCT showed mixed benefit results and significant local skin toxicity.

Outcomes

The outcomes that are best studied are of reducing the frequency and severity of attacks. Thompson *et al* performed a meta-analysis of calcium channel blockers used to decrease the frequency and severity of Raynaud's attacks in patients with scleroderma.[43] The meta-analysis included 8 RCTs ($n = 109$). Six of 8 compared nifedipine (variable doses to a maximum of 30 mg o.d.) to placebo and two studied nifedipine versus active treatment with either

Table 12.11 Number needed to treat for calcium channel blockers versus placebo (pooled data, Thompson *et al*[43]

Outcome	Weighted mean difference (WMD) (95% CI)	Pooled standardized mean difference (95% CI)	% Benefiting (95% CI) with calcium channel blocker	NNT (95% CI)
Reduction in frequency of attacks (all calcium channel blockers – 6 trials)	−4·85 (−10·17, 0·47)	−0·45 (−0·82, −0·08)	21% (4–37)	5 (3, 26)
Reduction in frequency of Attacks (nifedipine – 5 trials)	−0·80 (−1·70, 0·10)	−0·51 (−0·94, −0·08)	24% (4–41)	5 (3, 26)
Reduction in severity of attacks (all calcium channel blockers – 3 trials)	−5·23 (−11·58, 1·13)	−0·69 (−1·21, −0·17)	32% (8–50)	4 (3, 13)
Reduction in severity of attacks (nifedipine – 2 trials)	−1·50 (−3·49, 0·48)	−0·99 (−1·74, −0·24)	43% (12–61)	3 (2, 9)

losartan (ARB) or IV iloprost. The exposure time to treatment was from 1 to 16 weeks and 7 were crossover designs. Primary outcome measurements included frequency and severity of attacks, digital skin temperature, digital ulcers, and physician and patient global assessments. The weighted mean difference (WMD) or standardised mean difference (SMD) was calculated for each continuous outcome variable (Table 12.11 and Figure 12.1).

Benefits: Results indicated that in six trials of all CCBs versus placebo and five trials of nifedipine alone versus placebo, the WMD for the reduction in frequency of ischaemic attacks over a 2-week period was −4·85 (−10·17, 0·47) and −0·80 (−1·70, 0·10), respectively. For the reduction of severity of attacks, the SMD for three trials for all CCBs versus placebo was −0·69 (95% CI: −1·21, −0·17) and for two trials of nifedipine alone versus placebo was −0·99 (95% CI: −1·74,−0·24), with an overall decrease in severity of 35% during a 2 week period[43] (Table 12.11).

Adverse effects: None of the trials included directly studied the occurrence of adverse effects. Other studies have reported effects such as hypotension, dizziness, flushing, oedema, and headaches [44,45]

Evidence summary: Silver

There is Silver evidence that calcium channel blockers are effective in the short term in reducing frequency and severity of symptoms of RP in subjects with scleroderma.

Recommendation for case presentation

This treatment is favourable for this patient and should be recommended as an option.

Reduction of frequency of attacks may be the only clinically relevant outcome (Figure 12.1).

Prostacyclins

Both intravenous and oral prostacyclins have been studied in randomised controlled trials in scleroderma-associated RP. The intravenous preparations have more bioavailability, and thus combining (in another analysis) oral and IV preparations may reduce the overall efficacy that is found in these studies.

In a meta-analysis, Pope *et al* investigated the efficacy of prostaglandin analogues compared to placebo for seven RCTs (n = 332).[46] Five of the trials had a parallel design, five studied IV iloprost, one studied oral iloprost and another oral

Comparison: 01 Calcium Channel Blockers *v* placebo
Outcome: 01 frequency of attacks

Study	Treatment n	Treatment mean (sd)	Control n	Control mean (sd)	Weight %	WMD (95% CI Random)
Ettinger 1984	8	29·00 (29·05)	8	36·60 (25·85)	3·5	−7.60 [−34·55, 19·35]
Kahan 1983	10	10·40 (16·13)	10	28·10 (15·50)	10·7	−17·70 [−31·57, −3·83]
Kahan 1985 (a)	7	10·29 (8·24)	7	18·00 (5·91)	21·8	−7·71 [−15·22, −0·20]
Kahan 1987	15	25·80 (17·35)	15	30·60 (14·00)	14·1	−4·80 [−16·08, 6·48]
Rodeheffer 1983	9	13·11 (15·20)	9	15·00 (12·57)	11·8	−1·89 [−14·78, 11·00]
Thomas 1987	10	1·30 (1·22)	10	1·60 (0·87)	38·1	−0·30 [−1·23, 0·63]
Total (95% CI)	59		59		100·0	−4·85 [−10·17, 0·47]

Chi-square 10·49 (df = 5) P: 0·06 Z = 1·79 P: 0·07

−10 −5 0 5 10
Favours treatment Favours control

Comparison: 01 Calcium Channel Blockers *v* placebo
Outcome: 02 severity of attacks

Study	Treatment n	Treatment mean (sd)	Control n	Control mean (sd)	Weight %	WMD (95% CI Random)
Kahan 1985 (a)	7	3·58 (2·08)	7	6·31 (1·57)	15·5	−2.73 [−4·66, −0·80]
Kahan 1987	15	1·93 (0·80)	15	2·20 (0·41)	46·9	−0·27 [−0·72, 0·18]
Rodeheffer 1983	9	−1·33 (1·00)	9	−0·66 (0·70)	37·6	−0·67 [−1·47, 0·13]
Total (95% CI)	31		31		100·0	−0·80 [−1·70, 0·10]

Chi-square 6·25 (df = 2) P: 0·04 Z = 1·74 P: 0·08

−10 −5 0 5 10
Favours treatment Favours control

Comparison: 02 Nifedipine *v* placebo
Outcome: 01 frequency of attacks

Study	Treatment n	Treatment mean (sd)	Control n	Control mean (sd)	Weight %	WMD (95% CI Random)
Ettinger 1984	8	29·00 (29·05)	8	36·60 (25·85)	4·9	−7.60 [−34·55, 19·35]
Kahan 1983	10	10·40 (16·13)	10	28·10 (15·50)	13·8	−17·70 [−31·57, −3·83]
Kahan 1985 (a)	7	10·29 (8·24)	7	18·00 (5·91)	25·9	−7·71 [−15·22, −0·20]
Rodeheffer 1983	9	13·11 (15·20)	9	15·00 (12·57)	15·2	−1·89 [−14·78, 11·00]
Thomas 1987	10	1·30 (1·22)	10	1·60 (1·22)	40·2	−0·30 [−1·23, 0·63]
Total (95% CI)	44		44		100·0	−5·23 [−11·58, 1·13]

Chi-square 9·94 (df = 4) P: 0·04 Z = 1·61 P: 0·11

−10 −5 0 5 10
Favours treatment Favours control

Comparison: 02 Nifedipine *v* placebo
Outcome: 02 severity of attacks

Study	Treatment n	Treatment mean (sd)	Control n	Control mean (sd)	Weight %	WMD (95% CI Random)
Kahan 1985 (a)	7	3·58 (2·08)	7	6·31 (1·57)	40·5	−2.73 [−4·66, −0·80]
Rodeheffer 1983	9	−1·33 (1·00)	9	−0·66 (0·70)	59·5	−0·67 [−1·47, 0·13]
Total (95% CI)	16		16		100·0	−1·50 [−3·49, 0·48]

Chi-square 3·74 (df = 1) P: 0·05 Z = 1·49 P: 0·14

−10 −5 0 5 10
Favours treatment Favours control

Figure 12.1 From Thompson *et al.*[43]

Table 12.12 Number needed to treat for IV iloprost versus placebo (Pope *et al*, 2002)[46]

Outcome	% Improved with placebo	% Improved with IV iloprost	Relative risk of improvement with IV iloprost (95% CI)	Absolute benefit increase (95% CI)	NNT (95% CI)
Number of digital ulcers Healed (one trial)	0/4 (0%)	6/7 (86%)	Not calculated	86% (24, 97)	2 (2, 5)
Physican global Assessment (one trial)	17/60 (28%)	32/62 (52%)	1·82 (1·14–2·91)	23 % (6, 39)	5 (13,17)

Table 12.13 Number needed to harm for IV iloprost versus placebo (Pooled Data, Pope *et al*, 2002)[46]

Outcome	% with placebo	IV IL % with iloprost	Relative risk with IV iloprost (95% CI)	Absolute risk increase (95% CI)	NNH (95% CI)
Side effects (not specified) in meta-analysis) (2 studies)	29/84 (35%)	72/82 (88%)	2·54 (1·87, 3·45)	53% (40, 64)	1 (1, 2)

Table 12.14 Number needed to treat oral iloprost 50 μg versus placebo (Black *et al*,1998)[47]

Outcome	Pooled standardized mean difference (95% CI)	% Benefiting (95% CI)	NNT (95% CI)
Frequency of attacks 12 wks	−0·78 (−1·32, −0·23)	35% (11–53)	3 (2–9)
Total daily duration of attacks 12 wks	−0·80 (−1·35, −0·26)	36% (13– 53)	3 (2–8)

cisaprost. Relative risks (RR) were determined for dichotomous variables and a WMD for continuous variables[46] (Tables 12.12 and 12.13). A more recent study of oral iloprost (50 or 100 micrograms twice daily for 6 weeks) compared to placebo was conducted by Black *et al* (n = 103 subjects with RP and SSc)[47] (Tables 12.14 and 12.15).

Benefits: For the iloprost versus placebo trials included in the Cochrane analysis, the severity of attacks decreased by a WMD of −0·69 (95% CI: −1·12, −0·26), $p < 0·05$; while the frequency of attacks was decreased by a WMD of −0·80 (95% CI: −4·71, 3·11), however, the decrease was not statistically significant. IV Iloprost was more effective than both oral iloprost and oral Cisaprost.[46]

In the trial conducted by Black *et al*, at 6 weeks the frequency ($p < 0·07$), total daily duration (40% shorter for iloprost 50 micrograms, 35% shorter for 100 micrograms; compared to 10% longer for placebo, $p < 0·03$), and severity ($p < 0·07$) of Raynaud's attacks were decreased in the groups taking active oral iloprost.[47] Thus only duration of attacks was statistically significant in this study of oral iloprost at 6 weeks. However, at the end of follow up (12 weeks), the total daily duration of attacks (60% shorter for iloprost 50 micrograms and 100 micrograms compared to 9% shorter for placebo, $p < 0·001$), frequency ($p < 0·07$), and severity (46% less severe for iloprost 50 micrograms, 50% less severe for 100 micrograms, compared to 15% less severe for placebo, $p < 0·007$) of attacks were all decreased[47] (Tables 12.14 and 12.15).

Treatment with cisaprost showed no significant benefit over placebo, with none of the outcome

Table 12.15 Number needed to treat oral iloprost 100 μg versus placebo (Black *et al*,1998)[47]

Outcome	Pooled standardized mean difference (95% CI)	% Benefiting (95% CI)	NNT (95% CI)
Frequency of attacks 12 wks	−0·88 (−1·43, −0·33)	39% (16–55)	3 (2–7)
Total daily duration of attacks 12 wks	−0·95 (−1·51, −0·39)	42% (19– 57)	3 (2–6)

Table 12.16 Number needed to harm oral iloprost 50 μg versus placebo (Black *et al*, 1998)[47]

Outcome	% with placebo	% with iloporst 50 mg	Relative risk of outcome with iloprost 50 mg (95% CI)	Absolute risk increase	NNH (95% CI)
Treatment discontinuation due to adverse event	2/35 (6%)	9/33 (27%)	4·77 (1·11, 20·48)	22% (4, 39)	4 (2, 26)

Table 12.17 Number needed to harm oral iloprost 100 μg versus placebo (Black *et al*,1998)[47]

Outcome	% with placebo	% with iloprost 100 mg	Relative risk of outcome with iloprost 100 mg (95% CI)	Absolute risk increase	NNH (95% CI)
Any adverse event (most frequent headache, flushing, nausea, flu)	28/35 (80%)	34/35 (97%)	1·21 (1·02, 1·45)	17% (2, 33)	5 (3, 55)
Treatment discontinuation due to adverse event	2/35 (6%)	18/34 (53%)	9·00 (2·26, 35·91)	47% (27, 63)	2 (1, 3)

measurements reaching a statistical significance at the $p < 0{\cdot}05$ level.

Adverse effects: Adverse effects were reported by 85% of subjects on iloprost 50 micrograms, 97% on iloprost 100 micrograms, and by 80% of subjects taking placebo[47] (Tables 12.16 and 12.17).

Prostaglandin E_1 (Excluded)

In a placebo controlled trial of prostaglandin E_1 (PGE_1) in 55 RP patients (31 with SSc), excluded from the Cochrane analysis (because data for subgroups were presented as combined), Mohrland *et al* observed that PGE_1 (10 ng/kg/min) administered intravenously over 72 hours resulted in a significant reduction of the number of daily attacks immediately following infusion in patients with primary RP compared to placebo; however, this reduction was not significant in patients with secondary RP when compared with the placebo group (54% reduction in the PGE_1 group versus 53% in the placebo group).[48] The remainder of the analyses combined primary and secondary subgroups and results indicated that PGE_1 decreased the severity of Raynaud's symptoms immediately after infusion; however, the decrease was also seen in the placebo group and did not persist at weeks 2 and 4. The authors report that the immediate decrease of severity was stronger in the secondary group. Similarly, skin temperature was significantly increased in the PGE_1 group following infusion (2·6 °C increase with PGE_1 *v*

Table 12.18 Number needed to treat ketanserin versus placebo – pooled data from 2 trials (Pope *et al*, 2002)[49]

Outcome	% with Placebo	% with ketanserin	Relative risk of outcome with ketanserin (95% CI)	ARR (95% CI)	NNT (95% CI)
Improvement	3/21 (14%)	10/20 (50%)	3·50 (1·12–10·90)	36% (7, 58)	3 (2, 5)

Table 12.19 Number needed to harm ketanserin versus placebo – pooled data from 2 trials (Pope *et al*, 2002)[49]

Outcome	% with Placebo	% with ketanserin	Relative risk of outcome with ketanserin (95% CI)	Absolute risk increase (95% CI)	NNH (95% CI)
Side effects	5/17 (29%)	16/22 (73%)	2·47 (1·13–5·39)	43% (12, 65)	2 (1, 18)
Note: nature of side effects not specified					

0·7 °C with placebo), but this effect did not persist at weeks 2 and 4. The authors concluded that there is no lasting benefit from PGE_1 for treatment of RP.[48]

Intravenous prostacyclins

Evidence summary: Silver

There is Silver evidence from a systematic review with five trials that IV prostacyclins can be effective in RP. In some of these trials subjects had already failed on standard therapy with calcium channel blockers. Thus, there is strong evidence that these treatments are effective in scleroderma-associated RP.

Recommendation for case presentation

This option is one which could be considered for this patient. It should be considered as an option.

Oral prostacyclins

Evidence summary: Silver

Silver level evidence from two RCTs found that oral prostacyclin agents do not produce consistent benefit.

5-HT antagonists

Ketanserin

Ketanserin, a selective 5-HT2 serotonin receptor blocker, has been studied in RP and for potential disease modification of scleroderma. The trials are unimpressive.

A meta-analysis of ketanserin for RP associated with SSc included three RCTs ($n = 66$), all of which were placebo controlled and double blinded.[49]

Benefits: The ketanserin group had a higher percentage improvement (RR: 3·15, 95% CI: 1·07–9·32) (Table 12.18). However, the severity of attacks favoured placebo. Although not statistically significant, the active group had a decreased frequency of attacks, with a WMD of −12·20 (95% CI: −39·09, 14·69). Duration of attacks was decreased in the active group (WMD: −25·4; CI: −48·6, −2·2).[49]

Adverse effects: Adverse effects were more common in those taking ketanserin (RR: 2·47, 95% CI: 1·13–5·39) (Table 12.19).

Excluded study

An additional study by Coffman *et al* was excluded from the Cochrane analysis because data were not presented for subgroups.[50] This was a large, placebo controlled trial ($n = 222$; 79 had RP secondary to SSc) with results that indicated the frequency of attacks was decreased by 16% with ketanserin therapy ($p < 0.011$) and that both patient and physician global assessments were improved with ketanserin ($p < 0.01$ and $p < 0.03$, respectively). There were no changes in finger total blood flow, and the most common adverse effect was headache in 17% receiving active drug. The authors reported that both secondary and primary RP subjects responded similarly to ketanserin.[50]

Evidence summary: Silver

Three RCTs showed inconsistent benefit from ketanserin.

Naftidrofuryl

There are no included studies providing evidence for this intervention.

Excluded study

The only RCT had 15 out of 102 patients with secondary RP. Davinroy and Mosnier showed, in a trial of different doses of naftidrofuryl versus placebo ($n = 102$; 15 with secondary RP) that the active drug group had: reduced attack duration ($p < 0.05$), reduced severity of pain ($p < 0.001$), and reduced impact of symptoms on daily activity ($p < 0.05$). Patient and physician global assessments were also improved ($p < 0.02$).[51] Nilson reported a crossover study of naftidrofuryl in which cases with primary ($n = 6$) and secondary ($n = 8$; 5 with SSc) RP were compared to placebo. Basal blood flow was increased in subjects taking naftidrofuryl therapy (6.6 ± 2.8 ml/min/100 g on naftidrofuryl versus 4.4 ± 1.5 ml/min/100 g on placebo, $p < 0.05$).[52]

Benefits: Those subjects in the active drug group saw a reduced symptom impact, and an increased basal blood flow versus those in the placebo group. Also, global assessment, both patient and physician, improved.[51,52]

Adverse effects: Thirty-six per cent of subjects on active drug experienced epigastric discomfort. Results for primary versus secondary were not indicated.

Evidence summary

There are no RCTs with data on secondary RP.

Alpha blockers (prazosin, phenoxybenzamine)

Prazosin, a selective α_1-adrenoreceptor blocker, has been studied in idiopathic and secondary RP. Phenoxybenzamine is a non-selective α-adrenoreceptor blocker.

Two randomised placebo controlled crossover trials of prazosin were analysed in a Cochrane meta-analysis ($n = 40$). Outcomes were decreased frequency and severity of Raynaud's attacks,[53–55] and finger skin temperature and blood flow.[54]

Benefits: In one study by Surwit *et al*, the frequency of attacks was decreased in the active prazosin group by a SMD of -1.20, 95% CI: -2.17, -0.22 (Table 12.20).[53] In the other study, the percentage improvement was poor in both groups (1/5 in the active group *v* 0/5 in the placebo group).[55]

Adverse effects: Adverse effects were only reported by Surwit *et al,* and were observed in the active group only ($n = 2/11$, OR: 6.82, 95%

Table 12.20 Number needed to treat prazosin versus placebo (From Pope meta-analysis – 1 study – Surwit *et al*, 1984)[53]

Outcome	Standardized mean difference (95% CI)	% Benefiting (95% CI) with prazosin	NNT (95% CI)
Frequency of attacks	−1·20 (−2·17, −0·22)	49% (11, 66)	3 (2, 10)

CI: 0·39, 119·27).[53] For the excluded studies, adverse effects were mentioned by 50% of those receiving prazosin.[54]

Excluded study

In an additional randomised, double blind, placebo controlled crossover study of prazosin (1 mg t.i.d.) in both primary (n = 14) and secondary RP (n = 10; 5 SSc), Wollersheim *et al* reported that the daily number of Raynaud's attacks and the duration of attacks were decreased in subjects taking prazosin compared to placebo ($p < 0·003$ and $p < 0·02$ respectively).[54] During finger cooling tests, subjects on active prazosin had improved finger skin temperature and blood flow ($p < 0·0001$ for both), and reported subjective efficacy of prazosin was high ($p < 0·000001$). Sixty per cent of subjects responded to prazosin. Analyses showed that there were no differences in the scleroderma group compared to the other patients in response to treatment.[54]

Another group, Cleophas *et al*, examined the effects of phenoxybenzamine (10–20 mg/day) compared to placebo (washout) and phenoxybenzamine in conjunction with beta-blocker sotalol (40–80 mg/day) in a 24-week crossover trial (n = 31; 5 with SSc).[56] Results indicated that finger temperature recovery after cooling was significantly increased in both the phenoxybenzamine and the phenoxybenzamine + sotalol groups, compared to baseline (24·5 ± 3·2 and 25·3 ±4·3 compared to placebo 19·8 ±1·7, $p < 0·001$). The addition of beta-blockade decreased the adverse effects of increased body weight and heart rate.[56]

Evidence summary: Silver

In two small RCTs, prazosin is more effective than placebo, but the benefit is modest and considerable adverse effects have occurred in trials of RP secondary to scleroderma. The potential for adverse effects outweighs the benefits derived from active treatment.

No conclusions can be drawn with respect to phenoxybenzamine in RP secondary to scleroderma.

Recommendation for case presentation

This is not a very likely treatment and should not be recommended.

Beta-blockers

Beta-blockers have been studied, often in conjunction with calcium channel blockers in primary RP, for treating Raynaud's. The common adverse effect of cold hands and feet may affect compliance.

No randomised controlled trials of beta-blockers specifically in RP secondary to scleroderma were revealed in our literature search.

Excluded study

Our literature search revealed one placebo controlled crossover study of penbutolol (acebutolol) 20 mg b.i.d. in hypertensive patients with RP (n = 10; five with RP secondary to connective tissue disease).[57] Following 2 weeks of penbutolol treatment, the mean time required to induce an ischaemic attack was 4 minutes compared to 2 minutes and 55 seconds with placebo ($p < 0{\cdot}05$). There was no significant difference between groups in mean digital temperature.[57] The outcome measurements may not be clinically relevant.

Evidence summary: Bronze

In the one RCT, there is insufficient data from the subgroup with scleroderma-associated RP.

> ***Recommendation for case presentation***
> This is not a recommended option due to the lack of evidence supporting it.

Endothelin receptor blockers

Endothelin-1 is a protein, expressed in many tissues, that is stimulated by stress and ischaemia; serum levels of ET-1 are elevated in the blood vessels and interstitium of SSc patients. Endothelin receptor blockers have been used to treat SSc-associated pulmonary hypertension and are being investigated in trials of digital ulcers with encouraging results. The prevention of the occurrence of new digital ulcers may indicate a possible prophylactic effect of endothelin receptor antagonists in treating digital ulcers associated with RP secondary to SSc.

A randomised placebo controlled trial by Black *et al* studied the role of bosentan in prevention and healing of digital ulcers secondary to SSc. The trial lasted 16 weeks and involved 122 subjects (43 on placebo, 79 on active treatment).[58]

Benefits: Using Poisson regression analysis, the decrease in number of new ulcers at 16 weeks from baseline was –48% for active drug versus placebo, $p < 0{\cdot}008$. Time to onset of the first new digital ulcer was increased in the active group, though not statistically significant; however, time to onset of the fourth new digital ulcer was significantly decreased in the bosentan group ($p < 0{\cdot}004$). No differences were found between groups for healing time of ulcers. Subjects taking bosentan reported improved global disease severity, compared to those on placebo ($p < 0{\cdot}05$). Bosentan appeared to be well tolerated.

Adverse effects: Side effects in both groups included headaches, respiratory infection, and vomiting. With the exception of increased liver enzymes (14%, $n = 11$), adverse effects were not significantly increased in the treatment groups, and transaminase elevations were reversible upon discontinuation of bosentan.[58]

Evidence summary: Silver

In one RCT bosentan reduced the number of new ulcers.

> ***Recommendation for case presentation***
> This is a favourable treatment that could be considered for this patient, although it is very expensive.

Cyclofenil (anti-oestrogen)

A Cochrane review of cyclofenil for RP secondary to SSc included one randomised, double blind, placebo controlled crossover study ($n = 25$),[59] in which subjects had 6 months of one treatment, no washout, and then crossed over to 6 months of the alternate treatment in random order.

Benefits: Non-significant trends in favour of cyclofenil were found for digital ulcer healing (OR 2·22; 95% CI: 0·53, 9·26) and physician assessment (OR 1·26; 95% CI: 0·33, 4·73).[59]

Adverse effects: Subjects taking cyclofenil were more likely to drop out due to adverse effects (OR 1·58; 95% CI: 0·42, 5·91).

Evidence summary: Silver

In one RCT there was a non-significant trend in digital ulcer healing and physician assessment.

Recommendation for case presentation

This is not a treatment to be recommended to this patient due to the lack of proven efficacy.

Nitroglycerine

Nitrates have strong vasodilatory effects, often acting both systemically and locally. Topical and slow-release patches have been investigated for use in primary and secondary RP.

Our search found two studies of nitrates in secondary RP; both were randomised, placebo controlled crossover studies: one of topically applied nitroglycerine, 5 mg (Nahir *et al*)[60], and one of a slow-release transdermal glyceryl trinitrate (GTN), 0·2 mg/h patch (Teh *et al*).[61] In the Nahir trial ($n = 18$; 8 with SSc) the design was 2 weeks on each treatment (random order) interrupted by a 1 week washout period. A positive response was defined as a 25% reduction in the number of attacks.[60] The Teh study used a 1 week treatment A/1 week treatment B crossover design (no washout) with 15 SSc subjects.[61]

Benefits: Of those with secondary RP in the trial by Nahir *et al*, 64% had an improved response to nitroglycerine (this did not reach statistical significance), while 72% of the total subjects improved ($p < 0{\cdot}005$). Similarly, 54% of secondary RP subjects experienced decreased attack severity (p = NS), while 61% of total subjects did the same ($p < 0{\cdot}02$). Four of the five subjects who did not respond to active drug had scleroderma.[60] Teh *et al* found that GTN patches reduced the frequency and severity of RP attacks ($p < 0{\cdot}05$ for both). However, objective thermography studies did not show a significant difference between treatment groups.[61]

Adverse effects: Headaches, the most common adverse effect, were experienced in 56% of subjects.[60] Eighty per cent of subjects in the study by Teh *et al* also experienced headaches ($p < 0{\cdot}00$).[21]

Evidence summary: Silver

Two RCTs showed that nitroglycerine improves symptoms of RP. The common headache adverse effect may limit the clinical use or compliance.

Recommendation for case presentation

The adverse effects are far too intrusive to make this a very practical suggestion for this patient.

Dazoxiben (selective thromboxane synthetase (prostaglandin) inhibitor)

Dazoxiben is a selective inhibitor of the prostaglandin thromboxane A_2 (TXA_2), a protein involved in platelet aggregation and vasoconstriction. Thromboxane B_2 (TXB_2) is the stable metabolite of TXA_2. Dazoxiben also has benefit over cyclo-oxygenase inhibitors, in that it may enhance production of antiplatelet and vasodilatory prostacyclins (PGI_2).

Three of the four randomised controlled trials for dazoxiben were of crossover design, one of which also used nifedipine as active comparator.[62] All four trials had patients with both primary and secondary RP. Ettinger *et al* conducted a crossover study in which all subjects ($n = 22$, including four with systemic and four with limited scleroderma) had 2 weeks of nifedipine, dazoxiben or placebo following an initial 2 week washout period and interspersed by a 1 week washout prior to the treatment switch.[62]

Benefits: No significant differences were found between subjects' ratings of nifedipine, dazoxiben, and placebo; however, subjects preferred nifedipine over dazoxiben. The mean rate of Raynaud's attacks was 30·4 ± 4·5 (placebo), 24·7 ± 5·6 (nifedipine), and 32·0 ± 4.9 (dazoxiben), p = NS. No significant differences were found between treatment groups for severity, pain or duration of Raynaud's episodes as assessed by patients using a three-point scale. The mean temperature at which critical closure of the digital arteries occurred was 4·71 ± 1·2 °C (placebo), 4·11 ± 1·5 °C (nifedipine), and 6·47 ± 2·4 °C (placebo), p = NS.[62] In a randomised, placebo controlled, crossover trial (n = 21: 16 with secondary RP, of whom 13 had scleroderma), Luderer *et al* found that in *ex vivo* studies dazoxiben significantly increased the ratio of 6-keto $PGF_{1\alpha}$ to TXB_2 (from 3·57 ± 0·16 to 48·03 ± 6·2, p-value not given),[63] Whereas, *in vivo* serum concentrations collected at the end of each treatment and washout period indicated that the ratio was not significantly increased in subjects taking dazoxiben (100 mg four times per day). Digital blood flow was not significantly increased in the dazoxiben groups in either the earlier crossover group (3·57 ± 9·73 on dazoxiben versus 5·03 ± 15·16 on placebo) or the later group (6·65 ± 1·38 on dazoxiben versus 4·33 ± 0·89 on placebo, p-value not given). No improvement in any subjective variables (symptoms, frequency, severity, and duration of Raynaud's attacks) could be related to use of dazoxiben.[63] In a similar study (n = 25; 12 with secondary RP), Coffman and Rasmussen found that for patients with secondary RP, there were no significant differences in digital haemodynamics between drug and placebo periods.[64]

Belch *et al* conducted a case–control, randomised, placebo controlled, double blind study of dazoxiben 100 mg four times per day (n = 20) over a 6 week period in which three cases and three controls had RP secondary to SSc.[65] Results indicated that subjects taking dazoxiben had increased the finger temperature at week 2 ($p < 0·05$), but by week 4 the temperature had decreased significantly (versus controls), $p < 0·05$; however, by week 6 there were no differences in digital temperature of those on active drug versus controls. Patients on dazoxiben differed in their rating of symptoms at week 6 only (the majority felt symptoms had "definitely improved") while the active and placebo groups were similar at weeks 2 and 4. By week 6, plasma TXB_2 levels were decreased in subjects taking dazoxiben compared to controls (96 ± 42 pg/ml *v* 123 ± 32 pg/ml, $p < 0·01$, paired *t* test of baseline).[65]

Adverse effects: None were reported.

Evidence summary: Silver

Four RCTs showed no consistent benefits from dazoxiben for patients' symptoms of RP.

Another four RCTs were included. Fewer than 50 SSc patients per group were treated.

Other agents

Antiplatelet agents

Antiplatelet drugs have been investigated for efficacy in controlling idiopathic and secondary RP.

There are no randomised controlled trials studying solely scleroderma.

Evidence summary: Bronze

There are no data that support ticlodipine in the treatment of RP secondary to SSc.

Excluded study: In a trial of ticlopidine 250 mg b.i.d. versus placebo (n = 58; 12 with SSc), Destors *et al* found that the frequency of attacks was not reduced in 59% of subjects on active drug versus 44% on placebo, $p < 0·28$.[66] Similarly, no significant differences were found between the groups for subjective improvement of RP; however, a significant increase in triglyceridaemia (adverse effect) was noted in those on ticlopidine (1·59 mmol/l versus 0·93 mmol/l, $p < 0·006$).[66]

Butyrophenone (buflomedil)

Butyrophenone is a dopamine antagonist that also may have anti-adrenoreceptor as well as H1-receptor blocking activity.

Excluded study: One trial of RP with buflomedil involved only 6 of 398 subjects with secondary RP.[67]

Evidence summary: Bronze

There are no data to support treatment of scleroderma-associated RP with buflomedil.

References

41 Kelley W, Harris E, Ruddy S, Sludge C. *Textbook of Rheumatology, 5th edn.* Philadelphia: W.B. Saunders Company, 1997.

42 Freedman R, Ianni P, Wenig P. Behavioral treatment of Raynaud's phenomenon in scleroderma. *J Behav Med* 1984;**7**(4):343–53.

43 Thompson AE, Shea B, Welch V, Fenlon D, Pope JE. Calcium-channel blockers for Raynaud's phenomenon in systemic sclerosis. *Arthritis Rheum* 2001;**44**(8):1841–7.

44 Weber A, Bounameaux H. Effects of low-dose nifedipine on a cold provocation test in people with Raynaud's disease. *J Cardiovasc Pharmacol* 1990;**15**:853–5.

45 Sarkozi J, Bookman A, Mahon W, *et al.* Nifedipine in the treatment of idiopathic Raynaud's syndrome. *J Rheumatol* 1986;**13**:331–6.

46 Pope J, Fenlon D, Thompson A, *et al.* Iloprost and cisaprost for Raynaud's phenomenon in progressive systemic sclerosis (Cochrane Review). In: Cochrane Collaboration. *Cochrane Library.* Issue 1, 2002. Oxford: Update Software.

47 Black CM, Halkier-Sorensen L, Belch JJF, *et al.* Oral Iloprost in Raynaud's phenomenon secondary to systemic sclerosis: A multicentre, placebo-controlled, dose-comparison study. *Br J Rheumatol* 1998;**37**(9): 952–60.

48 Mohrland JS, Porter JM, Smith EA, Belch J, Simms MH. A multiclinic, placebo-controlled, double-blind study of prostaglandin E1 in Raynaud's sydrome. *Ann Rheum Dis* 1985;**44**(11):754–60.

49 Pope J, Fenlon D, Thompson A, *et al.* Ketanserin for Raynaud's phenomenon in progressive systemic sclerosis (Cochrane Review). In: Cochrane Collaboration. *Cochrane Library.* Issue 1, 2002. Oxford: Update Software.

50 Coffman J, Clement D, Creager M, *et al.* International study of ketanserin in Raynaud's phenomenon. *Am J Med* 1989;**87**:264–8.

51 Davinroy M, Mosnier M. Evaluation clinique en double-insu du naftidrofuryl dans le phenomene de raynaud. *Actualite Therapeutique* 1993;**69**:1322–26.

52 Haavik Nilson K. Effects of naftidrofuryl on microcirculatory cold sensitivity in Raynaud's phenomenon. *Br Med J* 1979;**1**(6155):20–21.

53 Surwit RS, Gilgor RS, Allen LM, Duvic M. A double-blind study of prazosin in the treatment of Raynaud's phenomenon in scleroderma. *Arch Dermatol* 1984;**120**(3):329–31.

54 Wollersheim H, Thien T, Fennis J, Van Elteren P, Van't Laar A. Double-blind, placebo-controlled study of Prazosin in Raynaud's phenomenon. *Clin Pharmacol Ther* 1986; **40**(2):219–25.

55 Russell IJ, Lessard JA. Prazosin treatment of Raynaud's phenomenon: a double-blind, single-crossover study. *J Rheumatol* 1985;**12**(1):94–8.

56 Cleophas T, Van Lier H, Fennis J, Van't Laar A. Treatment of Raynaud's syndrome with adrenergic alpha-blockade with or without beta-blockade. *Angiology* 1984;**35**(1):29–37.

57 Holti G. A double-blind study of the peripheral vasoconstrictor effects of the beta-blocking drug penbutolol in patients with Raynaud's phenomenon. *Curr Med Res Opin* 1979;**6**(4):267–70.

58 Black C, Korn J, Mayes M, *et al.* Prevention of ischemic digital ulcers in systemic sclerosis by endothelin receptor antagonism. *Arthritis Rheum* 2002;**46**:3414.

59 Blom-Bulow B, Oberg K, Wollheim FA, *et al.* Cyclofenil versus placebo in progressive systemic sclerosis. A one year double-blind crossover study of 27 patients. *Acta Med Scand* 1981;**210**(5):419–28.

60 Nahir AM, Schapira D, Scharf Y. Double-blind, randomised trial of Nitroderm TTS in the treatment of Raynaud's phenomenon. *Isr J Med Sci* 1986;**22**(2): 139–42.

61 Teh LS, Manning J, Moore T, Tully MP, O'Reilly D, Jayson M. Sustained-release transdermal glyceryl trinitrate

patches as a treatment for primary and secondary Raynaud's phenomenon. *Br J Rheum* 1995;**34**(7):636–41.

62 Ettinger W, Wise RA, Schaffhauser D, Wigley FM. Controlled double-blind trial of Dazoxiben and Nifedipine in the treatment of Raynaud's phenomenon. *Am J Med* 1984;**77**(3):451–6.

63 Luderer JR, Nicholas GG, Neumyer MM, *et al.* Dazoxiben, a thromboxane synthetase inhibitor in Raynaud's phenomenon. *Clin Pharmacol Ther* 1984;**36**(1):105–15.

64 Coffman JD, Rasmussen HM. Effect of thromboxane synthetase inhibition in Raynaud's phenomenon. *Clin Pharmacol Ther* 1984;**36**(3):369–73.

65 Belch JJ, Cormie J, Newman P, *et al.* Dazoxiben, a thromboxane synthetase inhibitor in the treatment of Raynaud's syndrome: a double-blind trial. *J Clin Pharmac* 1983;**15**(suppl 1):113S–116S.

66 Destors J, Gauthier E, Lelong S, Boissel J. Failure of a pure anti-platelet drug to decrease the number of attacks more than placebo in patients with Raynaud's phenomenon. Angiology 1986;**37**:565–9.

67 Maurel A, Betrancourt J-C, Van Frenkel R, Thuillez C. Action du buflomedil sur la microcirculation cutanée etudiée par un test de provacation au froid. Etude multicentrique, double aveugle versus placebo. *J Maladies Vasculaires* 1995;**20**:127–33.

Systemic sclerosis
Summaries and decision aids

Scleroderma and methotrexate
Summaries and decision aid

How well does methotrexate (MTX) work for treating scleroderma (also known as systemic sclerosis) and how safe is it?

To answer this question, scientists found and analysed 2 high quality studies testing 100 people who had scleroderma. People received either injections or pills of methotrexate or a placebo or sugar pill and were monitored for 6 months or a year. These studies provide the best evidence we have today.

What is scleroderma and how can methotrexate help?

Scleroderma or systemic sclerosis is a condition where skin, joints, and blood vessels are replaced with thick, hard, fibrous tissue. It is thought that scleroderma is caused by the body's immune system attacking its own tissues. The tissues become inflamed or swollen and produce too much collagen (a tough fibre-like tissue). People with scleroderma will likely have patches of hard skin and pain, swelling and stiffness in their joints and/or damage in their organs, such as the heart, lungs, and kidneys. Disease modifying antirheumatic drugs (DMARDs) can be prescribed to reduce pain and inflammation and to slow the progress of the disease. Methotrexate is a DMARD that may stop scleroderma from getting worse by controlling the immune system.

How well did methotrexate work?

Two studies showed that more people receiving methotrexate injections had improved skin thickness by 30% and could breathe better by 15% than people receiving a placebo or sugar pill.

When asked, people said that they felt better overall in one study but not in the other study when receiving methotrexate injections.

What side effects occurred with methotrexate?

Studies of people with scleroderma and studies of people with other diseases have shown that mouth ulcers, nausea, heartburn, rash, and lung problems may occur with methotrexate. Changes in liver enzymes and death may also occur.

What is the bottom line?

There is "Silver" level evidence that methotrexate decreases skin thickness and symptoms of scleroderma, such as problems breathing.

Stomach and intestinal side effects, and high liver enzyme levels may occur when taking methotrexate. But these side effects may not last long and so many people keep receiving methotrexate.

Based on Pope J, Furst D, Clements P, Ottawa Methods Group. Systemic sclerosis. In: *Evidence-based Rheumatology*. London: BMJ Books, 2003.

How well does methotrexate (MTX) work for treating scleroderma or systemic sclerosis and how safe is it?

What is scleroderma and how can methotrexate help?

Scleroderma or systemic sclerosis is a condition where skin, joints, and blood vessels are replaced with thick, hard, fibrous tissue. It is thought that scleroderma is caused by the body's immune system attacking its own tissues. The tissues then become inflamed or swollen and produce too much collagen (a tough fibre-like tissue). There are two types of scleroderma: localised – which affects mainly the skin but can affect the muscles and joints; and generalised – which affects the skin and organs, such as the heart, lungs and kidneys. Localised scleroderma may develop slowly and not cause severe problems, but generalised scleroderma may get worse over time.

Painkillers or analgesics are often prescribed to improve joint pain and swelling. Disease modifying antirheumatic drugs (DMARDs) can be prescribed to reduce pain and inflammation and also to slow the progress of the disease. Methotrexate is a DMARD that may stop scleroderma from getting worse by controlling the immune system. Methotrexate can also cause side effects and therefore it is important to know how well methotrexate works and how safe it is.

How did the scientists find the information and analyse it?

The scientists searched for studies that examined the treatment of scleroderma. Not all studies found were of a high quality and so only those studies that met high standards were selected.

Studies were randomised controlled trials where a group of patients received methotrexate and were compared to patients who received a placebo or a sugar pill.

Which high quality studies were examined in this summary?

Two high quality studies were examined. A total of 100 patients with scleroderma received either an injection of methotrexate or a placebo and were followed for about 6 to 12 months.

One study tested 29 patients for 24 weeks: 17 patients received a weekly injection of 15 mg of methotrexate and 12 received a placebo injection.

One study tested 71 patients for 1 year: 35 patients received methotrexate pills weekly and 36 received a placebo.

Improvement was measured by testing skin thickness or whether the skin could be pinched into a fold, general wellbeing, presence of ulcers or sores on the skin, and breathing.

How well did methotrexate work?

One study showed that more patients receiving methotrexate injection had improved skin thickness by 30%, could breathe better by 15%, and felt better overall by 30%, compared to patients receiving a placebo:

- 10 out of 100 patients had improved with a placebo
- 53 out of 100 patients had improved with methotrexate.

The other study showed that more patients receiving methotrexate pills had improved skin thickness and breathing compared to patients receiving a placebo:

- 24 out of 100 more patients benefited from receiving methotrexate than a placebo (sugar pill).

But in this study, improvement in overall wellbeing as measured by the patients themselves and as measured by their doctor was the same when receiving methotrexate or a placebo.

What side effects occurred with methotrexate?

Studies of people with scleroderma and studies of people with other diseases have shown that mouth ulcers, nausea, heartburn, rash, and lung problems may occur. Changes in liver enzymes and death may occur when receiving methotrexate:

- 65 out of 100 patients had abnormal liver enzyme levels or other side effects with methotrexate
- 17 out of 100 patients had the same side effects as above while receiving a placebo.

What is the bottom line?

There is "Silver" level evidence that methotrexate decreases skin thickness and symptoms of scleroderma, such as problems with breathing.

Stomach and intestinal side effects, and high liver enzyme levels may occur when taking methotrexate. But these side effects may not last long and so many people keep receiving methotrexate.

Based on Pope J, Furst D, Clements P, Ottawa Methods Group. Systemic sclerosis. In: *Evidence-based Rheumatology.* London: BMJ Books, 2003.

Information about scleroderma and treatment

What is scleroderma?

Scleroderma or systemic sclerosis is a condition where skin, joints, and blood vessels are replaced with thick, hard, fibrous tissue. It is thought that scleroderma is caused by the body's immune system attacking its own tissues. People with scleroderma will likely have patches of hard skin and have pain, swelling, and stiffness in their joints.

There are two types of scleroderma: localised – which affects mainly the skin but can affect the muscles and joints; and generalised – which affects the skin and organs, such as the heart, lungs, and kidneys. Localised scleroderma may develop slowly and not cause severe problems. But generalised scleroderma may get worse over time. If scleroderma is not treated, it may result in:

- ulcers or sores on toes and/or fingers
- trouble swallowing
- heartburn
- problems breathing well
- problems digesting food
- problems with your heart and kidneys
- surgery

What can I do on my own to manage my disease?

✓ moisturise skin ✓ exercise ✓ protect skin and joints ✓ rest and relax ✓ avoid smoking

What treatments are used for scleroderma?

Five kinds of treatment may be used alone or together. The common (generic) names of treatment are shown below.

1. *Pain medicines and non-steroidal anti-inflammatory drugs (NSAIDs)*
   - Acetaminophen
   - Acetylsalicylic acid
   - Celecoxib
   - Diclofenac
   - Ibuprofen
   - Indomethacin
   - Nabumetone
   - Naproxen
   - Piroxicam
   - Rofecoxib
   - Sulindac
2. *Disease modifying antirheumatic drugs (DMARDs)*
   - Methotrexate
   - Cyclophosphamide
   - 5-Fluorouracil
3. *Corticosteroids*
   - Dexamethasone
4. *Prostacyclins*
   - Epoprostanol
   - Treprostinil
5. *Miscellaneous therapies*
   - Stem cell transplantation
   - Bovine type I collagen
   - Bosentan
   - Angiotensin-converting enzyme inhibitors (ACE inhibitors)

What about other treatments I have heard about?

There is not enough evidence about the effects of some treatments. Other treatments do not work. For example:

- Acetylsalicylic acid
- Alpha interferon
- Anti-TGF beta
- Anti-oxidants
- Chlorambucil
- Cyclofenil
- Dipyridamole
- Gamma interferon
- Ketotifen
- N-acetylcysteine
- Penicillamine
- Potassium aminobenzoate (POTABA)
- Relaxin

What are my choices? How can I decide?

Treatment for your disease will depend on your condition. You need to know the good points (pros) and the bad points (cons) about each treatment before you can decide.

Scleroderma (systemic sclerosis) decision aid

Should I take methotrexate?

This guide can help you make decisions about a treatment your doctor is asking you to consider. It will help you to:

1. Clarify what you need to decide.
2. Consider the pros and cons of different choices.
3. Decide what role you want to have in choosing you treatment.
4. Identify what you need to help you make the decision.
5. Plan the next steps.
6. Share your thinking with your doctor.

Step 1: Clarify the decision

What is the decision?

Should I take methotrexate to decrease pain and slow the progress of scleroderma/systemic sclerosis?

Methotrexate can be taken as a pill daily or as an injection received weekly.

When does this decision have to be made? Check ✓ one

☐ within days ☐ within weeks ☐ within months

How far along are you with this decision? Check ✓ one

☐ I have not thought about it yet

☐ I am considering the choices

☐ I am close to making a choice

☐ I have already made a choice

Step 2: Consider the pros and cons of different choices

What does the research show?

Methotrexate is classified as: Likely beneficial

There is "Silver" level evidence from 2 studies of 100 people with scleroderma testing methotrexate. The studies lasted up to 1 year. These studies found pros and cons that are listed in the chart below.

What do I think of the pros and cons of methotrexate?

1. Review the common pros and cons that are shown below.
2. Add any other pros and cons that are important to you.
3. Show how important each pro and con is to you by circling from one (*) star if it is a little important to you, to up to five (*****) stars if it is very important to you.

PROS AND CONS METHOTREXATE TREATMENT

PROS (number of people affected)	How important is this to you?	CONS (number of people affected)	How important is this to you?
Decreases skin thickness in 53 out of 100 people with methotrexate in 10 out of 100 without methotrexate	* * * * *	Side effects: mouth ulcers, nausea, heartburn, rash, lung problems in 65 out of 100 people with methotrexate in 17 out of 100 people without methotrexate	* * * * *
Makes breathing easier in 53 out of 100 people with methotrexate in 10 out of 100 without methotrexate	* * * * *	Long term side effects are rare but include liver damage	* * * * *
May improve overall well-being in 53 out of 100 people with methotrexate in 10 out of 100 without methotrexate	* * * * *	Monthly clinic visits and blood tests are needed	* * * * *
Other pros:	* * * * *	**Personal cost of medicine**	* * * * *
		Other cons:	* * * * *

What do you think of taking methotrexate? Check ✓ one

☐ Willing to consider this treatment
Pros are more important to me than the Cons

☐ Unsure

☐ Not willing to consider this treatment
Cons are more important to me than the Pros

Step 3: Choose the role you want to have in choosing your treatment Check ✓ one.

☐ I prefer to decide on my own after listening to the opinions of others

☐ I prefer to share the decision with: ______________________

☐ I prefer someone else to decide for me, namely: ______________

Step 4: Identify what you need to help you make the decision

What I know	Do you know enough about your condition to make a choice?	☐ Yes ☐ No ☐ Unsure
	Do you know which options are available to you?	☐ Yes ☐ No ☐ Unsure
	Do you know the good points (pros) of each option?	☐ Yes ☐ No ☐ Unsure
	Do you know the bad points (cons) of each option?	☐ Yes ☐ No ☐ Unsure
What's important	Are you clear about which **pros** are most *important to you?*	☐ Yes ☐ No ☐ Unsure
	Are you clear about which **cons** are most *important to you?*	☐ Yes ☐ No ☐ Unsure
How others help	Do you have enough support from others to make a choice?	☐ Yes ☐ No ☐ Unsure
	Are you choosing without pressure from others?	☐ Yes ☐ No ☐ Unsure
	Do you have enough advice to make a choice?	☐ Yes ☐ No ☐ Unsure
How sure I feel	Are you clear about the best choice for you?	☐ Yes ☐ No ☐ Unsure
	Do you feel sure about what to choose?	☐ Yes ☐ No ☐ Unsure

If you answered No or Unsure to many of these questions, you should talk to your doctor.

Step 5: Plan the next steps

What do you need to do before you make this decision?

For example – talk to your doctor, read more about this treatment or other treatments for scleroderma.

Step 6: Share the information on this form with your doctor

It will help your doctor understand what you think about this treatment.

Raynaud's from scleroderma and calcium channel blockers Summaries and decision aid

How well do calcium channel blockers, such as nifedipine, work to treat Raynaud's from scleroderma?

To answer this question, scientists found and analysed one review including 5 high quality studies testing over 40 people who had Raynaud's from scleroderma. People had nifidepine (up to 30 mg per day) or a placebo or sugar pill. These studies provide the best evidence we have today.

What is Raynaud's and how can calcium channel blockers help?

Raynaud's is a condition in which the small blood vessels narrow and slow the flow of blood to the skin. The most common sign is cold, pale (white), numb fingers and toes. Attacks can occur when blood flow returns to the fingers and toes and is painful. Raynaud's can occur on its own or with another condition called scleroderma. Scleroderma is a condition in which the skin, joints, and blood vessels are replaced with thick, fibrous tissue. Drugs, such as calcium channel blockers, are often prescribed in Raynaud's to decrease the number of attacks and pain during the attacks. Calcium channel blockers, such as nifidepine, open blood vessels to let blood flow better through the body. Unfortunately, the increased blood flow may also cause other side effects.

How well did calcium channel blockers work?

The five studies showed that people had fewer attacks during 2 weeks when taking nifedipine than when taking a placebo or sugar pill.

Two studies measured pain during the attacks. The studies showed that nifedipine decreased the amount of pain that people had during the attacks.

What side effects occurred with calcium channel blockers?

Some studies have shown that side effects that can occur are low blood pressure, dizziness, flushing, water retention or swelling in the feet and legs, and headaches. Other studies testing calcium channel blockers in other diseases show that they are fairly safe over the long term.

What is the bottom line?

There is "Silver"' level evidence that in people who have Raynaud's from scleroderma, calcium channel blockers, such as nifidepine work well to decrease the number of attacks and amount of pain during the attacks in the short term (2 to 12 weeks). Calcium channel blockers, however, do not change the progress of the disease.

In most people the pros of taking calcium channel blockers outweigh the cons (or side effects). Calcium channel blockers also appear to be safe in the long term.

Based on Pope J, Furst D, Clements P, Ottawa Methods Group. Systemic sclerosis. In: *Evidence-based Rheumatology*. London: BMJ Books, 2003.

How well do calcium channel blockers, such as nifidepine, work to treat Raynaud's from scleroderma?

What is Raynaud's and how can calcium channel blockers help?

Raynaud's is a condition in which the small blood vessels narrow and slow the flow of blood to the skin. The most common sign is cold, pale (white), numb fingers and toes. When blood flow returns, the fingers and toes may be painful. These attacks usually occur when you are cold, emotionally stressed or when taking certain drugs. There are two types of Raynaud's: Primary Raynaud's, which is the most common and has no known cause; and Secondary Raynaud's, which occurs with other conditions such as scleroderma. Scleroderma is a condition where skin, joints, and blood vessels are replaced with fibrous (thick) tissue. It is thought to be caused by the body's immune system attacking its own healthy tissues.

Drugs are often prescribed in Raynaud's to decrease the number and severity of the attacks. Calcium channel blockers are one type of drug called "vasodilators". Calcium channel blockers, such as nifidepine, open blood vessels to improve blood flow through the body. The increase of blood flow may also cause other side effects and therefore it is important to know whether calcium channel blockers work well.

How did the scientists find the information and analyse it?

The scientists searched scientific journals for studies and reviews of the literature testing calcium channel blockers in patients with Raynaud's. Not all studies and reviews found were of a high quality and so only those studies and reviews that met high standards were selected.

- Studies had to be randomised controlled trials where a group of patients who received a calcium channel blocker was compared to another group of patients who received a placebo or sugar pill or another drug.
- Some studies were of medium quality. These studies tested smaller groups of patients or were studies where one group of patients first received a calcium channel blocker and then switched to receive a placebo and another group of patients first received a placebo and then switched to receive a calcium channel blocker.

Which studies and reviews were examined in the summary?

One review was examined in this summary and it included 6 studies comparing calcium channel blockers to a placebo or sugar pill. Five studies tested 44 patients with scleroderma. The patients received nifidepine (at no more than 30 mg per day) or a placebo or sugar pill for up to 12 weeks. The studies were of medium or high quality.

Studies measured how often attacks occurred during a 2 week time period and how severe or painful the attacks were.

How well did calcium channel blockers work?

The review showed that the effects of calcium channel blockers are modest. Patients had a lower number of attacks during a 2 week time period. The five studies showed that patients receiving nifedipine had on average 10 fewer attacks during 2 weeks than patients receiving a placebo. The studies also showed that 24 out of 100 more patients benefited from receiving nifedipine than a placebo.

The review also showed that calcium channel blockers decreased the amount of pain that patients had during the attacks. Two studies showed that 43 out of 100 more patients had less pain during attacks while receiving nifedipine than when receiving a placebo.

What side effects occurred with calcium channel blockers?

Other studies have shown that side effects that can occur are low blood pressure, dizziness, flushing, water retention or swelling in the feet and legs, and headaches.

The more common side effects which occur in 10 out of 100 patients are:

- water retention or swelling in the feet, legs and hands
- dizziness or lightheadedness
- nausea
- headache and flushing, weakness.

A less common side effect which occurs in 5 out 100 patients is:

- low blood pressure that goes back to normal when you stop taking nifedipine.

Other studies testing calcium channel blockers in other diseases show that they are fairly safe over the long term.

What is the bottom line?

There is "Silver" level evidence that in people who have Raynaud's from scleroderma, calcium channel blockers, such as nifidepine, work well to decrease the number of attacks and amount of pain during the attacks in the short term (2 to 12 weeks). Calcium channel blockers, however, do not change the progress of the disease.

In most people the pros of taking calcium channel blockers outweigh the cons (or side effects). Calcium channel blockers also appear to be safe in the long term.

Based on Pope J, Furst D, Clements P, Ottawa Methods Group. Systemic sclerosis. In: *Evidence-based Rheumatology*. London: BMJ Books, 2003.

Information about Raynaud's from scleroderma and treatment

What is Raynaud's?

Raynaud's is a condition in which the small blood vessels narrow and slow the flow of blood to the skin. The most common sign is cold, pale (white), numb fingers and toes. As blood flow returns, the fingers and toes may be painful. These attacks usually occur when you are cold and may also occur if emotionally stressed or from some drugs.

There are two types: primary and secondary. Primary Raynaud's is the most common and has no known cause. It often occurs in women aged 15 to 35 without any other symptoms. Secondary Raynaud's occurs along with other conditions such as scleroderma. Scleroderma is a condition where skin, joints, and blood vessels are replaced with fibrous (thick) tissue. It is thought to be caused by the body's immune system attacking its own tissues. It usually occurs in women or men older than age 35.

A painful attack of Raynaud's from scleroderma sometimes occurs and then gets better on its own. If Raynaud's continues to get worse and is not treated, it may result in:

- damage to blood vessels
- ulcers or sores on toes and/or fingers
- in the worst situations, it could lead to gangrene in fingers and toes that need to be surgically removed.

What can I do on my own to manage my disease?

✓ limit caffeine, nicotine (tobacco) ✓ keep warm ✓ avoid stressful situations

What treatments are used for Raynaud's from scleroderma?

The treatments may be used alone or together. The common (generic) names of treatment are shown below.

- captopril
- diltiazem
- felodipine
- nicardipine
- nifedipine
- nitroglycerine
- prostacycline

What about other treatments I have heard about?

There is not enough evidence about the effects of some treatments. Other treatments do not work. For example:

- Biofeedback
- Ketanserin
- Clofenil
- Dazoxiben
- Anti-platelet treatment
- Aaftidrofuryl
- Alpha blockers
- Beta blockers

What are my choices? How can I decide?

Treatment for your disease will depend on your condition. You need to know the good points (pros) and the bad points (cons) about each treatment before you can decide.

Raynaud's decision aid

Should I take calcium channel blockers, such as nifedipine?

This guide can help you make decisions about a treatment your doctor is asking you to consider. It will help you to:

1. Clarify what you need to decide.
2. Consider the pros and cons of different choices.
3. Decide what role you want to have in choosing you treatment.
4. Identify what you need to help you make the decision.
5. Plan the next steps.
6. Share your thinking with your doctor.

Step 1: Clarify what you need to decide

What is the decision?

Should I take calcium channel blockers, such as nifedipine, for fewer attacks and less painful attacks in Raynaud's from scleroderma?

Calcium channel blockers are pills that are taken every day.

When does this decision have to be made? Check ✓ one

☐ within days ☐ within weeks ☐ within months

How far along are you with this decision? Check ✓ one

☐ I have not thought about it yet

☐ I am considering the choices

☐ I am close to making a choice

☐ I have already made a choice

Step 2: Consider the pros and cons of different choices

What does the research show?

Calcium channel blockers are classified as: Beneficial

There is "Silver" level evidence from 5 studies of 44 people with Raynaud's from scleroderma testing nifedipine. The studies lasted up to 12 weeks. These studies found pros and cons that are listed in the chart below.

What do I think of the pros and cons of calcium channel blockers?

1. Review the common pros and cons that are shown below.
2. Add any other pros and cons that are important to you.
3. Show how important each pro and con is to you by circling from one (*) star if it is a little important to you, to up to five (*****) stars if it is very important to you.

PROS AND CONS OF CALCIUM CHANNEL BLOCKERS, SUCH AS NIFEDIPINE

PROS (number of people affected)	How important is it to you?	CONS (number of people affected)	How important is it to you?
Fewer painful attacks in the short term people had 10 less attacks during a 2 week period with nifedipine	* * * * *	Side effects: water retention or swelling in the feet, dizziness or lightheadedness, nausea, headache, flushing, weakness may occur in 10 of out 100 people	* * * * *
Less severe pain during an attack in the short term	* * * * *	It is not known whether nifedipine decreases the number of painful attacks over a long period of time	* * * * *
Long term safety is known in other diseases and appears very safe	* * * * *	**Personal cost of medicine**	* * * * *
Other pros:	* * * * *	Other cons:	* * * * *

What do you think about taking calcium channel blockers? Check ✓ one

☐	☐	☐
Willing to consider this treatment Pros are more important to me than the Cons	Unsure	Not willing to consider this treatment Cons are more important to me than the Pros

Step 3: Choose the role you want to have in choosing your treatment Check ✓one

☐ I prefer to decide on my own after listening to the opinions of others

☐ I prefer to share the decision with: ______________________

☐ I prefer someone else to decide for me, namely: ______________

Step 4: Identify what you need to help you make the decision

What I know	Do you know enough about your condition to make a choice?	☐ Yes ☐ No ☐ Unsure
	Do you know which options are available to you?	☐ Yes ☐ No ☐ Unsure
	Do you know the good points (pros) of each option?	☐ Yes ☐ No ☐ Unsure
	Do you know the bad points (cons) of each option?	☐ Yes ☐ No ☐ Unsure
What's important	Are you clear about which **pros** are most *important to you?*	☐ Yes ☐ No ☐ Unsure
	Are you clear about which **cons** are most *important to you?*	☐ Yes ☐ No ☐ Unsure
How others help	Do you have enough support from others to make a choice?	☐ Yes ☐ No ☐ Unsure
	Are you choosing without pressure from others?	☐ Yes ☐ No ☐ Unsure
	Do you have enough advice to make a choice?	☐ Yes ☐ No ☐ Unsure
How sure I feel	Are you clear about the best choice for you?	☐ Yes ☐ No ☐ Unsure
	Do you feel sure about what to choose?	☐ Yes ☐ No ☐ Unsure

If you answered No or Unsure to many of these questions, you should talk to your doctor.

Step 5: Plan the next steps

What do you need to do before you make this decision?

For example – talk to your doctor, read more about this treatment or other treatments for Raynaud's from scleroderma.

Step 6: Share the information on this form with your doctor

It will help your doctor understand what you think about this treatment.

13
Primary systemic vasculitis

Richard A Watts, Suzanne E Lane, David GI Scott, Ottawa Methods Group

Introduction

The primary systemic vasculitides – Wegener's granulomatosis (WG), Churg–Strauss syndrome (CSS), microscopic polyangiitis (MPA), and classical polyarteritis nodosa (PAN) – are a group of conditions characterised by inflammation and necrosis of blood vessel walls. The conditions share clinical features and are sometimes (excluding PAN) referred to as the "ANCA-associated vasculitides". The overall annual incidence in the UK during 1988–98 was 18·9/million – WG 10·6/million, MPA 8·1/million and CSS 3·1/million.[1] The aetiology is generally unknown, but systemic vasculitis has been described in patients with viral infections (especially Hepatitis B) and is associated with a variety of potential environmental triggers. Early studies of untreated systemic vasculitis reported 80% 1 year mortality,[2] which improved to around 20% following the introduction of corticosteroids and cyclophosphamide (CYC).[3,4] A 75% 10 year survival has been reported for WG and 55% for MPA.[5] Diagnosis is based on clinical suspicion supported by positive histology. The presence of antineutrophil cytoplasmic antibodies (ANCA) is strong supportive evidence but should not replace histology for confirmation of diagnosis. cANCA with proteinase 3 specificity is strongly associated with WG and pANCA with myeloperoxidase specificity with MPA (reviewed in Wiik, 2002[6]).

Methodology

The general search strategy was to look for all evidence synthesis in the Cochrane Library and Medline (Ovid). There are few systematic reviews of the treatment of primary systemic vasculitis. The MEDLINE database was also searched for randomised controlled trials and non-randomised trials. No time or language limits were placed on the search. The reference lists of identified papers and previous reviews were also searched. The search terms are outlined with the answers to each question in the text.

Outcomes

The aim of therapy is to induce and maintain remission with a minimum of tissue damage due to either disease activity or therapy. Several scoring systems have been devised to assess disease activity accurately (reviewed in Bacon and Luqmani, 2002[7]). However, these have only recently been introduced and many trials have not reported outcomes using these tools. Drug-induced toxicity is a major concern but has not been reported consistently.

Summary

For the purposes of this review we are considering WG, CSS, MPA, and PAN as a group of related conditions, which require a similar therapeutic approach. Where significant differences exist we will highlight them. The rarity of the conditions means that large clinical trials have been difficult to perform. There is a paucity of randomised controlled trials. To date, no Cochrane Reviews have been published and there are few formal meta-analyses.

We will present a summary of recent meta-analyses and randomised trials of therapies for primary systemic vasculitis including cyclophosphamide (both oral and pulsed intravenous), azathioprine, methotrexate, intravenous immunoglobulin, and plasma exchange. We discuss toxicities and strategies to minimise these, including trimethoprim/ sulphamethoxazole as prophylaxis against pneumocystis carinii infection and mesna for bladder prophylaxis against haemorrhagic cystis and cancer.

We use the following case to illustrate the questions surrounding the treatment of individual patients with new onset systemic vasculitis.

Case presentation

A 51-year-old Caucasian woman presents with a 2 month history of malaise, arthralgias, fever, and 4 kg weight loss. She had developed a rash over the extensor surface of the arms. Urinalysis showed red cell casts and 4+ proteinuria. Serum creatinine was 300 micromol/l, with a protein excretion of 3·2 g/24h. A renal biopsy showed a focal segmental necrotising glomerulonephritis; she was also cANCA positive with a PR3 level of 98% (normal < 6%).

Evaluating the evidence

Question 1

In a patient with active newly diagnosed systemic vasculitis (population), does cyclophosphamide (intervention) improve the survival (outcome) compared with corticosteroids alone (therapy)

Literature search

Database: MEDLINE <1966 to May Week 2 2002>

1. exp vasculitis
2. (vasculitis or angiitis).tw.
3. (aortitis or arteritis or phlebitis).tw.
4. (Behcet's syndrome or Churg–Strauss or Shwartzman phenomenon).tw.
5. mucocutaneous lymph node syndrom$.tw.
6. (thromboangiitis obliterans or Wegener$ granulomatosis).tw.
7. or/1–6
8. exp cyclophosphamide/
9. (ifosfamide or cyclophosphamide).tw,rn.
10. (cyclophosphane or cytophosphan or cytoxan or endoxan or neosar or procytox or sendoxan).tw.
11. or/8–10
12. 7 and 11
13. clinical trial.pt.
14. randomised controlled trial.pt.
15. tu.fs.
16. dt.fs.
17. random$.tw.
18. (double adj blind$).tw.
19. placebo$.tw.
20. or/13–19
21. 12 and 20
22. 13 or 14 or 17
23. 12 and 22

Evaluating the evidence

The natural history of untreated primary systemic vasculitis is of a rapidly progressive, usually fatal disease. Prior to the introduction of corticosteroids in WG, Walton observed a mean survival of 5 months, with 82% of patients dying within 1 year and more than 90% dying within 2 years.[2] The introduction of corticosteroids resulted in an improvement in survival in PAN to 50% at 5 years.[8] The median survival in WG was only 12·5 months using corticosteroids alone, with most patients dying of sepsis or uncontrolled disease.[9]

There are no meta-analyses or RCTs addressing this question. In the 1970s, at the National Institutes of Health (NIH, USA), the introduction of cyclophosphamide (CYC) combined with

Table 13.1 Number needed to treat for corticosteroids and plasma exchange plus CYC versus corticosteroids and plasma exchange (Guillevin, 1991)[11]

Outcome	With corticosteroids and plasma exchange	With corticosteroids and plasma exchange plus CYC	Relative risk with corticosteroids and plasma exchange plus CYC (95% CI)	ARR (95% CI)	NNT(95% CI)
Relapse	15/39 (38%)	3/32 (9%)	0·24 (0·08, 0·77)	29% (9, 46)	4 (3, 12)

prednisolone resulted in a significant improvement in the mortality of WG with a 5 year survival rate of 82%.[3,4] The NIH regimen combines low dose oral CYC (2·0 mg/kg/day) with prednisolone, initially at a dose of 1·0 mg/kg/day. Cyclophosphamide was continued for at least one year after the patient achieved complete remission and was then tapered. Prednisolone was continued daily for at least 4 weeks and changed to alternate day dosing prior to tapering. Patients were then maintained solely on CYC. In a prospective open study of 133 patients who received this regimen 75% achieved a complete remission and an 80% survival rate was observed over a mean follow up of 8 years. Relapse was observed in 50% of patients and drug toxicity was observed in 42%.[10] Corticosteroids were withdrawn at a median interval of 12 months. This regimen was designed to minimise exposure to corticosteroids and avoid neutropenia.

The only prospective randomised trial to assess the efficacy of CYC was performed in 71 patients with PAN or CSS who were randomised to treatment with corticosteroids and plasma exchange alone or with the addition of CYC.[11] A power calculation suggested that to achieve a 75% recovery in the CYC group (together with corticosteroids and plasma exchange) and 50% in the control group (corticosteroids and plasma exchange), 160 patients would be required. Oral CYC was given at 2·0 mg/kg/day for one year. A planned interim analysis at 3 years demonstrated better disease control in the CYC group but no difference in survival. The trial was therefore stopped after recruitment of 71 patients. The relapse rate was also lower in the CYC group (Table 13.1).

This group has recently analysed the results from four of their prospective trials carried out between 1980 and 1993.[12] These four trials were: (1) corticosteroids and plasma exchanges versus corticosteroids and plasma exchanges plus oral CYC in patients with PAN, CSS or MPA; (2) corticosteroids alone versus corticosteroids and plasma exchanges in patients with PAN (without HBV), MPA or CSS; (3) corticosteroids and pulse CYC versus corticosteroids and pulse CYC and plasma exchanges in patients with poor prognosis (Five Factor Score ≥ 1) PAN (without HBV), CSS, MPA; good prognosis patients (FFS = 0) received corticosteroids and either pulse or continuous CYC; (4) corticosteroids and anti-viral therapy in patients with PAN associated with HBV. The 278 patients were reclassified using current definitions for PAN, MPA and CSS. Overall survival was the same in the 215 patients who received CYC plus corticosteroids or corticosteroids alone. Stratification for disease severity suggested that patients with more severe disease (FFS ≥ 2) had prolonged survival when treated with CYC. In this analysis 15 of the 22 patients who died of severe vasculitis had not received corticosteroids. CYC did not, however, appear to reduce the relapse rate. They concluded that CYC should be used for patients with severe disease at presentation.

The NIH regimen is the basis against which further developments have been compared. Because of concerns regarding CYC toxicity

Table 13.2 Prospective studies of pulse versus oral cyclophosphamide in primary systemic vasculitis

Study	Disease	Patients (*n*)	Cumulative CYC at 6 mth (g)	Cumulative GC at 6 mth (g)	Mortality	Remission	Infections (serious)	Comment
Gayraud[15]	PAN, CSS	25	Oral 25·6	Oral 8·3	0	9/12	2/12	Good prognosis
			Pulse 5·8	Pulse 8·3	1	10/13	3/13	
Guillevin[16]	WG	50	Oral 23·8	Oral 9·6	20% at 6 th		40·7%	
			Pulse 10·1	Pulse 9·6			69·6%	
Adu[17]	PAN (8)	54	Oral 25·6	Oral 5·3	10% at 1 yr	8/24	1·6/pt*	
	MPA (17)		Pulse 9·0	Pulse 6·3	16% at 1 yr	7/30	1·7/pt*	
	WG (29)							
Haubitz[18]	WG	47	Oral 25·5	Oral 4·2	16% at 2 yr	84%	10/25	
	MPA		Pulse 7·2	Pulse 4·2	0% at 2 yr	100%	3/22	

Cumulative dose calculations based on a 70 kg person with a surface area of 1·6m^2, using the described protocols.

* = all infections.

there has been a trend towards shorter duration CYC (see below). In a consensus statement from the European Vasculitis Study Group, the combination of CYC for one year and a tapering dose of prednisolone was regarded as the standard treatment for patients with generalised/renal vasculitis.[13]

Adverse effects: Cyclophosphamide-associated adverse effects were frequent[10] – cystitis (43%), bladder cancer (2·8%), and myelodysplasia (2%). Serious infections (those requiring hospitalisation and intravenous antibiotics) occurred in 46% of patients (0·11 infections per patient year).

Evidence summary

Silver: RCT analyses show patients with more severe disease have prolonged survival with the use of cyclophosphamide in addition to corticosteroids as induction therapy for patients with primary systemic vasculitis.

Bronze: The consensus from the European Vasculitis Study Group is that the patient should receive cyclophosphamide and corticosteroids as induction therapy.

Question 2

In a patient with severe active primary systemic vasculitis (population) is pulse intravenous CYC (intervention) as effective and less toxic (outcome) than continuous daily CYC (therapy)?

Literature search

This was conducted as for Question 1.

Evaluating the evidence

Benefits: This is one of the most controversial areas in the treatment of vasculitis. CYC therapy is associated with significant toxicity, much of which is dose dependent (see below). The total dose of CYC can be reduced either by shortening the duration of therapy (Question 5) or by intermittent administration. A meta-analysis of three randomised trials considering only ANCA-associated vasculitis has been published.[14] In addition, there is one RCT in patients with PAN and CSS[15] (Table 13.2). In addition, there are 11 non-randomised trials with more than 5 patients (reviewed in De Groot, 2001[14]).

De Groot and colleagues performed a meta-analysis on the 143 patients in the three RCTs of

Table 13.3 Number needed to treat for continuous versus pulse CYC (De Groot, 2001) meta-analysis[14] (pooled data from three RCTs)

Outcome	With pulse CYC	With continuous CYC	Relative risk with pulse CYC	ARR (95% CI)	NNT
Failure to induce remission	5/69 (7%)	17/73 (23%)	0·33 (0·13, 0·82)	16% (41, 28)	7
Leucopenia	12/69 (17%)	26/73 (36%)	0·49 (0·28, 0·87)	18% (4, 31)	6
Infections	27/69 (39%)	42/73 (58%)	0·68 (0·49, 0·95)	18% (2, 34)	6

ANCA-associated vasculitis and concluded that pulsed CYC was less likely to fail to induce remission than continuous oral cyclophosphamide (RR 0·33 (0·13, 0·82)) and had a significantly lower risk of infection (RR 0·68 (0·49, 0·95)) and leucopenia (RR 0·49 (0·28, 0·87)) (Table 13.3). Relapses occurred slightly more frequently with pulsed CYC treatment (OR 1·79; 95% CI 0·85–3·75). The 11 non-randomised studies comprised 202 patients receiving pulse CYC. Pulses of CYC were given at doses of 375–1000 mg/m^2/pulse at 1–4 week intervals with variable steroid and adjuvant therapy regimens. Remission was achieved in 112/191 evaluable patients. Relapse occurred in 68/135 patients. Leucopenia, infection, haemorrhagic cystitis, and death were rare.

The RCTs are considered in some detail below as there are significant methodological differences which make interpretation difficult. Guillevin *et al*[16] randomised 50 patients in a multicentre trial with newly diagnosed WG (within one week of diagnosis) and prior to beginning therapy (Table 13.2). The primary endpoint was achievement of complete or partial remission or death. A power calculation based on 60% survival at 5 years of oral CYC and 85% for pulse therapy suggested that 66 patients would be needed in each arm. A planned interim analysis at 3 years demonstrated a statistically significant difference between the two groups. There was an increase in infectious complications (Pneumocystis carinii infection, PCP) in the continuous oral group and relapse in the pulse group. Both these were secondary endpoints of the trial. The rate of infectious complication was high in both arms – 40·7% in the pulse group and 69.6% in the continuous group. Mortality was high, with 20% dying in the first 6 months. This high morbidity and mortality might reflect different disease severity but also the more intense immunosuppression used by the French, who, unlike the NIH group, aimed to reduce the granulocyte count below 3x10^9/l and used higher doses of daily corticosteroids and for longer periods of time.

Gayraud *et al*[15] studied patients with good prognosis PAN (without HBV) and CSS (defined as an FFS equal to zero (Table 13.2)). The study was not blinded and there was no power calculation. Complete recovery (no manifestations of vasculitis for 18 months after the end of treatment) was achieved in 9/12 patients in the continuous group and 10/13 patients in the pulse group. Two patients in each group relapsed after completion of treatment and one in each group failed to respond. Toxicity was greater in the continuous group but not significantly. Adverse effects attributable to CYC (neutropenia, haemorrhagic cystitis, and alopecia) were seen in the continuous group only.

Adu and colleagues[17] conducted a randomised controlled trial of 54 patients with systemic vasculitis (Table 13.2). Remission was defined as a BVAS (Birmingham Vasculitis Activity Score)

score of 0–1, partial remission as a BVAS reduction of > 50%, and relapse as a rise in BVAS score. The primary endpoint was drug toxicity and secondary endpoints were survival and relapses. The steroid doses in the two arms were different. Neutropenia was less common in the oral group but the difference was not significant. The incidence of infection was comparable in the two arms. Remission induction was similar in both groups, as was survival. A power calculation was performed, suggesting that to detect a reduction in toxicity from 70 to 40% with a power of 80% and a 5% significance, 42 patients were required in each arm. It is unclear whether this calculation was performed before the study began or why the study was stopped early.

Haubitz and colleagues[18] performed a multicentre study of patients with new onset WG and MPA and renal involvement (Table 13.2). Sixty-five patients were eligible for the study, of whom 56 were randomised. The remaining 9 patients were not entered due to previous therapy with CYC or prolonged dialysis. Data from 47 patients were analysed. In 4 patients the protocol was not completed as the trial was stopped early, and 5 patients were found to be inelligible after randomisation. CYC was stopped after 1 year, if remission had been achieved for at least 6 months and the ANCA titres were below 1:64. During the 12 months of the study the mean prednisolone dose was not significantly different in the two groups. The mean monthly dose of CYC was significantly lower in the pulse group ($1{\cdot}3 \pm 0{\cdot}3$ g) compared with $2{\cdot}8 \pm 0{\cdot}8$ g ($p < 0{\cdot}001$) in the oral group. There were no significant differences in patient survival, remission rate, relapse rate, renal function or renal survival between the two groups. The trial was terminated prematurely as toxicity (leucopenia and severe infections) occurred substantially less frequently in the pulsed group.

None of the four trials was powered adequately to detect significant differences in efficacy. Two of the trials were stopped early due to an excess of adverse events in the continuous limb.[16,18] Differences in CYC regimen (in particular the interval between pulses ranging from 2 to 4 weeks) and corticosteroid dosing make direct comparisons difficult and it is not possible to clearly advocate one regimen. De Groot concluded in her meta-analysis of patients with ANCA-associated vasculitis that pulse CYC was more effective than oral CYC but was less effective in preventing relapse.[14] This is probably due to the lower cumulative doses of CYC used in the pulse regimens. A multicentre European trial (CYCLOPS) is currently under way to answer the question whether pulsed therapy is as effective, and safer than continuous oral CYC in terms of induction and maintenance of remission, and adverse effects.[19]

Adverse effects: In the De Groot meta-analysis on the 143 patients in the three RCTs of ANCA-associated vasculitis the authors found that pulsed CYC had a significantly lower risk of infection (OR 0·45; 95% CI 0·23–0·89) and leucopenia (OR 0·36; 95% CI 0·17–0·78).

Evidence summary: Silver

There are mixed results in four trials. Post hoc analysis of three trials suggests that pulse CYC was more effective in inducing remission than oral CYC, had lower toxicity but was less effective in preventing relapse.

Route of administration should be discussed with the patient, with particular reference to the trade-offs between increased efficacy at remission induction with lower toxicity and increased relapse rate.

Question 3

In a patient with active newly diagnosed systemic vasculitis (population), is methotrexate (intervention) as effective as CYC (outcome)?

Literature search

Database: MEDLINE <1966 to May Week 2 2002>

1. exp vasculitis/
2. (vasculitis or angiitis).tw.
3. (aortitis or arteritis or phlebitis).tw.
4. (Behcet's syndrome or Churg–Strauss or Shwartzman phenomenon).tw.
5. mucocutaneous lymph node syndrom$.tw.
6. (thromboangiitis obliterans or Wegener$ granulomatosis).tw.
7. or/1–6
8. methotrexate/
9. methotrexate.tw,rn.
10. (amethopterin or mexate).tw.
11. or/8–10
12. 7 and 11
13. clinical trial.pt.
14. randomised controlled trial.pt.
15. tu.fs.
16. dt.fs.
17. random$.tw.
18. (double adj blind$).tw.
19. placebo$.tw.
20. or/13–19
21. 12 and 20
22. 13 or 14 or 17
23. 12 and 22

Evaluating the evidence

Benefits: Methotrexate is the only other immunosuppressant to have been studied in the induction of remission in patients with active but not life threatening disease. There is one prospective RCT (NORAM – published in abstract) addressing this question. There are three prospective open studies.

The NIH group described, in an open study of 41 WG patients, the use of combined daily steroids and methotrexate (MTX).[20] Patients were excluded if serum creatinine levels exceeded 2·5 mg/dl due to concerns about the increased risk of MTX toxicity in renal failure or if they had significant lung disease. The dose of corticosteroids was similar to that used in the CYC studies with methotrexate: 20–25 mg once per week. Remission was achieved in 71% of patients in a median period of 4 months and prednisolone could usually be discontinued by 7 months. However, this protocol was not without toxicity; 9·5% developed opportunistic infection, including PCP, which contributed to 2–3 deaths. In addition, although cystitis and bladder cancer are not associated with MTX there is a small increased risk of other malignancies. MTX can also cause pneumonitis, dose-related bone-marrow suppression, and liver dysfunction, and may affect fertility.

De Groot reported a prospective open label study of 17 patients with non-life threatening generalised WG fulfilling the ARC (1990) criteria and CHCC definitions for WG.[21] Methotrexate was given intravenously – 0·3 mg/kg weekly. Fifteen out of seventeen patients received concomitant corticosteroids. Remission was achieved in 59%, but there was a 20% relapse rate. This remission rate is less than that achieved with CYC using the original NIH regimen and also that of Sneller[20] with MTX (71%). Toxicity was less, in particular opportunistic infection, which was not seen in this study, compared with 46% using CYC (Fauci[4]) and 10% in the NIH study. The NIH study used significantly more corticosteroids (initially 50–70 mg/day) compared with 10·0 mg/day.

Stone *et al*[22] described the use of MTX and prednisolone in a study of 19 patients with non-life-threatening WG. Seventeen patients showed improvement and 14 achieved remission but all relapsed.[22]

Methotrexate has generally been considered inappropriate for patients with renal involvement because it is renally excreted. Langford *et al*[23] recently re-analysed the 42 patients treated with methotrexate in the Sneller open label study; 21 patients had active glomerulonephritis with normal or near normal serum creatinine, 20 of whom achieved a renal remission. After a median follow up of 76 months only 2/20 patients had shown a rise in serum creatinine, 12 had stable renal function, and 6 had shown an improvement. Thus glomerulonephritis should not preclude the use of methotrexate if the serum creatinine is normal or near normal.

Preliminary data from the NORAM trial comparing MTX with CYC in early non-renal vasculitis show that at the primary endpoint (remission at 6 months) equal numbers were in remission (84% *v* 86%). MTX patients took longer to achieve remission. The relapse rate after 1 year (when the trial medications stopped) was unacceptably high (74% MTX and 42% CYC). Mean time to relapse was 13·3 months, suggesting that even non-renal AAV therapy should not be rapidly tapered.[24]

Adverse effects: Opportunistic infections appear more related to the dose of corticosteroids. In addition, although cystitis and bladder cancer are not associated with MTX there is a small increased risk of other malignancies. MTX can also cause pneumonitis, dose-related bone-marrow suppression, and liver dysfunction and may affect fertility. Concerns had been expressed about the use of methotrexate in patients with renal disease; however, the analysis by Langford *et al*[23] suggests that there is not unacceptable renal toxicity from methotrexate. Complete toxicity data from the NORAM trial are not yet available.

Evidence summary: Silver

There is no placebo controlled RCT. In a head-to-head RCT preliminary analysis found that CYC and MTX had equal remission rates in non-renal vasculitis patients.

Recommendation for case presentation
The patient in this case has significant renal involvement and therefore should not receive MTX as first line therapy.

Question 4

In patients with generalised vasculitis (population) do high dose corticosteroids (intervention) improve the mortality (outcome)?

Literature search

The literature search was conducted as for Question 1.

Evaluating the evidence

Benefits: The combination of corticosteroids and CYC is standard therapy for systemic vasculitis. Most studies of therapies have concentrated on the CYC dose (or alternatives) rather than on the dose of corticosteroids. The NIH regime was designed to minimise the use of corticosteroids to reduce steroid associated toxicity. There are therefore no trials or meta-analyses designed specifically to answer this question.

Adverse effects: Some trials, however, especially from the French group, have used much higher doses of corticosteroids and these studies have been associated with a much greater rate of infectious complications. In the multicentre study by Guillevin *et al*[16] of 50 WG patients the patients in both treatment groups were still receiving approximately 55 mg/day (assuming a body weight of 70 kg) after 3 months. The infection rate was very high (54%), with an overall mortality of 38% over 3 years. Eighteen per cent of their patients died from infection compared with 3% in the NIH series. Pneumocystis carinii infection occurred in 20% compared with 4% at the NIH. Cyclophosphamide was used more intensively in the Guillevin study and this may have contributed to the high morbidity.

Evidence summary: Bronze

Steroids given in higher doses and for longer than the original NIH regimen are associated with increased morbidity and mortality. The patient should receive the minimum dose of corticosteroids and consideration should be given to using alternate day dosing.

Question 5

In a patient with generalised systemic vasculitis (population) is short duration cyclophosphamide (intervention) associated with less toxicity and similar relapse rate than the traditional NIH CYC regimen (outcome)?

Literature search

The literature search was conducted as for Question 1.

Evaluating the evidence

Benefits: There are no meta-analyses addressing this question. One RCT (CYCAZAREM) to directly address this question has so far only been published in abstract form.[25]

Langford *et al*[26] at the NIH performed an open label prospective study using a staged approach to the treatment of Wegener's granulomatosis. Thirty-one patients with active WG were included. All patients received an induction regimen consisting of oral continuous CYC (2·0 mg/kg/day) and corticosteroids (1·0 mg/kg/day). Once disease remission had been achieved MTX was substituted for CYC. The initial dose of MTX was given within 1–2 days of the last CYC dose if the WBC was acceptable. Methotrexate was started at a dose of 0·3 mg/kg and gradually escalated to a maximum of 20–25 mg/week. Remission was induced in all patients. Comparison with historical controls treated with the standard NIH regimen of daily oral CYC for >1 year suggests that the relapse rate was no greater in the MTX treated patients. The relapse rate (16%) is similar to that reported by Guillevin16 in a randomised trial of oral versus pulse CYC and to that from De Groot.[26] Toxicity was low, but two patients developed MTX pneumonitis. All patients received prophylaxis with **trimethroprim/ sulphamethoxazole** (Septrin). No adverse events were observed in relation to the combination of MTX and **trimethroprim/ sulphamethoxazole** prophylaxis. Two patients developed cystitis (6%), a rate much lower than observed with the standard NIH regimen.

The CYCAZAREM trial used a similar approach but azathioprine (AZA) was used as maintenance therapy.[25] A total of 155 patients with ANCA-associated vasculitis were studied. Oral cyclophosphamide and corticosteroids resulted in remission in 145 patients. Ten patients were either intolerant of therapy or died. After remission induction at 3–6 months patients were randomised to either continue CYC for 12 months or switch to AZA. There was no difference in relapse rates (17%) up to the end of the study at 18 months after treatment outset. There was a trend to fewer adverse events in the AZA group. It is worth noting that in the NORAM trial there was a high relapse rate after therapy was withdrawn at 12 months.

A staged approach using CYC and corticosteroids is very effective at inducing remission in patients with ANCA-associated vasculitis. When remission has been induced a switch to less toxic drugs such as azathioprine and MTX should be undertaken for long term maintenance therapy.

Adverse effects: The NIH CYC regimen was associated with significant toxicity, including bone marrow suppression, haemorrhagic cystitis, bladder malignancy, and infection. Toxicity is predominately associated with total dose. Over the years there has been a trend towards reducing the length of CYC therapy with a switch to less toxic alternatives for maintenance therapy. The two drugs most commonly used for maintenance therapy are azathioprine and methotrexate (MTX), usually combined with corticosteroids.

In the Langford NIH study using a staged approach in WG, toxicity was low, but two patients developed MTX pneumonitis. All patients received prophylaxis with **trimethroprim/ sulphamethoxazole** and no adverse events were observed in relation to the combination of MTX and **trimethroprim/ sulphamethoxazole** prophylaxis. Two patients developed cystitis (6%), a rate much lower than observed with the standard NIH regimen.

In the CYCAZAREM trial there was a trend to fewer adverse events in the AZA group. Reversible leucopenia was the most commonly observed adverse effect of azathioprine. Azathioprine hypersensitivity was observed in 5/70 patients and needs to be distinguished from relapse of vasculitis.

Evidence summary: Silver

A cohort study plus an RCT found a staged approach using CYC and corticosteroids is effective at inducing remission in patients with ANCA-associated vasculitis; then when remission has been induced , it can be maintained with the same success rate but less toxicity with a switch to drugs such as azathioprine and MTX.

Question 6

In a patient in whom remission has been successfully achieved with cyclophosphamide (population) is azathioprine (treatment) the best drug to maintain remission (outcome)?

Literature search

1. exp vasculitis/
2. (vasculitis or angiitis).tw.
3. (aortitis or arteritis or phlebitis).tw.
4. (Behcet's syndrome or Churg–Strauss or Shwartzman phenomenon).tw.
5. mucocutaneous lymph node syndrom$.tw.
6. (thromboangiitis obliterans or Wegener$ granulomatosis).tw.
7. or/1–6
8. exp cyclophosphamide/
9. (ifosfamide or cyclophosphamide).tw,rn.
10. (cyclophosphane or cytophosphan or cytoxan or endoxan or neosar or procytox or sendoxan).tw.
11. or/8–10
12. azathioprine/
13. azathioprine.tw,rn.
14. (immuran or azothioprine or imuran or imurel).tw.
15. or/12–141
16. 11 and 15
17. 7 and 16
18. clinical trial.pt.
19. randomised controlled trial.pt
20. tu.fs
21. dt.fs.
22. random$.tw.
23. (double adj blind$).tw.
24. placebo$.tw.
25. or/18–24
26. 17 and 25

Evaluating the evidence

Benefits: There have been no meta-analysis addressing this question. Azathioprine and MTX are the two drugs usually used in this situation and they have not been compared directly. Fauci *et al* in their original report on cyclophosphamide in WG noted that azathioprine might be an effective agent to maintain remission in WG.[4] The recently completed CYCAZAREM trial suggests that up to 18 months there is no difference in relapse rates between patients switched to AZA as soon as remission is achieved and those in which CYC is continued for one year.[25] Langford and colleagues compared 31 patients who received MTX for remission maintenance after induction with oral CYC with 60 historical controls treated with CYC for more than one year.[26] There was no difference in relapse rate. De Groot *et al*[27] performed a four limb study in 65 patients with generalised WG. They compared MTX with and without concomitant prednisolone versus trimethoprim/sulphamethoxazole with and without prednisolone.[26] This was not a randomised trial. Remission was maintained in 86% patients receiving MTX alone and 91% in those receiving MTX and prednisolone. Trimethoprim/ sulphamethoxazole was not effective at maintaining remission.

There is probably no significant difference between AZA and MTX for maintenance of remission but no direct comparisons have been made, nor is there long term data beyond 18 months for azathioprine.

Adverse effects: The overall long term risks of AZA and MTX are probably similar and relate to myelosuppression, infection, and malignancy. Long term data over many years are not available from vasculitis studies and long term toxicity of these agents may be different from that observed in other conditions such as rheumatoid arthritis.

Evidence summary: Silver

Methotrexate and azathioprine for maintenance give similar results.

Question 7

In a patient in remission (population) does a rise in ANCA titre (test) predict relapse (outcome)?

There have been several prospective studies addressing the utility of serial ANCA testing in prediction of relapse of vasculitis.

Literature search

Database: MEDLINE <1966 to June Week 2 2002>

1. exp vasculitis/
2. (vasculitis or angiitis).tw.
3. (aortitis or arteritis or phlebitis).tw.
4. (Behcet's syndrome or Churg–Strauss or Shwartzman phenomenon).tw.
5. mucocutaneous lymph node syndrom$.tw.
6. (thromboangiitis obliterans or Wegener$ granulomatosis).tw.
7. or/1–6
8. antibodies, antineutrophil cytoplasmic/bl [Blood]
9. (anca or antineutrophil cytoplasmic or anti-neutrophil cytoplasmic).tw.
10. bl.fs.
11. 9 and 10
12. 8 or 11
13. 7 and 12
14. clinical trial.pt.
15. randomised controlled trial.pt.
16. tu.fs.
17. dt.fs.
18. random$.tw.
19. (double adj blind$).tw.
20. placebo$.tw.
21. or/14–20
22. 13 and 21

Evaluating the evidence

Following discovery of the association between WG and ANCA, several groups have studied the use of serial measurements of ANCA in predicting relapse of WG. Cohen-Tervaert[28] randomised 20 patients with a rising ANCA titre to either therapy at the time of clinical relapse or treatment with CYC and corticosteroids at the time of ANCA increase. Nine of 11 untreated patients subsequently relapsed. The treated patients did not sustain any relapses. Patients in the untreated group who subsequently required therapy needed more CYC and prednisolone than the treated group. In a pooled analysis only 48% of rises in ANCA titres as measured by indirect immunofluorescence were followed by relapse[29] and only 51% of relapses were preceded by rising titres.

Boomsma *et al*[30] prospectively assessed the value of serial determinations of ANCA (by indirect immunofluorescence and PR3/MPO by enzyme linked immunoassay, ELISA). One hundred patients with WG were studied and ANCA determined every 2 months together with disease activity using the Birmingham Vasculitis Activity Score. Thirty-seven patients relapsed during follow up (median 1054 days); 34/37 (92%) patients showed a rise in ANCA level preceding relapse determined by either ELISA or IIF. The predictive value of an increase in ANCA titres for relapse was 57% (17/30) for cANCA by IIF, 71% (27/38) for PR3-ANCA and 100% (3/3) for MPO-ANCA. Forty-three per cent of patients who showed a rise in cANCA and 29% with a rise in PR3-ANCA did not subsequently relapse. Only 39% of patients with an increase in ANCA relapsed within 6 months of the rise in ANCA, thus a rise in PR3-ANCA is not usually an indicator of imminent relapse. In this study serial measurements of ANCA were useful in prediction of relapse in patients with WG, and measurement of ANCA by PR3/MPO ELISA was superior to determination by IIF for prediction of subsequent relapses.

Girard *et al*[31] retrospectively analysed ANCA titres in a prospective trial of continuous versus pulse CYC in 55 WG patients. ANCA positivity was associated with relapse, but there was no correlation between cANCA and disease activity. Proteinase 3 levels were not measured in this study.

Evidence summary: Silver

Low predictive values predicting relapse were found, so it is not justified to escalate immunosuppressive therapy solely on the basis of an increase in ANCA level, as determined by PR3/MPO ELISA. An increase should be taken as a warning and the patient observed more closely.

Question 8

In patients receiving cyclophosphamide and corticosteroids (population) does oral trimethroprim/sulphamethoxazole (intervention) prevent infection with *Pneumocystis carinii* pneumonia (outcome)?

Database: MEDLINE <1966 to May Week 4 2002>

Literature search

1. exp vasculitis/
2. (vasculitis or angiitis).tw.
3. (aortitis or arteritis or phlebitis).tw.
4. (Behcet's syndrome or Churg–Strauss or Shwartzman phenomenon).tw.
5. mucocutaneous lymph node syndrom$.tw.
6. (thromboangiitis obliterans or Wegener$ granulomatosis).tw.
7. or/1–6
8. pneumocystis carinii/
9. pneumocystis carini$.tw.
10. 8 or 9
11. 7 and 10
12. clinical trial.pt.
13. randomised controlled trial.pt.
14. tu.fs.
15. dt.fs.
16. random$.tw.
17. (double adj blind$).tw.
18. placebo$.tw.
19. or/12–18
20. 11 and 19

Evaluating the evidence

Benefits: There are no meta-analysis or RCTs to answer this specific question. Data is available from the meta-analysis of the randomised and non-randomised trials of pulse cyclophosphamide in ANCA-associated vasculitis.

Pneumocystis carinii pneumonia (PCP), a common infectious complication in immuno-compromised patients, is associated with significant morbidity and mortality. Trimethoprim/ sulphamethoxazole (Septrin) 960 mg thrice weekly is widely used as prophylaxis. The rate of PCP infection reported in vasculitis patients receiving CYC and corticosteroids has been reported by Guillevin *et al* to be as high as 20%,[16] compared with 6% in the NIH cohort[32] and 1% in a German cohort.[33] This difference may be explained by the much higher doses of prednisolone used in the French study[16] and many patients in the German study received trimethoprim/sulphamethoxazole as part of their therapeutic regimen. Haubitz, in a study of 47 patients receiving either continuous oral or pulse CYC together with corticosteroids,[18] did not observe a single case of PCP. These patients did not receive trimethoprim/sulphamethoxazole, but the cumulative doses of CYC were low. Gayraud,[12] in his analysis of four French trials (CSS, MPA, PAN), noted only a single patient with PCP, but used slightly lower doses of prednisolone and CYC than Guillevin[16] in WG. De Groot noted in a meta-analysis of pulse cyclophosphamide for ANCA-associated vasculitis that in 11 non-randomised trials comprising a total of 167 evaluable patients that no cases of PCP occurred.[14]

Ognibene and colleagues[32] reviewed the NIH experience in an open retrospective study of 180 WG patients and noted that the overall incidence of PCP was 6%. PCP developed during therapy with corticosteroids and a second immunosuppressive agent. Lymphopenia was noted in all patients developing PCP. They concluded that these risk factors together with the functional abnormalities of lymphocytes and monocytes caused by corticosteroids were the major factors predisposing to PCP in WG. Godeau *et al* retrospectively compared a group of 12 patients with WG and PCP with 32 WG patients without PCP.[34] The mean cumulative dose of CYC was greater in the PCP group and the lymphocyte count was significantly lower during treatment in the PCP group (244/mm^3 *v* 738/mm^3) in the control group. Following multivariate analysis the severity of lymphopenia before and during immunosuppressive therapy was the best predictor of PCP infection in WG.

A cost–benefit analysis by Chung *et al* suggested that trimethoprim/sulphamethoxazole prophylaxis increased life expectancy and reduced overall costs.[35]

Adverse effects: The toxicity of prophylaxis with trimethoprim/sulphamethoxazole is due to the sulphonamide moiety. There is also an interaction with methotrexate resulting in an increased risk of myelosuppression.

Evidence summary: Bronze

The risks of PCP are related to the doses of CYC and corticosteroids, so the current use of lower cumulative doses of both drugs probably reduces the risk. Although there is no RCT data, observational data from trials and case series supports the approach that patients receiving CYC and corticosteroids should receive trimethoprim/sulphamethoxazole 960 mg thrice weekly as prophylaxis against PCP.

Question 9

In patients receiving cyclophosphamide (population) does mesna (intervention) prevent bladder toxicity (cancer or haemorrhagic cystitis) (outcome)?

Literature search

Database: MEDLINE <1966 to June Week 2 2002>

1. exp cyclophosphamide/
2. (ifosfamide or cyclophosphamide).tw,rn.
3. (cyclophosphane or cytophosphan or cytoxan or endoxan or neosar or procytox or sendoxan).tw.
4. or/1–3
5. bladder neoplasms/
6. (bladder adj2 (cancer or neoplasm$ or tumor$ or tumour$)).tw.

7. exp cystitis/ or cystitis.tw.
8. or/5–7
9. 4 and 8
10. clinical trial.pt.
11. randomised controlled trial.pt.
12. tu.fs.
13. dt.fs.
14. random$.tw.
15. (double adj blind$).tw.
16. placebo$.tw.
17. or/10–16
18. 9 and 17

Evaluating the evidence

Benefits: There are no meta-analyses or RCTs to answer this question. Data from several long term follow up studies and RCTs of continuous oral versus pulse CYC are available and from the meta-analysis of pulse CYC in ANCA-associated vasculitis.

The NIH regimen is associated with significant CYC-induced bladder toxicity. A retrospective study of 145 patients followed for a median of 8·5 years reported non-glomerular haematuria in 73 (50%).[36] Sixty patients underwent cystoscopy and there were macroscopic changes consistent with CYC-induced bladder damage. The median total dose of CYC was 124 g. Seven patients (5%) developed transitional cell carcinoma. In 6 out of 7 patient the total cumulative dose of CYC was > 100 g and duration of therapy was >2·7 years. The interval between CYC therapy and development of bladder cancer ranged from 7 months to 15·3 years. The risk of bladder cancer was estimated to be 5% at 10 years and 16% at 15 years. Compared with the general population there was a 31-fold increase in risk of bladder cancer in CYC-treated patients.

Stilwell and colleagues reported an open study of 111 patients with WG treated with CYC and followed for a mean of 6 years. In this study there was a 15% rate of haemorrhagic cystitis and 4% rate of bladder cancer.[37]

A retrospective open study of 142 patients with WG followed for a median of 7 years treated with CYC and mesna reported a 12% rate of cystitis.[33] The majority of these patients received daily oral cyclophosphamide and the median dose of CYC was 129 g in the cystitis patients compared with 75 g in all their patients. Nineteen per cent of patients who received a CYC dose >100 g developed cystitis compared with the 50% rate reported by the NIH.[36] In the German study[33] one patient developed bladder cancer after a total dose of 350 g CYC, one year after stopping CYC because of cystitis. This compares with a 5% rate of bladder cancer at 10 years in the NIH cohort. The German study also had a longer cumulative follow up (2144 patient years) compared with the NIH (1333 patient years)[32].

In a recent report of a staged approach to the therapy of WG with short duration CYC followed by MTX a 6% frequency of bladder toxicity was noted.[26] These patients did not receive mesna but the duration of follow up is only 16 months from remission. The mean CYC dose is not stated but would, from the protocol, be significantly less than the standard NIH regimen.

The trials of pulsed CYC have all reported much lower rates of bladder toxicity but have used much lower cumulative CYC doses. Gayraud *et al* in their review of four trials in PAN, CCS, and MPA[12] only observed one bladder cancer after a mean follow up of 88 months. These patients only received CYC for approximately one year. Similarly Haubitz *et al*[18] did not observe bladder cancer in either the oral or pulsed CYC group in their study. De Groot in the meta-analysis of non-randomised trials of pulse cyclophosphamide in ANCA-associated vasculitis noted that 3 of 146 evaluated patients developed haemorrhagic cystitis.[14]

Mesna (sodium 2-mercaptoethane sulphonate) protects against the urothelial toxicity of cyclophosphamide by scavenging the toxic metabolite acrolein. There are no RCTs reporting its use in reducing the urothelial toxicity of cyclophosphamide in vasculitis.

Adverse effects: Mesna is generally well tolerated but may cause skin eruptions, which must be distinguished from relapse of the original disease.

Evidence summary: Silver

Historical cohort data show the risk of bladder toxicity in patients receiving CYC is related to the cumulative dose administered and is greatest in patients receiving >100 g. Mesna reduces the risk of toxicity in these patients. The current use of much lower cumulative CYC doses and early change to alternative immunosuppressive agents for maintenance of remission is associated with a lower risk of bladder toxicity. However, bladder cancer may develop many years after CYC therapy and it is not known what the long term risk is for patients treated in these newer protocols. Current evidence suggests that all patients should continue to receive mesna to minimise the risk of bladder toxicity. Surveillance with regular (3–6 monthly) urinalysis should be continued indefinitely after a course of CYC. Haematuria (microscopic and macroscopic) should be investigated with urine cytology and cystoscopy.

Questions 10

In a patient with refractory systemic vasculitis (population) does plasma exchange (intervention) improve mortality (outcome)?

Literature search

Database: MEDLINE <1966 to May Week 4 2002>

1. exp vasculitis/
2. (vasculitis or angiitis).tw.
3. (aortitis or arteritis or phlebitis).tw.
4. (Behcet's syndrome or Churg–Strauss or Shwartzman phenomenon).tw.
5. Mucocutaneous lymph node syndrom$.tw.
6. (Thromboangiitis obliterans or Wegener$ granulomatosis).tw.
7. or/1–6
8. Plasma exchange/
9. (plasma exchange or plasmapheresis or exchange transfusion).tw.
10. 8 or 9
11. 7 and 10
12. clinical trial.pt.
13. randomised controlled trial.pt.
14. tu.fs.
15. dt.fs.
16. random$.tw.
17. (double adj blind$).tw.
18. placebo$.tw.
19. or/12–18
20. 11 and 19

Evaluating the evidence

Benefits: There have been several RCTs addressing this question. However, different patient groups have been studied.

Guillevin *et al*[38] compared corticosteroids alone with corticosteroids and plasma exchange in 78 patients with PAN and Churg–Strauss syndrome. The endpoints of the study were disease control or death. In both groups disease control was similar and there was no benefit in preventing relapse. The cumulative 7 year survival was 83% in the plasma exchange group and 79% in the control group. The same group compared corticosteroids and cyclophosphamide with corticosteroids, cyclophosphamide, and plasma exchange in 62 patients with poor prognosis PAN and Churg–Strauss syndrome.[39] There was no difference in initial control of disease or relapse rate between the two groups. The addition of plasma exchange to immunosuppressive therapy with prednisolone, cyclophosphamide, and azathioprine was studied in 48 patients with rapidly progressive glomerulonephritis. No difference in outcome was observed in patients presenting with a creatinine of < 500 micromol/l. Patients who were initially dialysis-dependent (19 cases) were more likely to recover renal function if they received plasma exchange (10/11) than if they did not (3/8) ($p = 0.041$).[40]

Recently an RCT (MEPEX) comparing plasma exchange and pulsed methylprednislone as adjunctive therapy in biopsy proven ANCA-associated vasculitis with acute renal failure (creatinine > 500micromol/l has been reported in abstract.[41] A total of 151 patients received either seven plasma exchanges (60 ml/kg) or three pulses of methylprednislone (15 mg/kg) in addition to standard therapy with cyclophosphamide and tapering prednisolone. Preliminary data suggest that renal outcome was better in the plasma exchange-treated group when expressed as either dialysis independence in surviving patients or overall rate of dialysis-free survival. Death rates were similar in both groups.

Adverse effects: Generally plasma exchange is well tolerated, but adverse event data is not yet available from the largest controlled trial to date.

Evidence summary: Silver

The fully reported RCTs suggest that plasma exchange is only of benefit in patients with a serum creatinine > 500 micromol/l or initial dialysis dependence. Preliminary data from the European MEPEX trial seems to confirm this. Plasma exchange should be considered in patients with a creatinine > 500 micromol/l or dialysis dependence.

Question 11

In a patient with refractory systemic vasculitis (population) does intravenous immunoglobulin (intervention) improve mortality (outcome)?

Literature search

Database: MEDLINE <1966 to May Week 4 2002>

1. exp vasculitis/
2. (vasculitis or angiitis).tw.
3. (aortitis or arteritis or phlebitis).tw.
4. (Behcet's syndrome or Churg–Strauss or Shwartzman phenomenon).tw.
5. mucocutaneous lymph node syndrom$.tw.
6. (thromboangiitis obliterans or Wegener$ granulomatosis).tw.)
7. or/1–6 (57642)
8. immunoglobulins, intravenous/
9. intravenous immunoglobulins.tw.
10. (intravenous antibodies or iv ig or alphaglobin or endobulin or gamimmune or gamimune or intraglobin or intravenous ig or venoglobulin).tw.
11. 8 or 9
12. 7 and 11
13. clinical trial.pt.
14. randomised controlled trial.pt.
15. tu.fs.
16. dt.fs.
17. random$.tw.
18. (double adj blind$).tw.
19. placebo$.tw.
20. or/13–19
21. 12 and 20

Evaluating the evidence

Benefits: The literature to date has included a number of open cohort studies on intravenous immunoglobulin in vasculitis with small numbers of patients. There has been one randomised, placebo controlled trial which investigated the efficacy of a single course of IV immunoglobulin (Ig) (total dose 2 g/kg) in previously treated primary systemic vasculitis patients with persistent disease in whom there was an intention to escalate therapy. Vasculitis activity was monitored using BVAS, CRP, and ANCA levels. Treatment response was defined as a reduction in BVAS of more than 50% after 3 months and there was an intention to keep doses of current immunosuppressive drugs unchanged. Follow up was up to 12 months. Seventeen patients were randomised to receive IV Ig and 17

Table 13.4 Number needed to treat for IV Ig versus placebo (Jayne, 2000)[42]

Outcome	With placebo	With IV Ig	Relative risk (95% CI)	ARR (95% CI)	NNT (95% CI)
Reduction of BVAS > 50% after 3 months	6/17 (35%)	14/17 (82%)	2·33 (1·18, 4·61)	47% (14, 68)	3 (2, 8)

Table 13.5 Number needed to harm for IV Ig versus placebo (Jayne, 2000)[42]

Outcome	With placebo	With IV Ig	Relative risk	Absolute risk increase (95% CI)	NNH (95% CI)
Any adverse effect	4/17 (24%)	12/17 (71%)	3·00 (1·21, 7·45)	0·47 (0·14, 0·68).	2 (1, 7)
Rise in serum creatinine	0/17 (0%)	4/17 (24%)	Cannot calculate	0·24 (0·004, 0·47)	2. (4, 250)

received placebo. Treatment responses were found in 14/17 and 6/17 in the IV Ig and placebo groups respectively ($p = 0{\cdot}015$, OR 8·56, 95% CI 1·74–42·2) (Table 13.4). Following infusion of IV Ig there were greater falls in CRP at 2 weeks in the IV Ig group but no differences between ANCA levels or cumulative exposure to immunosuppressive drugs. Also, there was no difference in CRP levels or disease activities after 3 months. Adverse effects were common but mild, including reversible rises in serum creatinine in four of the IV Ig group.[42]

Two open studies of IV Ig involving 26 and 14 patients with vasculitis have observed sustained reductions in disease activity in 75% and 40% respectively.[43,44] When given alone without concurrent immunosuppression as first line treatment for otherwise untreated vasculitis, 4 out of 6 patients in an open study had a sustained remission of their symptoms.[43]

Adverse effects: IV Ig may be associated with an increase in serum creatinine, especially in patients with impaired renal function (Table 13.5). Otherwise IV Ig is well tolerated. There are risks associated with transmission of infections (such as hepatitis B, C or HIV) or potentially other unknown agents.

Evidence summary: Silver

In an RCT a single course of IV Ig was shown to reduce serum antibodies and to have a short lived (3 months) beneficial response. Open studies found clinical improvement.

Recommendation for case presentation

Your patient has a diagnosis of WG with major organ involvement. Treatment with cyclophosphamide, corticosteroids, **trimethoprim/sulphamethoxazole** (Septrin), and mesna resulted in prompt resolution of systemic symptoms and rash. Renal function gradually returned to normal. The BVAS score became zero, indicating remission, and after 6 months azathioprine was substituted for cyclophosphamide and corticosteroids were tapered. The patient continues to be monitored and to receive treatment with oral azathioprine and low doses of corticosteroids.

Future research needs

There is still a lack of controlled trial evidence to guide therapy of systemic vasculitis. The results of the EUVAS trials will provide a solid basis for progress. Future trials need to include:

Box 13.1 Summary

Question	Type of evidence	Results	Comments
Does CYC improve survival?	Cohort studies 1 RCT Review 4 trials	Survival improved with CYC compared with prednisolone alone	Only RCT used plasma exchange in both limbs
Is pulse CYC as effective as continuous oral CYC?	Meta-analysis of 3 RCTs 1 other RCT	Remission induction rates are similar Relapse rates possibly higher with pulse Lower toxicity with pulse therapy	2 trials stopped early, due to increased toxicity in oral limb. Data on remission/relapse incomplete. Multicentre trial under way
Is MTX as effective as CYC at remission induction?	3 prospective non-randomised trials 1 RCT	Effective at remission induction in patients with non-renal disease	Suitable for patients with non-life-threatening disease. RCT (NORAM) reported in abstract only
Do high dose steroids improve mortality?	Cohort studies	Possibly, but toxicity significant	
Optimum duration CYC for induction?	1 RCT 1 open study	CYC can be stopped as soon as remission has been consolidated	CYCAZAREM trial
Is AZA the best drug to maintain remission?	Observation	AZA and MTX both effective at maintaining remission	No RCTs to answer question
Does rise in ANCA titre predict relapse?	3 trials	Rise in ANCA titre precedes relapse	Treatment should not be changed solely on basis of rise in ANCA titre
Does trimethoprim/ sulphamethoxazole prevent PCP?	Observational studies Cost–benefit analysis	Appears to be effective	Risks PCP reduced by decreasing dose of prednisolone and CYC
Does mesna prevent CYC induced bladder toxicity?	Observational studies	Risk reduced with mesna Risk associated with total CYC dose	Risks with modern low dose CYC regime unknown, especially as cancer can develop many years after therapy
Role of plasma exchange	4 RCTs	May be of use in patients presenting with creatinine > 5000 micromol/litre	MEPEX trial only in abstract; 2 negative trials in PAN, CSS
Does IV Ig improve disease activity when added to standard therapy?	1 RCT open study	Short term improvement in disease activity	Effects last 3 months, alternative in patients at high risk of infection

- the role of MTX in remission;
- duration of maintenance therapy;
- **trimethoprim/sulphamethoxazole** both as a therapeutic agent and as prophylaxis against PCP;
- role of biologics (for example, TNF-α blocking drugs).

References

1 Watts R, Lane S, Bentham G, Scott D. Epidemiology of systemic vasculitis – a 10 year study in the United Kingdom. *Arthritis Rheum* 2000;**43**:422–7.

2 Walton EW. Giant cell granuloma of the respiratory tract. *Br Med J* 1958;**2**:265–70.

3 Fauci A, Wolff S. Wegener's granulomatosis: studies in 18 patients and a review of the literature. *Medicine* 1973;**52**:535–61.

4 Fauci AS, Haynes BF, Katz P, Wolff SM. Wegener's granulomatosis: prospective clinical and therapeutic experience with 85 patients for 21 years. *Ann Intern Med* 1983;**98**:76–85.

5 Gordon C, Luqmani R, Adu D. Relapses in patients with a systemic vasculitis. *Q J Med* 1993;**86**:779–89.

6 Wiik A. The rational use of ANCA in the diagnosis in the diagnosis of vasculitis. *Rheumatology* 2002;**41**:481–3.

7 Bacon PA, Luqmani. Assessment of Disease, Activity and Damage. In: Ball GV, Bridges SL, eds. *Vasculitis*. Oxford: Oxford University of Press, 2002:246–54.

8 Frohnert PP, Sheps SG.Long term follow-up of periarteritis nodosa. *Am J Med* 1967;**43**:8–14.

9 Hollander D, Manning RT. The use of alkylating agents in the treatment of Wegener's granulomatosis. *Ann Intern Med* 1967;**67**:393–8.

10 Hoffman GS, Kerr GS, Leavitt RY *et al.* Wegener granulomatosis: an analysis of 158 patients. *Ann Intern Med* 1992;**116**:488–98.

11 Guillevin L, Jarrousse B, Lok C, *et al.* Long term follow-up after treatment of polyarteritis nodosa and Churg Strauss angiitis with comparison of steroids, plasma exchanges and cyclophosphamide to steroids and plasma exchange. A prospective randomised trial of 71 patients. *J Rheumatol* 1991;**18**:567–74.

12 Gayraud M, Guillevin L, Toumelin PL, *et al.* Long-term follow up of polyarteritis nodosa, microscopic polyangiitis, and Churg Strauss syndrome: analysis of 4 prospective trials including 278 patients. *Arthritis Rheum* 2001;**44**:668–77.

13 Rasmussen N, Abramowicz D, Andrassy K, *et al.* European therapeutic trials in ANCA-associated vasculitis: disease scoring, consensus regimens and proposed clinical trials. *Clin Exp Immunol* 1995;**101**(Suppl 1):29–34.

14 De Groot K, Adu D, Savage COS. The value of pulse cyclophosphamide in ANCA-associated vasculitis: meta-analysis and critical review. *Nephrol Dialysis Transplant* 2001;**16**:2018–27.

15 Gayraud M, Guillevin L, Cohen P, *et al.* Treatment of good-prognosis polyarteritis nodosa and Churg–Strauss syndrome: comparison of steroids and oral or pulse cyclophosphamide in 25 patients. French Cooperative Study Group for Vasculitides. *Br J Rheumatol* 1997;**36**:1290–7.

16 Guillevin L, Cordier JF, Lhote F, *et al.* A prospective, multicenter, randomised trial comparing steroids and pulse cyclophosphamide versus steroids and oral cyclophosphamide in the treatment of generalised Wegener's granulomatosis. *Arthritis Rheum* 1997;**40**: 2187–98.

17 Adu D, Pall A, Luqmani RA, *et al.* Controlled trial of pulse versus continuous prednisolone and cyclophosphamide in the treatment of systemic vasculitis. *Q J Med* 1997;**90**:401–9.

18 Haubitz M, Schellong S, Gobel U, *et al.* Intravenous pulse administration of cyclophosphamide versus daily oral treatment in patients with antineutrophil cytoplasmic antibody-associated vasculitis and renal involvement: a prospective, randomised study. *Arthritis Rheum* 1998;**41**: 1835–44.

19 Jayne D. Update on the European Vasculitis Study Group trials. *Curr Opin Rheumatol* 2001;**13**:48–55.

20 Sneller MC, Hoffman GS, Talar-Williams C, Kerr GS, Hallahan CW, Fauci AS. An analysis of forty-two Wegener's granulomatosis patients treated with methotrexate and prednisone. *Arthritis Rheum* 1995;**38**:608–13.

21 De Groot K, Muhler M, Reinhold-Keller E, Paulsen J, Gross WL. Induction of remission in Wegener's granulomatosis with low dose methotrexate. *J Rheumatol* 1998;**25**:492–5.

22 Stone JH, Tun W, Hellman DB. Treatment of non-life threatening Wegener's granulomatosis with methotrexate

and daily prednisone as the initial therapy of choice. *J Rheumatol* 1999;**26**:1134–9.

23 Langford CA, Talar-Williams C, Sneller MC. Use of methotrexate and glucocorticoids in the treatment of Wegener's granulomatosis. Long term renal outcome in patients with glomerulonephritis. *Arthritis Rheum* 2000;**43**:1836–40.

24 DeGroot K, Rasmussen N, Cohen-Tervaert JW, Jayne DRW for EUVAS. Randomised trial of cyclophosphamide versus methotrexate for induction of remission in non-renal ANCA-associated vasculitis. *Clev Clin J Med* 2002;**69** (Suppl I2): 116 (abstract).

25 Jayne D, Rasmussen N, Andrassy K, for the European Vasculitis Study Group. A randomised trial of maintenance therapy for vasculitis associated with antineutrophil cytoplasmic autoantibodies. *N Engl J Med* 2003;**349**:36–44.

26 Langford CA, Talar-Williams C, Barron KS, Sneller MC. A staged approach to the treatment of Wegener's granulomatosis: induction of remission with glucocorticoids and daily cyclophosphamide switching to methotrexate for remission maintenance. *Arthritis Rheum* 1999;**42**:2666–73.

27 de Groot K, Reinhold-Keller E, Tatsis E, *et al.* Therapy for maintenance of remission in sixty-five patients with generalized Wegener's granulomatosis. Methotrexate versus trimethoprim/sulfamethoxazole. *Arthritis Rheum* 1996;**39**:2052–61.

28 Cohen-Tervaert JW, Huitma MG, Hene RJ, *et al.* Prevention of relapses in Wegener's granulomatosis by treatment based on antineutrophil cytoplasmic antibody titre. *Lancet* 1990;**336**:709–11.

29 Cohen-Tervaert JW, Stegeman CA, Kallenberg CGM. Serial ANCA testing is useful in monitoring disease activity in patients with ANCA associated vasculitides. *Sarcoidosis Vasc Dif Lung Dis* 1996;**13**:246–8.

30 Boomsma MM, Stegeman CA, van der Leij MJ, *et al.* Prediction of relapses in Wegener's granulomatosis by measurement of antineutrophil cytoplasmic antibodies. A prospective study. *Arthritis Rheum* 2000; **43**:2025–33.

31 Girard T, Mahr A, Noel LH *et al.* Are anti-neutrophil cytoplasmic antibodies a marker predictive of relapse in Wegener's granulomatosis? A prospective study. *Rheumatology (Oxford)* 2001;**40**:147–51.

32 Ognibene FP, Shelhamer JH, Hoffman GS, *et al.* *Pneumocystis carinii* pneumonia: a major complication of immunosuppressive therapy in patients with Wegener's granulomatosis. *Am J Resp Crit Care Med* 1995;**151**:795–9.

33 Reinhold-Keller E, Beuge N, Latza U, *et al.* An interdisciplinary approach to the care of patients with Wegener's granulomatosis: long-term outcome in 155 patients. *Arthritis Rheum* 2000;**43**:1021–32.

34 Godeau B, Mainardi JL, Roudot-Thoraval F *et al.* Factors associated with *Pneumocystis carinii* pneumonia in Wegener's granulomatosis. *Ann Rheum Dis* 1995;**54**:991–4.

35 Chung JB, Armstrong K, Schwartz JS, Albert D. Cost-effectiveness of prophylaxis against *Pneumocystis carinii* pneumonia in patients with Wegener's granulomatosis undergoing immunosuppressive therapy. *Arthritis Rheum* 2000;**43**:1841–8.

36 Talar-Williams C, Hijazi YM, Walther MM, *et al.* Cyclophosphamide-induced cystitis and bladder cancer in patients with Wegener granulomatosis. *Ann Intern Med* 1996;**124**:477–84.

37 Stilwell TJ, Benson RC, DeRemee RA, McDonald TJ, Weiland LH. Cyclophosphamide-induced bladder toxicity in Wegener's granulomatosis. *Arthritis Rheum* 1988;**31**:465–70.

38 Guillevin L, Fain O, Lhote F, *et al.* Lack of superiority of steroids plus plasma exchange to steroids alone in the treatment of polyarteritis nodosa and Churg–Strauss syndrome. A prospective, randomised trial in 78 patients. *Arthritis Rheum* 1992;**35**:208–15.

39 Guillevin L, Lhote F, Cohen P, *et al.* Corticosteroids plus pulse cyclophosphamide and plasma exchanges versus corticosteroids plus pulse cyclophosphamide alone in the treatment of polyarteritis nodosa and Churg–Strauss syndrome patients with factors predicting poor prognosis. A prospective, randomised trial in sixty-two patients. *Arthritis Rheum* 1995;**38**:1638–45.

40 Pusey CD, Rees AJ,Evans DJ, Peters DK, Lockwood CM. Plasma exchange in focal necrotizing glomerulonephritis without anti-GBM antibodies. *Kidney Int* 1991;**40**:757–63.

41 Luqmani RA, Jayne D, Gaskin G on behalf of EUVAS. Adjunctive plasma exchange is superior to methylprednisolone in acute renal failure due to ANCA-associated glomerulonephritis. *Arthritis Rheum* 2002 Suppl. S207 (abstract).

42 Jayne DR, Chapel H, Adu D *et al.* Intravenous immunoglobulin for ANCA-associated systemic vasculitis with persistent disease activity. *Q J Med* 2000;**93**(7): 433–9.

43 Jayne D, Esnault V, Lockwood C. ANCA anti-idiotypic antibodies and the treatment of systemic vasculitis with intravenous immunoglobulin. *J Autoimmunity* 1993;**6**: 207–19.

44 Richter C, Schnabel A, Csernok E, *et al.* Treatment of anti-neutrophil cytoplasmic antibody (ANCA)-associated systemic vasculitis with high dose intravenous immunoglobulin. *Clin Exp Immunol* 1995;**101**:2–7.

Primary systemic vasculitis
Summaries and decision aids

Vasculitis and azathioprine
Summaries and decision aid

Should people with vasculitis who go into remission with cyclophosphamide change over to azathioprine?

To answer this question, scientists found 1 study and analysed it. People received cyclophosphamide and prednisone until they were in remission and then received pills of cyclophosphamide or azathioprine to stay in remission. This study provides the best evidence we have today.

What is vasculitis and how is it treated?

Vasculitis is a group of diseases, including Wegener's granulomatosis, Churg–Strauss syndrome, microscopic polyangiitis, and polyarteritis nodosa, in which blood vessels are inflamed. The inflammation or swelling can occur anywhere in the body causing the walls of blood vessels to thicken, weaken, narrow, scar or break. Blood clots may form and blood may not be able to flow well to the tissues and organs in the body. With low blood supply, the tissues may die and organs may not work well. When the disease is severe, cyclophosphamide and a corticosteroid (such as prednisone) are used to help people go into remission (a period of no symptoms) and stay in or maintain remission. Even though cyclophosphamide works to get people into remission, it has serious side effects that can permanently damage the body. It is thought that using cyclophosphamide for a short time until people are in remission and then changing to another drug (such as azathioprine or methotrexate) may decrease the chances of flare-ups in the future and the chances of permanent damage caused by cyclophosphamide.

Did taking cyclophosphamide and corticosteroids to go into remission and then changing to a different drug (azathioprine) for maintenance work well?

People went into remission with cyclophosphamide and corticosteroids and then to maintain the remission took azathioprine or kept on taking cyclophosphamide. After going into remission, the number of people who had flare-ups while taking azathioprine was about the same as the number of people who had flare-ups while continuing to take cyclophosphamide.

What were the side effects?

The study showed that both drugs caused side effects, such as temporarily decreasing the number of white blood cells that fight infection. Taking cyclophosphamide over a long period of time causes bladder cancer, but this does not happen with azathioprine. But cyclophosphamide and azathioprine are known to increase the chances of other cancers, such as lymphoma. The study included in this review was only 18 months long which is too short a time to determine the chances of cancer.

What is the bottom line?

There is "Silver" level evidence that after remission, cyclophosphamide should be stopped and other drugs such as azathioprine should be started to stop flare-ups in the future and to avoid the chances of serious side effects that cyclophosphamide over a long period might cause.

Based on Watts R, Scott DGI, Lane SE, Ottawa Methods Group. Primary systemic vasculitis. In: *Evidence-based Rheumatology*. London: BMJ Books, 2003.

Should people with vasculitis who go into remission with cyclophosphamide change over to azathioprine?

What is vasculitis and how is it treated?

Vasculitis is a group of diseases, including Wegener's granulomatosis, Churg–Strauss syndrome, microscopic polyangiitis, and polyarteritis nodosa in which blood vessels are inflamed. The inflammation or swelling can occur anywhere in the body and can cause the walls of blood vessels to thicken, weaken, narrow, scar or break. Blood clots may form and blood may not be able to flow well to the tissues and organs in the body. With low blood supply, the tissues may die and organs may not work well. Vasculitis can be mild or more severe and life-threatening.

Some types of vasculitis may only occur once and go away on their own, while others will need to be treated. Other types may occur in cycles, where there are flare-ups and then periods with no symptoms (remission). When the disease is severe, cyclophosphamide and prednisone are used to help people go into remission and stay in or maintain remission. Even though cyclophosphamide works to get people into remission, it may not maintain remission (stop flare-ups in the future) and it has serious side effects that can permanently damage the body. It is thought that using cyclophosphamide for a short time until people are in remission and then changing to another drug (such as azathioprine or methotrexate) may decrease the chances of flare-ups in the future and the chances of permanent damage caused by cyclophosphamide.

How did the scientists find the information and analyse it?

The scientists searched for studies and reviews of the medical literature that examined the treatment of vasculitis. Not all studies and reviews found were of a high quality and so only those studies that met high standards were selected.

The study selected was a randomised controlled trial – where one group of patients continued to receive cyclophosphamide and another group switched to azathioprine.

Which high quality studies were examined in this summary?

There was 1 study examined in this summary: 155 patients with vasculitis received oral (by mouth) cyclophosphamide and prednisolone and 144 went into remission. After remission, 73 patients continued to take cyclophosphamide and 71 patients stopped taking cyclophosphamide and received azathioprine instead. The study lasted for 18 months.

Did taking cyclophosphamide and corticosteroids to go into remission and then changing to a different drug (azathioprine) for maintenance work well?

People went into remission with cyclophosphamide and corticosteroids. Then to maintain the remission people took azathioprine or kept on taking cyclophosphamide. After going into remission, the number of people who had flare-ups while taking azathioprine was about the same as the number of people who had flare-ups while continuing to take cyclophosphamide after going into remission.

Specifically, the study showed that:

- 15 out of 100 patients who switched to azathioprine had a flare-up
- 13 out of 100 patients who continued to take cyclophosphamide had a flare-up

Were there side effects?

The study showed that both drugs caused side effects, such as temporarily decreasing the number of white blood cells that fight infection. Taking cyclophosphamide over a long period of time causes bladder cancer, but this does not happen with azathioprine. But cyclophosphamide and azathioprine are known to increase the chances of other cancers, such as lymphoma. The study included in this review was only 18 months long, which is too short a time to determine the chances of cancer.

The study showed that:

- about 10 out of 100 patients taking azathioprine or cyclophosphamide had serious side effects
- about 55 out of 100 patients taking azathioprine or cyclophosphamide had fewer white blood cells that fight infection
- 4 out of 100 patients who kept taking cyclophosphamide and 1 out of 100 patients who switched to azathioprine had blood in the urine caused by an infection in the bladder
- 7 out of 100 patients who switched to azathioprine had fevers, chills, and a rash that could have been due to a reaction to azathioprine.

What is the bottom line?

There is "Silver" level evidence that after remission, cyclophosphamide should be stopped and other drugs such as azathioprine should be started to stop flare-ups in the future and to avoid the chances of serious side effects that cyclophosphamide over a long period might cause.

Based on Watts R, Scott DGI, Lane SE, Ottawa Methods Group. Primary systemic vasculitis. In: *Evidence-based Rheumatology*. London: BMJ Books, 2003

Information about vasculitis and treatment

What is vasculitis?

Vasculitis is a group of diseases, including Wegener's granulomatosis, Churg–Strauss syndrome, microscopic polyangiitis and polyarteritis nodosa, in which blood vessels are inflamed. The inflammation or swelling can occur anywhere in the body and can cause the walls of blood vessels to thicken, weaken, narrow, scar or break. Blood clots may form and blood may not be able to flow well to the tissues and organs in the body. With a poor blood supply, the tissues may die and organs may not work well. Vasculitis can be mild or more severe and life-threatening.

Some types of vasculitis may occur once and go away on their own, while others will need to be treated. Other types may occur in cycles, where there are flare-ups and then periods with no symptoms (remission). Treatment is used to stop flare-ups and to make sure blood vessels are not damaged. If vasculitis is not treated, inflammation or swelling in blood vessels can lead to permanent damage to tissues or organs and cause:

- loss of vision
- heart attack, kidney failure, lung damage
- gangrene
- death.

What can I do on my own to manage my disease?

✓ exercise when possible ✓ avoid alcohol ✓ rest and relax ✓ dress warmly in cold weather

What treatments are used for vasculitis?

Three kinds of treatment may be used alone or together. The common (generic) names of treatment are shown below:

1. *Oral or IV corticosteroids*
   - Prednisone
   - Prednisolone
   - Methylprednisolone
2. *Immunosuppressive agents (cytotoxics)*
   - Azathioprine
   - Ciclosporin
   - Methotrexate
   - Cyclophosphamide
3. *Other therapies*
   - Plasma exchange
   - Intravenous immunoglobulin

What about other treatments I have heard about?

There is not enough evidence about the effects of some treatments. Other treatments do not work. For example:

- Acupuncture
- Electropuncture
- Ultrasound
- Electrical stimulation
- Thermotherapy

What are my choices? How can I decide?

Treatment for your disease will depend on your condition. You need to know the good points (pros) and the bad points (cons) about each treatment before you can decide.

Vasculitis decision aid:

Should I switch to azathioprine after going into remission with cyclophosphamide?

This guide can help you make decisions about the treatment your doctor is asking you to consider.

It will help you to:

1. Clarify what you need to decide
2. Consider the pros and cons of different choices.
3. Decide what role you want to have in choosing your treatment.
4. Identify what you need to help you make the decision.
5. Plan the next steps.
6. Share your thinking with your doctor.

Step 1: Clarify what you need to decide

What is the decision?

Should I continue to take cyclophosphamide or take a different drug (such as azathioprine) after going into remission?

Cyclophosphamide can be taken as a pill or as an infusion into the veins (IV); azathioprine is usually taken as a pill.

When does this decision have to be made? Check ✓ one

☐ within days ☐ within weeks ☐ within months

How far along are you with this decision? Check ✓ one

☐ I have not thought about it yet.

☐ I am considering the choices

☐ I am close to making a choice

☐ I have already made a choice

Step 2: Consider the pros and cons of different choices

What does the research show?

Taking azathioprine after going into remission is classified as: **Likely beneficial**

There is "Silver" level evidence from 1 study of people with vasculitis who stopped taking cyclophosphamide and started another drug after going into remission. These studies found pros and cons that are listed in the chart below.

What do I think of the pros and cons of azathioprine?

1. Review the common pros and cons.
2. Add any other pros and cons that are important to you.
3. Show how important each pro and con is to you by circling from one (*) star if it is a little important to you, to up to five (*****) stars if it is very important to you.

PROS AND CONS OF AZATHIOPRINE TREATMENT

PROS (number of people affected)	How important is it to you?	CONS (number of people affected)	How important is it to you?
Less flare-ups and lower chances of dying than if stopped taking medications for vasculitis	* * * * *	Side effects: lowers white blood cells in about 55 out of 100 people taking azathioprine or cyclophosphamide	* * * * *
Same number of people had a flare-up of vasculitis in the 18 months after going into remission with azathioprine or cyclophosphamide about 14 out of 100 people had a flare-up	* * * * *	Can cause fever, chills or rash 7 out of 100 people taking azathioprine	* * * * *
No chances of bladder cancer with azathioprine	* * * * *	Personal cost of medicine	* * * * *
Less people have blood in urine 1 out of 100 people with azathioprine have blood in urine 4 out of 100 people with cyclophosphamide have blood in urine	* * * * *	Other cons:	* * * * *
Other pros:	* * * * *		

What do you think about taking azathioprine? Check ✓ one

☐ Willing to consider this treatment
Pros are more important to me than the Cons

☐ Unsure

☐ Not willing to consider this treatment
Cons are more important to me than the Pros

Step 3: Choose the role you want to have in choosing your treatment
Check ✓ one

☐ I prefer to decide on my own after listening to the opinions of others

☐ I prefer to share the decision with: ______________________

☐ I prefer someone else to decide for me, namely: ______________

Step 4: Identify what you need to help you make the decision

What I know	Do you know enough about your condition to make a choice?	☐ Yes	☐ No	☐ Unsure
	Do you know which options are available to you?	☐ Yes	☐ No	☐ Unsure
	Do you know the good points (pros) of each option?	☐ Yes	☐ No	☐ Unsure
	Do you know the bad points (cons) of each option?	☐ Yes	☐ No	☐ Unsure
What's important	Are you clear about which **pros** are most *important to you?*	☐ Yes	☐ No	☐ Unsure
	Are you clear about which **cons** are most *important to you?*	☐ Yes	☐ No	☐ Unsure
How others help	Do you have enough support from others to make a choice?	☐ Yes	☐ No	☐ Unsure
	Are you choosing without pressure from others?	☐ Yes	☐ No	☐ Unsure
	Do you have enough advice to make a choice?	☐ Yes	☐ No	☐ Unsure
How sure I feel	Are you clear about the best choice for you?	☐ Yes	☐ No	☐ Unsure
	Do you feel sure about what to choose?	☐ Yes	☐ No	☐ Unsure

If you answered No or Unsure to many of these questions, you should talk to your doctor.

Step 5: Plan the next steps
What do you need to do before you make this decision?
For example – talk to your doctor, read more about this treatment or other treatments for vasculitis.

Step 6: Share the information on this form with your doctor
It will help your doctor understand what you think about this treatment.

Index

Page numbers in **bold** refer to figures, those in *italics* refer to tables/boxed material. Abbreviations used in this index are the same as those listed on pages xxviii to xxix.

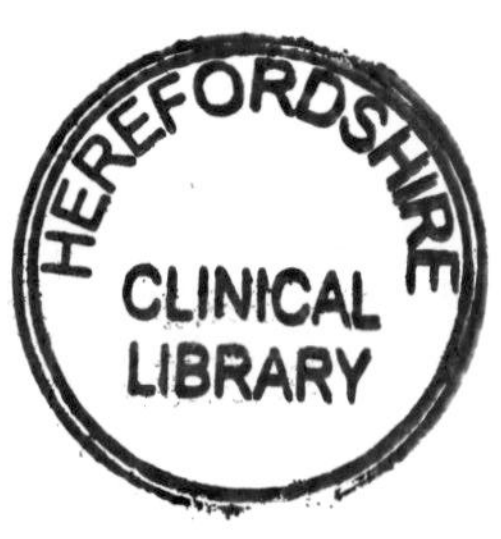